Pediatric Nephrology and Urology THE REQUISITES IN PEDIATRICS

SERIES EDITOR **LOUIS M. BELL,** M.D.
Patrick S. Pasquariello, Jr. Chair in General Pediatrics
Professor of pediatrics
University of Pennsylvania School of Medicine
Chief, Division of General Pediatrics
Attending Physician, General Pediatrics and
   Infectious Diseases
The Children's Hospital of Philadelphia
Philadelphia, Pennsylvania

OTHER VOLUMES IN
**THE REQUISITES IN PEDIATRICS
SERIES**

Orthopaedics and Sports Medicine

Endocrinology

COMING SOON IN
**THE REQUISITES IN PEDIATRICS
SERIES**

Toxicology

Pulmonology

Cardiology

Infectious Diseases

Hematology and Oncology

Gastroenterology

Pediatric Nephrology and Urology

THE REQUISITES IN PEDIATRICS

Bernard S. Kaplan, M.B., B.Ch.
Director of Pediatric Nephrology
Professor of Pediatrics
The Children's Hospital of Philadelphia
The University of Pennsylvania
Philadelphia, Pennsylvania

Kevin E. C. Meyers, M.B., B.Ch.
Pediatric Nephrologist
Assistant Professor of Pediatrics
The Children's Hospital of Philadelphia
The University of Pennsylvania
Philadelphia, Pennsylvania

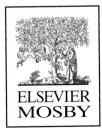

ELSEVIER
MOSBY

ELSEVIER
MOSBY

The Curtis Center
170 S Independence Mall W 300 E
Philadelphia, Pennsylvania 19106

NOTICE

Pediatric nephrology/urology is an ever-changing field. Standard safety precautions must be followed, but as new research and clinical experience broaden our knoweldge, changes in treatment and drug therapy may become necessary or appropriate. Readers are advised to check the most current product information provided by the manufacturer of each drug to be administered to verify the recommended dose, the method and duration of administration, and contraindications. It is the responsibility of the treating physician, relying on experience and knowledge of the patient, to determine dosages and the best treatment for each individual patient. Neither the Publisher nor the editors assume any liability for any injury and/or damage to persons or property arising from this publication.

The Publisher

Library of Congress Cataloging-in-Publication Data

Pediatric nephrology and urology: the requisites in pediatrics/[edited by] Bernard S.
    Kaplan, Kevin Meyers.—1st ed.
        p. ; cm.
    Includes bibliographical references.
    ISBN 0-323-01841-6
        1. Pediatric nephrology. 2. Pediatric urology. 3. Children—Diseases. 4. Pediatrics.
I. Kaplan, Bernard S., II. Meyers, Kevin
    [DNLM: 1. Kidney Diseases—Child: 2. Kidney Diseases—Infant 3. Urologic
Diseases—Child. 4. Urologic Diseases—Infant. WS 320 P3715 2005]
RJ476.K5P4347 2005
618.92'61—dc22   2004059748

Printed in the United States of America
Last digit is the print number: 9   8   7   6   5   4   3   2   1

THE REQUISITES ™
THE REQUISITES
THE REQUISITES
THE REQUISITES
THE REQUISITES

THE REQUISITES is a proprietary trademark
of Mosby, Inc.

This book is dedicated to our wives *Paige* and *Shiralee*

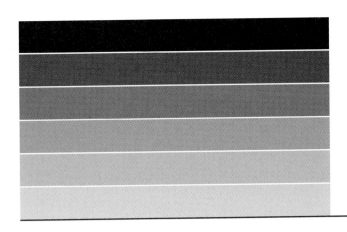

Contributors

Kristin Andolaro, RD, LDN
Clinical Dietician
Division of Nephrology
The Children's Hospital of Philadelphia
Philadelphia, Pennsylvania

H. Jorge Baluarte, MD
Professor of Pediatrics
Department of Pediatrics
The Children's Hospital of Philadelphia
Medical Director, Renal Transplant Program
Division of Nephrology
Department of Pediatrics
The Children's Hospital of Philadelphia
Philadelphia, Pennsylvania

Richard D. Bellah, MD
Associate Professor of Radiology and Pediatrics
Department of Radiology
University of Pennsylvania School of Medicine
Staff Radiologist
The Children's Hospital of Philadelphia
Philadelphia, Pennsylvania

Michael C. Braun, MD
Assistant Professor
Division of Pediatric Nephrology and Hypertension
University of Texas Health Science Center at Houston
Center for Immunology and Autoimmune Diseases
The Brown Foundation Institute of
Molecular Medicine
Houston, Texas

Chris Breen, RN, BSN, CNN
Clinical Nurse 4, Staff Nurse
Department of Dialysis
The Children's Hospital of Philadelphia
Philadelphia, Pennsylvania

Jon M. Burnham, Jr., MD
Instructor
Department of Pediatrics
The University of Pennsylvania School of Medicine
Fellow
Department of Rheumatology and General Pediatrics
The Children's Hospital of Philadelphia
Philadelphia, Pennsylvania

Douglas A. Canning, MD
Associate Professor of Urology
Department of Surgery
Hospital of the University of Pennsylvania
School of Medicine
Chief, Pediatric Urology
The Children's Hospital of Philadelphia
Philadelphia, Pennsylvania

Russell W. Chesney, MD
Le Bonheur Professor and Chair
Department of Pediatrics
University of Tennessee Health Sciences Center
Vice President of Academic Affairs
Administration Department
Le Bonheur Children's Research Hospital
Memphis, Tennessee

Anne Mette Christensen, MD
Attending Nephrologist
Division of Nephrology
Children's Hospital of Philadelphia
Philadelphia, Pennsylvania

John P. Conery, MD
Fellow-Physician
Department of Radiology
University of Pennsylvania
Children's Hospital of Philadelphia
Philadelphia, Pennsylvania

Katherine MacRae Dell, MD
Assistant Professor
Department of Pediatrics
Case Western Reserve University
Attending Pediatric Nephrologist
Division of Pediatric Nephrology
Rainbow Babies and Children's Hospital
Cleveland, Ohio

Barbara A. Fivush, MD
Professor of Pediatrics
Department of Pediatrics
Johns Hopkins University
Chief of Pediatric Nephrology
Department of Pediatrics
Johns Hopkins Hospital
Baltimore, Maryland

Joseph T. Flynn, MD, MS
Associate Professor of Clinical Pediatrics
Department of Pediatrics
Albert Einstein College of Medicine
Director, Pediatric Hypertension Program
Section of Pediatric Nephrology
Children's Hospital of Montefiore
Bronx, New York

Stuart L. Goldstein, MD
Assistant Professor
Department of Pediatrics
Baylor College of Medicine
Medical Director
Renal Dialysis Unit
Texas Children's Hospital
Houston, Texas

Cynthia Green, MSS, LSW
Social Worker
Division of Nephrology
The Children's Hospital of Philadelphia
Philadelphia, Pennsylvania

Marta Guttenberg, MD
Assistant Pathologist
Department of Pathology and Laboratory Medicine
The Children's Hospital of Philadelphia
Philadelphia, Pennsylvania

Bernard S. Kaplan, MB, BCh
Director of Pediatric Nephrology
Professor of Pediatrics
The Children's Hospital of Philadelphia
The University of Pennsylvania
Philadelphia, Pennsylvania

Thomas F. Kolon, MD
Assistant Professor
Department of Urology
University of Pennsylvania School of Medicine
The Children's Hospital of Philadelphia
Philadelphia, Pennsylvania

Jennifer Kolu, MSN, RN-CS, PNP
Department of Urology
The Children's Hospital of Philadelphia
Philadelphia, Pennsylvania

Kevin E.C. Meyers, MB, BCh
Pediatric Nephrologist
Assistant Professor of Pediatrics
The Children's Hospital of Philadelphia
The University of Pennsylvania
Philadelphia, Pennsylvania

Mini Michael, MBBS, FRACP
Post Graduate Fellow, Pediatric Nephrology
Department of Pediatrics
Baylor College of Medicine
Texas Children's Hospital
Houston, Texas

Dawn S. Milliner, MD
Professor of Pediatrics and Medicine
Division of Nephrology
Department of Pediatrics and Adolescent Medicine
Mayo Clinic
Rochester, Minnesota

Lawrence S. Milner, MD
Associate Professor
Department of Pediatric Nephrology
Tufts University School of Medicine
Floating Hospital For Children
New England Medical Center
Boston, Massachusetts

Julie Petro Mongiello, MSN, CRNP
Department of Nephrology
The Children's Hospital of Philadelphia
Philadelphia, Pennsylvania

Alicia M. Neu, MD
Associate Professor
Division of Pediatric Nephrology
Department of Pediatrics
Johns Hopkins University School of Medicine
Baltimore, Maryland

Jo-Ann Palmer, MSN, CRNP
Renal Transplant Coordinator
Department of Nephrology
Children's Hospital of Philadelphia
Philadelphia, Pennsylvania

Madhura Pradhan, MD
Clinical Assistant of Pediatrics
Department of Pediatrics
University of Pennsylvania
Attending Nephrologist
Department of Pediatrics
Division of Nephrology
The Children's Hospital of Philadelphia
Philadelphia, Pennsylvania

Pierre Russo, MD
Associate Professor
Department of Pathology and Laboratory
Medicine
University of Pennsylvania School of Medicine
Chief, Division of Anatomic Pathology
Department of Pathology and Laboratory Medicine
The Children's Hospital of Philadelphia
Philadelphia, Pennsylvania

Ann E. Salerno, MD
Fellow
Department of Pediatrics
University of Pennsylvania School of Medicine
Children's Hospital of Philadelphia
Philadelphia, Pennsylvania

Seth L. Schulman, MD
Associate Professor
Department of Pediatrics and Surgery
University of Pennsylvania
Attending Physician
Department of Pediatric Nephrology and Urology
The Children's Hospital of Philadelphia
Philadelphia, Pennsylvania

Kathy Shaw, MD
Professor of Pediatrics
Children's Hospital of Philadelphia
Chief, Division of Emergency Medicine
University of Pennsylvania School of Medicine
Philadelphia, Pennsylvania

Jonathan M. Sorof, MD
Associate Professor
Department of Pediatric Nephrology and
Hypertension
University of Texas–Houston Medical School
Houston, Texas

Lisa J. States, MD
Pediatric Radiologist
Department of Radiology
The Children's Hospital of Philadelphia
Philadelphia, Pennsylvania

Kimberly J. Sterner-Stein, MSW, LSW
Social Work Consultant
Division of Nephrology
The Children's Hospital of Philadelphia
Philadelphia, Pennsylvania

C. Frederic Strife, MD
Professor of Pediatrics
Division of Nephrology and Hypertension
University of Cincinnati College of Medicine
Cincinnati Children's Hospital Medical Center
Cincinnati, Ohio

Peter D. Thomson, MB, BCh (Wits), FCPaed (SA)
Professor in Paediatric Nephrology
Clinical Head of Paediatrics
University of Witwatersrand Donald Gordon Medical
Centre
Johannesburg, Gauteng, South Africa

Howard Trachtman, MD
Professor
Department of Pediatrics
Albert Einstein College of Medicine
Chief, Division of Nephrology
Department of Pediatrics
Schneider Children's Hospital of NS & LIJ Health System
New Hyde Park, New York

Rebecca Vereb, MEd
Doctoral Candidate
School Psychology Program
Lehigh University
Bethlehem, Pennsylvania

Aileen P. Walsh, PhD
Fellow
Department of Psychology
The Children's Hospital of Philadelphia
Philadelphia, Pennsylvania

Nataliya Zelikovsky, PhD
Assistant Professor
Department of Pediatrics
Division of Nephrology
University of Pennsylvania School of Medicine
Psychologist
Division of Nephrology
The Children's Hospital of Philadelphia
Philadelphia, Pennsylvania

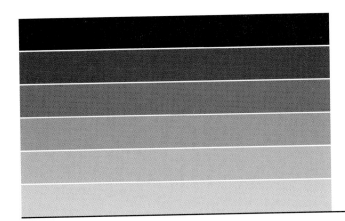

Foreword

The third volume of the **Requisites in Pediatrics** entitled, *Pediatric Nephrology and Urology* surpasses expectations in the choice of topics and the clarity of the information provided. Recall that the goal of this series was to ask leading pediatric subspecialists to edit a book that would include the essential fund of pediatric knowledge in their subspecialty area. Each book was to discuss the common pediatric conditions with accessible practical information that would guide primary care providers, resident physicians, nurse practitioners, and students in the care of their patients. The editors and authors were asked to include information about appropriate referrals to the specialist and to outline the laboratory testing that should be performed prior to the referral to assist the subspecialist in her or his search for the difficult diagnosis.

The book edited by Bernard S. Kaplan and Kevin E. C. Meyers is filled with practical information and the wisdom of expert clinicians and educators. One finds the information presented in a concise and readable manner. I particularly appreciated the "clinical pearls" that are highlighted throughout the text. It is easy for the reader to re-discover that lost, yet important clinical bit of information about the child with proteinuria or have that murky concept about peritoneal dialysis focused in a logical manner.

Another added value in this volume is that the concepts found in this book apply not only to the Nephrology or Urology patient but enrich the approach to all patients and families who may struggle with chronic disease. For example, Part I stresses the importance of the *pediatric nephrology team,* each with a vital role as care-provider, family supporter and advocate. Reading these first eleven chapters allows the primary care provider, nurses, resident physicians, and others to anticipate what the challenges will be for children and families. The reasons may then "talk the same language" as the pediatric nephrology team and thereby clarify,

support and reinforce the challenges and complex management regimes that are often required in the multi-dimensional approach to children with renal disease.

Part II of the book begins discussion of the most common diseases diagnosed and managed by pediatric nephrologists and urologists. *Hematuria, Proteinuria* and *Hypertension: Principles for the Practitioner* were especially welcome discussions. "HUS in not TTP" is another discussion that I have had the pleasure of hearing Dr. Kaplan speak about in clinical conference and was happy to see it so nicely written in Chapter 27 for those in the larger community. In Part IV, Jorge Baluarte and co-authors, takes the reader through the issues facing children and families undergoing renal transplantation. Part V of the book, shifts gears a bit to urologic problems, including an excellent discussion of *Urinary Tract Infections in Childhood* (Chapter 40). The clinical pearl that "fever is often the only sign of UTI in young infants" demands an understanding of the sensitivity and specificity of the rapid diagnostic screening tests available (Fig. 40-4). Douglas Canning's (Chapter 41) discussion about the urological evaluations in the child is an excellent contribution, especially for primary care providers.

As a general pediatrician and educator, I extend my deep appreciation to the editors and authors of this book. They have provided the reader with a clinical pearl of a book on Pediatric Nephrology and Urology. We hope you enjoy the third volume in the **Requisites in Pediatrics** series.

Louis M. Bell, MD
Chief, Division of General Pediatrics
The Children's Hospital of Philadelphia
The Patrick S. Pasquariello, Jr. Professor of Pediatrics
University of Pennsylvania School of Medicine
Philadelphia, PA

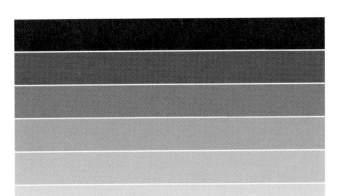

Contents

Color insert provided by Marta Guttenberg and Pierre Russo.

EXAMPLES OF RENAL PATHOLOGICAL ABNORMALITIES IN CHILDREN

Provided by Marta Guttenberg and Pierre Russo

1. Urological abnormalities

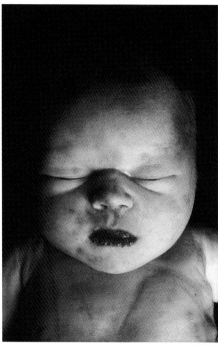

1. a. Abnormal facies associated with oligohydramnios: Note beaked nose, flat uncurled ears, and suborbital folds.

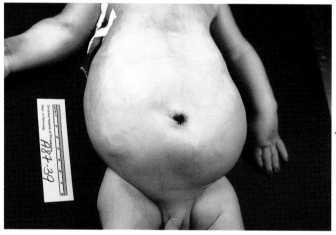

1. b. Prune belly syndrome: The absent anterior abdominal wall muscles results in a distended abdomen with a puckered surface.

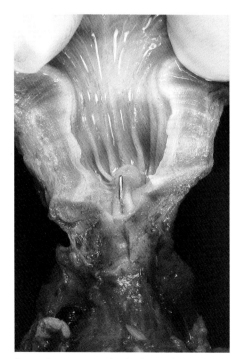

1. c. Posterior urethral valves: The urethra is obstructed and the bladder wall is markedly thickened.

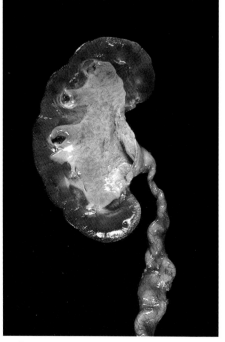

1. d. Hydronephrosis: Cross-section of a kidney showing the dilated pelvis secondary to ureteropelvic junction obstruction.

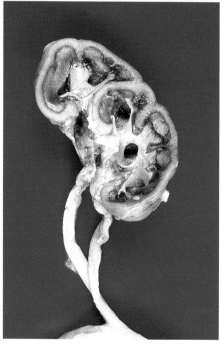

1. e. Duplicated collecting system: Both the upper and the lower systems are hydronephrotic secondary to obstruction.

2. Tubulo-interstitial diseases

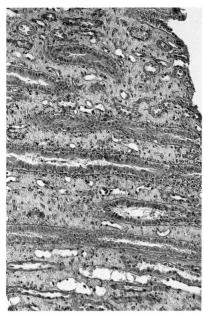

2. a. Pyelonephritis: Note encroachment of neutrophils on the tubular epithelium (H&E staining; original magnification, ×100).

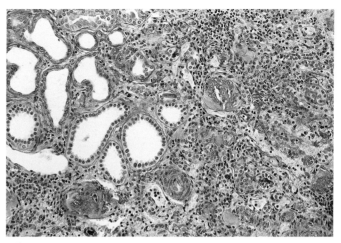

2. b. End-stage kidney disease: Note the interstitial inflammation, glomerular scarring, and cystic tubule dilatation (H&E staining; original magnification, ×40).

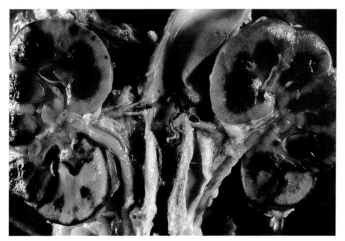

2. c. Renal infarction: There is marked congestion of the medulla.

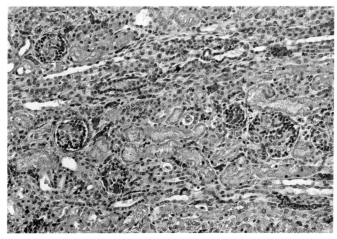

2. d. Acute tubular necrosis: There is loss of nuclei in the proximal tubular epithelial and mitotic figures representing cell regeneration (H&E staining; original magnification, ×40).

3. Cystic and dysplastic conditions

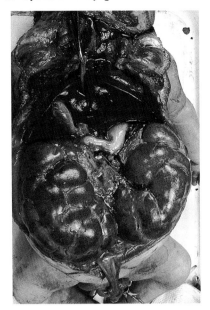

3. a. Autosomal-recessive polycystic kidney disease: The kidneys are massively enlarged, symmetrical, and reniform.

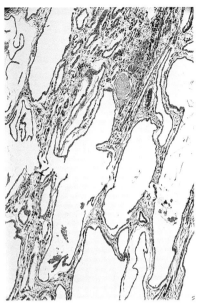

3. b. Autosomal-recessive polycystic kidney disease: Note the diffuse tubular ectasia by low-power microscopic examination (H&E staining; original magnification, ×10).

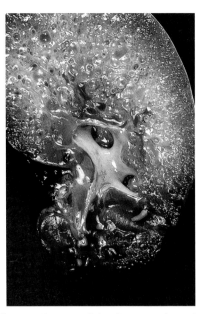

3. c. Autosomal-dominant polycystic kidney disease: There are numerous cysts on the surface of the kidney.

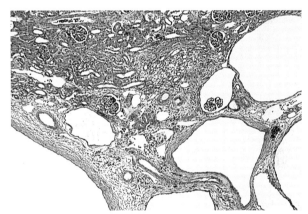

3. d. Autosomal-dominant polycystic kidney disease: The cysts are rounded. Note the glomerular cyst with the rudimentary glomerulus (H&E staining; original magnification, ×10).

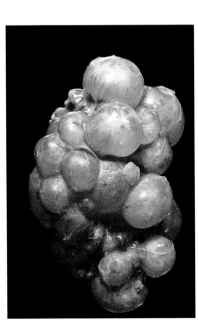

3. e. Multicystic kidney disease. The large cysts produce the appearance of a bunch of grapes.

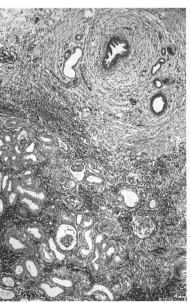

3. f. Renal cystic dysplasia. Note the dysplastic tissue consisting of mesenchymal condensation around primitive tubules.

4. Acute glomerulonephritis

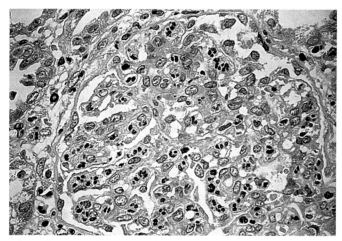

4. a. Acute post-infectious glomerulonephritis. Note the numerous infiltrating neutrophils and several closed capillary loops (H&E staining; original magnification, ×40).

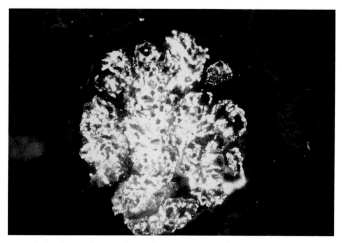

4. b. Acute post-infectious glomerulonephritis. Immunofluorescence microscopy. There are abundant, large, deposits of C3 in the mesangium and along the capillary walls. IgG is deposited in a similar distribution (original magnification, ×40).

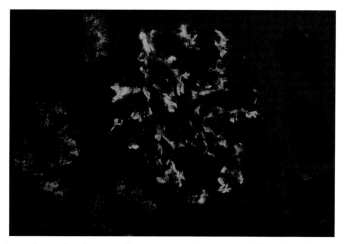

4. c. IgA nephropathy. Immunofluorescence microscopy. Note the characteristic mesangial deposition of IgA (original magnification, ×40).

5. Membranoproliferative glomerulonephritis

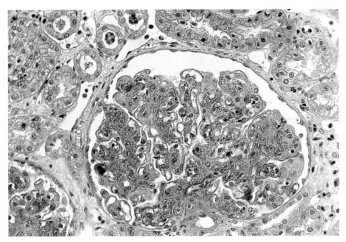

5. a. Membranoproliferative glomerulonephritis. The glomeruli are large, there is accentuation of the lobules, and the lumens are closed. There is expansion of mesangial matrix and an increase in mesangial cells.

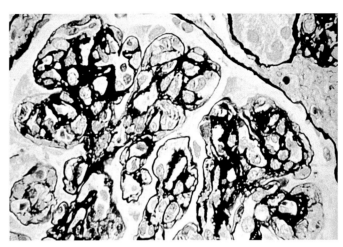

5. b. Membranoproliferative glomerulonephritis Type I: Reduplicated capillary basement membranes with mesangial sclerosis are demonstrated (Jones Silver staining; original magnification, ×40).

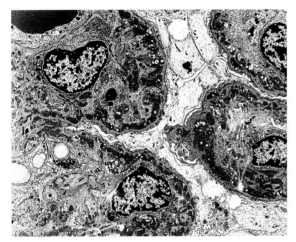

5. c. Membranoproliferative glomerulonephritis Type I: There are subendothelial electron dense deposits between the endothelial cell and glomerular basement membrane (electron microscopy).

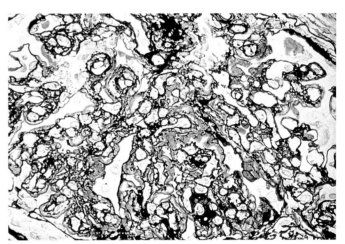

5. d. Membranoproliferative glomerulonephritis Type II: Splitting (reduplication) of the glomerular basement membrane is shown (Jones Silver staining; original magnification, ×40).

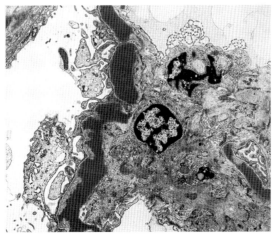

5. e. Membranoproliferative glomerulonephritis Type II: Note the ribbon-like, electron-dense deposits in the glomerular capillary basement membrane (electron microscopy).

6. Rapidly progressive glomerulonephritis

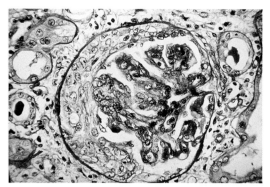

6. a. Rapidly progressive glomerulonephritis. Note the formation of a crescent of epithelial cells and histiocytes (Periodic acid-Schiff staining; original magnification, ×40).

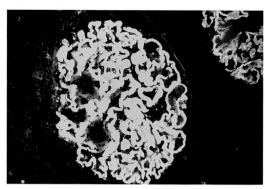

6. b. Rapidly progressive glomerulonephritis. Immunofluorescent microscopy from a patient with anti-glomerular basement membrane disease. Note the linear deposits of IgG along glomerular capillary loops (original magnification, ×40).

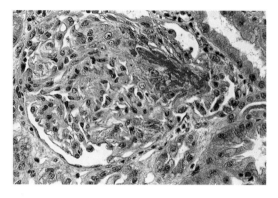

6. c. Wegener granulomatosis. Note the focal necrosis in the glomerulus of a patient with C-ANCA positive disease (H&E staining; original magnification, ×40).

7. Lupus nephritis

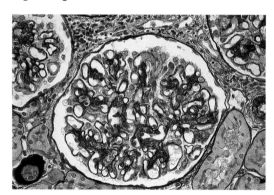

7. a. Class II: Note the mesangial hypercellularity.

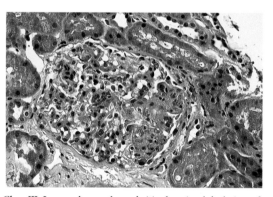

7. b. Class III: Lupus glomerulonephritis showing lobulation of capillary tufts with intracapillary cellular proliferation.

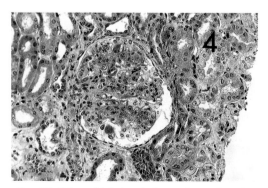

7. c. Class IV. Enlarged lobulated glomerulus with endocapillary proliferation (H&E staining; original magnification, ×40).

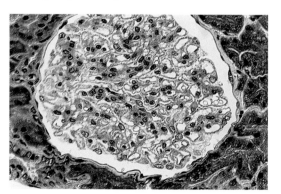

7. d. Class V. Thickened basement membranes.

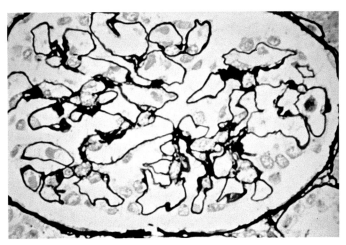

8. a. Minimal change disease: The findings are normal by light microscopy (Jones Silver staining; original magnification, ×40).

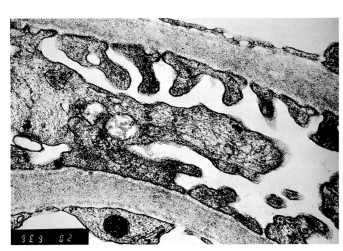

8. b. Minimal change disease: Normal foot-processes are seen by electron microscopy. The only abnormality may be effacement of the podocytes.

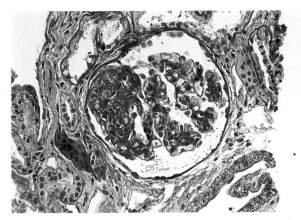

8. c. Focal segmental glomerulosclerosis: Note collapse and sclerosis of some of the capillary loops in this glomerulus. Throughout the biopsy specimen, less than 50% of glomeruli were involved (Periodic acid-Schiff staining; original magnification, ×40).

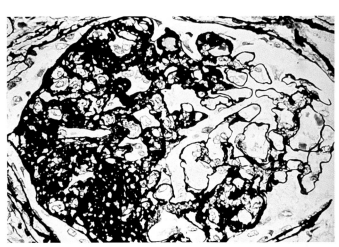

8. d. Focal and segmental glomerulosclerosis: There is expansion of the mesangial matrix (Jones Silver staining; original magnification, ×40).

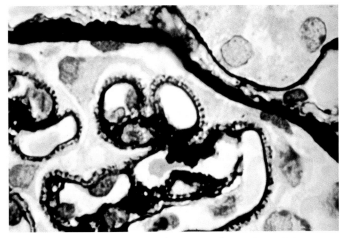

8. e. Membranous nephropathy: Note the spikes of basement membrane that have grown between the subepithelial deposits. (Jones Silver staining; original magnification, ×40).

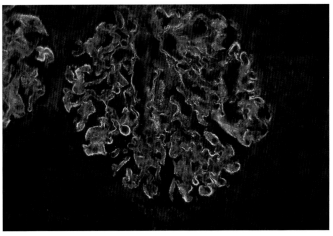

8. f. Membranous nephropathy: Immunofluorescence microscopy. Note the subepithelial deposits of IgG (original magnification, ×40).

9. Hemolytic uremic syndrome

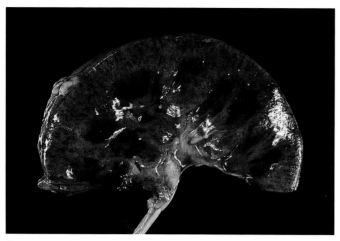

9. a. Hemolytic uremic syndrome: Punctate hemorrhages are noted throughout the cortex in a child who had severe disease.

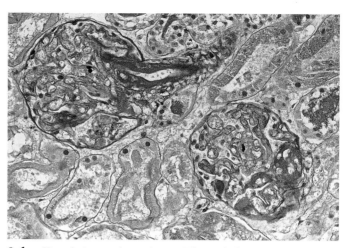

9. b. Hemolytic uremic syndrome: Fibrinoid changes of the afferent arterioles, endothelial swelling and tubular necrosis.

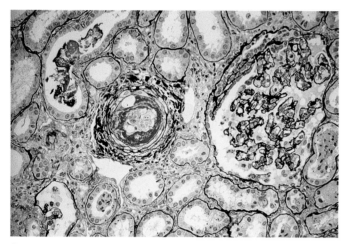

9. c. Hemolytic uremic syndrome. Note injury to an extraglomerular arteriole with fibrinoid changes of the intima.

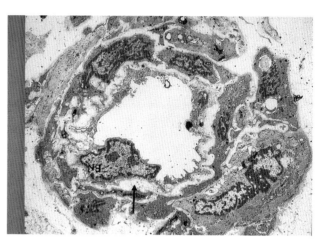

9. d. Hemolytic uremic syndrome. Endothelial damage and disruption (arrow) are shown by ultrastructural studies (electron microscopy).

10. Alport syndrome

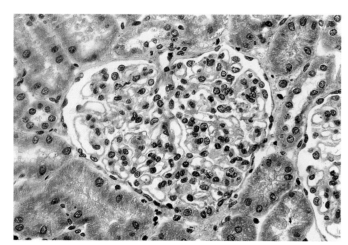

10. a. Alport syndrome: Non-specific changes as typified by mesangial hyperplasia and focal thickening of the basement membrane (Masson Trichrome staining; original magnification, ×40).

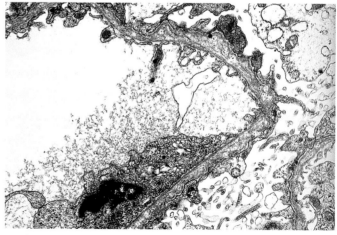

10. b. Alport syndrome: Note the thin, split and/or laminated glomerular basement membranes (electron microscopy).

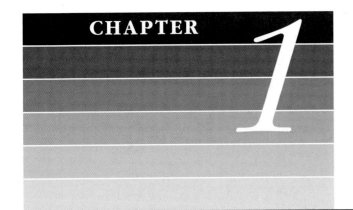

Introduction

BERNARD S. KAPLAN, M.B., B.Ch. AND
KEVIN E.C. MEYERS, M.B., B.Ch.

There are so many texts of nephrology, so many journals of nephrology, and so much information that one has to ask "why bother to edit yet another one?" Although there is no easy answer, we believe that none of these texts clearly enunciates the principles of team work in the care of pediatric nephrology patients and their families. Like the philosopher, Walter Kaufmann, who wrote *Religion in Four Dimensions*, we try to teach the important concept that the proper practice of pediatric nephrology requires an appreciation that patients and their afflictions must be seen in many dimensions. These include – in no particular order – the historical, religious, social, financial, geographic, psychological, economic, and biological aspects of a person. We cannot hope to cover each of these, but have included important discussions on some of the social, psychological, and biological problems in this discipline. By design and necessity we have chosen not to include anatomical and physiological descriptions of the kidneys; these are taught so well in other texts. Nor have we included an exhaustive or exhausting list of conditions because we have chosen to whet the appetite rather than satiate and bloat the reader.

We have had the privilege of training and working in several different political, economic, social, geographic, and medical worlds. We both obtained our medical educations at the University of the Witwatersrand in Johannesburg, South Africa. Our great teacher, mentor, and friend Philip Tobias impressed upon us the importance of never forgetting that the dissection of a human being allowed us to peer into the very core of that being's body, and that this was a sacred act. We recognize that taking care of another person's sick child is the most sacred and important responsibility with which anyone can be entrusted. According to Barton Childs, "Sir William Osler taught us how to practice medicine. Garrod taught us how to think about it. Osler conjured with facts, Garrod with ideas. Oslerian thinking is organized around treatment and management. It is a practical approach in which the student is perceived as an apprentice who is learning what he needs to know to practice medicine. It is pretty much what we do in residency training. Garrodian thinking in contrast is about concepts; what diseases are and why they exist." In the Johannesburg and Baragwanath Hospitals, we were trained at the bedside in the Oslerian tradition. We were trained to take a history, examine the patient painstakingly, develop a differential diagnosis, and judiciously use the limited technologies that were available.

At The Montreal Children's Hospital and The Children's Hospital of Philadelphia we entered the world of Garrod. Osler had come from McGill University in Montreal in 1884 to the University of Pennsylvania where we now work in elegant new buildings that have risen over the sites where Osler had taught, taken care of patients, and worked in "Ol' Blockly." The best of all worlds is attained, according to Barton Childs, in the doctor who cleaves to the Oslerian ideal in practice and the Garrodian in thinking.

We have another distinction, which is uncommon in this age of great population dispersals. Tony Meyers, Professor of Nephrology, taught Bernard Kaplan nephrology in Johannesburg. Kaplan in turn taught Tony's son, Kevin Meyers, nephrology in Philadelphia. In this way, one of the Hippocratic oath's injunctions, "to impart a knowledge of the Art to my own sons, and those of my teachers," has been fulfilled. We have also tried to impart knowledge of this art "to disciples bound by a stipulation and oath according to the law of medicine," but in a break with the oath, have ignored the injunction not to teach others. For, in this day and age of increasing specialization and complexity, patients and their families can be taken care of only by integrated teams of skilled professionals. In pediatric nephrology, a team must include at a minimum, nephrologists, surgeons, urologists, anesthesiologists, radiologists, nurses, social workers, nutritionists, psychologists, secretarial staff, and coordinators.

Pediatric nephrology can and should be taught in many different ways. None is exclusive of another. The basic requirements are knowledgeable teachers who love to teach, and learners who are avid for knowledge and instruction. Never before has so much information been so readily available to so many people in real time. No one can read all that needs to be read, understand all that is read, remember all that has been read, apply all that needs to be applied, as well as take care of extremely sick patients and their anxious families, contribute to the torrent of new knowledge, and teach. And yet, we must read much that needs to be read, understand enough of what is read, remember important and useful parts of what has been read, apply what needs to be applied, and take care of extremely sick patients and their anxious families, and make contributions to the torrent of new knowledge, and teach. In addition, and most importantly, we have to take care of our families and ourselves, have friends and hobbies, and try to avoid depleting our mental, psychic, and physical resources.

Although Stephen Jay Gould admired his friend Oliver Sacks extravagantly as a writer, he felt that he could never hope to match him in general quality or human compassion. Oliver, on the other hand, envied Gould because although they had both staked out a large and generous subject for their writing (Sacks on the human mind and Gould on evolution), Gould had devised and developed a general theory that allowed him to coordinate all his work into a coherent and distinctive body, whereas Sacks had only written descriptively. Gould thought Sacks had sold himself short because of his attempt to reintroduce the case study method of attention to irreducible peculiarities of individual patients in the practice of cure and healing in medicine. This is a long and poetic way of stating the obvious: the proper study of medicine must begin with attention to individual patients followed by a review of groups of similar cases, and then proceed to prospective, randomized, and well-designed clinical studies with appropriate controls and protection for human subjects. And all the while, attempts must be made to develop new knowledge at the bench and then to do translational research.

Much is required of a pediatric nephrologist, and of all other physicians, but our attentions are directed at those who want to know something of pediatric nephrology as well as those who may want to become pediatric nephrologists. J.D. Salinger noted that, "close on the heels of kindness, originality is one of the most thrilling things in the world, also the most rare." Kindness is an absolute requirement. Originality has provided us with an impressive range of treatment modalities that include medications, technological marvels that support and sustain life, and the ability to transplant the kidney from one human being to another, but none of this should be done in the absence of kindness. Close on the heels of *kindness* is the important understanding that one needs to be able to listen carefully to others and to avoid being dogmatic. As noted by Kierkegaard, "you are most likely to be in mortal sin when you are sure you are in the right."

Fox and Swazey's advice, modified slightly for the purposes of context, to physicians who take care of renal transplant patients, applies to all physicians.

"The final gatekeeper is the physician. Acting on behalf of the team, the patient, as well as for himself, he makes the ultimate judgment. The physician's role here is sociological and moral as it is medical. He acts as mediator and interpreter in the complex social system called into play by the situation. In this capacity he weaves his way back and forth among the patient, families, and the wide range of specialists who constitute the team. The physician is not free to abnegate his responsibility, nor may he exercise it arbitrarily or coercively. He must base his decision[s] on biomedical, psychological, and sociological criteria that are acceptable within his profession."

These wise words remain valid even today as pediatric nephrologists struggle to maintain their equanimity in a complex world of HMOs, insurance companies, bioethics committees, HIPAA regulations, institutional review boards, and endless levels of Kafkaesque bureaucracies. One must always try to remember, however, that these are relative difficulties that pale in contrast to the poverty of body and spirit, political repression, total lack of resources and other apocalyptic problems that bedevil less fortunate countries. And above all, one must always remember whom we serve: our patients and their families.

SUGGESTED READINGS

Childs B. In: Scriver CR, Beaudet AL, Sly WS, Valle D. *The Metabolic and Molecular Bases of Inherited Disease.* 7th edn. McGraw-Hill, New York, 2001, Chapter 3.

Fox RC, Swazey JP. *The Courage to Fail. A Social View of Organ Transplants and Dialysis,* 2nd edn. University of Chicago Press, Chicago, 1978, p. 9.

Gould SJ. *The Structure of Evolutionary Theory.* Belknap, Harvard, 2002, p. 37.

Kaufmann W. *Religions in Four Dimensions: Existential and Aesthetic, Historical and Comparative.* Reader's Digest Press, Thomas Y. Cromwell, New York, 1976.

CHAPTER 2

The History of Pediatric Nephrology

RUSSELL W. CHESNEY, M.D.

INTRODUCTION

Although the description of the formation of bubbles on a fluid surface, as a result of an edematous patient voiding into water, dates to Hippocrates (fifth century B.C.), the first substantial texts on urinary tract disease in children were published in the 16th to 19th centuries.[24] Remarkably, the first published observation concerning the formation of urine by the fetus, thereby producing amniotic fluid, appeared in the drawings of Leonardo di Vinci. Probably the most important early text mentioning childhood renal disease was "De Morbis puerorum" of Hieronymus Mercurialis (1583). This tract divides urinary disease into: (a) de incontinentia urinae; (b) de urinae suppressione; and (c) de calculo vescicae. This text recognizes the clinical differences between oligoanuria and reduced urine flow due to obstruction. Mercurialis also recognized the association between renal stones and infection and hereditary factors in stone disease. Another 10 texts during the 17th and 18th centuries briefly cover

Portions of this chapter are reproduced, with permission, from: Chesney RW. The history of pediatric discipline series: a history of pediatric specialties: the development of pediatric nephrology. Pediatr Res 2002;52:770-778.

nephrology topics. Edema and anasarca were described in the 1500s. Descriptions of anaphylactoid purpura date from the 19th century and of the nephrotic syndrome ('nephrosis') from the early 20th century.[5,13] The distinction between nephritis and the nephrotic syndrome was made during the 1940s.

ORIGINS OF SCHOLARSHIP IN CHILDHOOD RENAL DISEASES, 1820–1950

An examination of the history of pediatric nephrology (Table 2-1) shows that the main scientific focus, and the initial precise clinical observations, concerned fluid and electrolyte balance. A discipline develops when a scientific, clinical, or technical body of information allows unique observations to be made, and therefore the ability to measure electrolytes in body fluids was essential in the study of renal disease. German clinical scientists in the 19th century measured electrolytes in urine and blood using titrimetric methods and established norms for the excretion of electrolytes in neonates, infants and

Table 2-1 Early Founders of Pediatric Nephrology	
Organization	**Founders**
Fluid and Electrolyte Metabolism (United States)	J. Howland, D.C. Darrow, L. E. Holt, R.E. Cooke, E.A. Park, H.E. Harrison, A. Hess, A. Butler, M. Marriot, W. Wallace
Glomerular Diseases, Nephrotic Syndrome (Germany, Austria)	J. Schönlein, O. Heubner, E. Henoch, F. Volhard, T. Fahr, C. Munck
Urine Flow Rate, Infantile Urine Patterns (Germany)	O. Langstein, F. R. von Ruess

children.[10,11,25] They also demonstrated the value of the precise measurement of body fluid chemicals in relation to a clinical situation, and this theme dominated the research base of pediatric nephrology until the late 1950s.[8,10,14,16] Therefore, pediatric nephrology developed around questions of fluid and electrolyte metabolism, the balance of tonicity and volume, and the mechanisms of metabolic acidosis. The importance of these studies was that they were both quantitative and reproducible.[16]

The initial descriptions of glomerular disorders were case reports. Johan L. Schönlein and his student Edmond Henoch described parts of the syndrome that bears their names.[24] Textbooks of the late 19th and early 20th centuries described Bright disease in children, uremia, renal tuberculosis, post-scarlet fever renal disease, and albuminuria.[5] Otto Heubner, the professor of pediatrics in Berlin following Schönlein, described orthostatic proteinuria and its benign prognosis.[25] The term 'lower nephron nephrosis' defined a renal disease in children (the pale, edematous child with proteinuria and hypoalbuminemia with lipid-laden vacuoles in the tubules), and was replaced in the 1960s by the nephrotic syndrome.[5] Bright disease, a term which is no longer used, described late features of chronic glomerulonephritis in a patient with renal insufficiency and hypertension.[9]

Metabolism is the field of study of the founding scholars[8,10,11,14] who are the intellectual forefathers of modern pediatric nephrology, particularly in their belief in hypothesis-based quantitative science.[5] Their approach later influenced the study of glomerular diseases. Remarkably, nephrology, endocrinology, nutrition, and biochemical genetics emerged from the broad discipline of metabolism. The founders of neonatal nephrology evaluated normal and pathophysiologic renal-related processes in neonates (composition of urine, urine volume excretion), and described a disorder termed urate nephropathy[4,25] in the late 19th and early 20th centuries.

Henoch, Heubner, Langstein, and Addis made observations regarding the nephritis associated with scarlatina, diphtheria and congenital syphilis.[1,25] An early monograph by Karel de Leeuw described, in detail, the prognosis of various forms of nephritis, which was far less optimistic than today.[9] Addis' influential textbook *Glomerular Nephritis* (1950) was a paradigm shift[1] with brilliant and precise descriptions of childhood renal syndromes. His description of acute and chronic glomerulonephritis included extensive, thorough, long-term follow-up studies of chronic glomerulonephritis. These early scholars may be criticized for lumping most forms of nephritis into a few entities. Addis recognized that this limitation arose from the examination of thick sections of kidney tissue at autopsy, and from the fact that some children recovered with bed rest and diet. Early schemes for disease progression were not always accurate. What was required were means of precisely defining renal diseases and safe and effective treatments.

Those requirements became possible in the 1950s because of the development of percutaneous renal biopsy and the insistence on precision in the histological evaluation of renal tissue (Table 2-2).

EMERGENCE OF PEDIATRIC NEPHROLOGY AS A DISTINCT DISCIPLINE: 1950–1970

The term *pediatric nephrology* first appeared in 1963 in the book *Current Problems in Childhood Nephrology* written by the French pediatric nephrologists Pierre Royer,[22] Renée Habib, and Henri Mathieu of the Hôpital des Enfants-Malades in Paris. The advent of this term distinguished a topic in pediatric care deserving of it own in-depth texts.[17,23] The period up to the founding of the European Society of Pediatric Nephrology (ESPN) in 1966 and the American Society of Pediatric Nephrology (ASPN) in 1969 was marked by six fundamental scientific and/or technologic advances pertaining to kidney function and disorders. These advances were so pivotal that pediatric nephrology could never again be considered part of any other discipline (Box 2-1). The seminal event was the observation that ACTH or glucocorticoids could induce remission in children with nephrotic syndrome and prevent death due to infection and malnutrition.

> **Clinical Pearl**
>
> The mortality rate from the nephrotic syndrome of childhood, which was as high as 40–50%, was halved by using antibiotics to treat life-threatening infections, particularly peritonitis.

Shortly after the discovery of adrenocorticotropic hormone (ACTH) and cortisol in the 1940s, ACTH was used in a series of clinical trials in nephrotic children in relapse; when administered together with antibiotics, mortality was reduced to less than 10%.[20,21] This capacity to induce remission led to questions of why some children responded rapidly and why others failed to respond. The examination of renal tissue, obtained by renal biopsy, by light, immunofluorescence and electron microscopy provided the tools that answered some of these questions.[6]

In 1948, a forerunner of the National Kidney Foundation sponsored the Annual Conference on the Nephrotic Syndrome that was later changed to The Annual Conference on the Kidney. These meetings focused on renal physiology, renal metabolism, and kidney diseases and were organized by Jack Metcoff, a student of Gamble. Major input to these conferences came from M. Rubin, M. Rappaport, W. Heymann, H. Barnett, and P. Calcagno. The meetings were selective, with seldom

Table 2-2 Dates of Historical Significance in Pediatric Nephrology

1880s-present	German and Viennese interest in urinary flow rates and excretion in neonates; studies in glomerulonephritis: Langstein and Henoch
1906-	Studies of acidosis: Howland and Holt
1910-1940	Studies of rickets: Park and Hess
1930-1950	Insight into fluid and electrolyte balance; acid–base physiology; potassium divalent minerals: Gamble, Darrow, Cooke, Harrison
1948	Annual Conference on Nephrotic Syndrome (precursor of NKF, ASN, ASPN)
1950s	Percutaneous renal biopsy comes into use
1955	Description of hemolytic uremic syndrome (HUS): von Gasser
1961	Peritoneal dialysis in infants: Segar, Etteldorf
1966	European Society of Pediatric Nephrology founded
1968-1971	Peritoneal dialysis dramatically improves survival of HUS: Gianantonio, Kaplan
1968-1972	Hemodialysis in children: Metcoff, Fine, Potter, Mauer, Schärer, Broyer
1969	American Society of Pediatric Nephrology: Heymann is first president
1969	Use of alkylating agents in treatment of glomerular disease unresponsive to steroids: Good, Drummond, Michael, Grupe, West, Etteldorf
1968-1972	Transplantation in children
1971	International Society of Pediatric Nephrology begins: Arneil (Glasgow)
1972	Federal legislation to support end stage renal care: Greifer
1973	Synthesis of 1,25(OH)$_2$ vitamin D and use in children: DeLuca, Norman, Chan, Chesney
1973-1976	First textbooks of pediatric nephrology: Royer, Rubin, Barratt, Lieberman, James
1974	Sub-Board of Pediatric Nephrology: McCrory, Chair
1977	Workshop on Growth in Renal Failure, Carmel, CA: Holliday
1978	CAPD in children: Fine, Salusky
1979	Aluminum recognized as neurotoxin
1980	First Workshop on Developmental Renal Physiology, New York: Spitzer
1983	Beginning of lobbying efforts on behalf of pediatric nephrology research agenda: ASPN council and members
1986	AIDS nephropathy (Strauss)
1987	Workforce group report: ASPN appointees
1987	The journal *Pediatric Nephrology*: Chantler, Robson (eds)
1987	Erythropoietin for treatment of anemia of chronic renal failure
1990	National Kidney and Urology Diseases advisory board identifies need for more federal pediatric nephrology support
1992 on	Ion channel mutations responsible for many renal tubular syndromes, polycystic renal diseases, nephrogenic diabetes insipidus
1990s	Renal transplantation results improve with new therapeutic approaches; Quality goals in dialysis established
2000	Proteomics defines defects in congenital nephrotic syndrome, renal hypomagnesemia, variants of Alport syndrome

From Chesney RW: The history of pediatric discipline series: a history of pediatric specialties: the development of pediatric nephrology. Pediatr Res 2002;52:770-778.

Box 2-1 Six Critical Discoveries that Underline Pediatric Nephrology as a Discipline

- ACTH and glucocorticoids for treatment of idiopathic nephrotic syndrome
- Percutaneous renal biopsy in children permits classification of glomerular diseases
- Immunologic factors are essential, especially in glomerulopathies
- End-stage renal disease can be treated with dialysis
- Children can receive renal allografts from living or cadaveric donors
- Hypertension in children is the result of renal disease in 80% of cases

From Chesney RW: The history of pediatric discipline series; a history of pediatric specialities: the development of pediatric nephrology. Pediatr Res 2002;52:770-778.

more than 40 attendees. The International Study of Kidney Disease in Children (ISKDC) working group arose from the Kidney Conferences, and initiated important prospective renal biopsy studies of children with renal disease in many centers. This group designed defined, biopsy-based, prospective studies to elucidate the clinical features and prognosis of minimal lesion nephrotic syndrome, pediatric IgA nephropathy, focal sclerosing glomerulonephritis, membranous nephropathy, and mesangioproliferative glomerulonephritis. The use of light microscopy, immunofluorescence, and electron microscopy techniques by the ISKDC and other groups permitted the clinicopathologic identification of membranoproliferative glomerulonephritis;[26] IgA nephropathy (Berger disease);[2] and membranous nephropathy.[12] Pediatric nephrology moved rapidly into the realm of treatment of childhood renal disease by focusing on the structure and function of the kidney, renal biopsy, and dialysis and transplantation as essential components of the discipline. By 1970, the uremic child, *per se*, was becoming a focus for study and clinical care. From the 1970s new training programs emerged to train future pediatric nephrologists.

American pediatric nephrologists played key roles in the development of two societies based in internal medicine (90% of members of both societies are nephrologist internists). The Metcoff Annual Conference on the Nephrotic Syndrome was the forerunner of the National Kidney Foundation (NKF). In 1966, Henry Barnett, Robert Good, and Robert Vernier were among the founders of the American Society of Nephrology (ASN). Robert Vernier, Alfred Michael, and Norman Siegel served as Presidents of the ASN, the only pediatric nephrologists chosen for this prestigious position.

The ASPN was formed in Atlantic City in 1969 by Barnett, Heymann, Clark West, Edelmann, and others. The ASPN has held annual meetings with the American Pediatric Society-Society for Pediatric Research (APS-SPR) meetings. The ASPN has been important in formulating the agenda for pediatric nephrology in its roles as an educational society, in terms of public policy and in fostering its research agendas. The ASPN is also instrumental in recruiting trainees into the discipline using resident travel awards (Table 2-3). The International Pediatric Nephrology Association (IPNA) was founded in 1971 as a result of international cooperation engendered

among pediatric nephrologists. In Europe, the ESPN founded in Glasgow by Gavin Arneil in 1966 has been remarkably important to the development of the field of pediatric nephrology (Table 2-4). Members come from each European nation and the meeting site rotates from country to country. The ESPN has been essential in setting the standards for dialysis and transplantation in Europe as well as in developing transnational consortia of the study of numerous renal disorders. The ESPN frequently invites speakers from the US and Canada and, as well, plays an important role in the operations of IPNA. The close cooperation between the ASPN and the ESPN in the operation of IPNA has permitted interactions among American and European pediatric nephrologists and the rapid dissemination of new knowledge. The result has been several cross-Atlantic textbooks and numerous international studies.

DEVELOPMENT OF TRAINING PROGRAMS AND CERTIFICATION: 1970–1980

Research focused on animal models of glomerular disease, well-conducted clinicopathologic studies in children, and a fundamental immunologic experimental approach to understanding glomerulonephritis, including the role of complement pathway consumption and T-cell

Table 2-3 American Founders of Pediatric Nephrology and their Areas of Interest

Henry Barnett (Albert Einstein)	Developmental nephrology and clearance measurements in infants
Jay Bernstein (Albert Einstein)	Renal pathologist who defined developmental defects and cystic diseases
Philip Calcagno (Georgetown)	Developmental nephrology and drug handling by immature kidney
Daniel Darrow (Yale)	Metabolism expert and fluid and electrolyte therapy, especially the role of potassium
Chester Edelmann, Jr. (Albert Einstein)	Classification of renal tubular acidoses and renal function of the immature neonate
James Gamble (Harvard)	Metabolism and fluid and electrolyte therapy, parenteral fluid therapy
Robert Good, Jr. (Minnesota)	Immunologic mechanisms of renal disease and transplantation biology
Ira Greifer (Albert Einstein)	Treatment of nephrotic syndrome and organization of pediatric nephrology on national and global scale
Walter Heymann (Case Western)	Model of nephrotic syndrome, which resembles membranous nephropathy
Malcolm Holliday (University of California, San Francisco)	Renal nutrition and growth of uremic children
Charles Janeway (Harvard)	Studies on immune defects in children with nephrotic syndrome.
Wallace McCrory (Cornell)	Developmental nephrology and pathophysiology of glomerulonephritis. Chair of first Sub-Board of Pediatric Nephrology
Alfred Michael (Minnesota)	Pathogenesis and therapy of glomerular diseases
Jack Metcoff (Harvard, Michael Reese)	Pathogenesis and therapy of nephrotic syndrome. Conferences on the kidney
Mitchell Rubin (Buffalo)	Developmental nephrology. Editor of first textbook Pediatric Nephrology.
Adrian Spitzer (Albert Einstein)	Developmental nephrology and renal handling of phosphate. Organized workshops on development
Luther Travis (Galveston)	Diabetic nephropathy and fluid therapy for burns
Robert Vernier (Minnesota)	Mechanisms of glomerular disease and development of the glomerulus by use of electron microscope
Clark West (Cincinnati)	Immunologic mechanisms of glomerular disease and immunopathology

From Chesney RW: The history of pediatric discipline series: a history of pediatric specialties: the development of pediatric nephrology. Pediatr Res 2002;52:770–778.

Table 2-4 European Founders of Pediatric Nephrology and their Areas of Interest

Anita Aperia (Stockholm)	Renal handling of sodium by the preterm and term neonate kidney
Gavin Arneil (Glasgow)	Treatment of nephrotic syndrome and founder of ESPN and IPNA
T. Martin Barrett (London)	Pathogenesis of nephrotic syndrome. Editor of *Pediatric Nephrology* textbook
Horst Bickel (Heidelberg)	Supports large nephrology unit formation and discoveries in cystinosis
Johannes Brödehl (Hannover)	Develops large dialysis and transplant efforts; metabolic renal disease and renal phosphate handling
Michel Broyer (Paris)	Renal transplantation and dialysis; cystinosis; directs large Paris unit
Cyril Chantler (London)	Role of nutrition in renal disease; develops large dialysis and transplant unit, first co-editor of *Pediatric Nephrology*
Rosanna Coppo (Genoa)	Studies in IgA nephropathy and other glomerular diseases.
Louis Callis (Barcelona)	Studies on calcium disorders
Fabio Sereni (Milan)	Development of Italian pediatric nephrology – end-stage renal disease care. Developmental nephrology
Guido Fanconi (Zurich)	Described many pediatric nephrologic syndromes
Marie-Claire Gubler (Paris)	Pathophysiology of glomerulonephropathies with pathologic correlates
Jean-Pierre Guignard (Lausanne)	Studies of neonatal renal function
Renée Habib (Paris)	Preeminent renal pathologist whose classification of glomerular diseases is widely accepted
Niino Hallman (Helsinki)	Descriptions of congenital nephrotic syndrome of Finnish type
Edouard Henoch (Berlin)	Described Henoch–Schoenlein purpura
Ernst Leumann (Zurich)	Studies of childhood renal diseases including disorders of calcium metabolism
Leo Monnens (Groningen)	Metabolic and genetic studies in renal disease
H Ritter von Reuss (Vienna; Berlin)	Neonatal urinary excretion patterns
Juan Rodriquez-Soriano (Bilbao)	Studies of renal tubular acidosis
Pierre Royer (Paris)	Author of first textbook on pediatric nephrology, organizer of Paris School of Pediatric Nephrology; described many renal syndromes
Karl Schärer (Heidelberg)	Organizer of largest German unit and studies in hypertension, dialysis, transplantation and body composition
Harmen Tiddens (Utrecht)	A founder of Dutch pediatric nephrology involved in international pediatric nephrology trials and founding of ESPN
Richard White (Birmingham)	Clinicopathologic studies of glomerular disease
D Innes Williams (London)	Important figure in development of pediatric urology
Jan Winberg (Stockholm)	Studies of urinary tract infections

and B-cell interactions. Additional areas of focus were developmental renal physiology, including studies of glomerular filtration rate, acid–base physiology and handling of drugs, and fluid overload in glomerulonephritis.

All modern programs in the US, Canada, and Europe became involved in the use of renal biopsy techniques, dialysis and transplantation. Pediatric nephrologists conducted clinical research studies in uremic children with growth failure,[15] bone disease, acidosis, malnutrition, neurological impairment, depression, and hypertension. Recognition of the impact of chronic renal failure on growth was recognized by Lucas in 1883,[18] and has emerged as a dominant theme. Numerous groups worldwide have made important contributions to growth studies (see Box 2-1).

A remarkable and important legislation, Federal Act, Public Law 92-603, enacted in 1972, provided that Medicare would cover the cost and medical care for dialysis and transplantation for individuals, including children, with end-stage renal disease. This act expanded adult dialysis services and led to the development of chronic pediatric dialysis services and pediatric transplantation.[3,19] The importance of Public Law 92-603

is that it provides renal replacement care for "that stage of renal impairment that cannot be favorably influenced by conservative management alone and requires dialysis and/or kidney transplantation to maintain life or health." Because of universal health care coverage in Western Europe, the organization of pediatric dialysis and transplant centers, in general, occurred as part of each nation's health system.

FOCUSED RESEARCH THEMES SINCE 1970

By the late 1970s research had developed in the discipline of pediatric nephrology around several key themes. Several renal diseases are mostly found in children and were the subject of extensive inquiry: the hemolytic uremic syndrome (HUS), Henoch–Schönlein purpura, cystinosis, Lowe syndrome, minimal lesion nephrotic syndrome, congenital nephrotic syndrome, acute post-infectious glomerulonephritis, and posterior urethral valves. Other major areas of research focus have included pediatric hypertension, childhood renal osteodystrophy, cystic diseases of kidneys, renal dysplasia, hypoplasia, and agenesis, and renal venous thrombosis in neonates. These disorders have received attention and important advances have occurred. For example, the role of *Shigella*-like toxins produced by *Escherichia coli* O157:H7 and other *E. coli* strains in terms of the etiology and pathogenesis of HUS is now recognized. The role of renal parenchymal atrophy in the failure of the synthesis of $1,25(OH)_2$ vitamin D has been established. Pediatric nephrology, in collaboration with pediatric urology, is involved in research on infections of the lower urinary tract, renal parenchyma, obstruction, and vesicoureteric reflux. The emphasis on fetal renal physiology[4] has demonstrated the precursors of renal vascular formation, tubular development, renal hormone secretion, and developmental genes.

The American Board of Pediatrics offered the first certification examination in the sub-board of pediatric nephrology in 1974. The American Academy of Pediatrics developed an active section in pediatric nephrology and senior pediatric nephrologists who have made major contributions to the field are awarded the annual Henry Barnett award.

Because NIH study sections have little pediatric expertise, it became necessary for the ASPN to lobby intensively for more pediatric nephrology representation and to emphasize areas of important research. This same spirit has permitted the development of several multi-center networks aimed at enhancing research activities and improving the quality of patient care through prospective studies. This multicenter approach is important for conducting valuable research and defining best practices. Among these are regional groups (Southwestern Pediatric Nephrology Study Group, the New York-New Jersey Pediatric Nephrology Group) and national groups (North American Pediatric Renal Transplantation Cooperative Study [NAPRTCS]).

In 1985, a publications sub-committee of IPNA determined that a new pediatric nephrology journal should be established to serve the pediatric nephrologists of the world. This journal became the official publication of IPNA, ASPN, ESPN, Japanese Pediatric Nephrology Society, Asian Pediatric Nephrology Society, and Association of Latin American Nephrology in Pediatrics. Cyril Chantler (London) and Alan Robson (New Orleans) were its founding editors, and it is now in its eighteenth year and receives more than 350 manuscripts annually.

PEDIATRIC NEPHROLOGY IN A NEW CENTURY: 1990 INTO THE 21ST CENTURY

The research portfolio of pediatric nephrology is expanding as it enters the new century. Numerous groups are investigating the development of the renal vascular system, the ontogeny of the renin-angiotensin and aldosterone system, the mechanisms of cell recovery from hypoxic injury, transcription factors important in apoptosis and renal cell differentiation, and the elucidation of gene abnormalities in hereditary renal disorders. A large European multinational consortium successfully discovered mutations in many hereditary renal diseases. The role of molecular mechanisms is being examined as a basis for glomerular injury, as well as the importance of chronic inflammatory cytokine production. Newer modalities of anti-rejection therapy permit a one-year renal allograft graft survival rate of more than 95%. Pediatric nephrologists continue to employ contemporary molecular biologic tools, to define familial and genetic factors in renal diseases, to explore new technologies to enhance treatment of renal failure, to reexamine old 'truths' in the light of new information, and to reassess clinical issues in the light of current imaging techniques. Improvements in dialysis techniques and an understanding of adequacy continue to advance.

Pediatric nephrology has come a long way from its status 50 years ago. At that time, Robert E. Cooke stated that "the abysmal ignorance that exists in the field of clinical renal disease is illustrated by the deficiencies that exist, such as the inability to determine whether or not we are dealing with such obvious clinical conditions as glomerulonephritis or pyelonephritis, conditions that, as medical students, we are taught were clear-cut entities; likewise that nephrosis was a definite disease."[7] Technical methods such as organ culture, cell signaling, in-situ hybridization, transgenic and knockout mouse models, positional cloning, gene chips and elucidation of the human genome have begun to narrow this gap.

ACKNOWLEDGMENTS

The author is grateful for the comments and recent manuscripts of Dr. M.A. Holliday, and the reflections of W.E. Segar, C. West, I. Greifer, B.S. Kaplan, R. Fine, J. Lewy, P. McEnery, J. Robillard, and N. Siegel. I also appreciate the help of A.L. Friedman, B.S. Arant, D.P. Jones, A.B. Patters, R. Wyatt, and S. Roy. Any omissions are unintentional. A short history such as this requires severe selection, and not all important components or figures in the field are mentioned. I am also indebted to my father, the late Dr. Jack Chesney, for his collection of late 19th and early 20th century pediatric texts. Unlimited access to these volumes has been invaluable.

REFERENCES

1. Addis T. *Glomerular Nephritis: Diagnosis and Treatment.* McMillan, New York, 1950.

2. Berger J. IgA glomerular deposits in renal disease. Transplant Prac 1969;1:939-951.

3. Belzer FO, Schwertzer RT, Holliday MA. Renal homotransplantation in children. Am J Surg 1972;124:270-281.

4. Calcagno PL, Rubin MI, Weintraub DH. Studies in the renal concentration and dilating mechanisms in the premature infant. J Clin Invest 1954;33:91-99.

5. Chesney RW. The history of pediatric discipline series: a history of pediatric specialties: the development of pediatric nephrology. Pediatr Res 2002;52:770-778.

6. Churg J, Habib R, White RH. Pathology of the nephrotic syndrome in children. Lancet 1970;1:1299-1304.

7. Cooke RE. Introductory remarks in hereditary development, and immunologic aspects of kidney disease. In: Metcoff J (ed.), XIII Annual Conference on the Kidney. Northwestern University Press, Evanston, 1962, p. 3.

8. Darrow DC, Yannet H. The changes in the distribution of body water accompanying increase and decrease in extracellular electrolyte. J Clin Invest 1935;14:266-275.

9. de Leeuw K. The prognosis of nephritis in children. Acta Paediatr 1937;20 Suppl 1(2):1-24.

10. Gamble JL. *Chemical Anatomy, Physiology and Pathology of Extracellular Fluid*. Harvard University Press, Cambridge, 1950.

11. Gamble JL, Ross GS. The factors of dehydration following pyloric obstruction. J Clin Invest 1925;1:403-423.

12. Habib R, Kleinknecht C, Gubler MC. Extramembranous glomerulonephritis in children. J Pediatr 1974;82:754-761.

13. Henoch EH. *Verlesungen Uber Kinderkrankheiten*, 11th edn. Hirschwald, Berlin, 1903.

14. Howland J, Marriot M. Acidosis occurring in diarrhea. Am J Dis Child 1916;11:309-325.

15. Kaskel FJ, Powell DR, Tönshoff B. The Sixth Symposium on Growth and Development in Children with Chronic Renal Failure: The molecular basis of skeletal growth. Pediatr Nephrol 2000;14:535-706.

16. Langstein L. Diseases of the urinary apparatus. In: Pfaundler M, Schlossmann A (eds), *The Diseases of Children*. Philadelphia, 1908, pp. 12-23.

17. Liberman E. *Clinical Pediatric Nephrology*. JB Lippincott, Philadelphia, 1976.

18. Lucas RC. On a form of late rickets associated with albuminuria, rickets of adolescents. Lancet 1883;1:993-995.

19. Najarian JS, Simmons RL, Tallent MB, et al. Renal transplantation in infants and children. Ann Surg 1971;174:583-591.

20. Rappaport M, McCrory WW, Barbero G, et al. Effect of corticotropin (ACTH) on children with the nephrotic syndrome. JAMA 1951;147:1101-1106.

21. Riley CM. Nephrotic syndrome: effect of adrenocorticotrophic hormone. Pediatrics 1951;7:457-471.

22. Royer P, Habib R, Mathieu H, Broyer M, Walsh A. *Pediatric Nephrology: Major Problems in Clinical Pediatrics*. WB Saunders, Philadelphia, 1974.

23. Rubin MI, Barratt TM. *Pediatric Nephrology*. Williams & Wilkins, Baltimore, 1975.

24. Sereni F. Pediatric nephrology in Europe from the 16th to the 19th Century. Am J Nephrol 2002;22:207-212.

25. von Reuss AR. Der harn des neugeborenon kindes. In von Reuss AR, (ed): *Die Krankheiten des Neugeborenen*. Springer Verlag, Berlin, 1914, pp. 22-26.

26. West CD, McAdams AJ, McConville JM, et al. Hypocomplementemic and normocomplementemic persistent (chronic) glomerulonephritis: clinical pathologic characteristics. J Pediatr 1965;67:1089-1098.

PART I

11

CHAPTER 3

Clinical Evaluation of a Child with Kidney Disease

KEVIN E.C. MEYERS, M.B., B.Ch. AND

MADHURA PRADHAN, M.D.

Reasons for Referring Children with Suspected Kidney Disease for Evaluation

> Antenatal Imaging Findings
>
> Polyuria
>
> Oliguria and Anuria
>
> Abnormal Urine
>> Color
>>
>> Odor
>>
>> Incontinence
>>
>> Poor Urinary Stream
>>
>> Frequency, Dysuria, and Urgency
>
> Renal Calculi
>
> Edema
>
> Dehydration
>
> Evaluation, Screening, and Other Indications
>> Routine Neonatal Examination
>>
>> Screening for Bacteriuria
>>
>> Screening for Hypertension
>>
>> Family Studies
>>
>> Biochemical Evaluations
>
> Non-specific Symptoms that may Indicate Kidney Disease
>> Malaise and Fatigue
>>
>> Failure to Thrive

History

> Family History
>
> Pregnancy and Birth History
>
> Nutritional History
>
> Medications and Drugs
>
> Review of Systems
>
> Psychosocial History

Examination

> General Assessment
>> Physical Clues
>>
>> Head and Neck: Hair, Ears, Eyes, Nose, Mouth, and Neck
>>
>> Cardio-Respiratory
>>
>> Abdomen and External Genitalia
>>
>> Neurological
>>
>> Musculoskeletal
>>
>> Skin

Indications for Referral to a Pediatric Nephrologist or Urologist

---

> **Clinical Pearl**
>
> Antenatal ultrasonography detects increasing numbers of individuals with pre-symptomatic urogenital abnormalities.

Renal and urological disorders may present with obvious clinical symptoms and signs, as part of a systemic disease, or are diagnosed during screening of urine or blood pressure for well-child visits or other illnesses. Renal disease should be excluded in all sick children who have no obvious cause for their illness.

REASONS FOR REFERRING CHILDREN WITH SUSPECTED KIDNEY DISEASE FOR EVALUATION

Antenatal Imaging Findings

Renal disorders may be diagnosed antenatally. Polyhydramnios or oligohydramnios can be signs of a renal disease (Table 3-1). Oligohydramnios occurs in 4% of pregnancies, and polyhydramnios occurs in 1% of pregnancies in the USA. The Potter sequence (oligohydramnios sequence) in a neonate consists of combinations of sloping forehead, posterior set ears, small compressed nose, pulmonary hypoplasia, dislocated hips, flexural deformities, and talipes. This deformation sequence occurs as a result of bilateral renal adysplasia, autosomal recessive polycystic kidney disease (ARPKD) and obstructive uropathies. Routine antenatal ultrasonography may

Table 3-1	Renal Disorders Associated with Alterations in Amniotic Fluid Volume	
Oligohydramnios	**Polyhydramnios**	
Adysplasia	Partial obstruction	
Hypoplasia	Bartter's syndrome	
Polycystic kidneys	Nephrogenic diabetes insipidus	
Obstruction	Congenital nephrotic syndrome	
ACE inhibitors		

Table 3-2	Nephrogenic Diabetes Insipidus may be Primary or Secondary	
Primary Nephrogenic Diabetes Insipidus	**Secondary Nephrogenic Diabetes Insipidus**	
X-linked NDI (VP2 receptor)	Fanconi syndromes	
Autosomal recessive NDI (Aquaporin 2)	Bartter syndromes	
	Electrolyte abnormalities	
	Medications (diuretics, lithium)	
	Partial urinary tract obstruction	
	Chronic tubulointerstitial nephritis	
	Nephronophthisis	
	Early stages of chronic renal insufficiency	
	Psychogenic	

disclose unilateral hypoplasia and/or dysplasia, obstructive uropathy with hydronephrosis and/or pelviectasis, unilateral multicystic kidney or polycystic kidneys. Pelviectasis suggests a uretero-pelvic junction (UPJ) obstruction. However, an antenatal finding of pelviectasis is often not confirmed on postnatal examination and even when present, the correct treatment is not always obvious. First and early second trimester antenatal ultrasound (US) may fail to detect posterior urethral valves (PUV).

Polyuria

Polyuria results from excessive intake of fluid, absence of central release of antidiuretic hormone (ADH), tubular insensitivity to ADH, or an osmotic diuresis. Primary polydipsia can be distinguished by comparing the urine to plasma osmolalities after careful water deprivation and ADH challenge. Central and renal causes of excess water loss can be distinguished by measuring plasma ADH and by the renal concentrating response to administered ADH (Table 3-2). Progressive polyuria with polydypsia most frequently heralds new-onset insulin-dependent diabetes mellitus, but can also occur with renal tubular dysfunction. In infants, a defect in the urinary concentrating ability is suspected when there is irritability, lethargy, failure to thrive, and unexplained dehydration. These infants often prefer water to milk feeds. In children there may be thirst, excessive fluid ingestion, and nocturnal enuresis. Nephrogenic diabetes insipidus may be either primary or secondary (see Table 3-2).

Oliguria and Anuria

Anuria is the complete cessation of urine flow; oliguria is a reduction of urine volume such that homeostasis is no longer maintained. Oliguria is defined as a decrease in volume below 500 ml/day/1.73 m². This corresponds to approximately 1 ml/kg/hour in infants. Oliguria and anuria may occur as a result of prerenal factors (hypovolemia), intrinsic renal diseases or post-renal cause (urinary tract obstruction). An abrupt decrease in urine volume with tea- or cola-colored urine suggests acute glomerulonephritis.

Abnormal Urine

Color

Normal urine is light yellow when dilute, and dark orange-yellow when concentrated. The first morning urine is normally the most concentrated, and provides useful information about the concentrating capacity of the kidneys and protein loss. There are numerous reasons for a change in the color of urine (Table 3-3). Tea- or cola-colored urine suggests blood of glomerular origin, whereas bleeding from the lower urinary tract produces bright red urine. Blood in the urine is identified most readily on a dipstick, using a peroxidase assay that reacts with hemoglobin to turn green; greater than 1+ is considered positive. It is important to note that the dipstick tests for hemoglobin, not red blood cells (RBC). Because any chemical that reacts with peroxidase will produce a positive test, all positive dipstick screens of urine should be followed by microscopic examination to confirm the presence of RBC. Two important causes of a positive dipstick with a negative microscopic examination are free hemoglobin from hemolysis, and myoglobinuria from rhabdomyolysis. Medications and toxins that cause red urine are heme-negative. The presence of more than 10 RBC per high-power field (400×) of urine sediment from a centrifuged 10 ml urine sample is abnormal. Changes in urine color unique to children are associated with dyes (crayon ingestion, candies) and with inborn errors of metabolism (black-stained diaper with alkaptonuria, blue diaper syndrome). Medications that cause a change in urine color include rifampacin (orange) and pyridium (bright yellow).

Odor

A change in the urine odor, the uriniferous smell, is associated with concentrated urine and with the ingestion of certain foods (fish, asparagus). Cloudy offensive, malodorous urine suggests urinary tract infection, especially if

Table 3-3 Urine Color			
Dark Yellow	**Red/Orange**	**Dark Brown or Black**	**Abnormally Colored**
Concentrated	Porphyrins	Blood	Food coloring
Bile pigments	Beets	Homogentisic acid	Azathioprine
Blackberries	Rifampin	(Alcaptonuria)	Phenothiazines
Red food coloring	Melanin		Colored marking pens
Phenolphthalein	Tyrosinosis		*Serratia marcescens*
Hemoglobinuria	Methemoglobinemia		Urinary infection
Homogentisic acid			
Melanin			
Nitrofurantoin			
Salicylates			
Metronidazole			
Deferoxamine			
Urates			
Chloroquine			
Pyridium			
Myoglobinuria			
Methyldopa			
Porphyrin			
Sulfa			
Iron sorbitol			

associated with fever, frequency, urgency, lower abdominal or flank pain. Urine microscopy and culture are required to confirm a diagnosis of a urinary tract infection (UTI). A sweet urine odor occurs in maple syrup urine disease, whereas an odor of sweaty feet occurs in isovaleric acidemia.

Incontinence

Children are usually continent by 3 years of age, but 15% continue to have nocturnal enuresis at 5 years. Primary nocturnal enuresis is a nuisance but is usually benign. Persistence of daytime wetting is frequently a behavioral problem, or it may be a symptom of renal or urological disease. Secondary enuresis in a previously dry child must be evaluated for an organic or psychological problem. Daytime (diurnal) incontinence merits careful evaluation of the urinary system. This may be associated with an ectopic ureter below the bladder neck that results in daytime dribbling. More often, it is the result of bladder dysynergia with unstable bladder contractions, urgency, squatting, and urinary leak.

Poor Urinary Stream

It is important to ask about and to observe the urinary stream, especially in boys, with a suspected urinary tract abnormality. Causes of a poor urinary stream are a neurogenic bladder and posterior urethral valves.

Clinical Pearl
The mother of her first boy may not know how normal boys urinate.

Frequency, Dysuria, and Urgency

Changes in the voiding pattern or pain with urination is most frequently due to abnormalities of the bladder, urethra, and perineum. Children void four to eight times per day. Frequency of urination may be associated with small or large urinary volumes (polyuria). Dysuria, hesitancy, dribbling, or urgency often accompanies urinary frequency with small volumes. Causes of frequency with small volumes are reduced bladder capacity, bladder irritability (cystitis), dysfunctional voiding, hypercalciuria, caffeine, and behavioral problems. Frequency with dysuria is usually caused by urinary tract infections or urethritis. Vulvovaginitis in girls and balanitis in boys may present with dysuria.

Renal Calculi

Passage of a stone is associated with flank pain (renal colic) that may radiate to the groin. Frequently this is accompanied by hematuria and sometimes by a UTI.

Edema

Edema in children with renal disease occurs in the nephrotic syndrome, acute nephritis, and acute and chronic renal failure.

Clinical Pearl
Do not ascribe puffy eyes to an allergy before testing the urine for albumin!

Box 3-1   Causes of Generalized Edema

- Nephrotic syndrome
- Protein energy malnutrition (kwashiorkor)
- Protein-losing enteropathy (PLE)
- Cardiac failure
- Liver disease
- Generalized allergic reaction

In the nephrotic syndrome, puffiness is most evident around the eyes and face in the morning, is gravitational, and spreads to the lower part of the body later in the day. Ascites, sacral edema and pleural effusions also occur. The edema in nephrotic syndrome is primarily due to hypoalbuminemia, whereas in acute nephritis it is secondary to fluid retention. Other causes of generalized edema are listed in Box 3-1.

Dehydration

An inability to conserve water because of renal disease may result in dehydration despite relatively small losses of fluid by vomiting or diarrhea. Febrile children who have difficulty feeding develop hypernatremia. Thirst, dizziness, and postural hypotension are important clues. Infants with chronic salt loss caused by obstructive uropathy, dysplastic kidneys or Bartter syndrome can become rapidly dehydrated due to their inability to concentrate the urine. These children often have a history of salt craving.

Patients with a renal disease, especially if it is insidious, may have no obvious symptoms and a problem may only be identified at a well-child visit or when the child is seen for unrelated problems. Combinations of abnormal finding are high blood pressure, abnormal urinary sediment, or abnormal blood chemistries. The frequency of serendipitous findings of renal disease has led to proposals for population screening. This is a complex problem with no easy answers. We recommend routine blood pressure (BP) measurements and testing of urine at least twice a year for infants and children. Currently the American Academy of Pediatrics recommends checking BP starting at 3 years of age; urine screening is done prior to starting school.

Evaluation, Screening, and Other Indications

Routine Neonatal Examination

It is important to look for dysmorphisms on routine examination of a neonate (Table 3-4). There is an increased incidence of renal abnormalities in association with other congenital defects, especially those of the cardiovascular, gastrointestinal tracts and external genitalia. The prune belly syndrome is associated with absent anterior abdominal wall muscles, cryptorchidism, and urethral stenosis that result in hydroureteronephrosis. In the VATER association of anomalies, renal abnormalities include adysplasia and obstructive uropathy. Abnormalities of the ureters including duplication and ectopic ureter may occur with perineal hypospadias. Neurogenic bladder occurs with hydrocephalus, spina bifida, tethered cord and caudal regression. Preauricular pits may be familial, are more common in females and Blacks, and are not an indication for renal ultrasound when they are an isolated finding.

Screening for Bacteriuria

Screening for bacteriuria has been advocated because about 5% of children have at least one episode of UTI, and because UTI may be associated with vesicoureteric reflux and subsequent renal scarring. However, the treatment of asymptomatic bacteriuria in children is not established. Identification of mild abnormalities of the urinary sediment in otherwise well children requires rechecking of the urine on at least two more occasions. Those with persistent hematuria or proteinuria should be referred for further evaluation.

Screening for Hypertension

Most children with hypertension are asymptomatic, but symptoms may include headaches or seizures. Most are detected at routine child visits, physical sports examinations or through school screening programs.

Family Studies

It is important to obtain a careful family history of renal disease, hypertension, hematuria, proteinuria, deafness, renal calculi, urinary tract infection, cerebrovascular

---

Table 3-4   Examples of the Interplay of Renal Diseases and the Rest of the Body

Renal disorders may be part of other conditions	Renal adysplasia in the branchio-otorenal syndrome
	Cystic kidneys in tuberous sclerosis
Renal disorders may be a complication of other conditions	Glomerulonephritis in vasculitides
	Glomerulonephritis in bacterial endocarditis, hepatitis
Other systems may be affected by the complications of chronic renal failure	Renal osteodystrophy
	Congestive heart failure
	Peripheral neuropathy

accident, systemic lupus, and history of dialysis or renal transplantation.

Biochemical Evaluations

The kidney plays a central role in homeostasis. Therefore, laboratory evidence of renal dysfunction may be found by chance, especially when managing children with multi-system disorders.

> **Clinical Pearl**
>
> Elevated blood urea nitrogen (BUN) but normal serum creatinine is rarely indicative of a renal disease.

Non-Specific Symptoms that may Indicate Kidney Disease

Occasionally, children are found to have renal insufficiency when blood tests are performed for non-specific symptoms such as fatigue or malaise. Chronic renal failure may cause failure to thrive, lethargy, malaise, vomiting, loss of appetite, and failure in school. Some children present with bone pains and others with overt evidence of rickets.

Malaise and Fatigue

Chronic renal failure may present with a feeling of general ill health with malaise, fatigue and lethargy, and an increased need for sleep. The child may be unable to concentrate at school, and their grades may decline. Anemia contributes to this picture, and occasionally the patient presents to a hematologist for evaluation of pallor.

Failure to Thrive

Children with chronic renal failure and those with renal tubular disorders may fail to grow normally. The reasons for reduced growth are numerous, interact in complex ways, and include metabolic acidosis, renal osteodystrophy, abnormal growth hormone action, anemia, malnutrition, chronic salt and water losses, and treatment with corticosteroids. Initial evaluation of a child with failure to thrive (FTT) should include evaluation of the serum electrolytes, BUN, and serum creatinine. Typically, children with renal tubular acidosis begin to fail to thrive from age 6 to 9 months. Children whose heights decrease and cross percentiles, but who otherwise seem normal, should be evaluated with measurement of serum electrolytes, BUN, and serum creatinine. In a small child with poor muscle mass, the serum creatinine concentration may not reflect the true severity of renal insufficiency. When blood is drawn for electrolytes care must be taken to obtain a free-flowing blood sample and to process it immediately in order to prevent any spurious diagnosis of metabolic acidosis or hyperkalemia.

HISTORY

We cannot over-emphasize the importance of taking a careful history. The history is the key to making a correct diagnosis in over 80% of patients. A careful history enables one to focus on the physical examination and laboratory investigation. A history must be taken of the presenting symptom(s) (the main complaint) and should include a detailed enquiry about hematuria, dysuria, frequency, burning on micturition, nocturia, daytime wetting, urgency, voiding patterns, and enuresis. Details must be obtained of when and how the disorder began. It is useful to tabulate the chronological sequence of events as this often establishes a logical progression.

Family History

Important clues to the diagnosis are frequently revealed with detailed questioning about the family, as genetic factors are relevant to many renal diseases. A history of deafness and renal failure in immediate relatives suggests Alport syndrome (Box 3-2). Stroke and renal failure in succeeding generations is consistent with an autosomal dominant inheritance and suggests autosomal dominant polycystic kidney disease (ADPKD). Autosomal recessive conditions may occur more often in consanguineous unions. A family pedigree should be constructed and siblings, parents, grandparents and other relevant members should be included. This establishes the patient within the context of the family and helps to indicate the pattern of inheritance of genetic conditions. Specific direct questions should be asked about a family history of renal calculus, deafness and dialysis or renal transplant as this information is not always volunteered during open-ended questioning.

Pregnancy and Birth History

Neonates who are more likely to develop hypertension are those with reduced nephron mass as a result of

> **Box 3-2 Deafness and Renal Disorders**
>
> - Alport syndromes
> - Fechtner (Epstein) syndrome
> - Autosomal recessive renal tubular acidosis
> - Bartter syndrome
> - X-linked hypophosphatemic rickets
> - Branchio-otorenal syndrome
> - Townes–Brocks syndrome
> - 10p-syndrome (HHR or *h*ypoparathyroidism, *h*earing loss, vesicoureteric *r*eflux)

in utero growth retardation (IUGR), and those with an umbilical artery catheterization complicated by renal artery thrombosis. Maternal smoking, alcohol and drug use are associated with IUGR. Women who abuse alcohol while pregnant may deliver a child with fetal alcohol syndrome (FAS) that may be associated with renal hypoplasia. A history of a difficult delivery, maternal diabetes, or macroscopic hematuria suggests renal venous thrombosis; this can result in a small, scarred kidney and hypertension. Congenital nephrotic syndrome and maternal syphilis are causes of placentamegaly defined as a placenta that weighs more than 25% of the child's birth weight. Many medications may cross the placenta and damage the developing fetus. Angiotensin-converting enzyme (ACE) inhibitors, non-steroidal anti-inflammatory drugs (NSAIDs), and cocaine can affect fetal kidney development. The kidneys of neonates with severe perinatal hypoxia and acute respiratory failure (ARF) usually recover fully. A history of a single umbilical artery could indicate the presence of renal malformations such as renal dysplasia; however, most malformations are minor in nature and hence radiologic studies are not warranted in *asymptomatic* newborns with an isolated single umbilical artery.

Nutritional History

A careful dietary and feeding history must be taken. This should start with the neonatal period with inquiries about breast or bottle-feeding, and then progress to subsequent dietary preferences or difficulties. These include episodes of thirst, anorexia, vomiting and food preferences. Children with chronic renal failure secondary to obstructive uropathy, nephronophthisis and renal tubular causes of sodium wasting often have a preference for salty foods. In older children the dietary history should be taken together with an exercise history. Formal dietary assessment by a nutritionist skilled in the care of children is required in children with FTT or chronic renal failure.

Medications and Drugs

The history must include inquiries about use of prescription and over-the-counter medications such as NSAIDs. Teenagers should be asked whether they use recreational drugs, tobacco, and alcohol.

Review of Systems

Renal disorders may be part of, or a complication of, other conditions. So, because all systems may be affected by the complications of renal disorders, a careful enquiry must include the elicitation of symptoms from all of the major organ systems.

Psychosocial History

A social history includes the parents' ages, marital status, occupations and the child's position in the family, level and participation in school and sport, and whether or not he or she has friends. Answers to these questions help to understand relationships within the family and in society. It is often difficult to obtain and maintain medical insurance care for children with renal disorders, especially in low-income families, in families who do not have plans at work, and in those whose adolescent children earn below the minimum wage. Of greater importance is the effect that chronic illness has on the family. Even when adequate emotional and financial coping mechanisms are available, taking care of a child with a chronic renal illness is challenging. The support and involvement of a skilled social worker and psychologist play a crucial part in the care of these children (see Chapters 7, 8, and 9).

EXAMINATION

General Assessment

The general examination should begin while the patient and family are entering the consulting room. Much can be learned about the patient from initial observations prior to a formal introduction. For example, family dynamics and the patient's level of comfort with the visit are often immediately apparent. A rapid preliminary assessment should include the acuity of the illness, whether there is compromise of the circulatory or respiratory systems, whether the child is in pain, the level of consciousness and the child's mood.

Height and weight must be measured. In children it is preferable to use a stadiometer to measure height, and a digital scale that is accurate to 0.1 kg to measure weight. In children aged less than 1 year, length should be measured and the weighing scale must be accurate to 0.01 kg. Head circumference should be measured in children aged less than 3 years. The physical data should then be plotted on age- and sex-appropriate growth charts. These measurements give valuable information about the child's growth, state of nutrition and change in growth over time. These measurements have proved invaluable in helping with optimization of nutrition in infants with chronic renal failure. Additional features suggesting established chronic renal failure include pallor, a sallow skin color and skeletal deformity.

Hydration is assessed by initial consideration of total body water, and then by considering the intracellular fluid (ICF) and extracellular fluid (ECF) compartments. Clues to changes in total body water can be assessed from recent reviews of weight alteration. In situations

Table 3-5   Findings Frequently Associated with Structural and Biochemical Renal Disease

Somatic Region	Syndrome	Renal Abnormality
Deafness	Alport syndrome	Abnormal GBM
Preauricular pits	Branchiomotor renal (BOR)	Hypoplasia/Dysplasia
Eye colobomata		
Retinitis pigmentosa	Juvenile nephronophthisis	Medullary cystic disease
Characteristic facies	⎧Williams syndrome	Renal artery stenosis
	⎨Alagille syndrome	Adysplasia
	⎩Trisomy 21	Dysplasia
Short neck	Klippel–Feil syndrome	Adysplasia
Skin café-au-lait spots	Neurofibromatosis	Renal artery stenosis
Hypopigmented spots	Tuberous sclerosis	Angiomyolioma, polycystic
Dysplasia of nails	Nail-patella syndrome	Nephrotic syndrome
Chest: widely spaced nipples	Turner syndrome	Horseshoe kidney
Webbed neck	Turner, Noonan syndromes	Ectopia, adysplasia
Low hairline	Klippel–Feil syndrome	Adysplasia
Musculoskeletal		
Postaxial polydactyly	Bardet–Biedel syndrome	Cystic dysplasia
Patellae – absent/small	Nail-patella syndrome	Nephrotic syndrome
Short stature	Numerous conditions	

GBM = glomerular basement membrane.

where there is loss of water with normal serum sodium, mild dehydration is present with loss of 5% body weight, and severe dehydration with a loss of 15%. Changes in ICF occur with water gain or loss and are reflected in the serum by hyponatremia and hypernatremia, respectively. These changes affect mainly the brain because of its fixed volume, and either seizures (hyponatremia) or cerebral vein thrombosis (hypernatremia) may occur. The ECF is composed of the intravascular fluid (IVF) and interstitial fluid (IF) compartments. Expansion of the IF – for example in association with nephrotic syndrome (NS) – results in edema, and contraction decreases skin turgor. Expansion of the IVF volume is reflected clinically by hypertension, pulmonary congestion, elevated jugular venous pressure, hepatomegaly, and perhaps some pedal edema, whilst contraction (hypovolemia) is associated with hypotension. Occult hypovolemia can be diagnosed by looking for orthostatic changes in the blood pressure and pulse rate.

Physical Clues

Many physical changes are associated with structural and biochemical renal disease. Some of the more frequent associations are listed in Table 3-5. Preauricular pits or tags are associated with renal malformations if they occur with other malformations/dysmorphisms, a family history of deafness, auricular and/or renal malformations, or a maternal history of diabetes.

Head and Neck: Hair, Ears, Eyes, Nose, Mouth, and Neck

Inspection of the head and neck may reveal a low hairline, microcephalus, ear tags, and other dysmorphic features associated with renal disease (see Table 3-5). Deafness can occur in several syndromes (see Box 3-2). An eye examination (Table 3-6) may show coloboma, cataracts, retinitis pigmentosa, perimacular white specks, and the changes associated with hypertension.

Photophobia in a patient with renal dysfunction, FTT, and/or rickets, occurs in cystinosis. This can be confirmed by a slit lamp examination. Leisch nodules of the iris are present in neurofibromatosis. Treatment of secondary hyperparathyroidism may be complicated by hypercalcemia that may cause red eyes with episcleral calcification. Saddle nose deformity with nasal septal ulcers occur in Wegener's granulomatosis and systemic lupus erythematosus (SLE). Children with chronic renal failure often have an increased incidence of caries and tooth discoloration.

Cardio-Respiratory

The pulse must be assessed for rate, rhythm, and volume. Radio-femoral delay, weak femoral pulses and

Table 3-6   Eye Findings in Association with Renal Disorders

Coloboma	Tuberous sclerosis, Alport syndrome, Oculohepatoencephalo-renal syndrome, Lenz microphthalmia syndrome
Cataracts	Fabry's disease, Lowe syndrome
Retinitis pigmentosa	Bardet-Biedl syndrome Senior–Loken syndrome
Leisch nodules	Neurofibromatosis
Retinal phacomas	Tuberous sclerosis

reduced blood pressure in the lower limbs occur with coarctation of the aorta. When a vasculitis is suspected, the major vessels including the common carotid, vertebral, abdominal aorta, renal and femoral arteries must be auscultated for bruits and accessible vessels must be palpated for blood flow. Measurement of blood pressure is described in detail (see Chapter 15). Systemic hypertension, volume overload, pericardial effusion, and congenital heart disease can cause cardiomegaly. A gallop rhythm may occur in cardiac failure caused by volume overload, longstanding hypertension or congenital heart disease. The most frequent among the numerous causes of a heart murmur is the hyperdynamic state caused by the anemia of chronic renal failure. Pericardial rubs and effusions occur in uremia, but are rarely found in children because of early use of renal replacement therapy. However, pericardial rubs can occur in SLE and in infectious pericarditis. The respiratory rate, tachypnea and dyspnea as well as examination for cyanosis and clubbing, are important. The chest must be examined carefully to detect evidence of consolidation, pleural effusion, or pulmonary edema.

Abdomen and External Genitalia

The abdomen must be inspected to detect umbilical vessels, omphalocele (Beckwith-Wiedemann syndrome), umbilical hernia, absent abdominal muscles (prune belly syndrome), dilated veins (congenital hepatic fibrosis with portal hypertension in ARPKD), and flank masses. In children, flank masses are usually of renal origin, may be unilateral or bilateral and include multicystic kidney disease, hydronephrosis, ARPKD, and Wilms' tumor and (Table 3-7). The differential diagnosis of nephromegaly is shown in Box 3-3.

A palpable bladder and weak urinary stream are suggestive of posterior urethral valves, not only in a newborn boy but also in older males. There is a weak association between perineal hypospadias and urogenital malformations. Perineal hypospadias and cryptorchidism give the appearance of ambiguous genitalia. Nephrotic syndrome together with ambiguous genitalia occur in Denys-Drash syndrome. Undescended testes also occur in prune belly syndrome (Eagle-Barret syndrome). There are many

Box 3-3	Differential Diagnosis of Nephromegaly

- Multicystic kidney disease
- Hydronephrosis
- Autosomal recessive polycystic kidney disease
- Autosomal dominant polycystic kidney disease
- Wilms' tumor
- Renal venous thrombosis
- Acute pyelonephritis
- Lymphoma, leukemia
- Glycogen storage disease
- Tyrosinemia
- Beckwith-Wiedemann syndrome
- Perlman syndrome
- Amyloidosis
- Sarcoidosis
- Sickle cell anemia

syndromes and conditions in which hepatosplenomegaly is associated with renal disorders (Table 3-8). Imperforate anus occurs in the VATER association.

Neurological

The nervous system is usually grossly intact in children with urogenital disorders. Patients with systemic disorders, hypertension, uremia, hemolytic uremic syndromes, neuropathic bladder and patients in intensive care require careful neurological examinations. Focal deficits may be present with hypertension and systemic vascular disorders. Severe hypertension may cause facial nerve palsy, seizures, and hemorrhagic stroke. When a neuropathic bladder is suspected, the peripheral nervous system of the lower body must be examined carefully. Patients with microcephaly, mental abnormalities and nephrotic syndrome have the Galloway-Mowat syndrome.

Musculoskeletal

Muscle wasting occurs with advanced chronic renal failure. Muscle weakness occurs in rickets, hypokalemia, systemic lupus, and as a complication of corticosteroids. Mitochondrial disorders may be complicated by muscle weakness and renal tubular acidosis. Renal osteodystrophy, renal Fanconi syndrome, and renal tubular acidosis

Table 3-7	Incidence of Flank Masses by Age Distribution			
Age	Hydronephrosis (%)	Cystic (%)	Tumors (%)	Other (%)
Newborn	50	38		12
Less than 1 year	40		40	20
Over 1 year			70	30

Table 3-8	Liver-Kidney Associations
Congenital hepatic fibrosis	Autosomal recessive polycystic kidneys
	Nephronophthisis
	Jeune asphyxiating thoracodystrophy
	Biedl-Bardet syndrome
Cholestasis	Alagille syndrome

Table 3-9   Examples of Syndromes with Renal and Skeletal Anomalies

Syndrome	Renal Anomaly	Skeletal Anomaly
Acrorenal syndromes	Agenesis, dysplasia, hydronephrosis	Acrodactyly, oligodactyly, hemivertebrae
Bardet–Beidel syndrome	Dysplasia, hydronephrosis, VUR	Polysyndactyly
Caudal regression syndrome	Agenesis, horseshoe kidney, VUR, hypoplasia, hydronephrosis	Vertebral defects
Ellis van Creveld syndrome	Dysplasia, hydronephrosis	Polydactyly
Cornelia de Lange syndrome	Agenesis, hypoplasia, dysplasia	Small hands and feet
Meckel–Gruber syndrome	Dysplasia	Polydactyly
Nail-patella syndrome	Nephrotic syndrome	Absent patellae, iliac spurs
Schimke's syndrome	Nephrotic syndrome	Spondyloephiphyseal dysplasia
VATER association	Agenesis, horseshoe kidney, dysplasia	Vertebral anomalies
Townes–Brocks syndrome	Agenesis, dysplasia	Triphalangeal thumb
Fanconi anemia syndrome	Agenesis, horseshoe kidney, hypoplasia, hydronephrosis	Radial ray dysplasia

VUR = vesicoureteral reflux.

often present with clinical features of rickets (see Chapter 16). Congenital hip dislocation and limb deformations occur in newborns as complications of oligohydramnios. Slipped capital femoral epiphysis (SCFE) occurs more frequently than expected in chronic renal failure and after renal transplantation. Avascular necrosis of the femoral head is a complication of prolonged corticosteroid therapy, especially in children with systemic lupus. Deformities of the spine occur in spina bifida and VATER. Infants of diabetic mothers may have variable components of caudal regression that include sacral agenesis (Table 3-9). Hemihypertrophy occurs in the Beckwith-Wiedemann syndrome, and these children may have renal ectopia and are a risk of Wilms' tumor.

Skin

The skin and nails often give clues to an underlying systemic disorder. Skin manifestations of SLE are photosensitivity, malar rash, and discoid rash. In Henoch–Schönlein purpura the rash is a palpable purpura, mainly on the lower extremities and buttocks. Café-au-lait spots are found in neurofibromatosis. Skin manifestations of tuberous sclerosis are hypopigmented macules, adenoma sebaceum, periungual fibromas, shagreen patches. Dystrophic nails with absent lunulae and small or absent patellae are seen in the nail-patella syndrome. In patients with recurrent episodes of nephrotic syndrome nails may be pale with transverse lines (Beau's lines).

Longitudinal lines of the nails are seen in homocystinuria. Blue lunulae may indicate Wilson's disease or agyria.

INDICATIONS FOR REFERRAL TO A PEDIATRIC NEPHROLOGIST OR UROLOGIST

Children with hypertension (not related to coarctation of the aorta), hematuria, proteinuria or symptoms and/or signs of glomerulonephritis are referred to a nephrologist. Children who have a diagnosis of acute post-streptococcal glomerulonephritis should be referred if they have hypertension, or have increased serum creatinine or potassium concentrations. All children with chronic glomerular disease require nephrologic evaluation. Children with renal manifestations of a systemic disease also need a nephrologic evaluation. Parents may also request a referral to the nephrologist for reassurance, especially if there is a history of renal problems in the family.

Children with abnormal anatomy of the genitourinary tract, such as obstruction, tumors, non-glomerular gross hematuria, or obstructing renal calculi are referred to a pediatric urologist.

Some children are best managed together by a nephrologist and a urologist. These include children with renal calculi, reflux/urinary tract infections, and obstructive uropathy with compromised renal function.

CHAPTER 4

Pediatric Uroimaging

JOHN CONERY, M.D. AND

RICHARD BELLAH, M.D.

IMAGING MODALITIES

A variety of imaging modalities can be utilized in the evaluation of the pediatric urinary tract. The appropriate choice of imaging depends largely on the nature of the clinical question to be answered.

Ultrasound

Ultrasound (US) continues to be the mainstay of pediatric imaging for many conditions that require a morphologic assessment of the urinary tract. Availability, real-time imaging, lack of ionizing radiation, low cost, and excellent spatial/contrast resolution are advantages that US possesses. The most common indications for US of the pediatric urinary tract include: evaluation of the prenatal/neonatal hydronephrosis, identification and characterization of renal masses, initial assessment of the urinary tract for hematuria or hypertension, stone disease, and conditions that predispose a child to urinary tract infection (UTI).[16]

Technique

The standard US examination of the pediatric urinary tract includes views of both kidneys in terms of size, echotexture, and dilation. In the term infant, the average renal length is 4–5 cm; the kidneys grow, on average, approximately 3 mm per year to achieve a length of approximately 12 cm by young adulthood. Terms such as *echogenic*, *hyperechoic*, *hypoechoic*, and *anechoic* are commonly used when describing the appearance of the kidneys on US examinations; these are terms that describe the appearance of the renal cortex relative to adjacent structures, most often the liver. The pyramids – which are particularly prominent in newborns and infants – are normally of lower echogenicity (hypoechoic) compared to the adjacent renal cortex. The sonographic depiction of echogenic cortex relative to hypoechoic pyramids is referred to as *corticomedullary differentiation*. Normal corticomedullary differentiation is important because absence of this feature, although non-specific, may be indicative of underlying renal parenchymal disease. Doppler US imaging provides additional information to gray-scale US by evaluating vascular patency and vascular integrity of the kidneys.

Power Doppler US – a Doppler US technique to monitor blood flow, independent of flow direction – provides the ability to visualize tissue perfusion. The bladder is an integral part of every comprehensive renal US examination, and it should be examined for volume, wall abnormalities, wall thickness, calculi, distal ureters, and bladder emptying.

Appearance of the Kidneys

The sonographic appearance of the kidneys is dependent on age. In the neonate, the renal cortex is relatively more echogenic then that seen in older children and adults (Figure 4-1a and b). The marked cellularity of the neonatal renal cortex, as well as the heterogeneity in sizes of the glomeruli, account for the myriad of reflections that result in the relative increase in renal cortical echogenicity. In the premature infant, the cortex may be more echogenic than the adjacent liver and spleen. In preterm and healthy full-term infants, the cortical echogenicity of the kidney is slightly greater than or equal to that of liver and/or spleen. By about 12 months of age, cortical echogenicity is usually slightly less than that of the liver and spleen.

Voiding Cystourethrography

Voiding cystourethrography (VCUG) is a radiological or nuclear medicine study that provides an imaging depiction of bladder contour, compliance, and ability to empty. The radiological VCUG also provides the important anatomic depiction of the urethra. The VCUG procedure causes significant anxiety in both parents and children; careful preparation should, therefore, become

an integral part of every VCUG examination. The procedure involves sterile bladder catheterization, followed by instillation of water-soluble contrast. Radiation exposure is minimized by intermittent fluoroscopy. Images are obtained during bladder filling, as well as during voiding. The normal VCUG will usually demonstrate a rounded bladder with a smooth contour. Views of the urethra may be obtained in either the frontal (girls) or oblique (boys) position (Figure 4-2). The bladder capacity can also be estimated using this technique.

Low-dose radiological VCUG provides an excellent anatomic depiction of the bladder and urethra, but generally at a higher dosage than the radionuclide cystogram. Radionuclide cystography (RNC) is a sensitive method of detecting vesicoureteral reflux (VUR), but at the expense of resolution; the anatomic resolution is inferior to that of radiological VCUG. Traditionally, radiation doses for RNC have been lower than for fluoroscopic VCUG, but with the newer digital pulsed fluoroscopic units the doses are almost equal.[10]

Technique

The technique is similar to that used in VCUG, with sterile catheterization of the bladder. Saline containing Tc-99m pertechnetate is instilled into the bladder. There is continuous monitoring using a gamma camera to assess for VUR. The bladder is then filled to capacity, and the patient voids. Radiological VCUG can also be performed in conjunction with measuring intravesical/sphincter pressures (video urodynamics), and contributes information about bladder capacity, compliance, voiding function, and coordination of bladder/ urethral sphincter function.[1]

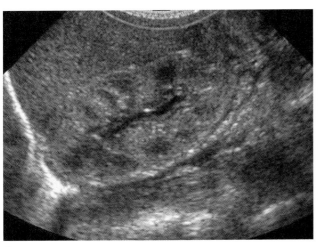
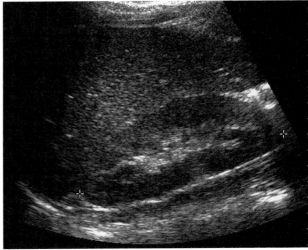

A   B

Figure 4-1   (a) Sagittal ultrasound of a normal right kidney in a 2-day-old male. The kidney is hyperechoic compared to the adjacent liver. (b) Sagittal ultrasound of a normal right kidney in a 4-year-old male. The renal parenchyma is hypoechoic compared to the adjacent liver.

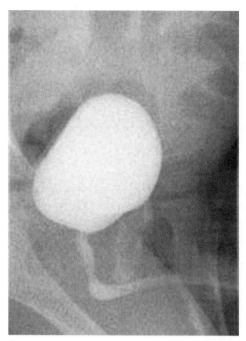

Figure 4-2   An oblique image from a voiding cystourethrogram in a 2-year-old male, showing a normal bladder and urethra.

Objectives of VCUG

One of the chief aims of VCUG is to identify the presence of VUR. RNC is an accepted modality for detecting VUR in the female with UTI, or in siblings of children with known VUR, whereas in males with UTI the radiological VCUG is the preferred method because details of the urethra are more clearly seen. Either method can be used for detection, grading, and follow-up of VUR. In pediatric patients with UTI, VCUG is used to evaluate whether the bladder empties properly. Conditions that affect bladder emptying include high-grade VUR, bladder outlet obstruction, and voiding dysfunction.

Intravenous Autography

Intravenous autography (IVU) has become a lost art in pediatric uroradiologic imaging. IVU provides excellent morphologic detail as well as semi-quantitative information about renal function, but has requirements of radiation and intravenous contrast administration. IVU should be performed in well-hydrated patients with normal renal function. After intravenous injection of iodinated contrast, only a limited number of images should be obtained. The morphologic assessment of the pediatric urinary tract has been largely replaced by less invasive cross-sectional imaging techniques, such as sonography and magnetic resonance (MR) urography. Some urologists still prefer IVU, however, as a way to integrate vertically the urinary tract and to help provide anatomic/functional information prior to or following urinary tract surgery (e.g., for hydronephrosis or stone disease). IVU is also occasionally

used for detection of the ectopic ureter in the female pediatric patient with constant wetting. Currently, IVU has no role in the evaluation of the child with urinary tract infection.

Computed Tomography

Computed tomography (CT) provides excellent morphologic as well as functional detail about the urinary tract. CT usually requires intravenous contrast volume similar to IVU, but more radiation than IVU; contrast CT should therefore be utilized in selected cases. At the expense of radiation, and because of its high sensitivity, non-enhanced (non-contrast) CT has emerged as the study of choice for the detection of urolithiasis in children and adolescents with renal colic, and in patients with difficult body habiti, for example with myelodysplasia. CT can readily identify urinary tract calculi of practically any composition, although small stones and even those composed of uric acid may occasionally be overlooked.[20]

Contrast-enhanced CT is the study of choice in the setting of trauma if acute renal injury is suspected. CT is far more sensitive than sonography in resolving acute pyelonephritis, and for determining if intervention is indicated for complications such as renal/perirenal abscess. CT further characterizes lesions identified by other techniques, such as renal cysts or angiomyolipomas. In evaluating hypertension, *CT angiography* – which requires a large volume of contrast and a rapid injection rate – is being used with greater frequency for anatomic depiction of renovascular disease (Figure 4-3a and b).

Magnetic Resonance Imaging

Magnetic resonance imaging (MRI) may be used to characterize and stage renal lesions. *MR urography* is a rapid MR technique that can provide anatomic details of the pyelocalyceal system and ureters, without exposing the patient to ionizing radiation or intravenous contrast. This technique can provide similar anatomic information to IVU. However, compared with IVU, spatial resolution is relatively poor in MR urography, and subtle abnormalities may not always be readily visualized. Image quality can also be significantly degraded by patient motion and/or respiration so that, despite the technique being rapid, sedation of the patient may still be required. Current indications for MR urography might include detection of ureteral ectopia in the female with 'continuous wetting,' complex duplicated renal collecting systems, and preoperative assessment of the pyelocalyceal system and ureteral abnormalities.[11]

Gadolinium-enhanced Functional Renal MR

This is now being used more frequently in a fashion similar to IVU and/or radionuclide renal scintigraphy.

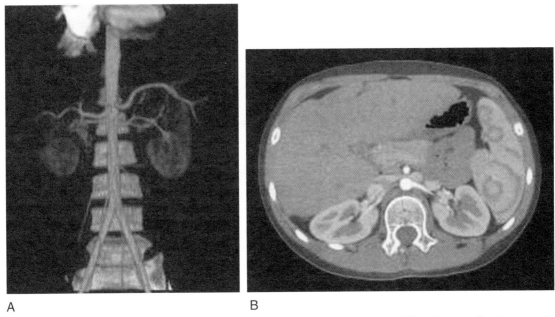

A   B

Figure 4-3   (a) A volume-rendered 3-D reconstructed image from a CT angiogram showing normal renal arteries. (b) Consecutive axial images from the same patient, showing normal left and right renal arteries.

Studies have shown that MR can also be used for the diagnosis for acute pyelonephritis. MRI and MR urography are of limited value, however, in evaluating urolithiasis, as small calcifications are difficult to visualize on MR. As these MR techniques evolve and refine, one might speculate that morphologic/functional assessment with MR urography could be performed in conjunction with MR angiography, and thus the need for multiple diagnostic imaging tests would be eliminated.[11]

Renal Angiography

Renal angiography is still regarded as the 'gold standard' in many children's hospitals, and has not yet been largely replaced by less invasive modalities, such as CT angiography or MR angiography. Furthermore, if therapeutic intervention is contemplated, conventional angiography is still a preferred diagnostic imaging method. In renal artery stenosis, for example, conventional angiography provides definitive diagnosis, a clear roadmap, as well as an opportunity for therapeutic angioplasty or stent placement. In many institutions, CT or MR angiography can be used as a screening tool in the young patient with hypertension, but conventional angiography remains the study of choice when renal artery stenosis is strongly suspected (i.e., abnormal screening MR angiogram, or abnormal renal US showing renal size disparity in a young patient with hypertension). A similar rationale applies for a diagnosis and potential treatment of a renal vascular malformation. Definitive or

preoperative embolization of vascular tumors is also possible with conventional angiography.

Nuclear Medicine Technetium-labeled Agents

These agents are commonly used for pediatric renal imaging. Radiation doses are relatively low, and technetium can be linked to various compounds that evaluate urinary system function. Diethylenetriamine-penta-acetic acid (DTPA) is cleared by glomerular filtration, and is therefore a good determinant of differential renal function, renal plasma flow, glomerular filtration, and renal clearance. Mercaptoacetyltriglycine (MAG 3) is actively excreted by the kidneys, and provides good information about collection system clearance. For example, either intravenous ^{99m}Tc-DTPA or MAG 3 can be used to evaluate renal function in a multicystic dysplastic kidney or in a renal transplant.

Diuretic Renography

Diuretic renography with ^{99m}Tc-MAG 3 or ^{99m}Tc-DTPA is commonly utilized to determine whether a dilated collecting system or ureter is either obstructive or non-obstructive. After intravenous administration of the radiotracer, continuous gamma camera monitoring documents renal uptake and filling of the collecting systems. When the collecting system is filled, furosemide is administered intravenously and a tracer washout tracing is obtained. The half-time clearance of tracer is used to determine if obstruction is present. Baseline absolute and relative renal function (split function) can be determined.

Captopril Nuclear Renography

Captopril nuclear renography is a non-invasive renal nuclear study which is used to detect renal artery stenosis in the patient with hypertension. If significant renal artery stenosis does exist, glomerular filtration rate (GFR) is maintained by constriction of the efferent arterioles. The angiotensin-converting enzyme (ACE) inhibitor, captopril, prevents this compensatory constriction, which results in a decrease in renal function after its administration. As the study is performed before and after its administration, the decreased function seen with captopril suggests renal artery stenosis, which can then be confirmed angiographically.

Radionuclide Cortical Scintigraphy

Radionuclide cortical scintigraphy (RCS) with ^{99m}Tc-labeled dimercaptosuccinic acid (DMSA) or ^{99m}Tc-labeled glucoheptonate is ideally suited for renal morphology evaluation, as these agents are concentrated in the cells of the proximal tubules. Indications for RCS include acute pyelonephritis, detection of renal scarring (in patients with hypertension), and identification of the occult/ectopic kidney. Following intravenous administration of the radiopharmaceutical, homogeneous uptake is normally seen within the renal cortex. Focal areas of tracer defect can be identified in acute pyelonephritis or in areas of focal parenchymal thinning due to reflux nephropathy. In the female with constant wetting and a solitary kidney, DMSA may identify the, otherwise, occult malpositioned kidney of which the ureter is ectopic.

URINARY TRACT INFECTION

Urinary tract infection (UTI) is one of the most common indications for urinary tract imaging in children. The significance of UTI rests not only on the acute morbidity but also on the potential for renal parenchymal scarring. The main goal of imaging in the work-up of UTI is to identify conditions that put the patients at risk for the development of pyelonephritis and scarring. In the acute setting, imaging can, at times, aid in the diagnosis of acute pyelonephritis, or its complications.

Imaging Techniques

The imaging work-up for children with a first UTI has long been a source of controversy. Recent studies have questioned the impact of imaging on patient management and outcomes, and the efficacy of antibiotic prophylaxis

in VUR.[8] At present, the American Academy of Pediatrics recommends a VCUG and US for infants and young children, aged between 2 and 24 months, after a first UTI.[15] These studies identify those patients with anatomic abnormalities, such as congenital obstruction and/or VUR that can predispose to pyelonephritis through stasis and/or ascending infection. In older children, an attempt may be made to distinguish upper UTI (pyelonephritis) from lower-tract infection (cystitis) on clinical grounds. If pyelonephritis is not clinically suspected in an older child (aged over 8 years), a normal renal US investigation may obviate the need for any further studies.[2]

Renal Ultrasound

Renal ultrasound is used to evaluate the morphology of the renal parenchyma and collecting system. The bladder is also included in the standard US examination, as abnormal bladder wall thickening can be seen with infection or bladder outlet obstruction. Dilatation of the pyelocaliceal systems and/or ureters can be secondary to obstructive uropathy or high-grade VUR, both of which may predispose the child to infection. US is less sensitive than contrast-enhanced CT or renal cortical scintigraphy in identifying acute renal parenchymal inflammation and/or renal scarring. However, in most cases, the diagnosis and treatment for acute pyelonephritis depends on clinical and laboratory findings as opposed to renal imaging. Furthermore, a normal renal US also does not exclude the presence of acute pyelonephritis or VUR.

VCUG, RNC, and RCS

VCUG and RNC are each utilized to evaluate the lower urinary tract for VUR. VUR is graded by severity (grades 1–5) (see Chapter 41), which provides the clinician with some idea of the likelihood of spontaneous resolution in cases of primary VUR. The ureteral insertion site can also be noted, although ureters will not be seen if VUR is not present. The bladder can be assessed for conditions that predispose to incomplete bladder emptying, such as high-grade reflux, bladder diverticula, and neurogenic bladder dysfunction. The urethra can be assessed for causes of bladder outlet obstruction, such as urethral valves or stricture. A 'spinning-top' urethra is a configuration due to bladder-sphincter dysynergia that can occasionally be seen with dysfunctional voiding. However, the urethra cannot be as equally or accurately assessed with RNC.

Since acute pyelonephritis is often diagnosed clinically, imaging studies are usually not recommended in the setting of suspected pyelonephritis. Studies, in addition to US, may be performed for complications of infection that are unresponsive to antibiotic therapy, such as renal abscess or persistent obstruction. US findings in uncomplicated acute pyelonephritis may be non-specific and, in many cases, appear normal. Less commonly, these gray-scale US findings may include focal or diffuse findings of swelling, as well as focal areas of increased and/or decreased echogenicity within the renal cortices. Color (power) Doppler US imaging may also show areas of decreased flow in areas of acute pyelonephritis.[7] If complicated infections, such as renal or perirenal abscesses form, US can show complex fluid collections within the renal parenchyma or extending beyond the renal capsule.

RCS using ^{99m}Tc-labeled DMSA can also be used in imaging acute pyelonephritis. Involved areas will appear as photopenic defects within the affected parts of the kidney.

Chronic changes of pyelonephritis result in focal or diffuse scarring, which can also be evaluated with imaging studies. In many institutions, because it is non-invasive, US remains the most commonly used initial modality for the evaluation of the child with recurrent infections. The sonographic features of chronic pyelonephritis can be manifested as focal areas of cortical thinning with loss of renal parenchyma. If the infection was diffuse, an overall decrease in renal volume can be seen. Cortical scintigraphy is still regarded by many as the most sensitive method for evaluating scarring from chronic pyelonephritis. In some centers, the algorithm for prophylaxis of a child with UTI would begin with RCS. Regardless of whether reflux would be present, if scarring was not demonstrated by RCS, then no additional imaging studies (e.g., VCUG) would be considered necessary. Although more sensitive than US for detected small renal scars, nuclear medicine scintigraphy is now routinely used in the evaluation of children with UTI, but the detection of small scars by nuclear medicine, not seen at US, is of uncertain significance.

Computed Tomography

On contrast-enhanced CT, acute pyelonephritis appears as a focal area or areas of low attenuation, or as a striated nephrogram. The kidneys may be enlarged and surrounded by inflammatory stranding within the perinephric fat (Figure 4-4). In cases of complicated pyelonephritis, an abscess will appear as a hypoattenuating mass with rim

enhancement. CT provides excellent anatomic detail of the relationship of the abscess of the kidney or its extension into surrounding structures. This modality is therefore useful in determining the appropriate interventional management.

Renal obstruction can also result in infection within the collecting system of the kidney, without infection of the renal parenchyma. To date, the numbers of neonates who present with pyonephrosis secondary to congenital urinary obstruction have decreased significantly because of the increased utilization of fetal US and early detection of fetal hydronephrosis. At US, pyonephrosis will appear as a dilated collecting system of the kidney and/or ureter that contains multiple low-level echoes. US is probably more sensitive than the CT for resolving the purulent nature of the internal contents of the dilated pyelo-calyceal system, ureter and/or bladder.

Investigational Guidelines

In 1993, the American College of Radiology developed *Appropriateness Criteria* for the utilization of radiological procedures (US, VCUG, RCS, RNC, IVU, CT). The purpose of these criteria is to provide creditable guidelines for radiology decision-making. In the clinical setting of pediatric urinary tract infection, at least 16 clinical variants were included, with appropriateness rating for each radiological procedure, as determined by the specific clinical scenario.

HEMATURIA

Imaging Protocols

The protocols for imaging the pediatric patient with hematuria, no matter whether the condition is microscopic or gross, seem to vary from clinician to clinician, and from institution to institution. The diagnostic work-up is tailored to the clinical signs and symptoms, and may or may not involve imaging studies. Hematuria may originate from hemorrhage within the kidney itself, from

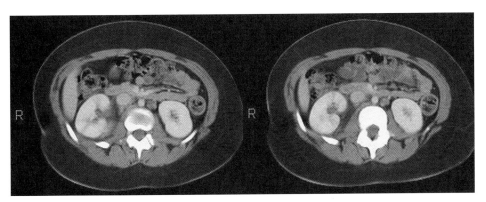

Figure 4-4   Two images from an enhanced CT scan in an 11-year-old female with pyelonephritis of the right kidney. There are thin linear hypodense areas (a 'striated nephrogram') within the right renal parenchyma, as well as inflammation in the perinephric fat.

anywhere along its vascular supply, or from any point along the collecting system.[13] In children, common causes for hematuria include UTI, urolithiasis, nephrocalcinosis, medical renal disease (nephritides), trauma, renal venous thrombosis, and renal tumors (both solid and cystic) (see Chapter 12).

Imaging Techniques

The investigational details relating to UTI have been discussed previously. CT and US are the modalities most commonly used to detect urolithiasis. At US, a urinary tract calculus appears as an echogenic, shadowing structure within the renal parenchyma, collecting system, ureter, or bladder. Sonography can also be used to assess for dilatation of the collecting system or ureters secondary to obstruction. Unlike CT, the identification of calculi on US does not depend on the stone's chemical composition, but rather on its density. Stones of certain chemical composition, not seen on CT (e.g., uric acid stones) may be visualized with US. The identification of ureteral calculi can at times be difficult with US because of the retroperitoneal location of the ureters.[4] At CT, calculi will more easily be visualized and appear as radiopaque foci within the collecting system, ureter(s), or bladder (Figure 4-5).

Pelvicalciectasis and ureterectasis can also be noted. Secondary signs of obstruction on CT include increased renal size and edema of the perinephric fat – findings that may not be quite as apparent on renal US examination. Unenhanced helical CT scanning can evaluate for both renal and ureteral calculi, or may disclose alternative causes of flank pain. CT is performed without contrast so as not to obscure any radiopaque stones. Nephrocalcinosis is most commonly caused by hypercalciuria, and results in calcium deposition within the renal parenchyma (cortical nephrocalcinosis) or medullary pyramids (medullary nephrocalcinosis). Urolithiasis and hematuria can occur in some cases. Renal calcification in nephrocalcinosis may be seen on plain film and CT as radiopaque areas conforming to the shape of the medullary pyramids or within the renal parenchyma. At US, these calcifications will appear as hyperechoic areas, typically within the medullary pyramids (Figure 4-6). Since most causes of nephrocalcinosis are systemic, calcifications are usually bilateral.

Causes of Hematuria

Hematuria can be caused by 'medical nephropathies,' including entities such as glomerulonephritis, metabolic disease, hypercalciuria, and interstitial nephritis.[13] Imaging is not required for the diagnosis of glomerulonephritis or interstitial nephritis. Sonographic findings are non-specific in these processes. The kidneys may be normal in size, or slightly enlarged. The echotexture of the renal cortices may be hyperechoic relative to liver or spleen, but the kidneys may also be normal in appearance (Figure 4-7).

Vascular causes of hematuria include trauma, sickle cell disease, renal venous thrombosis, and coagulopathies.[13] In the setting of trauma, hematuria is most concerning for renal parenchymal injury. However, depending on the extent and severity of trauma, hematuria can also be due to injury to an underlying or preceding condition, such as renal mass lesion or congenital hydronephrosis. In the former instance, contrast-enhanced

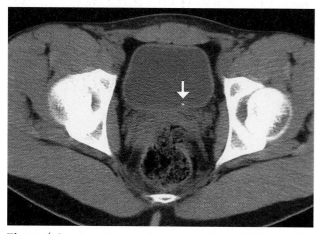

Figure 4-5 A single image from an unenhanced CT scan of the pelvis in a 15-year-old male with left flank pain. A 3-mm calculus is located at the ureterovesicle junction (arrow). Evaluation of the upper urinary tract showed no evidence of obstruction.

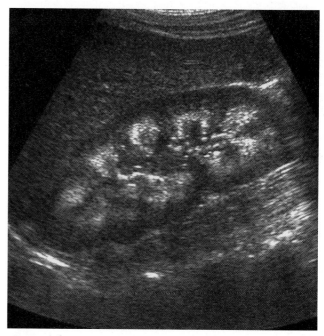

Figure 4-6 Sagittal view from an ultrasound of the right kidney in an 8-year-old male with nephrocalcinosis. The medullary pyramids are echogenic secondary to calcium deposition.

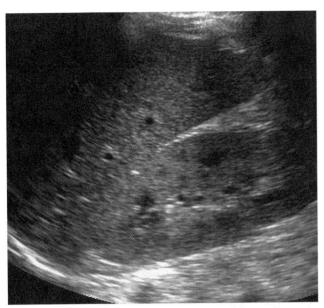

Figure 4-7   Ultrasound of the right kidney in the sagittal plane in a 14-year-old female with systemic lupus erythematosus. The renal parenchyma is hyperechoic relative to the adjacent liver.

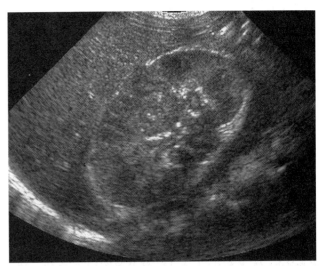

Figure 4-8   Sagittal image from a right renal ultrasound in a 10-day-old male. Linear echogenic areas in the renal parenchyma represent calcifications in intrarenal veins. There is also a loss of corticomedullary differentiation.

CT is the modality of choice for evaluating renal injury, and potential injury to the renal pedicle (vascular integrity) and collecting system. In the latter situation, in which the trauma may have only been relatively minor, US of the kidneys could be considered as the initial investigative modality. US is also the imaging study of choice when renal vein thrombosis is suspected. In the acute stages, the kidney itself may appear as enlarged and hypoechoic, secondary to venous congestion. Subsequently, areas of mixed echogenicity appear, followed in late stages by a decrease in renal size and an increase in cortical echogenicity. In neonates, intrarenal venous calcifications may develop (Figure 4-8).[4] Color and duplex Doppler findings may include decreased flow in the renal vein and high resistive flow in the renal artery.

CYSTIC DISEASE

Cystic renal disease in neonates and children can be classified as either genetic or non-genetic. Examples of non-genetic cystic disease would include multicystic dysplastic kidney (this is the most common), and obstructive cystic dysplasia. Genetic causes would include autosomal recessive polycystic kidney disease, autosomal dominant polycystic kidney disease, and cystic disease associated with syndromes.

Investigational Techniques

Multicystic dysplastic kidney (MCDK) is a mass of disorganized, non-functioning tissue. It is now often diagnosed with prenatal imaging. Post-natal sonography is performed to document the nature of the lesion, and will show multiple, non-communicating, anechoic cysts surrounded by abnormally echogenic parenchyma (Figure 4-9). The contralateral kidney is also evaluated, as there is a 15–25% incidence of contralateral renal abnormalities.[17] Both IVU and radionuclide imaging will show a non-functioning renal mass. Usually, radionuclide imaging is performed to document the lack of function and to confirm normal function in the contralateral kidney. Renal obstructive cystic dysplasia results from in-utero urinary tract obstruction. US will show anechoic

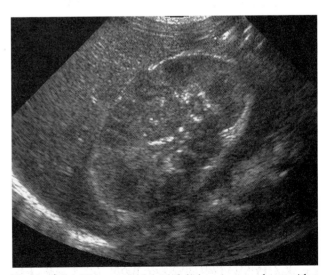

Figure 4-9   Ultrasound of the left kidney in a newborn with a multicystic dysplastic kidney. No normal renal parenchyma is visualized. Much of the kidney is replaced with non-communicating cysts.

cysts that are often subcapsular in location. The size and number of these cysts is variable, and is thought to depend on the timing of the obstruction during embryogenesis.[6]

Autosomal recessive polycystic kidney disease (ARPKD) is often diagnosed on prenatal sonography. In the classic case, post-natal imaging will show enlarged, echogenic kidneys with decreased corticomedullary differentiation.[18] The individual cysts are usually not resolvable by US. ARPKD is associated with hepatic fibrosis and biliary ductal plate malformation. In the neonatal/perinatal form, the renal disease predominates in the clinical picture, while in the juvenile form, the sonographic changes and effects of hepatic fibrosis (portal hypertension) may become evident.[5]

Prenatal diagnosis of *autosomal dominant polycystic kidney disease* (ADPKD) is uncommon. In some infants and young children, US will show enlarged, echogenic kidneys, similar in appearance to ARPKD. In cases when ARPKD and ADPKD are difficult to distinguish on US, CT may be helpful. ARPKD will show delayed excretion and a streaky enhancement pattern; ADPKD will usually show prompt excretion and uniform parenchymal enhancement.[9] In older children with ADPKD, multiple, large cysts will often become apparent (Figure 4-10). Asymmetrical renal involvement is also not uncommon.

SOLID RENAL MASSES

Mesoblastic nephroma, or fetal renal hamartoma, is the most common solid renal mass in neonates, particularly those aged less than 6 months. Sonography will show a solid tumor with varying echogenicity. Necrotic or cystic areas may be present. CT will also show a heterogeneous mass, which sometimes contains cystic

areas. US, CT, and MRI are the most commonly employed modalities in the evaluation of a child with *Wilms' tumor*. Sonography of Wilms' tumor will usually show a predominantly solid mass. The adjacent vascular structures, such as renal veins and inferior vena cava, can be interrogated with color and duplex Doppler to assess for tumor thrombus. A large tumor can obscure and distort vascular anatomy, making adequate evaluation difficult. In these cases, it becomes necessary to assess the vascularity with CT or MRI.[3] The primary tumor will appear as a heterogeneously enhancing mass on both CT and MRI (Figure 4-11). US, CT, and MRI can all be used to evaluate local extension and lymphadenopathy, as well as metastatic disease to solid abdominal organs, such as the liver. Although originally thought to represent subtypes of Wilms' tumor, clear cell sarcoma and rhabdoid tumor of the kidney are now recognized as distinct tumor types that do have similar imaging features to Wilms' tumor.

Angiomyolipomas are benign tumors that can be associated with tuberous sclerosis, or can be present as an isolated abnormality. Because of their fat content, these tumors tend to be hyperechoic on US (Figure 4-12) and low attenuation on CT. However, lesions containing smaller amounts of fat may be less distinctive. MRI sequences that highlight fat signal may be helpful in these cases.

Renal cell carcinoma is a rare tumor in children. When present, it usually occurs in older children or adolescents. Those patients with von Hippel–Lindau disease also have an increased incidence of this tumor compared to the general population. Renal cell carcinoma will usually appear as a solid tumor on all cross-sectional imaging modalities. It may be isoechoic to renal parenchyma on US. Small tumors that do not distort the renal architecture may be difficult to visualize. A small tumor may be more discernible on contrast-enhanced CT or MRI, as these lesions usually show contrast

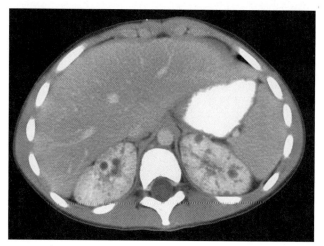

Figure 4-10 An image from an enhanced CT scan in a 6-year-old male with autosomal dominant polycystic kidney disease. Multiple hypodense cysts of various sizes are present in both kidneys.

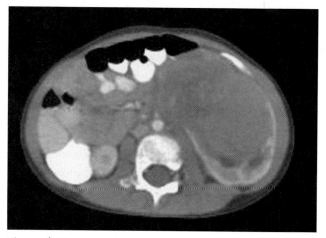

Figure 4-11 A single image from an enhanced CT scan in a 3-year-old male with Wilms' tumor. A large, heterogeneously enhancing mass in the left kidney splays the renal parenchyma.

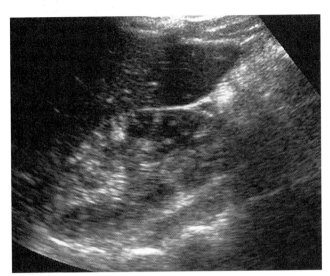

Figure 4-12 A sagittal ultrasound image of the right kidney in a patient with tuberous sclerosis. Multiple echogenic masses represent angiomyolipomas.

enhancement. The renal vein should be evaluated, as invasion by tumor is considered to be a poor prognostic sign.[19] CT and MRI can also evaluate local tumor spread, lymphadenopathy and metastases.

HYPERTENSION

In hypertensive pediatric patients, imaging studies are used most commonly to aid in the diagnosis of the renal or renovascular causes of hypertension. Renal US is usually performed as part of the initial work-up to evaluate the renal size, focal cortical thinning, parenchymal echotexture, and for adrenal masses. A unilateral small kidney can contribute to hypertension, and may be secondary to renovascular disease, congenital hypoplasia, and previous infection or obstruction. A normal renal US, along with an appropriate medical history, family history and laboratory tests, contributes to the diagnosis of essential hypertension. In these cases, no further imaging is necessary.

In patients with a normal renal US, but a history of urinary tract infection(s), cortical scintigraphy with ^{99m}Tc-labeled DMSA may be performed to assess for areas of scarring.[12] Renal cortical scintigraphy is more sensitive than US in assessing renal scarring; lesions may be visualized on RCS that were not detectable on sonography. As discussed previously, VUR is thought to predispose to pyelonephritis and renal scarring; therefore, hypertensive patients with renal scarring or a history of UTI may also be evaluated for reflux with a VCUG.

Investigational Techniques

Renal artery lesions, such as fibromuscular dysplasia and renal artery stenosis, may cause hypertension and can be imaged in a variety of ways. Non-invasive modalities include Doppler US, CT angiography, MR angiography and captopril renography. Color and duplex Doppler US evaluation of the renal vasculature can be performed at

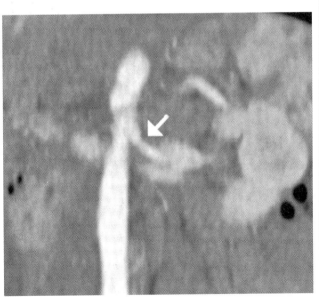

A

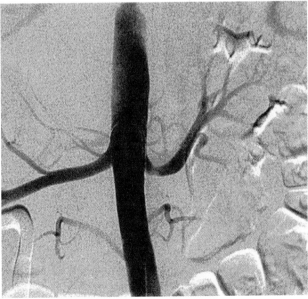

B

Figure 4-13 (a) A reconstructed coronal image from a CT angiogram in a 14-year-old male with left renal artery stenosis. There is a mild narrowing of the proximal left renal artery (arrow). (b) A single image from a renal angiogram in the same patient, showing mild narrowing of the proximal left renal artery.

the time of the initial US. Results are operator-dependent, and mild or distal lesions are difficult to evaluate with this modality.[12] MR and CT angiography can also provide excellent images of the renal vasculature, although patient movement can degrade detail on these modalities and are dependent on the timing of the contrast bolus (Figure 4-13a). Captopril renography is performed using either ^{99m}Tc-labeled MAG 3 or DTPA. Scanning is performed with and without dosing of captopril. A decreased renal function, following the administration of captopril, suggests the diagnosis of renal artery stenosis. The 'gold standard' for imaging renal vasculature is conventional angiography, which includes renal vein renin sampling. Conventional contrast angiography provides the most detailed image of the renal vasculature (Figure 4-13b). It also allows the opportunity for therapeutic intervention, such as angioplasty, if a stenotic lesion is seen. In patients with suspected pheochromocytoma, useful imaging modalities include CT, MRI, US, and radionuclide imaging with meta-iodobenzylguanidine (MIBG). MIBG is labeled with either I-123 or I-131, and localizes to neuroectodermal tumors, including pheochromocytoma. Since MIBG is used in whole-body scans, it can show tumors in areas not scanned during routine cross-sectional imaging. It may also show tumors that are too small to be resolved with the other modalities. MIBG is poor at specific anatomic localization. MRI, CT, and ultrasound can all show an adrenal or extra-adrenal mass. MRI has become the cross-sectional imaging study of choice because of improved conspicuity of pheochromocytomas compared to other modalities secondary to extreme hyperintensity on T2-weighted images.[14]

REFERENCES

1. Barnewolt C, Paltiel HJ, Lebowitz RL, et al. Genitourinary tract. In: Kirks D (ed), *Practical Pediatric Imaging.* Lippincott, Williams & Wilkins, Philadelphia, 1998, p. 1010.

2. Barnewolt C, Paltiel HJ, Lebowitz RL, et al. Genitourinary tract. In: Kirks D (ed), *Practical Pediatric Imaging.* Lippincott, Williams & Wilkins, Philadelphia, 1998, p. 1066.

3. Barnewolt C, Paltiel HJ, Lebowitz RL, et al. Genitourinary tract. In: Kirks D (ed), *Practical Pediatric Imaging.* Lippincott, Williams & Wilkins, Philadelphia, 1998, pp. 1116-1125.

4. Barnewolt C, Paltiel HJ, Lebowitz RL, et al. Genitourinary tract. In: Kirks D (ed), *Practical Pediatric Imaging.* Lippincott, Williams & Wilkins, Philadelphia, 1998, pp. 1150-1151.

5. Bellah RD. Renal sonography in neonates and infants. In: Merritt CR (ed), *Diagnostic Ultrasound: Categorical Course Syllabus.* American Roentgen Ray Society, Leesburg, VA, 1998, pp. 19-30.

6. Blanc CE, Barr M, DiPietro MA, et al. Renal obstructive dysplasia: ultrasound diagnosis and therapeutic implications. Pediatr Radiol 1991;21:274-277.

7. Dacher JN, Pfister C, Monroc M, et al. Power Doppler sonographic pattern of acute pyelonephritis in children: comparison with CT. Am J Roentgenol 1996;166: 1451-1455.

8. Hoberman A, Charron M, Hickey RW, et al. Imaging studies after a first febrile urinary tract infection in young children. N Engl J Med 2003;348:195-202.

9. Kaarianen H, Jaakelainen J, Kivisarri L, et al. Polycystic kidney disease in children: differential diagnosis between the dominantly and recessively inherited forms. Pediatr Radiol 1988;18:45-50.

10. Kraus SJ. Genitourinary imaging in children. Pediatr Clin North Am 2001;48:1381-1424.

11. Nolte-Ernsting CCA, Staatz G, Tacke J, et al. MR urography today. Abdom Imag 2003;28:191-209.

12. Norwood VF. Hypertension. Pediatr Rev 2002;23:197-208.

13. Patel HP, Bissler JJ. Hematuria in children. Pediatr Clin North Am 2001;48:1519-1537.

14. Quint LE, Glazer GM, Francis IR, et al. Pheochromocytoma and paraganglioma: comparison of MR imaging with CT and I-131 MIBG scintigraphy. Radiology 1987;165: 89-93.

15. Roberts KB. The AAP practice parameter on urinary tract infections in febrile infants and young children. Am Family Phys 2000;62:1815-1822.

16. Siegel M. Urinary tract. In: Siegel M (ed), *Pediatric Sonography.* Lippincott, Williams & Wilkins, Philadelphia, 2002, p. 386.

17. Slovis TL, Sty JR, Haller JO. *Imaging of the Pediatric Urinary Tract.* WB Saunders, Philadelphia, 1989, p. 96.

18. Slovis TL, Sty JR, Haller JO. *Imaging of the Pediatric Urinary Tract.* WB Saunders, Philadelphia, 1989, p. 101.

19. Slovis TL, Sty JR, Haller JO. *Imaging of the Pediatric Urinary Tract.* WB Saunders, Philadelphia, 1989, p. 191.

20. Tamm EP, Silverman PM, Shuman WP. Evaluation of the patient with flank pain and possible ureteral calculus. Radiology 2003;228:319-329.

CHAPTER 5

Immunization of Children with Renal Disease

ALICIA M. NEU, M.D. AND

BARBARA A. FIVUSH, M.D.

INTRODUCTION

The ability of childhood immunizations to prevent disease is well documented, and vaccine delivery is often the focus of routine medical visits in healthy children. Unfortunately, children with chronic illnesses may require frequent hospitalization and repeated visits with sub-specialists, so that the delivery of routine well-child care – including immunizations – can be delayed or overlooked. This is especially true for children with chronic kidney disease, some of whom may require weekly visits with a pediatric nephrologist. However, because these children may be at increased risk for vaccine-preventable disease, either as a result of their underlying disease process or the medications needed to treat it, it is especially important that they receive standard childhood vaccinations in a timely fashion (Box 5-1).

This chapter will review the standard childhood immunization schedule, as well as supplemental vaccines needed for children with chronic kidney disease. In addition, data on the response to these vaccines, where available, will be presented. The chapter will focus on immunizations in children with chronic kidney failure, defined as an irreversible reduction in glomerular filtration rate below 75 ml/min/1.73 m^2, children who require renal replacement therapy with either peritoneal dialysis or hemodialysis, and children who are status-post renal transplantation. Special considerations for immunizing children with the idiopathic nephrotic syndrome will also be discussed.

STANDARD RECOMMENDATIONS FOR IMMUNIZATIONS IN CHILDHOOD

The Advisory Committee on Immunization Practices (ACIP), the Committee on Infectious Diseases of the American Academy of Pediatrics (AAP), and the American Academy of Family Physicians (AAFP) continuously revise and update the guidelines for delivering immunizations to children. The most recent guidelines are presented in Figure 5-1, and can also be found at the AAP and Centers for Disease Control (CDC) websites (www.aap.org, www.cdc.gov/nip).[3] Immunization against diphtheria, tetanus, pertussis, *Hemophilus* influenza type b, polio, measles, mumps, rubella, *Streptococcus pneumonia*, varicella-zoster virus (VZV) and hepatitis B is considered standard in the United States.[3] Recent changes to this schedule include the recommendation that only inactivated poliovirus vaccine (IPV) be given, based on the elimination of wild-type poliomyelitis viruses from the Western hemisphere and the risk for vaccine-associated paralytic poliomyelitis with oral poliovirus vaccine.[2] Thus, the only live-viral vaccines remaining on the schedule are VZV and measles, mumps, rubella (MMR).[3] Also relatively new to the schedule is the addition of the heptavalent conjugated pneumococcal vaccine, which is now recommended for all children under the age of 2 years.[3,4] In general, children with the idiopathic nephrotic syndrome, chronic kidney failure, those on dialysis, and those status-post transplant should receive all of the recommended childhood

---

Box 5-1   Children With Chronic Kidney Disease Requiring Adjustment in the Routine Schedule for Childhood Immunization

- Chronic kidney disease may result in abnormal response to routine childhood immunizations so that increased dose or monitoring of response may be necessary
- Some children may not be candidates for live-viral vaccines because of a state of relative immunosuppression
- Many children with chronic kidney disease may be susceptible to or at risk for more serious infection from pathogens that are not typically problematic in healthy children and, therefore, may benefit from additional or supplemental immunizations

---

immunizations according to the standard schedule, whenever possible. However, it is important to determine if the child is on immunosuppressive medications, as the live viral vaccines (VZV, MMR) should be avoided in these patients. In the following sections, each vaccine will be discussed separately, and special considerations for children with kidney disease will be pointed out.

Hepatitis B Vaccine

Two recombinant hepatitis B vaccines are currently licensed for use in the United States, namely Recombivax HB® (Merck & Co Inc, West Point, PA) and Engerix-B® (GlaxoSmithKline, Research Triangle Park, NC). Hepatitis B vaccine is to be given in three doses (5 μg Hepatitis B surface antigen (HbsAg) for Recombivax HB, and 10 μg HbsAg for Engerix-B), with the first dose ideally given in the first few days of life.[3] Children with chronic kidney failure, on dialysis and post-transplant are considered at high risk for this infection, because of the potential need for blood products. The inability to produce a reliable and long-lasting response with standard hepatitis B immunization has been well documented in adults on dialysis, and it is currently recommended that these patients receive an augmented dose of 40 μg of either Recombivax HB or Engerix-B.[23] Unfortunately, data on vaccine response in older children with kidney failure are less consistent. In a study of 62 children on dialysis or post-transplant who received three doses of 5 μg (age <10 years) or 10 μg (age >10 years) of HBsAg, 60 had protective antibody levels 2 months after the final immunization.[19] One of the remaining patients developed a protective antibody level after a fourth dose, and the last patient responded after a fifth dose of vaccine.[19]

In a multicenter study performed by the Southwest Pediatric Nephrology Study Group, 78 pediatric patients with chronic kidney failure, on dialysis or status-post renal transplant were given half of the adult dialysis dose of 20 μg HbsAg.[27] Overall, 91% of patients developed a protective titer of 10 mIU/ml or greater after a three-dose regimen.[27] A higher percentage of patients with chronic kidney failure and on dialysis had protective antibody levels than those immunized post-transplant (96.4% versus 66.7%).[27] In addition, patients with chronic kidney failure tended to have higher mean geometric mean antibody titers after three immunizations, than those patients on dialysis or post-transplant, and the authors suggested that whenever possible, at least two immunizations be given prior to the point at which dialysis or transplant is necessary.[27] Both of these studies were published relatively recently and it remains to be seen if the recommendations from the AAP and ACIP will be altered in response to these data. In addition, most children will now be receiving this vaccine in infancy and there are no data regarding response to this vaccine in infants with chronic kidney disease. Currently, the ACIP recommends that dialysis patients less than 20 years of age receive hepatitis B immunization according to the standard schedule (i.e., 5 μg Recombivax HB or 10 μg Engerix-B for three doses).[23] Post-vaccination testing should be performed 1 to 2 months after the primary series is completed and then annually.[23] Up to three additional doses may be given to patients who do not develop protective antibody levels (>10 mIU/ml), and patients whose antibody levels fall below the protective level should receive a booster immunization.[23] Patients with idiopathic nephrotic syndrome are not identified as high-risk with regard to hepatitis B infection and, therefore, monitoring of antibody levels in these patients is not indicated and these patients should receive hepatitis B vaccine according to the standard schedule.

Diphtheria, Tetanus and Pertussis Vaccine

Diphtheria, tetanus and acellular pertussis (DTaP) vaccine is currently recommended for all children at 2, 4, and 6 months of age, with booster doses at 15–18 months and again at 4-6 years of age.[3] In addition, tetanus and diphtheria toxoids (Td) are recommended at 11–12 years of age if at least 5 years have elapsed since the last dose of tetanus and diphtheria toxoid-containing vaccine, with subsequent Td boosters every 10 years.[3] Children with chronic kidney failure, on dialysis and status-post transplant can safely receive these vaccines according to the standard schedule.[11,18,23] Although studies in older children on dialysis and post-renal transplant suggest that the seroconversion rate after DTaP immunization is lower than in healthy children, a study in infants vaccinated while on dialysis revealed protective antibody titers to diphtheria and tetanus toxoids in most patients.[11,18,22,23] Data on response to or immunity after this vaccine in children with idiopathic nephrotic syndrome are not available. Thus, children with chronic kidney failure, on dialysis and status-post transplant as well as those with nephrotic syndrome should receive DTaP and Td booster according to the standard childhood schedule.

Hemophilus influenzae Type b Conjugate Vaccine

Hemophilus influenzae type b (Hib) conjugate vaccine is currently given at 2 and 4 months of age, with a third dose at 6 months, depending on which vaccine preparation is used.[3] A booster dose is also given at 12 to 15 months of age.[3] There are no data regarding response to this vaccine in children with chronic kidney failure, or those with idiopathic nephrotic syndrome; however, one study evaluated antibody levels in infants vaccinated while on dialysis and revealed protective antibody levels in 90% with persistence of immunity for as long as 22 months post-vaccination.[21] Another study measured antibody levels at 2 months after the third dose of Hib conjugate vaccine in 42 pediatric patients on dialysis or status-post renal transplant, and all had protective levels.[19] This vaccine is composed of bacterial polysaccharide conjugated to protein and, therefore, can safely be given to children who are on immunosuppressive medications. Thus, current recommendations are that children with kidney disease receive this vaccine according to the standard schedule.

Inactivated Polio Virus Vaccine

As mentioned previously, it is now recommended that only IPV vaccine be used for routine immunization in children.[2,3] This vaccine, which contains inactivated virus from the three serotypes responsible for paralytic polio, is routinely given at 2 months, 4 months, 6-18 months and 4-6 years.[3] There are no studies documenting response to this vaccine in infants with kidney disease; however, one study evaluated antibody levels in 49 older children on dialysis after vaccination with IPV and found that 86% of patients had protective levels to all three serotypes.[25] Because it is not a live viral vaccine, IPV can safely be given to children on immunosuppressive medications. Thus, children with chronic kidney failure, those on dialysis, status-post renal transplant and those with idiopathic nephrotic syndrome may be vaccinated according to the standard schedule.

Measles, Mumps, Rubella Vaccine

Measles, mumps and rubella (MMR) vaccine is routinely given between 12 and 15 months of age, with a second dose at school entry (age 4-6 years).[3] This live, attenuated viral vaccine is contraindicated in patients receiving immunosuppressive medications post-renal transplant, and therefore, it is important to give MMR vaccine, and document protection against MMR prior to transplantation. To that end, several studies have evaluated response to MMR vaccine in children with kidney failure and on dialysis. Although an early study in 10 children on dialysis revealed that only 30% of patients had protective antibody levels to all three viruses, a subsequent study found that 88% of patients with chronic renal failure and/or on dialysis who were vaccinated in infancy had positive antibody titers to measles, mumps and rubella at the time of transplantation.[12,24] More recently, a study in 62 pediatric dialysis patients revealed that 100% of patients had positive antibody titers to measles, mumps and rubella 2 months after vaccination.[19] Although these data suggest that pediatric patients with chronic kidney failure and on dialysis respond well to MMR vaccine, because immunization post-transplant is contraindicated, it is reasonable to document antibody titers prior to transplantation, with repeat vaccination if necessary.[5] In addition, this live viral vaccine should be avoided in children with idiopathic syndrome while they are receiving immunosuppressive therapy, including corticosteroids, if possible. Specifically, delivery of MMR vaccine should be delayed in any patient treated with corticosteroids at a dose greater than 2 mg/kg body weight or 20 mg total daily or on alternate days for more than 14 days.[5] Once corticosteroids are discontinued, it is generally recommended that MMR vaccination be delayed for at least 1 month after cessation of the medication.

Varicella Zoster Vaccine

Since 1995, VZV vaccine has been recommended for all immunocompetent children at 12 to 18 months.[3] Children aged over 18 months without a history of having chickenpox can also be immunized. Because of the high risk for morbidity and mortality associated with varicella zoster infection in adulthood, children aged 13 years and more without a history of chickenpox infection should receive two doses of the vaccine, with the second dose at least 1 month after the first.[3] This live, attenuated virus vaccine is contraindicated in immunocompromised patients, including those on immunosuppressive medication status-post renal transplant.[9] In addition, this vaccine should be avoided in children with idiopathic nephrotic syndrome who are receiving immunosuppressive therapy, including those treated with corticosteroids at a dose greater than 2 mg/kg body weight or a total daily dose of 20 mg.[9] Children receiving lower doses of corticosteroids may receive VZV vaccination.[9] Because of the significant risk

RECOMMENDED CHILDHOOD AND ADOLESCENT IMMUNIZATION SCHEDULE
UNITED STATES, 2002

Vaccine ▼ / Age ▶	Birth	1 mo	2 mos	4 mos	6 mos	12 mos	15 mos	18 mos	24 mos	4–6 y	11–12 y	13–18 y
Hepatitis B[1]	Hep B #1 only if mother HBsAg (–)		Hep B #2			Hep B #3				Hep B series		
Diphtheria, Tetanus, Pertussis[2]			DTaP	DTaP	DTaP		DTaP			DTaP	Td	
Haemophilus influenzae Type b[3]			Hib	Hib	Hib	Hib						
Inactivated Polio[4]			IPV	IPV		IPV				IPV		
Measles, Mumps, Rubella[5]						MMR #1				MMR #2	MMR #2	
Varicella[6]						Varicella				Varicella		
Pneumococcal[7]			PCV	PCV	PCV	PCV				PCV / PPV		
Hepatitis A[8]										Hepatitis A series		
Influenza A[9]					Influenza (yearly)							

Vaccines below this line are for selected populations

Range of recommended ages / Catch-up immunization / Preadolescent assessment

Figure 5-1 This schedule indicates the recommended ages for routine administration of currently licensed childhood vaccines, as of December 1, 2001, for children through age 18 years. Any dose not given at the recommended age should be given at any subsequent visit when indicated and feasible. ▨▨▨▨▨ Indicates age groups that warrant special effort to administer those vaccines not previously given. Additional vaccines may be licensed and recommended during the year. Licensed combination vaccines may be used whenever any components of the combination are indicated and the vaccine's other components are not contraindicated. Providers should consult the manufacturers' package inserts for detailed recommendations.

1. **Hepatitis B vaccine (Hep B).** All infants should receive the first dose of hepatitis B vaccine soon after birth and before hospital discharge; the first dose may also be given by age 2 months if the infant's mother is HbsAg-negative. Only monovalent hepatitis B vaccine can be used for the birth dose. Monovalent or combination vaccine containing Hep B may be used to complete the series; four doses of vaccine may be administered if combination vaccine is used. The second dose should be given at least 4 weeks after the first dose, except for Hib-containing vaccine, which cannot be administered before the age of 6 weeks. The third dose should be given at least 16 weeks after the first dose, and at least 8 weeks after the second dose. The last dose in the vaccination series (third or fourth dose) should not be administered before age 6 months.

Infants born to HbsAg-positive mothers should receive hepatitis B vaccine and 0.5 ml hepatitis B vaccine series within 12 hours of birth at separate sites. The second dose is recommended at age 1-2 months, and the vaccination series should be completed (third or fourth dose) at age 6 months. Infants born to mothers whose HbsAg status is unknown should receive the first dose of the hepatitis B vaccine series within 12 hours of birth. Maternal blood should be drawn at the time of delivery to determine the mother's HbsAg status; if the HbsAg test is positive, the infant should receive HBIG as soon as possible (no later than age 1 week).

2. **Diphtheria and tetanus toxoids and acellular pertussis vaccine (DTaP).** The fourth dose of DTaP may be administered as early as age 12 months, provided that 6 months have elapsed since the third dose and the child is unlikely to return at age 15–18 months. Tetanus and diphtheria toxoids (Td) is recommended at age 11–12 years if at least 5 years have elapsed since the last dose of tetanus and diphtheria toxoid-containing vaccine. Subsequent routine Td boosters are recommended every 10 years.

3. ***Haemophilus influenzae* type b (hib) conjugate vaccine.** Three Hib conjugate vaccines are licensed for infant use. If PRP-OMP (PedvaxHib® or ComVax® (Merck)) is administered at ages 2 and 4 months, a dose at age 6 months is not required. DTaP/Hib combination products should not

for morbidity and mortality with varicella zoster infection in patients who are on immunosuppressive medication, there has been great interest in insuring adequate antibody response after VZV vaccination in children with chronic kidney failure and those on dialysis, with the goal of providing protection for these children before immunosuppressive medications are introduced post renal transplant. Similarly, children with idiopathic nephrotic syndrome may require intermittent therapy with immunosuppressive medications for many years, so vaccine response in this group has also been the focus of great attention. Because early studies of VZV vaccine in children with chronic kidney failure and on dialysis demonstrated a lower seroconversion rate than in healthy children after a single immunization, two multi-center, prospective studies evaluated antibody levels after a two-dose regimen of VZV vaccine in children with chronic kidney failure and on dialysis.[15,28] Both studies revealed that nearly all patients seroconverted after the second dose of vaccine, with a 98% seroconversion rate in one study and 100% in the other.[15,28] In children with idiopathic nephrotic syndrome, the reported seroconversion rates after a single dose of VZV vaccine have been 43–85%, while a study of 29 children with steroid-sensitive nephrotic syndrome demonstrated a 100% seroconversion rate after a two-dose regimen.[1,14,26] It should be noted that none of these studies included a large number of children between 12 and 18 months of age, which is currently the target age for VZV vaccination, and thus the ability of infants and toddlers with chronic kidney disease, on dialysis and those with idiopathic nephrotic syndrome to respond to this vaccination is not known. In light of this fact, and the data from the studies in older children, it is reasonable to measure antibody levels after VZV vaccination and provide a second vaccination to those patients who do not have a protective titer. In addition, antibody levels should be checked prior to proceeding to renal transplantation and supplemental vaccination considered if positive antibody titers are not demonstrated.

Pneumococcal Vaccine

Children with kidney disease, including those with chronic kidney failure, on dialysis, status-post renal transplant and the idiopathic nephrotic syndrome are considered high-risk for the development of invasive infection with *Streptococcus pneumoniae* and the AAP and ACIP recommend immunization with the 23-valent polysaccharide pneumococcal (23PS) vaccine in this high-risk group.[4,8] This vaccine is poorly immunogenic in infants and toddlers, and therefore, is only given to children 2 years of age and older.[8] Since 2000, the ACIP and AAP have recommended that the heptavalent pneumococcal conjugate vaccine (PCV7), which is highly immunogenic in infants, be given to all children, including those with kidney disease, at 2, 4, 6, and 12 to 15 months of age.[3,4] In addition, children between 2 and 6 years of age who are at high risk for invasive pneumococcal infection who have not been immunized previously, should receive

be used for primary immunization in infants at ages 2, 4, or 6 months, but can be used as boosters following any Hib vaccine.

4. **Inactivated polio vaccine (IPV).** An all-IPV schedule is recommended for routine childhood polio vaccination in the United States. All children should receive four doses of IPV at ages 2 months, 4 months, 6–18 months, and 4–6 years.

5. **Measles, mumps, and rubella vaccine (MMR).** The second dose of MMR is recommended routinely at age 4–6 years, but may be administered during any visit, provided that at least 4 weeks have elapsed since the first dose and that both doses are administered beginning at or after the age of 12 months. Those who have not previously received the second dose should complete the schedule by their 11- to 12-year-old visit.

6. **Varicella vaccine.** Recommended at any visit at or after age 12 months for susceptible children – that is, those who lack a reliable history of chickenpox. Susceptible persons aged ≥13 years should receive two doses, given at least 4 weeks apart.

7. **Pneumococcal vaccine.** The heptavalent pneumococcal conjugate vaccine (PCV) is recommended for all children aged between 2 and 23 months. It is also recommended for certain children aged between 24 and 59 months. Pneumococcal polysaccharide vaccine (PPV) is recommended in addition to PCV for certain high-risk groups.

8. **Hepatitis A vaccine.** Recommended for use in selected states and regions, and for certain high-risk groups; consult your local public health authority.

9. **Influenza vaccine.** Recommended annually for children aged ≥6 months with certain risk factors (including, but not limited to, asthma, cardiac disease, sickle cell disease, HIV, diabetes), and can be administered to all others wishing to obtain immunity. Children aged ≤12 years should receive vaccine in a dosage appropriate for their age (0.25 ml if aged 6–35 months or 0.5 ml if aged ≥3 years). Children aged ≤8 years who are receiving influenza vaccine for the first time should receive two doses, separated by at least 4 weeks.

(Data from American Academy of Pediatrics Committee on Infectious Diseases: Recommended childhood immunization schedule – United States, 2002. Pediatrics 2002;109:162.)

Table 5-1   Recommendations for Pneumococcal Immunization with PCV7 or 23PS in Children with Kidney Disease

Age	Previous Dose	Recommendations
≤23 months	None	PCV according to standard recommendations (see Figure 5-1)
24–59 months	4 doses of PCV7	1 dose of 23PS vaccine at 24 months, at least 6–8 weeks after the last dose of PCV7
		1 dose of 23PS vaccine, 3–5 years after the first dose of 23PS vaccine
24–59 months	1–3 doses of PCV7	1 dose PCV 7
		1 dose of 23PS, 6–8 weeks after the last dose of PCV7
		1 dose of 23PS vaccine, 3–5 years after the first dose of 23PS vaccine
24–59 months	1 dose of 23 PS	2 doses of PCV7, 6–8 weeks apart, beginning at least 6–8 weeks after the last dose of 23 PS vaccine
		1 dose of 23 PS vaccine, 3–5 years after the first dose of 23PS vaccine
24–59 months	None	2 doses of PCV7 6–8 weeks apart
		1 dose of 23PS vaccine, 6–8 weeks after the last dose of PCV7
		1 dose of 23 PS vaccine, 3–5 years after the first dose of 23PS vaccine

two doses of PCV7 6 to 8 weeks apart.[4] It is also recommended that high-risk children receive supplemental immunization with the 23PS vaccine, to expand serotype coverage.[4] The timing of this vaccine varies, depending on the age of the patient, and the number of previous immunizations with PCV7.[4] Specific recommendations for immunizing high-risk children with PCV7 and 23PS vaccine are given in Table 5-1, and can also be found at the AAP and CDC websites (www.aap.org, www.cdc.gov/nip).[4] Children with kidney disease older than 6 years should also receive vaccination with 23PS.[8] Revaccination should occur 3 years after the previous dose in those children who are 10 years old or younger at the time of revaccination, and at 5 years in children older than 10 years at the time of revaccination.[8] Revaccination is important as several studies have suggested that although response to vaccination in children with kidney disease is good, there may be a rapid decline in antibody levels.[13,16,19] However, these studies evaluated response to and long-term antibody levels after 23PS, and there are no data available on response to PCV7, or response to 23PS after previous immunization with PCV7 in children with chronic kidney failure, on dialysis, status-post renal transplant or the idiopathic nephrotic syndrome.[13,16]

Hepatitis A Vaccine

Since 2001 the recommended childhood immunization schedule has included two vaccines which are intended only for selected populations, hepatitis A and influenza vaccines.[3] Hepatitis A vaccine is recommended for children aged 2 years and older who live in areas with an average annual rate of hepatitis A disease of at least 20 cases per 100,000 population during the period of 1987–1997.[7] In the United States, this includes the states of Arizona, Alaska, California, Idaho, New Mexico, Nevada,

Oklahoma, Oregon, South Dakota, Utah, and Washington.[7] Children living in areas where the average annual rate of hepatitis A disease was at least 10 per 100,000 population during the 1987–1997 period should also be considered for vaccination.[7] This includes the states of Arkansas, Colorado, Mississippi, Montana, Texas and Wyoming.[7] Children living in these areas, including those with kidney disease, are to receive two doses of hepatitis A vaccine, again after the age of 2 years.[3] There are currently no data available on response to hepatitis A vaccine in children with chronic kidney failure, on dialysis, status-post renal transplant or with the idiopathic nephrotic syndrome.

Influenza Vaccine

Influenza vaccine is the second vaccine included on the recommended childhood immunization schedule, but intended only for selected populations.[3] In 2002, the schedule begins to focus on the expansion of routine influenza immunization for children other than those at high risk, and vaccination of otherwise healthy children aged from 6 to 23 months is now encouraged.[3,6] High-risk populations continue to be a priority for immunization, and this group includes children with chronic kidney failure, on dialysis, status-post renal transplant and the idiopathic nephrotic syndrome.[6] In addition, household contacts of high-risk individuals should receive immunization. The influenza vaccine is given annually in the autumn, and the vaccine composition changes each year based on the strains of influenza viruses likely to circulate in the upcoming year.[6] The vaccine is intended only for children older than 6 months of age. The dose and schedule of vaccine depend on the age of the child and whether previous influenza vaccination has occurred.[3,6] Specifically, children aged 6–35 months should receive

0.25 ml, while those 3 years or older receive 0.5 ml.[6] Because split-virus vaccines (labeled as split, subvirion, or purified-surface antigen vaccine) are associated with a decreased risk for causing febrile reactions, the ACIP currently recommends that children under the age of 13 years receive only split-virus vaccines.[6] While older children may receive either split- or whole-virus vaccines, whole-virus vaccine is not available in the United States.[6] Two doses of influenza vaccine, given at least 1 month apart, are recommended for children under the age of 9 years who are receiving the vaccine for the first time.[3,6] Because of the significant risk for influenza-related morbidity and mortality in pediatric patients with chronic kidney disease, there have been several studies evaluating vaccine response in this population. Although an early study of influenza vaccine in pediatric renal transplant patients revealed a lower seroconversion rate than in healthy siblings, two other studies have demonstrated seroconversion rates that are similar between transplant patients and controls.[10,17,20] One of the studies also vaccinated pediatric patients with chronic kidney failure and on dialysis, and revealed equivalent seroconversion rates between the study groups and controls.[17] These studies suggest that influenza vaccine produces a reasonable humoral response in patients with chronic kidney disease. Nevertheless, because of the significant risk for mortality from this disease in these patients, as pointed out above, household contacts should receive vaccination in an effort to decrease the risk for exposure to influenza.[6]

SUMMARY

Pediatric patients with chronic kidney failure and on dialysis should receive all of the vaccines currently recommended for healthy children according to the standard schedule, whenever possible. Children who are on immunosuppressive medications post-renal transplant should also receive all of the standard immunizations, with the exception of MMR and VZV vaccine, which are live, attenuated virus vaccines.[5,9] Because of this, every effort should be made to vaccinate children with chronic kidney failure and on dialysis with MMR and VZV vaccines prior to transplantation. In addition, protection against MMR and VZV should be documented prior to transplantation and revaccination considered in those patients without protective antibody titers. Children with the idiopathic nephrotic syndrome treated with immunosuppressive medication including corticosteroids at a dose of more than 2 mg/kg per day or a total dose of 20 mg per day should not receive MMR or VZV vaccines.[5,9] Ideally, these vaccines should be delayed until at least 1 month after immunosuppressive medications have been discontinued, although children

on maintenance corticosteroids at doses lower than those listed above may receive the VZV vaccine.[5,9]

Children with chronic kidney failure, on dialysis and status-post transplant are at high risk for infection with hepatitis B, and these patients may benefit from an augmented dose of this vaccine.[27] At the very least, antibody levels should be monitored and additional doses provided if an antibody level >10 mIU/ml is not achieved after completing the three-shot series.[23] In addition, antibody levels should be monitored yearly, with a booster dose if levels fall below 10 mIU/ml.[23] Because of the increased risk for invasive pneumococcal infection, children with chronic kidney failure, on dialysis, status-post renal transplant and the idiopathic nephrotic syndrome should receive supplemental immunization with the heptavalent conjugated and 23-valent polysaccharide pneumococcal vaccine.[4] The number and timing of these supplement vaccines depends on the patient's age and previous vaccinations (see Table 5-1). In addition, revaccination with 23PS is indicated every 3 years in patients aged ≤10 years of age at the time of revaccination, and every 5 years in patients older than 10 years of age at the time of revaccination.[4] Finally, because patients with chronic kidney failure, on dialysis, status-post renal transplant and with the idiopathic nephrotic syndrome are at increased risk for morbidity and mortality from influenza infection, these patients, their household contacts and their medical caregivers should receive influenza vaccine annually in the fall.

REFERENCES

1. Alpay H, Yildiz N, Onar A, et al. Varicella vaccination in children with steroid-sensitive nephrotic syndrome. Pediatr Nephrol 2002;17:181–183.

2. American Academy of Pediatrics Committee on Infectious Diseases. Prevention of poliomyelitis: Recommendations for use of only inactivated polio vaccine for routine immunization. Pediatr 1999;104:1404–1406.

3. American Academy of Pediatrics Committee on Infectious Diseases. Recommended childhood immunization schedule – United States, 2002. Pediatrics 2002;109:162.

4. American Academy of Pediatrics Committee on Infectious Diseases. Recommendations for the prevention of pneumococcal infections, including the use of pneumococcal conjugate vaccine (Prevnar), pneumococcal polysaccharide vaccine, and antibiotic prophylaxis. Pediatrics 2000; 106:362–366.

5. Centers for Disease Control and Prevention. Measles, mumps, and rubella vaccine use and strategies for elimination of measles, rubella, and congenital rubella syndrome and control of mumps. Recommendations of the Advisory Committee on Immunization Practices. MMWR 1998; 47:1–57.

6. Centers for Disease Control and Prevention. Prevention and control of influenza. Recommendations of the

Advisory Committee on Immunization Practices (ACIP). MMWR 2002;51:1–31.

7. Centers for Disease Control and Prevention. Prevention of hepatitis A through active or passive immunization. Recommendations of the Advisory Committee on Immunization Practices (ACIP). MMWR 1999;48:1–37.

8. Centers for Disease Control and Prevention. Prevention of pneumococcal disease. Recommendations of the Advisory Committee on Immunization Practices (ACIP). MMWR 1997;46:1–94.

9. Centers for Disease Control and Prevention. Prevention of varicella. Recommendations of the Advisory Committee on Immunization Practices (ACIP). MMWR 1996;45:1–25.

10. Edvaardsson VO, Flynn JT, Deforest A, et al. Effective immunization against influenza in pediatric renal transplant recipients. Clin Transplant 1996;10:556–560.

11. Enke BU, Bökenkamp A, Offner G, et al. Response to diphtheria and tetanus booster vaccination in pediatric renal transplant recipients. Transplant 1997;64:237–241.

12. Flynn JT, Frisch K, Kershaw DB, et al. Response to early measles-mumps-rubella vaccination in infants with chronic renal failure and/or receiving peritoneal dialysis. Adv Perit Dial 1999;15:269–272.

13. Fuchshuber A, Kühnemund O, Keuth B, et al. Pneumococcal vaccine in children and young adults with chronic renal disease. Nephrol Dial Transplant 1996;11:468–473.

14. Furth SL, Arbus GS, Hogg R, et al. Varicella vaccination in children with nephrotic syndrome: a report of the Southwest Pediatric Nephrology Study Group. J Pediatr 2003;142:145–148.

15. Furth SL, Hogg RJ, Tarver J, et al. Varicella vaccination in children with chronic renal failure: a report of the Southwest Pediatric Nephrology Study Group. Pediatr Nephrol 2003;18:33–38.

16. Furth SL, Neu AM, Case B, et al. Pneumococcal polysaccharide vaccine in children with chronic renal disease: A prospective study of antibody response and duration. J Pediatr 1996;128:99–101.

17. Furth SL, Neu AM, McColley SA, et al. Immune response to influenza vaccination in children with renal disease. Pediatr Nephrol 1995;9:566–568.

18. Ghio L, Pedrazzi C, Assael BM, et al. Immunity to diphtheria and tetanus in a young population on a dialysis regimen or with a renal transplant. J Pediatr 1997;130:987–989.

19. Laube GF, Berger C, Goetschel P, et al. Immunization in children with chronic renal failure. Pediatr Nephrol 2002;17:638–642.

20. Mauch TJ, Crouch NA, Freeze DK, et al. Antibody response of pediatric solid organ transplant recipients to immunization against influenza virus. J Pediatr 1995;127: 957–960.

21. Neu AM, Lederman HM, Warady BA et al. *Haemophilus influenza* type b immunization in infants on peritoneal dialysis. Pediatr Nephrol 1996;10:84–85.

22. Neu AM, Warady BA, Furth SL, et al. Antibody levels to diphtheria, tetanus and rubella in infants vaccinated while on peritoneal dialysis: a study of the Pediatric Peritoneal Dialysis Study Consortium. Adv Perit Dial 1997; 13:296–298.

23. Rangel MC, Coronado VG, Euler GL, et al. Vaccine recommendations for patients on chronic dialysis. Semin Dial 2000;13:101–107.

24. Schulman SL, Deforest A, Kaiser BA, et al. Response to measles-mumps-rubella vaccine in children on dialysis. Pediatr Nephrol 1992;9:566–568.

25. Sipilä R, Hortling L, Hovi T. Good seroresponse to enhanced-potency inactive poliovirus vaccine in patients on chronic dialysis. Nephrol Dial Transplant 1990; 5:352–355.

26. Quien RM, Kaiser BA, Deforest A, et al. Response to the varicella vaccine in children with nephrotic syndrome. J Pediatr 1997;131:688–690.

27. Watkins SL, Alexander SR, Brewer ED, et al. Response to Recombinant hepatitis B vaccine in children and adolescents with chronic renal failure. Am J Kidney Dis 2002;40:365–372.

28. Webb NJA, Fitzpatrick JJ, Hughes DA, et al. Immunization against varicella in end stage and pre-end stage renal failure. Arch Dis Child 2000;82:141–143.

CHAPTER 6

Social Issues in Children with Renal Disorders

CYNTHIA GREEN, M.S.S., L.S.W. AND
KIMBERLY STERNER-STEIN, M.S.W, L.S.W.

INTRODUCTION

The goals of this chapter are to detail the numerous social issues that affect, and are affected by, renal disease, so that medical professionals working in nephrology may be aware of the wide-ranging implications that their diagnoses and treatments may have for pediatric patients and their families. The role of the nephrology social worker as part of the team of clinicians is essential to providing optimal care for these patients. Effective interventions, which may be used in relation to specific social issues, can affect medical status and treatment outcomes.

TANYA'S STORY

When 12-year-old Tanya M. (names and some aspects of the history have been changed to protect confidentiality) was diagnosed with chronic renal failure secondary to focal segmental glomerulosclerosis, she and her parents were upset, yet somewhat relieved. At last they had an explanation for the increasing fatigue in a child who used to have boundless energy; the inattentiveness at school that had led to plummeting grades for a one-time straight-A student; and the swollen body of a once-willowy girl that had elicited merciless teasing from the boys in her class. Although dialysis and transplant loomed over their futures, her illness, however serious, could be treated. It now seemed that they could make plans and move forward.

Two years later, however, the family felt as though they had taken one step forward but two steps back. With all the time Mrs M. had needed to shuttle Tanya to and from medical appointments and to learn how to do home peritoneal dialysis, she had lost her secretarial job, and with it, the family's health insurance. Before they could obtain other coverage through the state Medicaid program, Tanya had required hospitalization, leaving the family with a $12,000 bill to pay out of its own pocket. Because Mr M.'s blood type was compatible with Tanya's, and Mrs M.'s was not, he had begun the process of evaluation to be a transplant donor. This required taking a number of unpaid days off from his construction job, with the result that the family's finances were stressed even further. He had no idea how they would manage during the six or more weeks he would need to take away from work for the surgery; at least three of those weeks would be without a salary.

Burdened by nightly dialysis and nagging abdominal pain that often kept her out of school, Tanya had been transformed from a sweet, cooperative youngster into an irritable, withdrawn teenager, testing her parents' patience at a time when they were already under stress. Mrs M. had no idea how she would be able to persuade Tanya to take the more than 20 pills a day she would need after the transplant, because Tanya frequently balked at taking the few she was currently prescribed. Tanya's siblings were starting to act up with too little parental energy and attention to go around, the 14-year-old sister hanging out with a rough crowd of friends who dabbled in drugs and vandalism, and the 5-year-old brother throwing tantrums and fighting with his kindergarten classmates.

Every chronic illness in childhood has psychosocial effects on the patient and those close to them.[6,16] For chronically ill children and adolescents, the major developmental tasks that are so crucial to maturing to well-adjusted, independent adulthood are often delayed and sometimes never mastered.[6,17] Nearly half of the parents and more than half of the well siblings of children with chronic illness report significant psychiatric symptoms and behavioral problems.[6] Even in this context, however, the personal and familial ramifications of renal disease, especially as kidney failure reaches end stage, are among the most far-reaching and devastating.[1,14,18] The severity of psychological, financial, vocational, educational, and relational issues faced by renal patients has been recognized in the fields of medicine and social work since the 1970s, when Congress decreed that patients receiving the newly established treatments of dialysis and transplantation would be eligible for health insurance coverage through the Medicare system. This is the only non-elderly population that receives this benefit. Furthermore, it was mandated that social work services be made available to all with end-stage renal disease (ESRD) being treated at hospitals or freestanding dialysis centers.[1,15]

Complexity of the Psychosocial Issues

Several theories attempt to explain the complexity of the psychosocial issues faced by renal patients and their families. Some kidney diseases disproportionately affect racial groups that have a history of social and economic deprivation in Western societies. Many renal diseases are inherited or familial, and therefore multiple family members of a seriously affected proband may also be ill (parent and child, more than one sibling). Poverty, ignorance, and lack of access to medical care among some populations can result in late detection and poor treatment of renal problems and precursor illnesses such as hypertension and diabetes. Kidney failure itself is one of the few diseases for which even the most successful available treatment, renal transplantation, is not a cure. Even with the best results it is a temporary respite from illness in which health may be restored at the price of significant impediments to normal functioning. Many ESRD

patients must miss work or school three times a week for hemodialysis, spend 10–12 hours a night connected to a peritoneal dialysis machine, and undergo more than one transplant during their lifetime.

Illness Intrusiveness

The extent to which illness and/or treatment interfere with other important facets of a person's life is well documented for renal disease. This high level of illness intrusiveness includes physiological effects, appearance changes, demanding treatment schedules, and decreased involvement in relationships and social and leisure activities.[10] Whatever the reason, it is clear that the types of challenges faced by the M. family are typical for those who have children with renal disease. The addition of single parenting, illiteracy, mental illness, developmental disability, substance abuse, unemployment, or any of a myriad other stressors can stretch any family to its breaking point. Therefore, it is apparent that social issues can have a profound impact on the well being of renal patients and their families. Numerous studies have shown that psychosocial interventions can increase patient adherence to treatment plans, improve patient-perceived quality of life and medical outcomes, and decrease medical costs by reducing hospitalizations.[4,15]

THEORETICAL UNDERPINNINGS: AN ECOLOGICAL PERSPECTIVE

Systems Theory

The ecological, or systems theory of human behavior is the fundamental premise behind nephrology social work and social work in general.[6,7] Systems theory holds that every individual is part of a system comprising the ecology, or environment, in which that person exists; the person and the environment constantly act upon each other in ways that produce changes in each.[7] An individual's ability to function depends on how well that person and his or her environment fit together. Since all parts of the ecology are interrelated, a change in functioning can be effected by introducing change at any part of the system.

Ecomap

This conceptual framework can be illustrated using what is called an *ecomap*, which shows in graphic form the various aspects of the environment with which a person may interact.[7] Family, friends, work, school, the healthcare system, religious institutions, hobbies, and the social welfare system are some of the environmental components that may be important to an individual's functioning. Each of these components takes on varying degrees of importance depending on the individual's history, current situation, motivation, and desires. A sample ecomap for a pediatric renal patient is shown in Figure 6-1. The child is pictured in the center of a constellation of environmental components that include household members (parents, siblings, and anyone else living in the same home); extended family (grandparents, aunts and uncles, other relatives); the living environment (the neighborhood in which the family resides, its safety, cleanliness, noise level, and types of neighbors living nearby); concrete resources available to the family (food, shelter, clothing, transportation, health insurance, income level); friends; school; recreation (sports, hobbies, other leisure activities); the social welfare system (Medicare/Medicaid, Social Security, child protective services in cases of abuse or neglect); religion; and the healthcare system (physicians, nurses, other medical professionals). Larger circles indicate the more influential spheres of an individual's life, and influences will vary from person to person. For some, the religion circle might be very large, while for a high-school football star, the recreation circle might dominate. Lines drawn from the central figure to the other circles can indicate the level of functioning experienced in each of the spheres. A double solid line to school would indicate the solid connection of a student who excels in academics, gets along with teachers, and enjoys her classmates' company; a jagged line to family would depict poor functioning at home and a high level of conflict between the child and other members of the household. For pediatric renal patients, the healthcare circle is often as large as or larger than those for school and friends.

The systems model can also be applied to the nuclear family unit.[6,7] The actions and beliefs of each family member – and this can include children, parents, stepparents, grandparents, aunts, uncles, cousins, lovers, and foster parents, depending on the make-up of the household – affect each other family member, to some extent determining their actions and beliefs. For example, the withdrawal from family life of a depressed parent can elicit acting-out behaviors from attention-starved children. Dealing with the drug abuse of a teenager can rip apart his or her parents' relationship with each other.

THE ROLE OF THE NEPHROLOGY SOCIAL WORKER

The ecological perspective is therefore the guiding principle that determines the role and functions of the social worker as part of the pediatric nephrology medical team. These functions generally fall into one of three categories: providing direct patient care; serving as consultant to the rest of the renal team; and acting as advocate for renal patients in general on a *macro* level with the hospital or medical facility, or out in the larger community. The overriding goal, however, is always the same: to provide or facilitate provision of any psychosocial services needed to help patients and families adjust to illness, so the patient's physical health can be restored as much as is medically possible and daily living can resume with minimum alteration.[5]

Psychosocial Assessment

Direct patient care by a social worker can take several different forms.[15] First and foremost is psychosocial

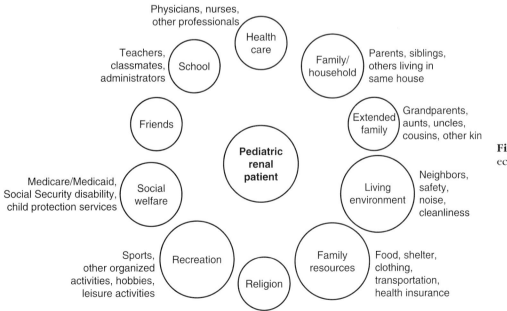

Figure 6-1 An example of an ecomap.

assessment. The importance of assessment in assisting patients and families in reaching an optimal level of functioning cannot be overstated. In the same way that the provision of proper medical treatment depends entirely upon accurate diagnosis, the provision of appropriate and effective social work interventions depends upon thorough and accurate gathering of information about the patient and family's situation, strengths, and needs. Assessment is an ongoing process, initially taking place in the early days and weeks following the diagnosis of a chronic renal disease, but continually being re-examined as the child's medical condition and treatment plan change and the child and family progress through life's developmental stages. It is important to note that assessment often uncovers multiple, contradictory needs. Social work clinicians must be prepared to help negotiate these dilemmas in the best interest of both patient and the family unit.

An example of an assessment is shown in Figure 6-2. Families should be helped to understand that the personal information gathered through this instrument, which may seem intrusive to some, remains confidential within the renal team and that its purpose is to allow the team to understand patient and family strengths and challenges that may affect the patient's medical care. The assessment includes such information as family composition, level of patient and family understanding of the medical situation, behavioral and mental health issues, school and learning issues, coping styles and supports, and insurance and financial situation (Box 6-1).

Regular reassessments are also important in keeping current with a patient and family's circumstances as they change over time.[12,15] Loss of employment, new problems in school, behavioral changes, and changes in marital status or family make-up are common over the course of a chronic illness and can create new needs for support.

Once a psychosocial assessment is completed, the renal social worker provides ongoing counseling to patients and family members regarding medical decision-making, care planning, and psychological coping. Some mental health issues are best managed by medication, and/or intensive talk therapy provided by a psychiatrist, psychologist, or social work clinician working as a psychotherapist. However, the nephrology social worker acts as the primary mental health practitioner for many patients and families.[15,19] For patients already overburdened by medical appointments and treatment regimens, the frequency of contact with a renal social worker who is conveniently available during clinic visits uniquely positions the social worker to act in this role. Close and intense relationships may develop over time between social worker and family. And since social workers receive intensive, 2-year postgraduate professional training in the principles of human

development and the skills needed to help people optimize functioning in their environment, they possess the essential tools needed to work as counselors in a medical setting.[19]

Clinical Pearl

Many mental health problems are situational and require only brief intervention. An example is the depression that new dialysis patients frequently experience when the impact of this treatment on their lives becomes fully understood.

Adjustment to newly diagnosed renal disease can lead to severe, clinical depression in some while others regain their equanimity after a short period of adjustment under a social worker's guidance. Early, intensive social work intervention with patients starting hemodialysis, for example, has been shown to have a significant, positive effect on patients' adjustment and quality of life.[2]

Coordinating Resources

Another key function of the renal social worker is to coordinate the many resources needed to support the care of a long-term renal patient. Transportation, financial considerations, health insurance, home nursing and medical equipment, special school or work accommodations, and the need to be followed by multiple medical specialists and/or mental health practitioners are just some of the issues that may impact a family's ability to care for a child with renal disease. Even the most capable family can become emotionally, physically, and financially depleted by the time and energy required managing so many responsibilities. Many of these specialized resources have not been a part of the family's life before the onset of illness, making education an important part of the social worker's job.

Box 6-1   Assessment Often Uncovers Multiple and Contradictory Needs

- The patient and family come to realize that kidney failure is irreversible
- Life must irrevocably change for every family member
- Decisions are made concerning the types and timing of treatments
- Lifestyle modifications must be made to accommodate additional responsibilities
- Severe illness reshapes family members' hopes, dreams, aspirations for the future
- Different family members' needs, desires, or rights clash

Psychosocial Assessment
Division of Nephrology, The Children's Hospital of Philadelphia

---

FOR OFFICE USE ONLY

Patient name_____

Date of Birth_____ Medical record #_____

Diagnosis_____

Family members present during assessment_____

Assessment admini tered by_____

---

1. Please list everyone who lives in your household

   Full name   Age   Relationship to patient

   a._____

   b._____

   c._____

   d._____

   e._____

   f._____

   g._____

2. Parent/guardian marital status

   ☐ Married ☐ Single ☐ Divorced ☐ Separated ☐ Widowed ☐ Living with partner

   ☐ Other (please describe)_____

3. Are parents/guardians currently employed?

   ☐ Both ☐ One (who?)_____ ☐ Neither

   Employer's name/work phone_____

   Employer's name/work phone_____

4. Why does your child see a nephrologist (kidney doctor)?_____

   _____

5. Does your child understand why he/she sees a nephrologist (kidney doctor)?

   ☐ Yes ☐ No (please explain) _____

6. Does your child attend school?

   ☐ Yes Grade_____ Name of school_____

   ☐ No (please explain)_____

7. Does your child receive special education services?

   ☐ No ☐ Yes (please describe)_____

Figure 6-2   Patient questionnaire used in the Division of Nephrology, The Children's Hospital of Philadelphia, as part of a psychosocial assessment.

8. Has your child ever been diagnosed with (if yes, please describe):

    a. Learning disability ☐ No ☐ Yes_____

    b. Developmental problems ☐ No ☐ Yes_____

    c. Emotional problems ☐ No ☐ Yes_____

    d. Behavioral problems (e.g., ADHD) ☐ No ☐ Yes_____

9. How would you describe your child's learning style?

    ☐ Learns by hearing ☐ Learns by seeing ☐ Learns by doing ☐ Don't know

10. Does anyone in your household have a history of/current problem with/see a therapist/counselor for:

a. Marital/family difficulties	☐ No ☐ Yes (who?)_____
b. Emotional problems	☐ No ☐ Yes (who?)_____
c. Mental illness	☐ No ☐ Yes (who?)_____
d. Drug or alcohol use	☐ No ☐ Yes (who?)_____
e. Learning/school problems	☐ No ☐ Yes (who?)_____
f. Behavioral problems	☐ No ☐ Yes (who?)_____
g. Developmental problems	☐ No ☐ Yes (who?)_____

11. How would you describe your child's temperament (behavior, reactions) compared with other children his/her age?

☐ More fearful	☐ Less fearful	☐ Average
☐ Less mature	☐ More mature	☐ Average
☐ More hyper/restless	☐ More calm/quiet	☐ Average
☐ More easily distracted	☐ More focused	☐ Average

12. How would you describe your child's attitude (check all that apply)?

☐ Highly sensitive	☐ Self-absorbed	☐ Outgoing/friendly
☐ Rigid/defiant	☐ Active/aggressive	☐ Inattentive
☐ Well-regulated	☐ Timid/shy	☐ Flexible/easygoing

13. Compared with other children the same age, does your child have:

☐ More friends	☐ Fewer friends	☐ An average number of friends
☐ Don't know		

14. How would you describe your relationship with your child?

☐ Warm/open	☐ Anxious/tense	☐ Angry/hostile
☐ Overly involved	☐ Distant	☐ Other (please describe)

15. Does your child have insurance or other health coverage? ☐ No ☐ Yes

    If yes, what kind (check all that apply)?

☐ Provided by parent/guardian employer	☐ Paid privately by family
☐ Medicaid (including CHIP)	☐ Medicare

Figure 6-2   Cont'd

Answer questions 16–18 ONLY IF ONE OR MORE PARENT IS EMPLOYED:

16. Do you anticipate any problems with employer(s) due to your child's illness/treatment?

     ☐ Yes   ☐ No   ☐ Not sure

17. Will parents/guardians have to stop work due to child's illness/treatment?

     ☐ Yes   ☐ No   ☐ Not sure

18. Would a change in parent/guardian employment jeopardize your child's health insurance?

     ☐ Yes   ☐ No

19. Is your family currently experiencing any financial difficulties?

     ☐ No ☐ Yes (please describe)_____

     _____

20. Are there other stresses in your life that could make your child's illness difficult for you and your family to manage?

     ☐ No ☐ Yes (please describe)_____

     _____

21. Who can you count on to provide the following (check all that apply):

     a. Emotional support

         ☐ Spouse/partner ☐ Other relatives ☐ Friends ☐ Work associates ☐ No one

     b. Financial support:

         ☐ Spouse/partner ☐ Other relatives ☐ Friends ☐ Work associates ☐ No one

     c. Information:

         ☐ Spouse/partner ☐ Other relatives ☐ Friends ☐ Work associates ☐ No one

     d. Help with everyday tasks:

         ☐ Spouse/partner ☐ Other relatives ☐ Friends ☐ Work associates ☐ No one

22. How will you get to CHOP for appointments?

        ☐ Own car ☐ Public transportation ☐ Rides from others ☐ Don't know

23. Is there anything else you would like to share about your child and/or your family that might make it easier for the medical team to assist you?

     _____

     _____

     _____

     _____

24. This form is intended for use only by members of the Division of Nephrology at The Children's Hospital of Philadelphia. The information helps us to provide your child and family with the best possible care. May we include this form in your child's medical chart?
     ☐ Yes   ☐ No

Figure 6-2   Cont'd

At the same time, obtaining these resources requires not only knowledge but also persistence and the ability to solve problems creatively. The advocacy of a social worker on behalf of a family with government agencies, managed-care insurance companies, and healthcare providers can make the difference between a patient receiving what he or she is entitled to receive or doing without. A good example is Supplemental Security Income, or SSI (Box 6-2).

The application process is lengthy and multi-step. It entails the gathering of documentation from medical sources regarding the child's disability and verification of income that is determined not only by the amount of the parents' paychecks but by other financial considerations such as number of people being supported by that income and level of debt. The social worker can ensure that all appropriate materials are submitted to the agency, and that the case is presented in a way that most clearly and forcefully demonstrates the family's eligibility.

A Voice at the Table

During interdisciplinary patient care conferences, it is the social worker's role to represent patient and family points of view and to help other team members understand how medical decisions may be affected by non-medical issues.[11]

> **Clinical Pearl**
>
> The social worker acts as patient and family advocate not only to the outside world but also within the renal team.

One such commonly held discussion centers around the choice families must make between in-center hemodialysis and home peritoneal dialysis. While medical constraints may determine the choice for some children, when there is a medical option, medical staff often recommend peritoneal dialysis, because its daily performance allows for gentler treatment and more liberal fluid and diet restrictions. But are the parents cognitively and emotionally capable of handling sophisticated medical equipment and making judgments about treatment that only physicians and nurses made just 20 years ago? Is there enough space in the home for the cycling machine and bulky dialysate bags? Do work schedules and other family members' needs allow the time to supervise dialysis for 10–12 hours each night? Would the parents simply prefer not to take on this responsibility, as is their right? A thorough examination up front of the many non-medical factors that affect treatment efficacy can help to prevent proceeding in a direction that is likely to fail, and the social worker can provide the family with anticipatory guidance regarding treatment choices.

Ethical Issues

Another area in which the nephrology social worker may serve as a consultant to the medical team involves ethical decisions. As mentioned earlier, patient and family desires and motivations can conflict at times, just as the goals, values, and opinions of members of the nephrology team can differ from those of the patient and family, or even those of other team members (Box 6-3).

When disagreements as to treatment direction occur, the social worker can act as a consensus-builder by helping patient, family, and professionals explain their viewpoints to one another and explore all of the implications of a decision.[11]

Macro-level Advocate

The nephrology social worker can and should act as a *macro*-level advocate for patients and families. This involves advocating for resources and services to be

---

Box 6-2 Supplemental Security Income (SSI)

- Children diagnosed with chronic, disabling conditions may be eligible for monthly payments, called 'SSI,' of up to several hundred dollars from the Social Security Administration if their families meet government-determined income guidelines

---

Box 6-3 Examples of Frequent Ethical Dilemmas in Pediatric Nephrology

- A family's desire to pursue a living-related transplant for the child despite a medical condition that puts the donor parent at unusual risk of complications
- An HIV-positive teenager's desire to withdraw from dialysis support during the final stage of her life while her caregivers wish to continue treatment
- A family's pursuit of alternative therapies such as homeopathy in opposition to the medical team's recommendation of dialysis
- A parent's wish to list her child for a cadaver kidney transplant despite the child having a developmental level that will remain below 12 months of age

made available by the hospital and medical staff; by community-based agencies; and by public policy. Macro-level advocacy could involve seeking funds from the hospital's budget to purchase computers to be used at each patient seat in dialysis, so children can do schoolwork during treatment; requesting insurance coverage for specific medications or equipment that are essential to renal patients' well-being but are not included as covered items by most managed-care companies; pushing school districts to provide homebound tutoring for children who are able to attend school only part-time due to health issues; or lobbying state legislatures not to lower the income limits for Medicaid, which serves as an insurance safety net for many pediatric renal patients. Providing this type of support to patients and families not only empowers them to advocate for themselves, raising self-esteem and bolstering self-sufficiency, but also gives them the tools they need to follow medical regimens and work together with physicians for the good of the patients' health.

Dialysis

At the start of dialysis, assessment should be revisited. The particular challenges involved in dialysis must be addressed. Many of these issues will be unfamiliar to families and hard for them to anticipate without previously having had the experience of dialysis, which is a good reason for exploring them in an assessment update with a team member who has expertise in these areas.[20]

1. The size and condition of the living quarters become important if a family is considering home administration of continuous cycling peritoneal dialysis.
2. Is there sufficient storage space for the bulky dialysate bags and other supplies?
3. Can a room, or at least a portion of a room, be dedicated as the patient's treatment area to insure hygiene and to accommodate the cycler?
4. Is there adequate cleanliness throughout the house to prevent frequent infections?
5. Are there household pets that should be restricted from wandering into the treatment room?
6. Transportation to and from the dialysis unit is of key importance for a patient starting hemodialysis.
7. Is there an adult available to accompany a younger child three times a week?
8. Does an adolescent who is old enough to travel alone have access to specialized medical transportation or know the public transportation route?
9. Is the patient's school aware that some classes may have to be missed on a regular basis to allow time for treatment, and how will this affect the youngster's academic performance?

Renal Transplantation

This is such a specialized form of treatment that most ESRD programs require an in-person meeting with a social worker to review the challenges likely to be encountered at the time of and following the surgery. The important information that must be discussed prior to embarking upon either a living-related or cadaveric transplant is outlined in Figure 6-3. The social work evaluation should be done in conjunction with a psychological evaluation that focuses on the mental health status and functioning level of patient and family. It is particularly important to highlight any issues that might impact on adherence to the post-transplant immunosuppressant medication regimen and thereby jeopardize the transplanted organ. Together, these assessment tools can predict areas of potential weakness and allow supports to be put in place prior to surgery to maximize the possibility of a successful transplant.

From a social perspective, familiarity with the following topics has proved especially useful in supporting transplantation:

1. Assessing the patient's and family's knowledge of the transplant surgery and short- and long-term post-transplant care.
2. Understanding the various roles assumed by different family members and exploring support that may be obtained from extended family, friends, neighbors, and other community members during the acute phase of surgery and recuperation.
3. Reviewing any history of mental health issues or substance abuse that may recur or be exacerbated by the stress of a transplant and stand as a barrier to optimal patient care.
4. Planning for a school absence of at least 6 weeks when the highly immunosuppressed transplant recipient should be shielded from exposure to infectious agents.
5. Determining the financial impact on the family of the many expenses not covered by medical insurance (transportation to and from hospital and follow-up clinic, loss of income during transplant donor's surgical recovery or time taken off from work by a parent to care for the recipient, medications excluded by the patient's insurance policy).

SOCIAL CHALLENGES AND INTERVENTIONS BY SYSTEM

This is a detailed look at the many social challenges faced by renal patients and their families, as well as the potential interventions members of the medical team may initiate to enhance patient care.

Pre-Transplant Social Work Evaluation (from Division of Nephrology, The Children's Hospital of Philadelphia)

Patient name_____

Date of birth_____ Medical record #_____

Date of evaluation_____ Length of time _____

Participants_____

_____

_____

Evaluation administered by_____

I.   **Introduction**

A. Purpose of evaluation
  a.   To assist families in assessing their social situation as it relates to successful planning for renal transplantation
  b.   To assist families and medical team in delineating plan to address identified social needs

B. Explanation of social work role
  a.   Helping families assess their knowledge base concerning diagnosis, treatment options and treatment plan
  b.   Helping families assess their support systems and needs prior to transplantation
  c.   Assessing risk factors to medical outcome and interventions needed
  d.   Assessing adherence history and planning interventions as needed
  e.   Assessing and coordinating resources throughout care
  f.   School transition planning
  g.   Assessing need for further emotional supports for patient/family members
  h.   Discussing boundaries of confidentiality

II.   **Medical situation**

A. Medical diagnosis

B. Plan for transplant (treatment options, alternatives, donation, timing of transplant)

C. Medical course to date

III.   **Family's knowledge surrounding transplantation**

A. Understanding of medical diagnosis

B. Understanding of treatment plan

C. Understanding of transplant plan

D. Understanding of transplant course
  a.   Pre-transplant evaluation
  b.   Transplant hospitalization
  c.   Post-transplant care
  d.   Kidney donation

IV.   **Family composition**

A. Immediate family

B. Extended family

C. Primary and secondary supports

D. Community/recreational supports

E. Spiritual supports

Figure 6-3   Pre-transplant social worker's evaluation form used in the Division of Nephrology, The Children's Hospital of Philadelphia.

V.   **Family health/mental health history**

    A. Other health problems in family and changing responsibilities

    B. Mental health history/problems in family

    C. Cognitive deficits/issues in family that affect ability to understand/carry out care plan

    D. Substance abuse/addiction history in family

VI.   **Post-transplant caregiving arrangement**

    A. Clinic visits and schedule

    B. Unexpected outpatient/inpatient visits

    C. Medication plan/adherence/supervision of patient's care

VII.   **Financial supports/insurance**

    A. Employment situation

    B. Employment supports/stability

    C. Time off for transplant care

    D. Time off for recovery of donor

    E. Financial situation

    F. Financial implications of transplant

    G. Insurance
        a.   Private insurance
        b.   Medical Assistance (Medicaid) entitlement
        c.   Social Security entitlement (SSI)
        d.   Medicare entitlement
        e.   Financial counseling available

VIII.   **Education situation/plan**

    A. Name of patient's school

    B. Grade

    C. Important contacts

    D. Special educational services/supports in place

    E. School staff's knowledge of transplant plan

    F. Plan for hospitalization

    G. Plan for homebound instruction following transplant

    H. Plan for transition back to school post-transplant

Figure 6-3   **Cont'd**

IX.   **Resources available for emotional issues**

    A. Social work

    B. Psychology/adherence specialist

    C. Psychiatry

    D. Local referrals

    E. Child life specialist services

    F. Hospital's family resource center

X.   **Educational literature available**

    A. Mailing lists for transplant community materials

    B. Pharmacy literature

    C. Insurance literature

    D. Magazines/newsletters for transplant patients

XI.   **Financial resources**

    A. Charitable funds

    B. Transportation assistance

XII.   **Discussed and agreed upon the following plan with family:**

Figure 6-3   Cont'd

Family

No system is more crucial to the well-being of a chronically ill child than the family. Research provides evidence that a positive family environment – one that is characterized by cohesiveness among members, low levels of conflict, and a place in which members feel comfortable directly expressing their emotions – can act as a buffer against the inevitable stress created by serious, long-term illness.[18] Yet the demands on caregivers of pediatric renal patients are immense, making the maintenance of a loving, conflict-free home life extremely difficult. The physical demands of home care are often exhausting.[12] Parents are expected to perform medical treatments at home that can be either painful or frightening to children:

- Giving growth hormone or erythropoietin injections
- Changing catheter dressings
- Administering nasogastric feedings or replacing the tubes
- Supervising peritoneal dialysis
- Policing their youngsters' dietary intake, depriving them of treats available to their siblings and peers
- Interrupting their routines several times a day to swallow unpleasant pills and liquid medications

Time must be found to accompany patients to medical appointments and to handle home care – time that is not being spent with the spouse or other children. Because of the intricacies of home medical regimens, it may be difficult to find relatives or paid babysitters who are willing and able to give the parents any respite.

The emotional demands of care-giving are equally burdensome. Decision-making can be wrenching when parents first learn about the challenges they and their child will face. During adolescence, acting-out behaviors may be most marked when limitations on independence and social life are most painfully realized.[3,12] Because the medical and ethical questions faced by families may have no right or wrong answers, these create nagging anxieties over the life-altering consequences of choosing one direction rather than another.[3] It may take years for a parent to accept the impaired child they have, rather than the idealized perfect child and future every new parent hopes for; indeed, this acceptance may never be achieved. The never-ending anxiety of monitoring a child's condition and being responsible for reporting symptom changes that could have major health implications takes its toll.[12] Guilt and grief reactions may be provoked by a poor outcome of a particular decision. If the parents have chosen hemodialysis rather than peritoneal dialysis and there are vascular access problems, this can cause guilt. A peritoneal membrane that does not function, the loss of an allograft, and especially death, can provoke guilt and grief reactions.

It is important to communicate medical information about diagnosis, prognosis, and treatment options (Box 6-4). The family must be taught how chronic illness in general and the child's particular renal disease can affect emotional development, behavior, and social functioning. They must be guided with strategies to restore balance and harmony to family life by reducing conflict, managing difficult behaviors, and taking advantage of all available support resources. Parents who are impeded from bonding with a sick infant by their own grief, for example, can be helped to understand that this reaction is normal and can be overcome with time and by focusing on the child's positive attributes. They can be referred for peer support to other parents who have been through similar situations and are willing to share their experiences.[16] Parents who are reluctant to place further demands on a sick child by disciplining inappropriate behaviors can be counseled that limit-setting makes a child feel secure and less prone to act out, and they can be helped to devise limits that make sense within the context of the child's physical condition.[11]

Mental Health

When conflict and poor functioning persist for a patient or family over time, despite education and short-term supportive counseling, more specialized mental health treatment may be warranted. A patient or parent may have such severe anxiety or depression that intensive support is needed through individual therapy or the prescription of psychotropic medication. Family therapy is advised when destructive relationship patterns among family members may be entrenched. This becomes particularly evident when adherence to medication or other treatment is affected and decreases to the point of endangering the patient's health.[9]

Again, education is an important form of intervention, helping patients and families to understand the source of their difficulties and why the care of a psychologist, psychiatrist, or other individual or family therapist is important. The renal social worker can assess which

type and level of mental health care is needed. An adolescent who has threatened self-harm requires inpatient psychiatric hospitalization, for example, and with the patient's and family's agreement can be referred to an appropriate provider. Families in crisis often have difficulty negotiating the mental health system on their own to find high-quality, affordable providers whose expertise matches their needs. An ongoing collaboration between this provider and the renal team throughout the course of treatment is essential in order to maximize the positive impact it can have on the renal patient's medical care. By regularly tracking the progress of mental health treatment, the team can determine the safety and efficacy of psychotropic medications in the context of the patient's renal disease and other medications; gauge the appropriate timing for new medical interventions or decision-making; and predict more accurately whether and how adherence to the medical treatment regimen is being affected.

School

Second only to family, school is the system of most importance to children and adolescents aged 5 to 18 years. Many spend more waking hours in school and school-related activities than they do with family members at home. School is the arena in which many developmental tasks are played out: mastering a skill; interacting with peers and developing a social milieu; establishing a personal identity; moving towards independence from family; preparing for sexual roles and relationships.[17] Chronic illness can impede these tasks in numerous ways. Research shows that ESRD patients' school adjustment is hindered by both poor academic achievement, which may be linked to subtle cognitive deficits resulting from long-term renal disease, and psychological factors.[13] Irregular school attendance may interfere with academic performance and formation of a peer group, thus setting up a cycle of school avoidance. Appearance abnormalities and other differences may prevent youngsters from identifying with peers or being accepted by them. Forced dependency due to physical setbacks may either prevent separation and individuation or provoke dangerous rebellion in the form of medical non-adherence. Relationships with the opposite sex may be delayed or non-existent.[17]

Care-giver attitudes are particularly important in maintaining optimal school attendance and performance.[8] Parents must be persuaded not to be too overprotective of children they perceive as vulnerable, as they may overtly or subtly indicate support for a child's staying out of school. At the same time, they should be educated about the special services to which their children may be entitled due to medical problems, learning disabilities, or psychological and emotional issues.

Box 6-4 Effective Intervention within the Family System

- Focus on education
- Provide information
- Encourage communication between the family and nephrology team

> **Clinical Pearl**
>
> Many teachers and school administrators may never have encountered a student who is a dialysis or transplant patient, and so may be unaware of the special needs that these conditions spawn.

Educators may either unduly restrict a child's participation in school activities out of ignorance or fear, or push a child to meet expectations that are not realistic considering the effects of his or her illness or treatments.[8] Many parents are unaware of the legal protections for children with special needs that are in place. This includes early intervention through physical, speech, and occupational therapies for pre-school-age infants and children with disabling conditions.

> **Clinical Pearl**
>
> In 1990, the Individuals with Disabilities Education Act passed into law, providing federal funding to states to provide mandated special school services for eligible students.

Perhaps the most effective intervention involving school is to hold a meeting with a medical team representative (social worker and/or nurse), parents, children who are old enough to participate, and school personnel including the classroom teacher, school nurse, any special education teachers or teachers of specialized curricula that may be affected (physical education, for example), and pertinent school administrators (principal, guidance counselor). Literature explaining the child's disease and treatment can be distributed at this time, and an appropriate academic plan can be devised. The medical representative can provide guidance regarding the child's expected attendance level, limitations, and needed supports, such as homebound or supplemental tutoring. Regular contact by the renal team with an identified point person at school can identify problems that need intervention at an early stage and keep school personnel informed as to the child's medical condition as it changes over time. In lieu of a meeting, correspondence outlining a child's medical issues and treatment plan as they relate to school can provide parents with sufficient validation to negotiate with school staff on their own. Success in school produces a domino effect of increased self-esteem, decreased depression, and better adherence to medical treatments, so the investment of time and energy can be parlayed into better medical outcomes.

Community Supports

Chronic illness, and particularly renal disease, can be isolating. Changes in appearance or poor growth can make children and adolescents reluctant to socialize; the large amount of time required for medical care can limit the entire family's involvement in school, extracurricular, community, or leisure activities. But isolation can breed further withdrawal, depression, and a lack of support for overburdened parents trying to go it alone.

Patients and families should be encouraged to maintain contacts with community groups that have provided support in the past. Family friends, neighbors, religious groups, or other organizations with which parents have been affiliated in the past can prove to be invaluable resources both emotionally and in terms of concrete services such as financial aid and transportation assistance. Youngsters should be encouraged to confide in friends about their condition, rather than keeping it secret. They should continue as much as is physically possible to participate in esteem-building activities in athletics, the arts, or community service. Maintaining as many avenues as possible in which a child or adolescent can excel fosters a sense of accomplishment and pride that can go a long way toward countering the feelings of inferiority and shame that illness can engender.

Finances, Insurance, and Employment

The expense of healthcare for chronic renal disease can be extremely onerous for many families, even those with adequate income and insurance. When a child is in medical crisis, money may be the last thing on a parent's mind. However, when the crisis has passed, families may find themselves in financial disarray. For those already living on a shoestring, missing the salary from even a few days off work in order to stay with a hospitalized child can result in catastrophe. Phone and electric services are shut off for non-payment, an employer may threaten to terminate employment, a landlord may even send an eviction notice. It is therefore important that all families be made aware early in the course of a child's illness of all financial supports and legal rights to which they are entitled.

In the private sector, employer-based group medical insurance is the mainstay support for paying medical bills that can, over the life of a renal patient, mount into millions of dollars. Parents should be advised to examine their policies to determine what, if any, lifetime limits on payment exist. A consultation with the employer's benefits specialist should help workers fully understand their child's coverage, as well as the employer's leave policies (Box 6-5).

If an employee qualifies for Family Medical Leave, the time does not have to be taken consecutively; employees can take a day here and two days there to accompany children to medical appointments, for example. The FMLA guarantees that the employee's job be kept open and that medical insurance continue throughout the leave period. It should be kept in mind, however, that this is unpaid time off. Parents should be urged to examine their personal resources and, if necessary, should be

Box 6-5 The Federal Family and Medical Leave Act (FMLA) of 1993

Employees of at least 12 months' standing at companies with more than 50 employees, in federal, state, and local government, or at public or private educational institutions are entitled to take up to 12 weeks of job-protected leave for every 12-month period of employment in order to take care of a seriously ill family member.

referred to a credit counselor or charitable organization for assistance.

Public-sector entitlements are more generous for ESRD patients than perhaps any other chronically ill population. All patients who are on any form of dialysis or who have had a transplant become eligible for Medicare, which provides federally funded medical insurance that can act as primary coverage for those who are uninsured or supplemental coverage for those already covered by an employer-based policy. Parents should be directed to the closest office of the Social Security Administration, which administers Medicare, in order to apply for coverage. Additionally, free, state-administered Medicaid insurance is available through local public welfare offices for those youngsters whose families meet income guidelines; low-income families can also apply for Supplemental Security Income (SSI), a federal program providing monthly cash payments to patients who are determined to be disabled and whose families meet income guidelines. All of these entitlements require detailed information to be submitted by health care providers in order to justify patients' eligibility. It is important that physicians meet requests for information in a timely way to make sure families receive the maximum support allowed.

Child Welfare Services

At times, family limitations or difficulties may warrant the involvement of child protective services. Each state has a child welfare agency whose charge is to intervene in cases of abuse or neglect, including medical neglect. Parents may voluntarily seek or accept services or may be involuntarily required to participate. Reporting to child protective services is not optional for healthcare providers, who are required by law to contact their state agency in cases involving suspicion of physical or sexual abuse, verbal and emotional abuse, physical neglect by not providing adequate food, shelter, clothing, or supervision, or medical neglect through failure to administer needed medications or follow up with a physician's recommendations for appointments or procedures.

Clinical Pearl

Reporting a family to child protective services is not an option for healthcare providers. They are required by law to do so in verified or suspicious circumstances.

It is important to view the reporting process not as a punitive measure or a way to assign blame, but as a means for obtaining assistance for families under stress. Only under the most egregious circumstances are children removed from the home. In the majority of cases, a state-designated caseworker will work with parents to improve organizational and parenting skills while the family remains intact. The medical team would be likely to continue to have regular contact with the patient and family and, therefore, should seek to preserve good relations with the parents, despite the referral to social services. Many families respond positively when child welfare involvement is framed as a way to help them handle what is clearly a difficult situation, when it is explained that legal obligations allow the medical team no other option, and when they are told of the referral in advance rather than surprised by a knock at the door. Ongoing collaboration between the medical team and state caseworker can then help ensure that the medical plan is followed to the benefit of the patient.

CONCLUSIONS

Should medical professionals care about or get involved with their patients' psychosocial issues? Does this involvement overstep boundaries? The demonstrated interplay between social well-being and medical outcome – particularly in the case of a lifelong, life-altering illness such as renal disease – argues otherwise. Paying attention to social issues as a component of patient care – and, if possible, utilizing the services of a nephrology social worker as part of the treatment team – is often the tipping point for producing a result that patients, families, and medical professionals agree is beneficial for the patient.

REFERENCES

1. Bare MR. Confronting a life-threatening disease: renal dialysis and transplant programs. In: Kerson TS (ed), *Social Work in Health Settings: Practice in Context*. Haworth Press, New York, 1989.

2. Beder J. Evaluation research on the effectiveness of social work intervention on dialysis patients: the first three months. Soc Work Health Care 1999;30:15–30.

3. Brady DK, Lawry K. Infants, families and end stage renal disease: strategies for addressing psychosocial needs in the first two years of life. J Nephrol Soc Work 2000;20: 17–20.

4. Callahan MB. The role of the nephrology social worker in optimizing treatment outcomes for end stage renal disease patients. Dialysis Transplant 1998;27:630-642.

5. Callahan MB, Moncrief M, Woodrow L. Working toward improved outcomes: nephrology social work indicators. J Nephrol Soc Work 1999;19:33-41.

6. Cohen MS. Families coping with childhood chronic illness: a research review. Families, Systems & Health 1999; 17:149-164.

7. Compton BR, Galaway B. *Social Work Processes*, 5th ed. Brooks/Cole, Pacific Grove, CA, 1994.

8. Davis ID. Pediatric renal transplantation: back to school issues. Transplant Proc 1999;31:61S-62S.

9. Davis MC, Tucker CM, Fennell RS. Family behavior, adaptation, and treatment adherence of pediatric nephrology patients. Pediatr Nephrol 1996;10:160-166.

10. Devins GM. Illness intrusiveness and the psychosocial impact of end-stage renal disease. In: Hardy M, Kiernan J, Kutscher AH, et al. (eds), *Psychosocial Aspects of End-stage Renal Disease: Issues of Our Times*. Haworth Press, Binghamton, NY, 1991.

11. Drotar D, Ganofsky MA, Makker S, et al. A family-oriented supportive approach to dialysis and renal transplantation in children. In: Levy NB (ed) *Psychological Factors in Hemodialysis and Transplantation*. Plenum, New York, 1981.

12. Fedewa MM, Oberst MT. Family caregiving in a pediatric renal transplant population. Pediatr Nursing 1996;22: 402-407.

13. Fukunishi I, Honda M. School adjustment of children with end-stage renal disease. Pediatr Nephrol 1995;9: 553-557.

14. Furr LA. Psycho-social aspects of serious renal disease and dialysis: a review of the literature. Soc Work Health Care 1998;27:97-118.

15. McKinley M, Callahan MB. Utilizing the case management skills of the nephrology social worker in a managed care environment. J Nephrol Soc Work 1998;18:35-42.

16. Paluszny MJ, DeBeukelaer MM, Rowane WA. Families coping with the multiple crises of chronic illness. In: Hardy M, Kiernan J, Kutscher AH, et al. (eds), *Psychosocial Aspects of End-stage Renal Disease: Issues of Our Times*. Haworth Press, Binghamton, NY, 1991.

17. Sexton S, Rubenow J. Transplants in children and adolescents. In: Craven J, Rodin G (eds), *Psychiatric Aspects of Organ Transplantation*. Oxford University Press, New York, 1992.

18. Soliday E, Kool E, Lande MB. Psychosocial adjustment in children with kidney disease. J Pediatr Psychol 2000;25: 93-103.

19. Tramo JG. The nephrology social worker as the primary psychological practitioner. In: Levy NB (ed), *Psychological Factors in Hemodialysis and Transplantation*. Plenum, New York, 1981.

20. Warady B, Alexander S, Watkins S, et al. Optimal care of the pediatric end stage renal disease patient on dialysis. Am J Kidney Dis 1999;33:567-583.

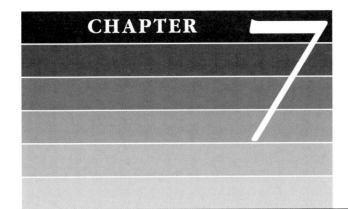

CHAPTER 7

Psychological Considerations in Renal Disease

NATALIYA ZELIKOVSKY, Ph.D. AND

REBECCA VEREB, M.Ed.

INTRODUCTION

Survival of children with renal disease has risen remarkably over the past 10 years, with the advancement of more effective medicines, improvement of dialysis treatments, and the viable option of renal transplantation. There is more of a focus on quality of life issues and the development of interventions to enhance the psychological adjustment of children with chronic health conditions, such as renal disease. Pediatric psychologists are increasingly being integrated in healthcare settings; in areas such as pediatric nephrology and organ transplant centers. The availability of pediatric psychologists and social workers on multi-disciplinary teams enhances patient care, particularly for patients with complex psychosocial issues. Integration of psychosocial colleagues highlights a biopsychosocial perspective and emphasizes the importance of treating the whole person – mind, body, and behavior.

FACTORS THAT AFFECT ADJUSTMENT

Although many children are resilient and prevail in spite of adverse conditions, there are many elements that can derail the path toward healthy adaptation. Factors associated with their medical condition, individual characteristics of the child, and the family/social context, all have significant impact on the adjustment process for children with a chronic illness. All experiences have the potential to increase the risk for maladjustment or alternatively, to buffer the effects of stress associated with chronic illness.

Although disease type or severity have not been consistently linked to adaptation, the combination of *poor functional* status and *illness chronicity* can increase frustration and impatience with the medical process. Children who have been hospitalized for a long time may have trouble focusing on the positive things that they left behind such as friends, hobbies, and their favorite playground. As their illness advances, children may develop a sense of hopelessness about the medical outcome and their future. It may become more challenging for physicians to instill an optimistic outlook in their patients. But despite frequent exposure to medical events, the *quality of children's experiences* in the hospital setting has been found to have an important impact on children's emotional and behavioral adjustment. Some patients seem to enjoy the time spent in the hospital despite having to undergo invasive medical procedures, because they may receive more attention and support from nurses, as compared to their home environment.

The child's *age at critical points* during the course of the illness – and particularly age at diagnosis – may affect the child's ability to tolerate medical stressors and to develop effective coping strategies. Certain *developmental transitions* are generally coupled with increased stress (adolescent–parent conflict, beginning high school, transitioning to adult facility) for healthy youngsters, but may overwhelm an already fragile family structure of chronically ill children. Becoming aware of the child's cognitive, emotional and behavioral development during critical ages will help the pediatricians determine the level of explanation necessary to make information digestible for each child.

Children's belief in the source of their health problems may moderate the extent to which medical stressors affect them psychologically. Indeed, children's belief that "powerful others" (physicians and parents) are primarily responsible for their health may result in feelings of helplessness and lack of control. Other children have an internal locus of control and a strong sense of self-efficacy (the belief that one can effect the environment to yield a beneficial or self-advantageous outcome). Physicians often perceive these youngsters as independent, confident, and responsible in managing their illness. Although a positive belief system is generally considered a personal strength, children who always feel in control may be at risk for maladjustment (anger, loss of hope, internalized anxiety) if their efforts do not result in a positive medical outcome. Children who have a strong sense of self-efficacy despite periodic disappointments, and take an optimistic, goal-oriented approach to deal with their concerns may be better adjusted.

The *family environment* is instrumental in foretelling the psychological outcomes for children. Children rely on their parents to help meet their medical needs (attending clinic appointments, purchasing medications, giving injections, assisting with peritoneal dialysis). In some instances, parental premorbid psychiatric histories (traumatic experiences, chronic depression or anxiety, marital discord, and family death) disrupt their child's healthy development. Even though families will experience periods of distress and disorganization during the course of their child's illness, most families will rebound and stabilize to promote the ongoing care of their child.[6] Thus, it is important that physicians view families not as generally dysfunctional, but rather as competent families that are experiencing severe stress and disruption associated with their child's illness and treatment.

Social support provided by the extended family, school, community, and medical team can buffer the potentially negative impact of both chronic illness and pre-existing psychopathology. Conversely, lack of social support has been associated with increased risk for maladjustment.[6] Children who grow up in a warm and caring support structure are more likely to feel competent and confident in being able to overcome the tragedies of a chronic illness, whereas children who do not have sufficient social support may feel isolated, afraid, and insecure in overcoming the burdens of illness.

PSYCHOLOGICAL ADJUSTMENT DURING THE COURSE OF RENAL DISEASE

Diagnosis to End Stage

Children diagnosed with renal disease and their families have to adjust to a number of changes in their daily life. As children move through the stages – from initial diagnosis to dialysis to transplant and beyond – they display a variety of emotional and behavioral reactions. Learning that your child has been diagnosed with a medical condition is difficult for most families, who are generally in shock and take time to process and accept the news. Some families become angry in disbelief while others become sullen and internalize their emotions. Similarly, some children are anxious as they await a transplant and seek a lot of information while others prefer not to think about it and do not want to hear the details. Physicians should be prepared for all types of reactions from patients and their families.

Reported rates of adjustment problems among children with renal disease are approximately 19 to 30%.[12] When comparing children with kidney disease to healthy controls, elevated behavioral problems, lower social competence, and higher levels of internalizing symptoms (anxiety or depression) have been noted.[4] Patients who are first starting dialysis may be at particular risk for psychological problems (66%) relative to non-dialysis patients and healthy control groups.[5] However, adjustment improves after about 1 year on dialysis and stabilization of the medical condition.

Parents of children diagnosed with renal disease face a number of stressors, which may disrupt the entire family structure. As many as 20% of mothers whose children were awaiting organ transplant reported clinically elevated levels of parenting stress.[9,12] Stressors experienced by parents are related to the child's deteriorating medical status and waiting for an organ match, management of complex treatment regimens, or being evaluated as a potential donor. Disruption to typical roles and routines, changes in financial and employment status, loss of social supports, and changes in future plans of the family are common stressors.[3,4]

> **Clinical Pearl**
>
> The diagnosis of chronic renal disease in a child has an impact on the whole family.

In response to these disruptive changes, parents may become anxious, depressed, guilty, or angry. Because families have such an important impact on their children, poor parental adjustment has been linked to increased psychiatric and behavior problems in their children and lower adherence to the medical regimen.[5,9] Parents who are overprotective and worry excessively may limit opportunities for peer interactions and school attendance, which compromises the child's cognitive and social development.

Alternatively, a stable family environment can buffer the stress of childhood chronic illness. Lower levels of parenting stress, family cohesion and expressiveness, and less family conflict influence children in positive ways. Children in more supportive and cohesive families display fewer behavior problems, lower rates of anxiety and depression, better adherence, and improved overall psychological adjustment.[12] A strong social support network can protect children by encouraging them to talk about their illness openly and model effective coping with stress.[3] Because parents are the primary source of social support for children, and supportive family environments are related to better outcomes in children, helping families identify additional supports is likely to benefit the child as well.

Post-Transplant

As the children's physical health improves after the kidney transplant and they have more energy, parents note positive emotional and behavioral changes in their children. Children have a renewed sense of hope for a 'normal' life full of school activities, social events, and academic achievement. Nonetheless, they face a new set of anxieties and stresses after the transplant, including adjustment to the strict medication regimen of immuno-suppressants and fears about possible organ rejection or infection. While families try to return to 'normal' adjust-ment in family roles and responsibilities occurs to accommodate the post-transplant care.[3]

Many parents also report improvement in their own mental health and better family functioning after their child's transplant.[7] However, 56% of mothers experi-ence clinically significant levels of stress at 1 month post-transplant, and as many as 41% continued to report distress approximately half a year after their child's surgery.[8] Mothers report financial and caretaker burden post transplant. Thus, even with notable improvements, parents continue to need psychological and social supports after their child has received an organ trans-plant.[7] Identification of families' psychosocial needs prior to transplantation helps target families who are at risk for maladjustment post-transplant for early intervention.

Transition back to school after a prolonged period of absenteeism is so overwhelming for some children that they refuse to attend school. Children may be concerned about catching an infection, anxious about separating from their parents, lack confidence in their academic and social abilities, or worry about how other children will perceive them, especially given changes in physical appearance.[11] Parents may contribute to the child's anxiety about separa-tion if they are overprotective and may allow the child to stay home. A school re-entry team should be formed to successfully transition the child back into school.[6]

Clinical Pearl

Physicians must send a strong message to parents that it is important for their child to return to school, so they can learn, interact with peers, and develop independence.[2]

For a child with a chronic illness, school may be the only place where they can be a child rather than a patient and have some control over their environment. The school re-entry team can educate school personnel about how the child's behavior and academic perform-ance may be impacted by the illness. Members of the medical team, particularly the renal social worker, can help parents advocate for the child's academic, social, and psychological needs.[2] Peers can be positive influences during this process, and assist the child in adjusting to school by being supportive and accepting. And yet, due to ignorance about the nature of renal disease, some peers may avoid the child who has just returned to school out of fear that they may 'catch' the illness.[2] Educating students in the classroom about the child's illness and making the child's differences (physical appearance, academic delay) acceptable can ease the child's transition back into school.

DEVELOPMENTAL CONSIDERATIONS

The child's developmental level will affect their abil-ity to participate in decision-making and the extent to which the parents remain involved in their treatment. Younger children and children who are cognitively delayed may have difficulty understanding medical infor-mation and articulating concerns about their care, whereas older children and adolescents are better able to comprehend the concept of illness.[10] For example, preschool children may believe that illness results from 'bad' behavior, which may lead the child to feel guilty and perceive treatment as punishment. Children in elementary school may believe that illness results from germs and not following health rules, such as washing your hands before eating. Adolescents understand their illness is more complex than simply resulting from germs but may still not fully appreciate medical implica-tions of health risk behaviors.

The cognitive effects of renal disease on child development and functioning will vary depending on age at disease onset, severity and duration of illness, and presence of other health conditions. Increases in urea can cause encephalopathy, which can result in reduced alertness, concentration, memory, and coordination. Infants and toddlers may have developmental delays that result from the neurological effects of renal disease and from limited opportunities to explore their environ-ment.[10,13] Repeated hospitalizations may also impede a young child's ability to form a secure attachment to the parents because the child frequently may be in the care of healthcare staff during the first few years of life.[14] Fatigue, frequent hospitalizations, clinic appointments, or dialysis treatments may interfere with school-aged children's academic development due to missed school days. Also, reduced peer interactions limits children's ability to learn age-appropriate social skills.[10] An adolescent's identity development and desire for autonomy may be impeded by social alienation due to school absenteeism, and the need for closer parental supervision due to increased risk for non-adherence.[14] Changes in physical appearance caused by medication side effects may also affect how an adolescent is accepted by peers.

Research suggests that children with renal disease perform as well as healthy controls on global measures of intelligence. Differences exist in specific areas, as children with renal disease perform lower on measures of abstract ability, visual-perceptual reasoning, visual-motor integration and immediate recall and memory.[10] When comparing children with acquired and congenital forms of renal disease, no differences were found on measures of intelligence, academic achievement, behavior, and immediate memory. However, children with congenital conditions had more difficulties with long-term memory and fine motor coordination.[1] Following transplantation, children with renal disease show gains on measures of cognitive functioning, such as improvements in memory and learning, and ability to pay attention as compared to pre-transplant functioning.[4,10,13]

PSYCHOLOGISTS' ROLE ON THE RENAL TRANSPLANT TEAM

Many transplant centers have integrated psychosocial screenings as part of their pre-transplant evaluation process. However, the inclusion of comprehensive, standardized psychological evaluations for every pediatric transplant recipient is far less common. Transplant psychologists play a critical role as members of a multidisciplinary team – they help to clarify the psychological needs, assess emotional and behavioral readiness for surgery, and prepare families for the potentially stressful process.

Psychologists also identify risk factors for medical non adherence and assess a patient's motivation for life-long behavior change. After all, a patient's involvement does not end with the transplant surgery. Patients must be ready – not just medically but also mentally, emotionally, and behaviorally – to accept the life-long commitment to manage the implications of renal disease. The consequences for transplanting patients who have not taken the process seriously can be devastating, at times leading to depression, non-adherence, and graft rejection.

A comprehensive psychological evaluation includes a psychosocial interview with the patient and family, an adherence assessment, and a battery of standardized psychological questionnaires. The key domains of a psychosocial evaluation are summarized in Table 7-1.

After the evaluation, psychologists make specific recommendations to the families and transplant team that may include but are not limited to:

- Psychotherapy to work through issues that may impact adjustment (e.g., parent–child conflict, adolescent depression, adjustment to divorce or a family loss).
- Intervention to improve adherence to medical regimen to ensure that they can handle the more complicated post-transplant regimen.
- Behavior management for parents of young children who are oppositional, uncooperative, and have frequent temper tantrums.
- Interventions to reduce anxiety about medical procedures.
- Working with renal social workers to identify additional resources or social supports for the family. Although the broad goal for a transplant psychologist is to prepare patients for transplantation, the specific treatment goals are individualized to meet the needs of each patient and family.

Following kidney transplantation, psychological services may be needed for a subset of patients. Even though the possibility of medical complications is relayed to all families, some have difficulty adjusting to unexpected complications. Children who are generally active and socially involved become frustrated if the recovery process is slower than they had anticipated. Children who were asymptomatic prior to transplantation have to suddenly adjust to the typical post-surgical physical discomforts and pain. Once discharged from the hospital, patients remain at home for a period of 6 weeks, during which time they receive much attention – in the form of gifts, visits from friends and family, and emotional support. With time, this level of attention dissipates and children must return to school. Some children have difficulty during this transition and may benefit from working with a psychologist to support them as they readjust to school.

In summary, a transplant psychologist's role is multifaceted and beneficial throughout the process – prior, during, and post transplant – depending on the needs of the child and family.

PSYCHOLOGICAL CONSULTATIONS AND INTERVENTION

Physicians are in a good position to identify children and families who need to be referred for psychological services. Families may report problems to and seek advice from physicians or physicians themselves may witness changes in the child or family unit that may need to be evaluated by a psychologist. Psychological consultations are warranted for, but are not limited to: significant

Table 7-1 Domains Assessed During a Psychological Evaluation

Domains	Sample questions for assessment
Knowledge	Age-appropriate understanding of diagnosis and treatment
	Accurate and realistic expectation for post-transplant care
Acceptance	Acceptance of medical diagnosis and treatment
	Denial or minimizing of symptom frequency or severity
Decision-making	Comfort with decision to pursue kidney transplant or
	Readiness to perform regimen tasks of dialysis treatment
Relationship with medical team	Quality of relationships (trust, empathy, support)
	Degree of communication (regular, open, honest)
Risk taking behaviors	Safe sexual behavior among pre-teens and adolescents
	Substance use (alcohol, drugs, history of rehab)
	Significant legal history (detention center, foster care)
Adherence behaviors	Adherence with medication regimen
	Adherence with special diets
	Clinic attendance
Patient adjustment	Emotion/Behavior (depression, anxiety, anger, acting out)
	Social (peers, siblings, other patients)
	School (attendance, academic performance)
Parent adjustment	Parental psychopathology (depression, anxiety)
	Care-taker burden out (physical, emotional)
	Substance use (alcohol, drugs)
Family functioning	Stressful life events (marital discord, recent move, death)
	Relationship with siblings (competition, attention-seeking)
	Family dynamics (supportive, available, stable, cohesive)
Coping styles	Active, problem-solving, information-seeking style
	Passive, avoidant, withdrawn style
	Parental modeling of coping at home
Social support	Perceived availability support when needed
	Breadth of support (friends, co-workers, community)
	Religious, recreational, and social activities

behavior problems on the inpatient unit; uncooperative behavior precluding administration of medical procedures; ineffective coping with acute or chronic pain; persistent symptoms of depression or anxiety; poor adherence with medical recommendations; and increased family strain. Deciding whether to refer a patient may be difficult, but medical staff should err on the side of caution and discuss their observations with the team's psychologist or social worker to determine whether further evaluation would be helpful. Identifying the family's strengths and psychosocial risks and referring for psychological intervention early is most helpful.

All children and families will have some difficulties managing the illness, but when the problems are so severe as to interfere with daily functioning or the problems continue longer than would be expected, then psychological services may be appropriate. A mother of a child recently diagnosed with chronic renal failure may develop signs of depression, such as trouble sleeping or changes in appetite. These symptoms are to be expected, given the trauma experienced by the mother. However, if a number of symptoms are occurring simultaneously, the degree of distress is concerning to the mother, or the symptoms are preventing the mother

from taking care of herself and/or her child, then psychotherapy for depression may be necessary. Another example would be a child who is exhibiting anxiety about possible kidney rejection following a transplant. Initial worry would be expected because of the potential threat that exists, but if the child's anxiety persists for several months without improvement, then a referral to a psychologist is warranted.

Convincing the family to seek a psychological evaluation and/or treatment is another challenge. Because of the social stigma associated with psychological services, many people react negatively to recommendations regarding mental health treatment. When introducing the idea of psychological services to the patient and family, the physician can alleviate negative feelings and perceptions. Emphasizing that the physician perceives the family as capable and competent (lowering resistance), but that adjusting to a child's illness is challenging for many families (normalizing feelings). Explaining that other families have benefited from psychological services may help parents to be more accepting of the referral.

An effective way to introduce a mental health professional to a family is to explain that as a nephrologist you have expertise in taking care of their child's renal disease, and that *you* are seeking consultation or advice of psychologist in order to help their child with emotions (e.g., sadness, worrying, pain); not an area of your expertise. Presenting a referral in this manner yields a less defensive and more open-minded attitude. The focus is on the process of consultation rather than telling the parents that they or their child 'need help', which may pull for insecurity and anger in the parents. This approach maintains the core responsibility of the child's care in the hands of the physician, whom the family trusts.

CONCLUSIONS

Children function within complex and overlapping systems, such as the family, school, community, and the hospital setting. These interrelated systems impose numerous demands and sometimes, conflicting expectations on pediatric patients and their families. In order ultimately to achieve excellence in patient care, it is important to consider the children's adaptation from a developmental biopsychosocial perspective. As pediatric nephrologists treat the physical aspects of the medical conditions, clinical psychologists and social workers can help to support the behavioral, developmental, social, and emotional adjustment of patients and families. Together, a well-integrated team can effectively manage the multifaceted impact of chronic renal disease on patients, families, and healthcare professionals.

REFERENCES

1. Crocker JF, Acott PD, Carter JE, et al. Neuropsychological outcome in children with acquired or congenital renal disease. Pediatr Nephrol 2002;17:908–912.
2. Davis ID. Pediatric renal transplantation: back to school issues. Transplant Proc 1999;31 (Suppl 4A):61S–62S.
3. Engle D. Psychosocial aspects of the organ transplant experience: what has been established and what we need for the future. J Clin Psychol 2001;57:521–549.
4. Fennell EB. End-stage renal disease. In: Yeates KO, Ris MD, Taylor HG (eds), *Pediatric Neuropsychology: Research, Theory, and Practice.* Guilford, New York, 2000, pp. 366–380.
5. Garralda ME, Jameson RA, Reynolds JM, et al. Psychiatric adjustment in children with chronic renal failure. J Child Psychol Psychiatr 1988;29:79–90.
6. Kazak AE, Segal-Andrews AM, Johnson K. Pediatric psychology research and practice: a family/systems approach. In: Roberts MC (ed), *Handbook of Pediatric Psychology,* 2nd ed. Guilford, New York, 1995, pp. 84–104.
7. Reynolds JM, Garralda ME, Postlethwaite RJ, et al. Changes in psychosocial adjustment after renal transplantation. Arch Dis Child 1991;66:508–513.
8. Rodrigue JR, MacNaughton K, Hoffman RG, et al. Transplantation in children: a longitudinal assessment of mother's stress, coping, and perceptions of family functioning. Psychosomatics 1997;38:478–486.
9. Rodrigue JR, Hoffman RG, MacNaughton K, et al. Mothers of children evaluated for transplantation: stress, coping resources, and perceptions of family functioning. Clin Transplant 1996;10:447–450.
10. Schweitzer JB, Hobbs SA. Renal and liver disease: end-stage and transplantation issues. In: Roberts MC (ed), *Handbook of Pediatric Psychology,* 2nd ed. Guilford, New York, 1995, pp. 425–445.
11. Sexson S, Madan-Swain A. The chronically ill child in the school. School Psychol Q 1995;10:359–368.
12. Soliday E, Kool E, Lande MB. Psychosocial adjustment in children with kidney disease. J Pediatric Psychol 2000;25:93–103.
13. Stewart SM, Kennard BD. Organ transplantation. In: Brown RT (ed), *Cognitive Aspects of Chronic Illness in Children.* Guilford, New York, 1999, pp. 220–237.
14. Streisand RM, Tercyak KP. Evaluating the pediatric transplant patient: general considerations. In: Rodrigue JR (ed), *Biopsychosocial Perspectives on Transplantation.* Kluwer, New York, 2001, pp. 71–92.

SUGGESTED READING

Roberts MC (ed), *Handbook of Pediatric Psychology*, 3rd ed. Guilford Press, New York, 2003.

Rodrigue JR. *Biopsychosocial Perspectives on Transplantation.* Kluwer Academic/Plenum Publishers, New York, 2001.

Resource For Families

Starbright Series. Living with Kidney Disease on CD-ROM. www.starbright.org.

CHAPTER 8

Patient-Physician Communication

AILEEN WALSH, Ph.D. AND

NATALIYA ZELIKOVSKY, Ph.D.

INTRODUCTION

Although speaking to patients is a daily activity for physicians, doing so well and effectively is often difficult. Communicating with children and their parents poses special challenges. Not only do pediatricians need to manage the anxieties, concerns, and questions of parents who have been told that their child is ill, but they must also work with children who vary widely in their ability to understand and cope with medical information. The pediatric nephrologist is in an optimal position to impact patient adjustment and adherence, and yet the importance of the doctor-patient relationship as a resource is often overlooked.[2] The purpose of this chapter is to highlight the components of effective communication so that useful, productive, and mutually beneficial doctor-patient relationships are fostered.

Clinical Pearl

'Communicating with patients' should not be another task added to the list of things that physicians have to do. Rather, clear communication should be woven into a physician's daily practice of diagnosis, treatment, and health promotion.

ESTABLISHING A POSITIVE RELATIONSHIP

It is important that physicians establish a strong rapport with the patient and family at an early stage, based on trust, openness, and a partnership to work toward common goals of diagnosis and treatment. Such a rapport is fostered through positive interactions between patients and their physicians. An important contribution to a good patient-physician relationship is the manner in which information is delivered. Conversations should not be rushed, and should be in lay terms. The information must be developmentally appropriate for the patient. No matter how difficult the family or the physician's day, empathy provided to families is necessary – and does not go unnoticed.

Research on the delivery of information to families in intensive care units or providing a diagnosis of cancer consistently indicates that families value the quality of the information as well as the manner in which it is delivered.[1,3] Additionally, the quality of the relationship between the family and the medical team, the physician's communication skills, and perceptions of the physician as warm and approachable are important influences on adherent behaviors.[4] For example, pediatric kidney transplant patients have attributed their non-adherence to insufficient information and communication about their illness, loss of trust in the physician, and feelings of dependence on the medical team.

Effective communication involves giving clear information, responding to the patient's reactions and their questions, and doing so in a context of openness and concern. Physicians should be cognizant of a family's cultural values, coping styles, and the supports available to the family when establishing a working relationship with them. These factors influence how information should be delivered, how the information is heard, and how families based on this information make medical decisions.

Cultural values influence the choices that families make with regard to treatment, depending on how illness, death, medication, and transplantation are viewed in their culture. A family's religious values may also strongly influence their willingness to accept a kidney transplant, and whether they would allow members of the family to be donors. The ethnic, cultural, and religious framework of each family may also dictate who is present to receive information and who is available to provide support. For some families, extended family members are as involved as nuclear family members; for others, families may value having a clergy member present when discussing difficult information. It is helpful for physicians to understand how the patient's cultural and religious values intersect with medical decision-making in the early stages of developing a relationship. This understanding and a focus on the family's strengths can help to minimize misunderstandings that can create tension within the patient–physician relationship.

Family dynamics, the personality style of each family member, and the coping skills on which each member relies during times of stress also influence communication between the family and the physician. As physicians come to know families over time, they learn about how families cope with difficult news, how they react to stressful situations, and how they make medical decisions. Some families or members of families become tearful while others become angry. It may be difficult to assess the reactions of those who remain quiet when hearing difficult news. These reactions should be interpreted in light of the seriousness of the discussions. For example, being told that their child has elevated blood pressure is different for parents from being told that their child is in kidney failure and will soon need a transplant.

Early in the relationship physicians should try to find out from families:

- How they like to receive information. Do they prefer to hear everything even if it creates anxiety, or would they like a summary of the main developments in the child's medical status?
- How do they typically react to stressful situations (e.g., withdraw, cry, take action)?
- What tends to be helpful at these times (e.g., obtain additional information, increase support)?

The physician can then ask other members of team (e.g., a nurse practitioner, psychologist, and/or social worker) to provide the necessary supports.

DEVELOPMENTAL CONSIDERATIONS

The relationship between healthcare professionals and patients evolves over time, often times coinciding with changes in the patient's medical, developmental, and cognitive status. Because of the chronicity of many renal diseases, the team sees the patients develop physically, emotionally, and socially, just as parents watch their children grow. Therefore, times of transition (e.g., adolescence, transplantation, or transfer to adult facility) are difficult periods not only for the patient's family but also for the medical team. Children's needs, goals, and abilities to process information and participate in their treatment changes over time, and so pediatricians should adjust the level of communication and interactive style accordingly.

Communicating effectively with children can be challenging, but it is important and can be done well if a developmental perspective is kept. The pediatrician must focus on the age-appropriate needs of the patient. Children experience the world and respond to the concept of illness and death in different ways at different developmental stages. The following summary outlines the key characteristics of each developmental stage.

Toddlers

Children at this age understand what hurts and what does not, what feels good, and what feels bad. They need honest reassurance and the use of words that are age-appropriate. For example, a dialysis team gave the names of popular cartoon characters to the dialysis catheter lumens of a 3-year-old patient so that she understood to what they were referring when they were hooking her up. Explain procedures in simple, concrete terms – for example, "This medicine is to help your tummy feel better." Children at this age need only to understand what is happening in the moment because they do not have any true sense of time, nor will they understand how what is happening currently fits into the 'big picture' of their care. The focus of communicating with toddlers is to generate trust so that they can understand what is happening at the moment when their cooperation is needed.

School-Age Children

Children at this age are concerned about practical issues (e.g., will they be home in time for the holidays, or can they play in the baseball game on Friday) and want to know when they will be 'normal' again. Some children may feel guilty or responsible for their illness, usually as a result of a misunderstanding about what causes the disease. Procedures should be explained to them before they occur in concrete terms. Whether the child will miss school is another important issue to address. It is helpful to emphasize to the child and the parent the importance of remaining in school and maintaining responsibilities at home. Encourage children of this age to ask questions so that any misconceptions can be clarified right away.

Adolescents

Most teenagers are able to understand the details of their illness, but how they react to or act on that information may vary, as teens do not always behave consistently. Teenagers struggle to balance their health needs against their social agendas and their increasing bids for independence. It should be recognized that, for many families, adolescence is when the responsibility for the day-to-day management of a chronic illness switches to the child. It is helpful to talk to adolescent patients with and without their parents present. Try to engage children of this age in their treatment. They are more likely to cooperate if they trust the physician and believe that the physician respects them. As children develop into teenagers, they may have new questions about their illness that reflect their advancing cognitive skills and the new priorities that accompany the developmental shift to adolescence. Physicians should not be surprised that they will have to repeat information previously given, and adjust the information for the more mature child now in front of them.

PRACTICAL SUGGESTIONS FOR IMPROVING COMMUNICATION

Whether the conversation is being held with patients or parents, there are some general guidelines that will help physicians to lay a solid foundation for effective communication. Common pitfalls that healthcare professionals encounter in their interactions with families are listed in Box 8-1, followed by strategies for improving communication.

Box 8-1 Common Pitfalls to Effective Communication

- Starting with 'medical talk' rather than first establishing rapport
- Focusing on the parents and ignoring the child in the room
- Not truly listening to the patient's experience, thoughts, and feelings
- Reacting emotionally, rather than responding to the patient's needs
- Being overly optimistic rather than instilling a realistic sense of hope
- Getting into a power struggle with the patient by disagreeing, threatening, or scaring
- Not stopping to assess if and what the patient heard and understood
- Delivering one-sided information rather than encouraging active involvement

One must avoid euphemisms when speaking to patients and families, and not be overly optimistic. Although instilling a sense of hope in patients is important, providing false hope or not specifying reasonable limits for hope can cause patients and their families to feel as though the physician has been dishonest with them. Even when done with the best of intentions, being unrealistic will erode the patients' trust. Trust is difficult to regain, and may result in an inability to relate effectively.

Similarly, one must not make promises that cannot be kept, whether promising a treatment outcome or unrealistically assuring a family that a procedure will be done at a specified time. Even if the care-giver believes there is control over those things, emergencies arise and schedules get rearranged. Families come to count on the physician, and if what is promised is not delivered they may be more skeptical when promises are made in the future.

One must assume that the information has not been fully understood, remembered, or accepted no matter how intelligent the person, particularly when giving upsetting news. Even information that seems straightforward or that seems clear at the time it is given will likely need to be repeated more than once. This is particularly true if the information is complicated, or requires the patient to do something differently such as changing the medical regimen, or is difficult for the patient to hear. The recipient of the information should be asked to summarize what he or she has been told to check understanding and correct any misconceptions and false hopes. Presenting the information in different forms including verbal explanations, written brochures, and drawings is helpful.

All healthcare professionals should be aware of their own reactions to patients before beginning any conversations. Hiding emotions may be difficult with some patients, but showing disappointment, anger, or frustration may leave the patient feeling inadequate, hopeless, or afraid that they have failed. Getting into a power struggle with a patient or using scare tactics generally has a detrimental affect on the relationship, even if it appears as if the patient is in agreement at the time of the discussion. Many patients want to appease their physician to gain approval or avoid a negative reaction, but may not necessarily follow-up with suggestions if they feel threatened.

Some patients develop a close bond with their nephrologist, and may not want to interact with anyone else. Others develop a tense, mistrustful relationship with their physician and welcome a fresh approach, preferring to work with other members of the team. It is important for a physician to be aware of the quality of the relationship that colleagues have with a particular patient. This can help to anticipate situations and be better prepared for a patient or family's reaction when walking into an examination or hospital room.

Clinical Pearl

Members of a medical team must agree on the treatment for a patient to ensure that clear, consistent messages are transmitted to the family.

DISCUSSING DIFFICULT TOPICS

Physicians have to talk to their patients about very difficult topics that require thought and sensitivity, including revealing a diagnosis and discussing a significant change in the course of treatment, such as the need for dialysis or transplant. At some point in their career, a pediatrician has to discuss end-of-life issues with a young patient. This is something no one would opt to do if given a choice. Even the most seasoned physicians may still have trouble talking through these issues with families. This difficulty can be related to anxieties about having to reveal the information, personal reactions to the information, or fear of the patient or family's reaction. It is helpful to have a plan or strategy for approaching conversations about difficult topics so that the stress related to them can be managed (Box 8-2).

There are basic considerations that can help structure these conversations and provide a map for getting through them.

- Where will this conversation be held? The setting must be in private. As few people as possible should be present. Unless there is an emergency, information that is potentially devastating to patients and families should never be given over the phone.
- Who should participate in the conversation? Consider which members of the family should be involved. Decide whether it is appropriate for the pediatric patient to be present for the discussion. In some instances, the physician should first meet with the parents and then meet with the patient. It may be helpful for a social worker or a psychologist to be present during the conversation to help facilitate the processing of the information.

Box 8-2 Useful Tips for Navigating through Difficult Conversations

- The family must have privacy
- The physician must be prepared for a strong emotional reaction
- The physician must speak frankly, warmly, and sensitively.

Box 8-3 Pace

- **P**lan the setting
- **A**ssess the family's knowledge or experience with the diagnosis and treatment
- **C**hoose strategies that best meet the needs of the family
- **E**valuate the family's understanding of what you have told them.

- How is the information delivered? The importance of body language cannot be underestimated. There is a difference between a physician who tells a family their child needs to transition to dialysis while standing up in the middle of the examination room, compared with a physician who sits down with the family while she or he gives the news. The family might perceive standing as an indication that the physician is rushed or is uncomfortable about discussing this issue. The family is more likely to believe they can ask the sitting physician questions. It is important to ask parents during these conversations about their understanding of what is being said, to encourage questions, and to summarize all of the major points of the conversation. It is suggested that physicians PACE themselves through difficult conversations (Box 8-3).[1]

A NEW DIAGNOSIS

Having to tell a family that their child has a chronic kidney condition, or that the disease has progressed to a new level, is difficult for both the physician and the family. Families may initially be in shock and non-responsive or alternatively, may have intense emotional reactions. It can be difficult to sit with a family who is experiencing such turmoil. Regardless of the type of chronic illness that was diagnosed in a child, families focus on the way in which they were informed of the diagnosis and the quality of the information given to them at that time.[1] It was found that families reacted most negatively to receiving the diagnosis over the phone while they were alone at home or at work, or heard the news in the presence of strangers such as hospital roommates, or received inadequate information.

Importantly for physicians, families are able to distinguish the intensity of their own reactions to the information presented from their impression of the physician who revealed that information, and the way the process unfolded.[1] That is, families can appreciate and benefit from supportive and sensitive responses from their physicians, even when it appears that they are too distraught to do so.

> **Clinical Pearl**
>
> It is important that physicians understand that the intensity of the reaction is usually to the news itself, and rarely to the messenger delivering it. Therefore, doctors should not personalize intensely emotional reactions from patients or parents.

It is essential for physicians to follow-up with patients and families after the initial conversation. As they get used to the news, families usually have more questions and may need to have misconceptions or misunderstandings clarified.

DISCUSSING TREATMENT OPTIONS

Clinical and laboratory data often indicate the best treatment course, but for families who must accept a treatment, decisions may not be clear-cut. It may be frustrating for a physician whose patients make choices that he or she is certain are not in their best interests. However, patients may do so because of cultural or religious beliefs. They may have a different set of priorities than their physician, such as balancing the needs of the whole family as compared to the needs of one child. Or their decision may be based on what they perceive to be unacceptable aversive components of the recommended treatment, such as sterility caused by cyclophosphamide. The physician's role is to provide patients and families with as complete and as accurate information as possible regarding the recommended treatment, its implications, and its side effects. The physician must also discuss alternative treatments and the possible outcomes of no treatment. The patient or family must be permitted to make the decision that is best for them, recognizing that it may not always fit with medical advice or the physician's personal beliefs. The physician must assess whether or not they are acting in the best interests of their child. In some instances of conflict over treatment it may be helpful to have an ethics conference to formulate an acceptable plan that is in the best interests of the child. In occasional cases it may be necessary to report the child and family to a youth protection agency.

HANDLING END-OF-LIFE ISSUES

One of the most difficult things that any physician ever has to do is to tell a child or her family that he or she is going to die. Using a developmental framework can help guide physicians through discussions about the terminal nature of an illness and to anticipate how children understand such information. For example, a 6-year-old tends to see the world simply in terms of good and bad, and may perceive death as a punishment for bad behavior. They are likely to blame themselves for what is happening and make attempts to 'avoid' death by being good – not understanding that the cause of death is medical and not behavioral, and that death is inevitable and irreversible. A child this young would try to hide their feelings but may regress, acting more immaturely and exhibiting signs of aggressive behavior.

A 14-year old girl may understand that death is universal and unavoidable in a terminal illness, but as a teenager she may see herself as invincible. Adolescents can simultaneously feel fearful and fascinated with the idea of death and may try to 'tempt' death. This developmental stage is characterized by inconsistent behavior and intense emotional reactions such as depression, anger, and guilt.

> **Clinical Pearl**
>
> It is extraordinarily difficult, but physicians must discuss death with their pediatric patients. Children need to be allowed to confront and prepare for death and to say goodbye to their loved ones.

Parents, siblings, and extended family also may exhibit a range of responses including disbelief, anger, and great sorrow. Some may have difficulty accepting the news and may 'bargain' with the physician for more time, or encourage the physician to search for yet another treatment option. The doctor must understand that these reactions – which may feel very personal at the time – are not usually directed at the physician but at the news that the doctor has revealed. It may be helpful for a doctor to consult with a clergy member, or other member of the healthcare team with whom the family has formed a relationship, or a social worker, nurse practitioner, or psychologist before giving the news. These people may help to assist the doctor while delivering the news and to provide additional support for the family. Families appreciate a doctor's ability to be empathic and sensitive and also his or her help with deciding among the end-of-life decisions that must be made.

For many families, the exact words used to convey information during difficult conversations are less important than how the news was delivered and how they were taken care of when they were in states of shock, anger, or grief. Some suggestions for facilitating these conversations with children and their families are listed in Box 8-4.

> **Box 8-4   Suggestions for Facilitating Difficult Conversations**
>
> - Be available
> - Don't avoid the child or the topic
> - Pay attention. Observe and listen
> - Face your own feelings of loss and grief before helping the child and family
> - Create an atmosphere that fosters support and invites questions
> - Encourage expression of grief as a normal process by talking, painting, writing
> - Acknowledge that this is difficult and that it hurts
> - Allow expression of emotions such as crying, yelling, resistance
> - Respect a child's need to grieve at any time
> - Keep in mind that the child's priorities during grief may not be same as yours
> - Do not single these children out or give special privileges
> - Age-appropriate reading materials may help open communication
> - Find support groups if it would be helpful to process and normalize feelings in a group setting

Although it is important that information be accurate and complete, it is equally important for the physician faced with the task of delivering difficult news to focus on how the information is delivered, and to respond empathically.

CONCLUSIONS

Although good communication should be a part of everyday practice, it is not something that should be assumed or taken for granted. It takes practice to integrate the strategies described above and to recognize the common pitfalls that impede the working relationship between doctors and their patients. It is worthwhile to remain cognizant of how one interacts with families and how they respond, as the better one's working relationship, the more likely families are to follow one's advice and to ask questions when they are confused. This enables a doctor to help and to treat patients and families more effectively and thereby optimize medical care and outcomes.

REFERENCES

1. Garwick A, Patterson J, Bennett FC, et al. Breaking the news: how families first learn about their child's chronic condition. Arch Pediatr Adolesc Med 1995;149:991-997.

2. Griffin KJ, Elkin TD. Nonadherence in pediatric transplantation: a review of the existing literature. Pediatr Transplant 2001;5:246-249.

3. Jurkovich GJ, Pierce B, Pananen L, et al. Giving bad news: the family perspective. J Trauma 2000;48:865-873.

4. Lemanek KL, Kamps J, Chung NB Empirically supported treatments in pediatric psychology: regimen adherence. J Pediatr Psychol 2001;26:253-275.

SUGGESTED READING

Speece MW, Brent SB. The development of children's understanding of death. In: Corr CA, Corr DM (eds), *Handbook of Childhood Death and Bereavement*. Springer, New York, 1996, pp. 29-50.

CHAPTER 9

Adherence to Medical Regimens

NATALIYA ZELIKOVSKY, Ph.D. AND

AILEEN WALSH, Ph.D.

INTRODUCTION

Non-adherence with medical regimens is a well-documented problem among pediatric patients. 'Adherence' is defined as the extent to which patients' behaviors such as medication-taking, following special diets, and modifying habits coincide with medical or health advice. The term has been modified from the previously used word 'compliance', which implied a judgment on a patient who "...did not comply with the doctor's orders." Children with chronic renal disease have to adhere to complex medication regimens, dietary restrictions, and clinic attendance. As patients progress to end-stage renal disease, they may have to add time-consuming dialysis treatments to their routines, which is often disruptive to regular social and family life. Whereas chronic dialysis treatment or even mortality was inevitable for children with renal disease several decades ago, transplantation is now a viable alternative with potential for improved quality of life. Transplantation is a more cost-effective treatment option for renal patients than is dialysis, but only if the kidney graft remains viable for more than 2 years.[3]

Although survival rates continue to rise for most pediatric renal transplant patients, the process of transplantation is far from simple. Transplant recipients are faced with the life-long responsibility of implementing medical regimens that are complex, demanding, and emotionally burdensome, often taking a toll on the child and family. Whereas optimal adherence can stabilize patients' medical condition, slow down the disease process and prevent organ rejection, poor adherence can result in graft loss and even mortality.[2,11] Non-adherence has also been associated with the overuse of healthcare services, including more frequent re-admissions, longer hospital stays, and increased hospital costs.[3] Additionally, non-adherence poses dilemmas when considering the shortage of available organs and the associated costs of transplantation, and also raises questions about the reliability of clinical trial data.[3,10] Despite the serious implications of erratic adherence, non-adherence rates among pediatric patients are estimated to be 50%.[15]

FACTORS AFFECTING NON-ADHERENCE

Adjusting to a novel and complicated medical regimen is expectedly overwhelming, time-consuming, and stressful. With time, many families are able to incorporate the regimen into their daily routine. For a subset of the families however, adjustment to change in routine and integration of a new regimen remains an enormous challenge. A number of empirically supported psychological, behavioral, physical, medical, and systemic correlates of non-adherence have been identified.

Specific aspects of the illness and treatment course play a significant role in adherence rates. *Disease-related factors* such as the duration and course of illness, symptom severity, and physical discomfort as well as type, complexity, and efficacy of the *medical regimen* can affect both a child's and family's acceptance of the treatment.[15] The *side effects* of medications (e.g., acne, weight gain, trembling) may lead to insecurities about appearance, and subsequent inconsistent adherence in an effort to minimize the side effects.[9] Children who are younger, developmentally and/or *cognitively* delayed, and patients with attentional difficulties may have trouble understanding or remembering specific aspects of the regimen.

Individual characteristics of each patient can influence their ability to follow through on recommendations. *Psychological* factors such as mood (i.e., depression, anxiety, pessimism), behavioral problems, denial of illness, or the need to minimize its severity, and differences in coping styles are sometimes related to low rates of adherence.[4,9] Children's general adaptive functioning and specifically, communication and socialization skills may affect the level of treatment adherence among children with renal disease, both prior to and post transplantation.[6]

Because children's needs, interests, concerns, and skills change, pediatricians must consider healthcare behaviors within the context of their patients' development. Adolescence in particular can be a tumultuous, conflict-ridden time, and adherence during this *developmental stage* tends to decline while the risk for behavioral and emotional maladjustment increases.[13] Normative developmental changes that make adherence a particular challenge for adolescents include increasing desire for independence, a sense of immortality, a decrease in parental influence on values and behaviors, and greater concern about appearance and social acceptance. Pediatricians can imagine how a teenage boy who is feeling invincible and rebellious may respond when asked to follow a structured and inconvenient plan, particularly if the immediate benefits are not clear to him. Early identification and prevention of factors that influence psychological adjustment and adherence need to be major goals for programs for transplant adolescents.

There has been a more recent focus on *racial and socioeconomic factors* related to poverty, unemployment, and limited insurance benefits and their influences on medication adherence and clinic attendance.[2,18] Associations between regimen factors (i.e., pill size, medication taste, and complexity of the regimen) and adherence were stronger and more consistent among African-American patients than European-American patients.[17] Differences among ethnic groups in motivation and perceived control as they relate to adherence affect adherence behaviors among different ethnic groups.[18] It is important that physicians are sensitive to the different struggles families of various ethnic backgrounds encounter when managing their child's medical care.

Finally, children with chronic illness function within several *systems* – the family, school, community, and medical team. The impact of these contexts, particularly the family, on patients' health-related behaviors could be enormous. Among pediatric kidney transplant recipients, *family* cohesion, expressiveness, and communication, and parenting stress have been shown to influence psychological adjustment and post-transplant adherence.[6,8] For dialysis patients too, poor adherence has been related to family stress and conflict over responsibilities.[5] In general, parental attention and regular monitoring of medication taking in a supportive manner can buffer the potentially negative impact of burdensome medical regimens.

MEASUREMENT CONSIDERATIONS

One of the main obstacles to the accurate and reliable identification of adherence problems is the shortage of appropriate assessment tools. Unfortunately, there is no available 'gold standard' in the measurement of adherence, leaving physicians and other healthcare providers to estimate non-adherence based on the means they find accessible, affordable, and convenient. Assets and liabilities of various types of adherence measures are listed in Table 9-1. Each approach has appealing qualities to the clinician, and yet all have their limitations.[14,15] There is no single measure that is sufficient to capture accurately the extent or the nature of adherence difficulties. Therefore, an integration of several methods into a multi-component assessment is highly recommended for healthcare providers working with youth with renal disease.

One way to assess adherence is through semi-structured interviewing, in combination with examination of objective adherence indicators. The Medical Adherence Measure (MAM) is a comprehensive semi-structured adherence interview developed by the primary author. It has four modules, which assess adherence to medication, diet, exercise, and clinic attendance, which are domains applicable across chronic illness groups. Each module includes structured questions about knowledge of the medical regimen, self-reported adherence, any organizational system used to ensure adherence and obstacles that may result in non-adherent behaviors. Sample items and responses that physicians may expect from their patients are listed in Table 9-2.

Although self-report tends to overestimate adherence, administering the measure after rapport has been established and presenting questions in a non-accusatory manner encourages truthful responding. For example, a physician may begin the conversation with "Jason, I would like to talk with you about your experiences in taking the medications I prescribed. I know that taking so many medications is hard, especially for someone as active as you are in school activities. I would like to learn which medications are easy for you to take and which ones you find difficult, so that we can work on it together." This introduction sets the stage for an open discussion by acknowledging the difficulty of the regimen, recognizing that the child is attempting to lead a developmentally appropriate life, and leaving room for the patient to share experiences and challenges. The tone

Table 9-1   Assets and Liabilities of Adherence Measures (Adapted from Rapoff[15]).

Measure	Assets	Liabilities
Drug assays	• Can verify drug ingestion • Permits adjustment of drug levels • It is a quantifiable measure	• Subject to variations in metabolic absorption • Provides short-term information only • More invasive and expensive
Pharmacy refills	• Objective measure of access to the medications • Can be repeated to collect data over time • Unobtrusive for the patient	• Patient may use multiple pharmacies • Time consuming to collect • Does not provide information on actual consumption
Diet diaries/phone interviews	• Can obtain information on multiple diets at the same time • Can obtain repeated measures • Provides consistent contact with the healthcare team	• Burdensome and expensive • Must rely on patient/parent recall • Difficult to use reliably with younger patients
Pill counts	• Feasible to conduct • Inexpensive • Can be used to validate patient's estimates	• Relies on patients to return unused medications • Overestimates adherence • Does not measure consumption
Provider report	• Feasible to conduct • More accurate than patient self-report • Correctly identifies only adherent patients	• Overestimates adherence • Accuracy not a function of provider training or experience • Good for global estimates but not specific non-adherence areas
Patient report	• Feasible to conduct • Accurate if patient asked in non-judgmental way • Allows for continuous report on their own behavior	• Overestimates adherence • Subject to reporting bias and memory problems • Not feasible for patients who are younger or delayed

of the discussion should be one of partnership between the physician and the patient – working together to improve adherence with the prescribed regimens.

It is important to use at least one measure based on more objective data to collaborate adherence information reported by patients and parents. Meyers and Zelikovsky developed the Biomedical Marker Adherence Score (BMAS) that allows a pediatric nephrologist to rate adherence based on clinical data. The recorded serum levels are compared to the range expected if a patient had been adherent to the prescribed dosage. When the actual laboratory value falls within 80 to 120% of the expected range, an adherence score of 0 is assigned, signifying that the patient's serum values do not differ

Table 9-2   Sample Adherence Questions in Each Domain

Domain	Sample Question	Sample Responses
Knowledge	• Can you tell me what medications you've been prescribed? • What is each one for?	• I'm bad with names. The little white pill is… The huge one that's hard to swallow…. • I'm not sure; my mom knows.
Behavior	• In the past week, how many times have you missed your prednisone? • What time of day are you most likely to forget your medication?	• A few…not sure (try to think back)…about four times because those days I play basketball. • I tend to miss my afternoon meds because no one is home. I do take my evening ones, but late because I'm out.
Obstacles	• What are some reasons you miss your medications? • What's difficult about the low-sodium diet?	• Sometimes, I go to my friend's house and forget to bring them. Plus, the prednisone…makes me fat! • Everything has salt…there's nothing I can eat. It's a pain.
Organization	• Where do you store your medications? • How do you keep track of what you have taken?	• They're all on the kitchen counter, but stuff gets piled on top of them. • I just remember. But sometimes I see that the one from the morning is still in the pillbox.
Support	• Who does the shopping and cooking for your special diet? • Does anyone accompany you to your clinic appointment?	• My mom does both. (Do you go with her?). Not really, and she forgets to get the snacks I like. • My mom. Sometimes my dad comes for important meetings. But usually just my mom.

substantially from the expected range. If the value falls 40–80% below the expected range, a score of –1 will be assigned. If the laboratory value falls 120–140% above the expected range, a score of +1 will be assigned. Similarly, if the observed values fall 0–40% below or 160–200% above the expected range, scores of –2 and +2 will be assigned, respectively.

Clinical Pearl

- Adherence is not a dichotomous concept – consider the degree of adherence on a spectrum.[1]
- Reports of missed doses may be more accurate than patients' reports of doses taken.[19]
- More accurate information can be obtained if a time frame is specified, preferably 7 days.

Table 9-3	Stages of Change Model
Pre-contemplation	Patient is not prepared to make changes or follow their regimen within the next 6 months
Contemplation	Patient more aware of the benefits of adherence – but also more aware of the costs involved. Resolve to make positive health-related changes may be tenuous
Preparation	Patient is prepared to do what is necessary as they believe the benefits of following their regimen outweigh the costs
Action	Patient has been following the regimen for less than 6 months
Maintenance	Patient has incorporated the regimen into their lifestyle

THEORIES THAT INFORM ADHERENCE INTERVENTIONS

There are multiple theories of adherence that drive assessment and intervention protocols. A thorough discussion of those theories can be reviewed in Rapoff.[15] The Health Beliefs Model (HBM) and the Stages of Change Model have been two of the most influential theories in the development of intervention strategies to improve adherence rates among children.

The HBM emphasizes that patients' beliefs have a significant impact on the actions they take with regard to their medical treatment. The HBM proposes that the probability of a patient following medical advice is a function of their perception of their disease severity and the risk it poses, the benefits and consequences of following the medical advice, the barriers to doing so, and the internal or external cues that prompt them to action. Therefore, adherence is not viewed as a given, or even necessarily expected outcome, because patients are viewed as individuals who will make choices. This model was adapted for pediatric populations to include recognition of the role that parental beliefs and attitudes play in influencing their children's health beliefs. Patients who perceive their treatment to have benefit to them are more likely to be adherent, while those who perceive more obstacles or threats are found to be more non-adherent.

A second vein of research focuses on the 'stages of change' associated with adopting a new health behavior.[12,16] The first emphasis of this model is that there are five stages that specify when changes in attitudes and beliefs are associated with changes in behavior, which are described in Table 9-3. The Stages of Change model is helpful in that it delineates the stages of readiness through which patients must navigate as they manage their illness, and provides medical staff with an understanding as to 'where the patient is' when it comes to their thought process and healthcare behaviors.

The second emphasis of this model is the process by which these changes occur. For instance, patients at the pre-contemplation stage are going to need a great deal of intervention in order to successfully follow their regimen. Being told that one must change one's behavior (e.g., start restricting fluid or change the diet) and that one must do so immediately is not likely to result in successful change for patients in the pre-contemplation stage. These patients have not started thinking about complying with such requests, and certainly have not prepared for the implications of these behavioral changes on their life. On the other hand, patients who are in the preparation stage need assistance developing a specific plan and problem-solving of potential obstacles to ensure that they are ready to adhere to their treatment recommendations. Regardless of the stage, patients need to be supported through the process of change and the type of intervention that will be effective will be dependent on their current stage in this process.[12]

Clinical Pearl

- Physicians must take into account patients' beliefs about their health status and medicine.
- Patients' readiness for change is a process – and one that can unfold slowly.
- Adherence changes over time. It is not a static condition.

INTERVENTIONS: HOW DO WE ENHANCE ADHERENCE?

Although the factors that influence adherence are increasingly understood, how to best respond to patients who are having adherence difficulties is an area that still requires extensive research. What is clear is that no one intervention is going to be a 'best fit' for all patients. A careful assessment of adherence behaviors and areas of difficulty for each patient is necessary in order to design and implement interventions that can successfully promote adherence.

There are three categories that encompass the majority of adherence interventions currently in use.[10] The first are *educational* interventions. These programs aim to improve adherence by teaching children and families about the nature of their disease and the routines associated with the treatment recommendations. The relationship between the illness and the treatment regimen prescribed, including the effects of non-adherence on the disease process is also addressed. Education requires more than simply telling patients what they must do – more complicated parts of the regimen should be modeled (i.e., administration of Epogen injections on an orange), and time allotted for the patient to practice those components. Repeating this process over several sessions is helpful for many patients, especially patients who are younger or cognitively delayed.

Even though physicians may have a solid working relationship with their patients, some families may be non-adherent simply because they misunderstand or do not recall the child's regimen. Patients, on average, recall two to three recommendations made by medical providers and sometimes 'remember' recommendations that had not actually been made. Therefore, another consideration for ensuring adherence is how the information is delivered. Instructions should be given in simple and explicit terms (i.e., "take – for – days, *even* if symptoms decrease"), and delivered in several forms (i.e., oral, written, visual representation). Instructions should be developmentally appropriate. For example, some children may benefit from a picture of a pill so that they can remember it by color and size, whereas adolescents may respond better to a computer program that educates them about medication-taking.

The second category guiding adherence interventions are *organizational* strategies, which focus on the regimen itself and altering it to promote adherence. Of course, such changes should take place within the context of a collaborative relationship between the patient, the family and the medical staff in order to formulate a treatment plan that is both feasible and medically appropriate. In an effort to minimize resistance and keep patients actively involved in their treatment, patients should participate in the decision-making process whenever medically reasonable. For example, providing adolescents with a range of options that are all medically sound may give them a sense of control over choosing the best option for him/her, and may thereby increase the chances that the patient will actually follow through on the recommendation.

Regimen complexity has been associated with non-adherence. Reducing the number of medications or altering the time of day at which they are to be taken may be helpful. Rates of non-adherence can increase from 10–15% for one drug to approximately 35–50% when up to five medicines are added to the regimen. Incorporating organizational strategies is often beneficial, particularly for families that are overwhelmed and disorganized. Simplifying the regimen when possible, limiting medications with severe side effects, and reducing patient discomfort by prescribing a different form (smaller pills, liquid form) may improve adherence for some patients. Requiring all patients to develop an organized system for storing and keeping track of their medications at home (i.e., weekly pill box, storage locations that will serve as visual reminders) is absolutely necessary to ensure optimal adherence.

Finally, *behavioral* interventions aim to improve adherence by targeting specific behaviors for change. Behavioral contracting between patients, parents, and their physician defines the patient's mutual participation and responsibility for achieving the goals of treatment. Behavioral interventions incorporate rewards and incentives to increase rates of adherence. Some programs that treat younger children have patients earn tokens for following treatment recommendations, which can be exchanged for gifts or movie rentals. Making privileges such as computer or phone time contingent upon responsible medical care is more appropriate for older children and adolescents.

For patients who tend to be forgetful about their medications, using stimulus cues or reminders in the patient's home and school environments can be an effective behavioral strategy. Such prompts should be individualized and may include notes on the refrigerator, watch alarms, and special calendars. Similarly, reminders may be helpful for families who frequently miss clinic appointments. Research suggests that adherence with scheduled appointments is significantly better when patients receive their scheduled appointment time before leaving clinic than when scheduling their own appointments after leaving clinic. Sending out appointment reminder cards, a common practice for dentists, is another way clinics can increase attendance.

Addressing psychological factors that may impact adherence (e.g., depression, low self-esteem due to medication side effects, ambivalence about transferring to an adult facility) is often a focus of behavioral interventions. Because children and adolescents function within a family system, maladaptive family interactions (i.e., family conflict, poor communication) must also be discussed when non-adherence with medical regimens is evident. A chronic illness in one member of the family impacts each of the other members in a variety of ways. Typical relational issues that emerge when children

---

Box 9-1 Top 10 Tips for Enhancing Adherence

1. Maintain an open and honest partnership.
2. Establish small realistic goals.
3. Provide a range of acceptable options from which to choose.
4. Take into account the family's daily schedule and routine.
5. Keep the prescriptions simple and concise.
6. Deliver instructions in clear, explicit form(s) and repeat them.
7. Evaluate the patient's understanding and recollection of the instructions.
8. Use gradual implementation for complex regimens in small manageable steps.
9. Identify reminders in patient's environment (alarms, phone calls, notes).
10. Involve all systems (family, psychosocial staff, school personnel).

---

become adolescents may be magnified. Interventions that sustain parent involvement, and at the same time minimize parent–child conflict are the interventions with the greatest likelihood of promoting treatment adherence.[7]

In summary, interventions for long-term health conditions tend to be complex and labor-intensive. Furthermore, not all of the interventions that are effective for improving adherence tend to have a positive impact on medical treatment outcomes. In a review of studies addressing adherence among children and adolescents, behavioral interventions were found to be most helpful, particularly when the interventions were linked to specific treatment components.[10] The educational, organizational, and behavioral strategies that are most effective in improving adherence with medical treatments are outlined in Box 9-1.

CONCLUSIONS

Non-adherence to medical regimens is a major public health concern as it has been linked to increased healthcare utilization, the loss of transplanted organs, and poor health outcomes for children. The effects for individual children and families – and the toll taken on the physicians who care for them in terms of time and frustration – can be considerable. Understanding the factors that contribute to non-adherence is critical if we are to develop interventions that will increase the likelihood that patients will be adherent. Although research in the field of adherence with children with renal disease is still developing, it is clear that the problem is one that must be addressed. Physicians should be cognizant of the medical, psychological, social and developmental factors that impact on adherence, the difficulties in accurately assessing rates of adherence, and the types of available interventions for patients with adherence difficulties. Although the field as a whole needs to spend time more thoroughly investigating these issues, individual physicians can make an impact by actively seeking to collaborate with their patients such that optimum healthcare is achieved.

REFERENCES

1. Alcazar CBD. The spectrum of adherence among hemodialysis patients. J Nephrol Social Work 1998;18:53–65.
2. Bittar AE, Keitel E, Garcia CD, et al. Patient noncompliance as a cause of later kidney graft failure. Transplant Proc 1992;24:2720–2721.
3. Brickman AL, Yount SE. Noncompliance in end-stage renal disease: a threat to quality of care and cost containment. J Clin Psychol Med Settings 1996;3:399–412.
4. Brownbridge B, Fielding D. An investigation of psychological factors influencing adherence to medical regime in children and adolescents undergoing haemodialysis and CAPD. Int J Adolescent Med Health 1989;4:7–18.
5. Cohen B, Kagan L, Richter B, et al. Children's compliance to dialysis. Pediatr Nursing 1991;17:359–420.
6. Davis MC, Tucker CM, Fennell RS. Family behavior, adaptation, and treatment adherence of pediatric nephrology patients. Pediatr Nephrol 1996;10:160–166.
7. Fennell RS, Foulkes LM, Boggs SR. Family-based program to promote medication compliance in renal transplant children. Transplant Proc 1994;26:102–103.
8. Foulkes LM, Boggs SR, Fennell RS, et al. Social support, family variables, and compliance in renal transplant children. Pediatr Nephrol 1993;7:185–188.
9. Griffin KJ, Elkin TD. Nonadherence in pediatric transplantation: a review of the existing literature. Pediatr Transplant 2001;5:246–249.
10. Lemanek KL, Kamps J, Chung NB. Empirically supported treatments in pediatric psychology: regimen adherence. J Pediatr Psychol 2001;26:253–275.
11. Meyers KEC, Thompson PD, Weiland H. Pediatric renal transplantation non-compliance. Pediatr Nephrol 1995;9:189–192.
12. Prochaska JO, DiClemente CC, Norcross JC. In search of how people change: applications to addictive behaviors. Am Psychol 1992;47:1102–1114.
13. Pucheu S, Antonelli P, Silla M. Psychodynamic aspects of adolescents' therapeutic compliance following a kidney transplant. In: Sugar M (ed), *Trauma and Adolescence*. International Universities Press, Madison, CT, 1999, pp. 125–141.
14. Quittner AL, Espelage DL, Ievers-Landis C, et al. Measuring adherence to medical treatments in children considering

multiple methods and sources of information. J Clin Psychol Med Settings 2000;7:41-54.

15. Rapoff MA. *Adherence to Pediatric Medical Regimens.* Kluwer, New York, 1999.

16. Robbins ML. Medication adherence and the transplant recipient: helping patients at each stage of change. Transplant Proc 1999;31(Suppl 4A):29S–30S.

17. Tucker CM, Fennell RS, Pederson T, et al. Associations with medication adherence among ethnically different pediatric patients with renal transplants. Pediatr Nephrol 2002;17:251-256.

18. Tucker CM, Peterson S, Herman KC, et al. Self-regulation predictors of medication adherence among ethnically different pediatric patients with renal transplants. J Pediatr Psychol 2001;26:455-464.

19. Wagner GJ, Rabkin JG. Measuring medication adherence: are missed doses reported more accurately than perfect adherence? Aids Care 2000;12:405-408.

SUGGESTED READING

Clinical Focus

Rapoff M. *Adherence to Pediatric Medical Regimens.* Kluwer Academic/Plenum, New York, 1999.

Research Focus

Drotar D (ed). *Promoting Adherence to Medical Treatment in Chronic Childhood Illness: Concepts, Methods, and Interventions.* Lawrence Erlbaum, Mawah, NJ, 2000, pp. 237-258.

CHAPTER 10

Nutritional Management of Pediatric Renal Diseases

KRISTIN ANDOLARO, R.D., L.D.N. AND

KEVIN E.C. MEYERS, M.B., B.Ch.

INTRODUCTION

Infants, children and adolescents with renal diseases require close nutritional management to optimize growth and development. This often requires dietary modifications, including the alteration of phosphorus, sodium, potassium, protein, and fluid intakes. Flexibility and resourcefulness are needed to achieve even partial adherence to these dietary changes in individual patients. The dietitian must establish a rapport with the child and with the primary care-givers, priorities within the diet must

be explained, and limit-setting techniques must be explained. Adherence with dietary modifications is enhanced through good communication with the family, simplification of regimens, concrete explanations and ongoing evaluation of the family's understanding.

> **Clinical Pearl**
>
> Nutrition assessment and ongoing evaluation of nutrition status is an integral and indispensable part of pediatric renal care.

ASSESSMENT OF NUTRITIONAL STATUS

Children with kidney disease require frequent nutrition assessments to analyze diet, assess growth parameters, and evaluate growth chart trends (Box 10-1).

The Medical History

This includes the principal diagnosis, list of problems, current renal replacement modality, and/or treatment.

> **Box 10-1 Requirements of a Comprehensive Nutrition Assessment**
>
> - Careful medical, social, and family history
> - Accurate anthropometric data
> - Diet recall
> - Review of gastrointestinal symptoms
> - List all medications
> - Evaluation of laboratory studies

Anthropometric Data

Growth parameters are measured on a regular basis. The use of wall-mounted stadiometers or length-boards is essential for accurate recording of height/length. The weight, height/length and head circumference (HC) (for all children aged under 36 months) are plotted on charts standardized for sex and age.[14] Additional parameters include percentage of standard height for age, ideal body weight (IBW), percentage of IBW, usual body weight (UBW), percentage of UBW, and body mass index (BMI). Mid-arm circumference (MAC), triceps skin fold (TSF), and mid-arm muscle circumference (MAMC) are compared with values from healthy children of the same age and sex (Box 10-2).

Social and Family Histories

Social and family issues must be addressed during the nutrition counseling process. Adherence to nutrition recommendations can be affected by income, time, and comprehension skills. (See section on patient education.)

Dietary History

Taking a 24-hour diet recall is one way to determine food intake. However, there are limitations to this method as the previous 24 hours may not represent typical intake; there may be difficulty remembering details or portions; and information may be omitted. Asking for the usual food intake may give a better idea of what is typically eaten in a day, but this has the same limitations as a 24-hour recall. When applicable, a 3-day food record can provide more detailed diet information, although patients may alter their usual eating habits because their intake is being recorded.

Gastrointestinal Issues

Gastrointestinal conditions that influence fluid and food intake are nausea, vomiting, constipation, diarrhea, gastroesophageal reflux, stool pattern and, in patients on peritoneal dialysis, abdominal fullness.

Box 10-2	Ways to Evaluate the Age of a Child
Chronological age	The age of the child in years and months
Height age	The age at which the child's height crosses the 50th percentile
Bone age	The epiphyseal maturation of the wrists and hands

Medications

All medications and the times they are taken should be noted. Their influence on dietary intake and the dietary intake's influence on the absorption of the medication should be evaluated. Medications that are often used by children with renal disease include sevelamer (Renagel®), calcium carbonate (Tums®), calcium acetate (Phoslo®), calcitriol (Rocaltrol®), ferrous sulfate, prednisone, bicarbonate or sodium citrate, Prilosec® (omeprazole), Reglan® (metoclopramide), Zantac® (ranitidine HCl), and Lasix® (furosemide). Recombinant erythropoietin (rhEPO; Epoetin®) and growth hormone (rhGH) are given by injections. Calcium acetate, sevelamer, and calcium carbonate are taken with meals for phosphate binding, and the latter is taken between meals for calcium supplementation. Children often dislike the taste of calcium carbonate and bicarbonate or sodium citrate. Bicarbonate and sodium citrate cause gastric bloating. Ferrous sulfate can cause constipation.

Laboratory Studies

All of the following must be noted: blood urea nitrogen (BUN); serum concentrations of sodium, potassium, chloride, bicarbonate, creatinine, calcium, phosphorus, and magnesium; and hemoglobin, hematocrit, serum cholesterol, and serum triglycerides. Serum cholesterol is elevated in patients with nephrotic syndrome and is often elevated in chronic renal insufficiency (CRI); it may also have serious potential effects on the heart. Serum albumin is decreased in patients with nephrotic syndrome, and its synthesis is decreased with inflammation and acidosis. The prealbumin is degraded by the kidney and may be falsely elevated in kidney disease.

NUTRITION INTERVENTION AND THE FORMULATION OF A DIETARY PRESCRIPTION

Recommendations are offered for age-appropriate increases in weight gain and length. Suggestions are made to help correct abnormal laboratory values. Advice is offered for enteral and parenteral nutrition concerning calorie, protein, fluid, vitamin, and mineral requirements.

Calorie Needs

The recommended dietary allowance (RDA) is used to determine calorie needs in infants less than 1 year of age (Table 10-1). The WHO equation (resting energy expenditure (REE) multiplied by an activity factor) (Tables 10-2 and 10-3) or RDA is used to determine the calorie needs for children aged more than 1 year

Group	Age (years)	Energy (kcal/kg/day)	Protein (g/kg/day)
Infants	0–0.5	108	2.2
	0.5–1.0	102	1.6
Children	1–3	98	1.2
	4–6	90	1.1
	7–10	70	1.0
Males	11–14	55	1.0
	15–18	45	0.9
Females	11–14	47	1.0
	15–18	40	0.8

Table 10-1 Recommended Daily Allowance (RDA) for Energy and Protein During Childhood

(Table 10-4). Calculation of the ideal energy intake can be achieved using a number of methods (Box 10-3).

Determining estimated caloric needs requires clinical judgment, and modifications are made depending on the response. Providing optimal calories from carbohydrate and fat helps to spare protein in CRI (Table 10-5).

> **Clinical Pearl**
>
> Modular supplements, such as Duocal® (SHS, North America) provide additional calories with a minimal increase in the renal solute load.

Additional data are needed to assess energy expenditure in children with renal failure. The RDA was devised for healthy children, and therefore may not be applicable to all children with renal insufficiency in whom height might be a better standard than weight or age for calorie needs.

Protein Needs

Protein is often restricted to preserve kidney function in adult patients with CRI. However, because children require protein for growth and development, protein allowances should not be less than the RDA for the child's age. And yet, for children who eat well, this may seem like a restriction.

> **Clinical Pearl**
>
> Intake of high biological value (HBV) protein with all of the essential amino acids is encouraged (chicken, beef, fish, eggs).

RENAL CONDITIONS THAT REQUIRE SPECIFIC NUTRITIONAL ADVICE

Acute Renal Failure (ARF)

Nutritional support is important to maintain lean body mass, stimulate repair and immune functions, and to decrease the mortality rate in ARF.[4] Malnutrition is an important contributing factor to the high mortality and morbidity associated with ARF in pediatrics.[20] Nutritional support is an important and accepted part of the management of ARF because ARF affects fluid balance, disturbs electrolyte and acid–base balance, and alters the metabolism of proteins, carbohydrates, and lipids (Box 10-4).

Table 10-2 WHO Equation for Resting Energy Expenditure (REE)

Age (years)	Kcal/day
Males	
0–3	60.9 W − 54
3–10	22.7 W + 495
10–18	17.5 W + 651
18–30	15.3 W + 679
Females	
0–3	61.0 W − 51
3–10	22.5 W + 499
10–18	12.2 W + 746
18–30	14.7 W + 496

Table 10-3 Activity/Stress Adjustment Factors

REE × 1.3	Well-nourished at bed rest; mild to moderate stress
REE × 1.5	Normally active child with mild–moderate stress
	Inactive child with severe stress (trauma, sepsis, cancer)
	Minimal activity and malnutrition requiring catch up growth
REE × 1.7	Active child requiring catch-up growth
	Active child with severe stress

REE = resting energy expenditure.

Table 10-4 Dietary Reference Intakes: Recommended Intakes for Individuals *Food and Nutrition Board Institute of Medicine, National Academies*

Life-Stage Group	Calcium (mg/d)	Phosphorus (mg/d)	Magnesium (mg/d)	Vitamin D (g/d)	Fluoride (mg/d)	Thiamin (mg/d)	Riboflavin (mg/d)	Niacin (mg/d)	Vitamin B6 (mg/d)	Folate (g/d)	Vitamin B12 (g/d)	Pantothenic Acid (mg/d)	Biotin (g/d)	Choline (mg/d)	Vitamin C (mg/d)	Vitamin E (mg/d)	Selenium (g/d)
Infants																	
0-6 mos	210*	100*	30*	5*	0.01*	0.2*	0.3*	2*	0.1*	65*	0.4*	1.7*	5*	125*	40*	4*	15*
7-12 mos	270*	275*	75*	5*	0.5*	0.3*	0.4*	4*	0.3*	80*	0.5*	1.8*	6*	150*	50*	6*	20*
Children																	
1-3 yr	500*	460	80	5*	0.7*	0.5	0.5	6	0.5	150	0.9	2*	8*	200*	15	6	20
4-8 yr	800*	500	130	5*	1*	0.6	0.6	8	0.6	200	1.2	3*	12*	250*	25	7	30
Male																	
9-13 yr	1300*	1250	240	5*	2*	0.9	0.9	12	1.0	300	1.8	4*	20*	375*	45	11	40
14-18 yr	1300*	1250	410	5*	3*	1.2	1.3	16	1.3	400	2.4	5*	25*	550*	75	15	55
19-30 yr	1000*	700	400	5*	4*	1.2	1.3	16	1.3	400	2.4	5*	30*	550*	90	15	55
Female																	
9-13 yr	1300*	1250	240	5*	2*	0.9	0.9	12	1.0	300	1.8	4*	20*	375*	45	11	40
14-18 yr	1300*	1250	360	5*	3*	1.0	1.0	14	1.2	400	2.4	5*	25*	400*	65	15	55
19-30 yr	1000*	700	310	5*	3*	1.1	1.1	14	1.3	400	2.4	5*	30*	425*	75	15	55

This table presents Recommended Dietary Allowances (RDAs) in bold type and Adequate Intakes (AIs) in ordinary type followed by an asterisk (*). RDAs and AIs may both be used as goals for individual intake. RDAs are set to meet the needs of almost all (97% to 98%) individuals in a group. (Reprinted with permission from National Academy of Sciences. Dietary Reference Intakes. Applications in Dietary Assessment. A Report of the Subcommittee on Interpretation and Uses of Dietary Reference Intakes and the Standing Committee on the Scientific Evaluation of Dietary Reference Intakes, p. 287. Washington, DC, National Academy Press, 2000.)

Box 10-3   Calculation of Energy Requirements

- Ideal calories for chronological age based on RDA
- RDA for calories for the height age
- Holiday–Segar method first 10 kg 100 kcal/kg; second 10 kg 50 kcal/kg; and 20 kcal/kg thereafter
- Catch-up growth (kcal/kg = RDA × IBW/Current weight)
- WHO equation for measurement of resting energy expenditure (REE) multiplied by an activity factor

Box 10-4   Factors Determining Metabolic Changes in Acute Renal Failure (ARF)

- Severity and type of ARF
- Type and intensity of renal replacement therapy
- Underlying disease process

Patients should be given enteral feedings whenever possible because this helps to support intestinal function. However, whenever this is not possible, parenteral nutrition must be given. Energy metabolism remains normal in patients with uncomplicated ARF, whereas oxygen consumption and resting energy expenditure increase by at least 30% when ARF is associated with sepsis or systemic inflammation. Hypercatabolism of protein is a central feature of ARF. Protein breakdown from muscle occurs because of insulin resistance, metabolic acidosis, and release of enzymes and cytokines from activated leucocytes. Prior malnutrition, if present, and renal replacement therapy, contributes to the increase in catabolism. Increased release of amino acids from muscle and impairment of production of some amino acid by the kidneys leads to increased hepatic gluconeogenesis and ureagenesis. The hyperglycemia associated with ARF is mainly the result of perturbations of the insulin–glucose axis. These changes include: peripheral insulin resistance with increased plasma insulin levels; decreased insulin-stimulated muscle uptake of glucose; increased hepatic gluconeogenesis; and defective muscle glycogen synthesis. Impaired lipolysis results in an increased triglyceride content of the plasma lipoproteins. The HDL-cholesterol levels are

decreased and LDL- and VLDL-cholesterol levels are increased. The intake of fluid, sodium, potassium, calcium and phosphorus often require modification, and are individualized according to the type of ARF and the patient's fluid and electrolyte status. Children with ARF require between 1.0 and 1.5 g/kg protein intake per day, depending on the catabolic state. The amount of protein must take into account losses incurred by dialysis.

Carbohydrates and lipids should act as the major energy sources; a glucose intake of up to 5 g/kg/day, and lipid intake of 0.5–1.0 g/kg/day are acceptable. This energy supply should have a carbohydrate to lipid ratio of 50–60%/40–50%, with a maximum total energy intake up to 45 kcal/kg/day. Children undergoing dialysis also require supplemental water-soluble vitamins.[5]

Chronic Renal Insufficiency

The primary objectives of nutritional management in children with CRI are to try to slow the progression of renal disease and to prevent the metabolic abnormalities of renal failure while supporting normal rates of growth and development.[9] Meticulous nutritional care of infants is of utmost importance, as CRI can severely impair growth and development. Most children have growth retardation, and many are malnourished when they present with CRI (Box 10-5; Table 10-6).

Table 10-5   Useful Modular Supplements

Supplement	Kcal	Carbohydrate	Protein	Fat
Duocal®	42 per tbsp	60% hydrolyzed corn starch	N/A	40% (65%) refined vegetable oil
Promod®	28 per scoop 17/per tbsp	<10%	>71% whey protein	19% soy lecithin
Polycose® liquid	2 per ml	100% glucose polymers	N/A	N/A
Polycose® powder	23 per tbsp	100% glucose polymers	N/A	N/A
Microlipid®	4.5 per ml	N/A	N/A	100% (50%) safflower oil emulsion
MCT oil	7.7 per ml	N/A	N/A	100% fractionated coconut oil
Rice cereal	12.8 per tbsp	89%	7%	4% safflower oil
Margarine/butter	102 per tbsp	N/A	N/A	100% LCT

LCT = long-chain triglyceride; NA = not applicable.

Box 10-5 Causes of Malnutrition in Children with Chronic Renal Insufficiency (CRI)

- Anorexia
- Altered taste sensation
- Feeding disorders
- Gastroesophageal reflux
- Medication-nutrient interactions
- Hormonal derangements
- Metabolic derangements

Table 10-6 Indicators of Malnutrition

Indicator	Change
Length or height	Decreased
Weight	Decreased
Weight to height ratio	Decreased
Head circumference	Decreased
Lean body mass	Decreased
Fat mass	Decreased
Extracellular water	Increased
Skeletal maturation	Delayed
Sexual development	Delayed
Protein turnover/muscle protein synthesis	Decreased
Muscle protein catabolism	Increased
Serum protein, albumin, and transferrin	Decreased

Clinical Pearl

- The current recommendations for calories and protein are to provide the RDA level for age and gender.
- A safety factor is included to provide the nitrogen that is needed for growth and for individual variability.

Optimal nutritional support does not fully correct the derangements in growth and body composition in CRI, but inadequate nutrition impairs growth and development. The level of renal impairment must be factored in when a nutritional prescription is formulated (Table 10-7).

The recommended energy intake as indicated by the RDA reflects the mean healthy population requirement for each age and gender group (see Tables 10-1 and 10-4). In children with CRI, the dietary prescription needs to provide adequate calories for optimal growth and development without exceeding the excretory limits of the kidneys for other nutrients.[11] An assessment of the energy and protein requirements requires an understanding of protein-energy interactions in growing children. Inadequate energy intake has a negative impact on nitrogen balance so that at intakes close to protein-energy balance, a 5% increase in energy intake has an effect on nitrogen retention equivalent to a 10% increase in protein intake. This is known as the 'protein-sparing effect'. The optimal energy intake for children with CRI is not known, but this should be equivalent to the RDA.[15] Additional energy intake is required if there is an intercurrent illness and/or poor weight gain. rhGH and rhEPO also enhance growth. Dietary protein intake is significantly greater in patients receiving rhGH, despite no change in nitrogen excretion.[13] Protein intake can be restricted to the RDA without compromising growth, as long as adequate energy is supplied.

Many infants with obstructive uropathy have tubular dysfunction that manifests with polyuria, acidosis, and salt wasting. Adequate fluid and salt intake must be provided, and acidosis must be corrected to prevent growth failure. Cow's milk is detrimental in infants because of a high solute and protein load that can cause intravascular volume depletion, hyperphosphatemia, acidosis, potential gastrointestinal bleeding and an inadequate nutritional profile.[19] Salt may need to be restricted, however, if there is a progressive decline in renal function, or if there is edema or hypertension.[6] The standard infant formulas can be used if the serum potassium or phosphorus concentrations are not elevated. Solid foods can be introduced in the usual manner. When salt restriction is required, foods high in salt content should be minimized, and 1-3 g of salt can be given per day. The judicious use of diuretics may allow less salt restriction and permit a more palatable diet. Potassium restriction is usually not required until the glomerular filtration rate (GFR) is below 10 ml/min/1.73 m^2.[2] With decreasing

Table 10-7 Levels of Glomerular Filtration Rate (GFR) and Associated Metabolic Changes

GFR (ml/min/1.73 m^2)	Renal Function	Growth Velocity	Acidosis	Secondary Hyperparathyroidism	Depletion of Muscle and Fat Stores
>60%	↓	±↓	±	±	0
25-60%	↓↓	↓	+	+	±
<25%	↓↓↓	↓	++	+	+/++

Table 10-8 High-potassium Foods to Avoid

Fruits	Vegetables	Others
Avocado – ¼	Artichoke	Bran/bran products
Banana – ½	Broccoli	Chocolate – 50–75 g
Cantaloupe	Brussels sprouts	Granola
Dates	Carrots – raw	Milk (all types) – 1 cup
Dried fruits (all types)	Dried beans/peas	Molasses – 1 tbsp
Figs	Escarole	Nutrition supplements – unless
Honeydew	Greens, except kale	recommended by your dietitian
Kiwi – 1	Kohlrabi	Nuts and seeds – 35 g
Mango – 1	Lentils/legumes	Peanut butter – 2 tbsp
Nectarine – 1	Lima beans	Salt substitute/lite salt
Orange – 1	Mushrooms – canned	Yogurt
Papaya – ½	Parsnips	
Prunes	Potatoes (all types)	
Raisins	Pumpkin	
Juices of these fruits (orange and prune)	Rutabagas	
	Tomatoes	
	Tomato products	
	Vegetable juices including salt free juice	
	Winter squash (acorn, hubbard)	

GFR, each intact nephron excretes a greater fraction of filtered potassium, and the secretion of potassium by the gut also increases. Loop diuretics and prevention of acidosis also helps to prevent hyperkalemia. Potassium intake must be restricted when the serum potassium concentration is constantly above 5 mEq/l (Table 10-8). In addition, low-potassium milk formulas, low-potassium foods (Table 10-9) and Kayexalate® (polystyrene sulfonate) are prescribed when the serum potassium concentration is elevated.

Table 10-9 Low-Potassium Foods

Fruits *Limit to 2–3 Servings/Day	Vegetables *Limit to 2–3 Servings/Day	Other *4 or More Servings/Day
Apples	Alfalfa sprouts	Biscuit
Apple sauce	Arugula	Cornbread
Apricots (fresh) – 1 medium; canned – ½ cup	Beans, green	Crackers
Blackberries	Bean sprouts	Donut
Blueberries	Beets, cooked	Rice
Cherries	Cabbage	Muffin
Cranberries	Carrots, cooked	Noodles
Fruit cocktail	Cauliflower	Pasta
Grapes	Celery – 1 stalk	Plain pancakes or waffles
Mandarin oranges	Cucumber	White bread and bread
Peaches (fresh) – 1 small; canned – ½ cup	Eggplant (aubergine)	Products – NOT whole grain
Pears (fresh) – 1 small; canned – ½ cup	Kale	Cereals – NOT bran or whole grain
Pineapple	Lettuce	Cake – NOT carrot or chocolate
Plums – 1	Mixed vegetables	Coffee – limit to 1 cup
Raspberries	Mushrooms – fresh	Cookies – without nuts or chocolate
Strawberries	Okra	Pies – without chocolate or
Tangerines – 1	Onions	high-potassium fruits
Watermelon – 1 cup	Parsley	Pretzels or popcorn without salt
Juices of these fruits - (apple, cranberry,	Radish	Tea – limit to 2 cups
grape, pineapple)	Rhubarb	Tortilla
	Squash (summer, zucchini)	

Lower than 200 mg per serving. A serving is ½ cup unless otherwise noted. To lower the potassium content of vegetables, soak overnight, boil in large amounts of water, rinse and drain.
*Information adapted from National Kidney Foundation.

Maintenance of normal serum calcium and phosphorus levels is important to prevent metabolic bone disease and to promote growth (see Chapter 32). Vitamins and other minerals are supplemented when protein or other restrictions become necessary. Children frequently require iron supplementation; this must always be provided when rhEPO is used.

Fluid requirements depend upon the cause of the renal disease and level of the GFR. Increased fluid intake is required in salt-losing states. If fluid restriction becomes necessary because of edema or hypertension, the required amount is based on measured urine output and insensible needs. Insensible needs are calculated as 500 ml/m^2/24 hours.

Hemodialysis

The calorie needs for children on hemodialysis are the same as those for CRI. The frequency of dialysis is increased for infants to allow for optimal nutrient intake. The intake is further optimized by enteral supplementation. In children and adolescents, adequate intake is maximized by limiting dietary restrictions and by focusing on their favorite foods whenever possible. Few data are available on the optimal protein needs for children on hemodialysis, and most information is based on adult studies. The Kidney Disease Outcome Quality Initiative (KDOQI) recommends that chronic hemodialysis patients require the RDA plus 0.4 g protein/kg/day to achieve a positive nitrogen balance.[9] There are no data available that demonstrate any advantage to providing supplemental protein above the RDA *and* protein lost via hemodialysis. Causes of a pre-dialysis BUN less than 100 mg/dl are dialysis-related issues, inadequate blood flow, recirculation of blood, infection with increased catabolism, and protein intake in excess of non-protein energy intake. Food diaries are useful for estimating total energy intake, the ratio of protein to non-protein energy intake, and the biological value of the ingested protein. The urea generation rate can be calculated (see Box 10-6).

The persistence of BUN concentrations <50 mg/dl may indicate inadequate calorie and protein intake. Food records, kinetic modeling (normalized protein catabolic rate, nPCR), arm anthropometric measurements, and serum albumin concentrations are useful for establishing and monitoring interventional strategies. Fats in the form of margarine, and appropriate oils, are a valuable source of calories for children on hemodialysis. Salt is restricted for hypertension or for inter-dialysis weight gains of >1 kg/day. Potassium usually can be controlled with appropriate dialysis and avoidance of high-potassium foods (see Table 10-9). If hyperkalemia persists despite these adjustments, Kayexalate® should be prescribed.

> **Clinical Pearl**
> Take into account the sodium load in Kayexalate® in edematous or hypertensive patients.

The guidelines for calcium and phosphorus intake are the same as in CRI. Hemodialysis-associated losses of water-soluble vitamins mandate that water-soluble vitamins, iron and vitamin D are routinely supplemented.[17] Fluid restriction is individualized, and encouraged through behavioral reward modification systems.

Peritoneal Dialysis (PD)

Most children on PD are treated with either continuous cycling peritoneal dialysis (CCPD) or continuous ambulatory peritoneal dialysis (CAPD) (see Chapter 34). Peritoneal dialysis allows for a more liberal fluid, protein, potassium, and sodium intake than hemodialysis. Unsupplemented calorie intake is inadequate for most children on PD, and averages about 80% of RDA. The reduced intake results from a feeling of fullness induced by the intraperitoneal fluid. In addition, the absorbed glucose causes a feeling of satiety via the appetite satiety center in the hypothalamus. Patients on PD have greater protein needs because of increased losses of protein through the peritoneal membrane. Recommendations for children are based on RDA, dialysate-related protein losses, and nitrogen balance studies. Protein loss during PD is inversely related to age and size, but there is a wide variability in children and therefore careful monitoring and adjustments are needed. Kinetic modeling is available and the nPCR can be used to estimate protein intake. Approximately 70% of protein must be of high biological value. Children maintained on PD are at greater risk of protein malnutrition compared to those treated with hemodialysis. The nPCR must be greater than 1 g/kg/day in order to maintain adequate nutrition.[1] Serum triglycerides and cholesterol concentrations tend to be elevated in patients on PD, and therefore poultry and fish are encouraged because of their lower saturated fat contents. Complex carbohydrates and unsaturated fats are also used to compensate for the high glucose content of PD fluid and to help control hyperlipidemia.

> **Box 10-6 Calculation of the Urea Generation Rate**
>
> - In a stable patient, the normalized protein catabolic rate (nPCR) equals or is slightly less than dietary protein intake.
> - In an unstable patient, measurement of the nPCR is a useful additional measure to determine dietary strategies and to monitor outcome.

Salt restriction is only required if there is residual renal function with nephrotic range protein losses, or for hypertension that is not volume-related. Infants require addition of sodium chloride to the dialysate to optimize growth. Most children on CCPD do not require potassium restriction. Constipation should be prevented, as excretion of potassium by the gut in children on PD comprises an important component of potassium loss. Recommendations for prevention of constipation are a diet high in fiber, adequate fluid intake, and stool softeners when necessary. Children on PD have higher phosphate ingestion because of increased protein requirements (Table 10-10). There is an ongoing need for calcium supplementation, phosphorus binding and vitamin D administration to prevent hypocalcemia and bone disease. Vitamin and mineral supplementation is the same as for hemodialysis. Little or no fluid restriction is required as long as ultrafiltration is adequate. High-calorie oral supplements can be given when the energy intake is suboptimal. Modular supplements can be added to provide additional calories (see Box 10-3).

Post-Transplantation

The nutritional needs after renal transplant with a well-functioning allograft are not well defined. The recommendations that follow are for a child with a functional graft. The same recommendations as for CRI and dialysis apply if the GFR is reduced.

> **Clinical Pearl**
>
> Important long-term nutritional problems after kidney transplantation are increased appetite, weight gain, obesity, hypercholesterolemia, and hyperlipidemia.

Table 10-10 Recommended Protein Intake for Children on Peritoneal Dialysis (PD)*

Age	Protein Intake for PD (g protein/kg/day)
0–0.5 months	2.9–3.0
0.6–1.0 months	2.3–2.4
1–3 years	1.9–2.0
4–6 years	1.0–2.0
7–10 years	1.7–1.8
Males (years)	
11–14	1.7–1.8
15–18	1.4–1.5 (based on growth potential)
19–21	1.3 (based on growth potential)
Females (years)	
11–14	1.7–1.8
15–18	1.4–1.5 (based on growth potential)
19–21	1.3 (based on growth potential)

From: The Kidney Disease Outcomes Quality Initiative (K/DOQI) Clinical Practice Guidelines for Nutrition of Chronic Renal Failure, 2001.

Many of these patients have a history of poor weight gain, and require enteral feeding for an adequate calorie intake. Prior to transplant, parents have been focused on weight gain. After a successful transplant, appetite increases because the patient is no longer uremic and is receiving corticosteroids. Corticosteroids and calcineurin inhibitors may increase insulin secretion and cause glucose uptake by adipocytes, impaired glucose tolerance, glycosuria and insulin resistance.

> **Clinical Pearl**
>
> Excessive weight gain after renal transplantation may cause cardiovascular disease and post-transplant diabetes mellitus.[3]

Although post-transplant weight gain is the result of an increase in body-fat mass[21] associated with reduced physical activity,[22] exercise alone is not sufficient to control the weight gain[16] because of rebound eating. Successful weight management requires dietary measures enhanced by exercise.[12]

Sugar and concentrated sweets are eliminated from the diet. Between 40–50% of the calorie intake should come from complex carbohydrates including fruits, vegetables, and whole grains. This strategy helps to eliminate non-nutritious calorie intake and also helps with weight management. Immunosuppressive agents increase protein metabolism by reducing muscle uptake and increasing liver uptake of amino acids. Children require 2–3 g/kg per day of protein immediately after the transplant, but this is reduced to the RDA by 3 months post transplant.

Salt and potassium restriction are no longer needed. Post-transplant hyperkalemia is the result of calcineurin inhibitor administration. Hypophosphatemia is a frequent problem after transplantation because of reduced hyperparathyroidism and tubular ischemia.[8] Supplementation of phosphate is often required for the first few months after transplant. Vitamins are not routinely supplemented. Patients are encouraged to increase their fluid intake to at least 2 l of water per day.

It is essential to prepare parents and patients for the possibility of obesity, and to educate them to eat a diet in which the intake of calories, fat, cholesterol, and sodium are controlled within the setting of a balanced diet. The parents are often excited to see their child eat, and so do not set limits. Counseling should be focused on weight management, because failure to set food limits often results in obesity. Continuing outpatient nutrition assessment is used to reinforce weight-management techniques.[18]

Nephrotic Syndrome

Sodium intake is restricted to <2 g per day for children with nephrotic syndrome who are in relapse or receiving corticosteroids. Protein intake is supplemented to the RDA with replacement of ongoing losses, but excessive intake is not encouraged because this increases the GFR. Hyperlipidemia in patients with chronic nephrotic syndrome should be treated with a low-saturated fat diet, statins, and angiotensin-converting enzyme inhibitors. The latter can decrease urinary protein losses and thereby improve hyperlipidemia.[19] The oligoantigenic diet is of no proven benefit.

NUTRITIONAL SUPPLEMENTATION

Enteral

Supplemental nutrition is recommended for patients with decreased height and/or weight velocity and/or failure to consume the RDA for calories and protein. Oral supplementation is preferred if patients are able to meet calorie needs and achieve optimal weight gain. Tube feedings are initiated when the oral route fails.[11] The choice of formula and volume depends on laboratory values, age, and degree of kidney function, pre-dialysis versus dialysis-dependent status, mode of dialysis, total fluid limit, and feeding tolerance. Carnation Good Start® is indicated when a low-sodium, -potassium and -phosphorus infant formula is needed. A modular supplement, such as Duocal®, is used if a patient requires a concentrated formula. Concentrating a formula by adding less water increases the renal solute load and must be avoided. Similac PM 60/40®, another low-sodium, -potassium and -phosphorus formula, may provide insufficient phosphorus for infant growth and cause phosphate-deficient rickets. Renal formulas include Suplena® and Renalcal® for predialysis and Neprol® and Magnacal® for dialysis children. Frequent adjustments of the feeding regimen may be necessary. Vitamin A levels must be monitored in dialysis patients who are taking fat-soluble vitamins because a reduced clearance of vitamin A metabolites by abnormal kidneys may lead to toxic levels of the vitamin. Zinc and copper may need to be supplemented because intake may be below the RDA in children on PD.

Parenteral

Parenteral nutrition is used when oral intake and tube feedings are not tolerated. Fluid limitations can make it difficult to provide estimated calorie needs. Parenteral nutrition is generally started with the minimum recommended requirements of electrolytes, but this also depends on laboratory results and oral intake. Protein, fat, and dextrose recommendations are based on patient needs. Intradialytic parenteral nutrition improves the nutritional status of malnourished adolescent hemodialysis patients who could not be corrected by enteral supplementation.[7,10]

PATIENT EDUCATION AND SOCIAL CONSIDERATIONS

Nutritional counseling for renal patients should be based on an individualized plan of care. Patients and care-givers often feel overwhelmed when introduced to the renal diet, and so have to learn about different nutrients and how they affect the body. Understanding which foods contain which nutrients can be difficult for many patients and care-givers. Patients and care-givers often require many nutrition education sessions to gain a good working knowledge of the renal diet. There are many psychosocial impediments to using a renal diet (Box 10-7).

REFERENCES

1. Brem AS, Lambert C, Hill C, et al. Prevalence of protein malnutrition in children maintained on peritoneal dialysis. Pediatr Nephrol 2002;17:527-530.
2. Brewer ED. Pediatric experience with intradialytic parenteral nutrition and supplemental tube feeding. Am J Kidney Dis 1999;33:205-207.
3. Clunk JM, Lin CY, Curtis JJ. Variables affecting weight gain in renal transplant recipients. Am J Kidney Dis 2001;38:349-354.
4. Drüml W. Protein metabolism in acute renal failure. Miner Electrolyte Metab 1998;241:47-54.
5. Drüml W. Nutritional management of acute renal failure. Am J Kidney Dis 2001;37(Suppl 2):89-94.
6. Feld LG, Springate JE, Waz WR. Special topics in pediatric hypertension. Semin Nephrol 1998;18:295-303.
7. Goldstein SL, Baronette S, Gambrell TV, et al. nPCR assessment and IDPN treatment of malnutrition in pediatric hemodialysis patients. Pediatr Nephrol 2002;17:531-534.
8. Green J, Debby H, Lederer E, Levi M, et al. Evidence for a PTH-independent humoral mechanism in post-transplant

hypophosphatemia and phosphaturia. Kidney Int 2001;60: 1182–1196.

9. Kopple JD. National kidney foundation K/DOQI clinical practice guidelines for nutrition in chronic renal failure. Am J Kidney Dis 2001;37(1 Suppl 2):S66–S70.

10. Krause I, Shamir R, Davidovits M, et al. Intradialytic parenteral nutrition in malnourished children treated with hemodialysis. J Renal Nutr 2002;12:55–59.

11. Kuizon BD, Nelson PA, Salusky IB. Tube feeding in children with end-stage renal disease. Miner Electrolyte Metab 1997;23:306–310.

12. Lopes IM, Martin M, Errasti P, et al. Benefits of a dietary intervention on weight loss, body composition, and lipid profile after renal transplantation. Nutrition 1999;15:7–10.

13. Mendley SR, Majkowski NL. Urea and nitrogen excretion in pediatric peritoneal dialysis patients. Kidney Int 2000;58: 2564–2570.

14. National Center for Health Statistics (CDC, National Center for Health Statistics: CDC growth charts: United States. http://www.cdc.gov/growthcharts/ May 30, 2000.

15. National Research Council, Food, and Nutrition Board. *Recommended Dietary Allowances*, 9th edn. Washington D.C., National Academy of Science, 1989.

16. Painter PL, Hector L, Ray K, et al. A randomized trial of exercise training after renal transplantation. Transplantation 2002;74:42–46.

17. Pereira AM, Hamani N, Nogueira PC, Carvalhaes JT. Oral vitamin intake in children receiving long-term dialysis. J Renal Nutr 2000;10:24–29.

18. Schonfeld-Warden N, Warden CH. Pediatric obesity. An overview of etiology and treatment. Pediatr Clin North Am 1997;44:339–361.

19. Sedman A, Friedman A, Boineau F, et al. Nutritional management of the child with mild to moderate chronic renal failure. J Pediatr 1996;129:S13–S18.

20. Star RA. Treatment of acute renal failure. Kidney Int 1998;54:1817–1831.

21. van den Ham EC, Kooman JP, Christiaans MH, et al. Posttransplantation weight gain is predominantly due to an increase in body fat mass. Transplantation 2000;70: 241–245.

22. van den Ham EC, Kooman JP, Christiaans MH, et al. Relation between steroid dose, body composition and physical activity in renal transplant patients. Transplantation 2000;69:1591–1594.

SUGGESTED READING

Hendricks KM, Duggan C, Walker WA. *Manual of Pediatric Nutrition*, 3rd edn. BC Decker, Lewiston, 2000.

Samour PQ, Helm KK, Lang CE. *Handbook of Pediatric Nutrition*, 2nd edn. Aspen Publishers, Gaithersburg, 1999.

Transitioning Pediatric Renal Patients to Adult Care

CYNTHIA GREEN, M.S.S., L.S.W.,

SETH SCHULMAN, M.D.,

JO-ANN PALMER, M.S.N., C.R.N.P., AND

CHRIS BREEN, R.N.

INTRODUCTION

The dilemma of how and when to transition chronically ill adolescents from pediatric to adult medical care is, in essence, a new and happy one. Transitioning – according to the American Society for Adolescent Medicine – refers to the "purposeful, planned movement of adolescents and young adults with chronic physical and medical conditions from child-centered to adult-oriented health care systems."[9] A generation ago, so few children with serious chronic medical conditions survived past their teenage years that any discussion of transitioning was irrelevant, but today the majority grows into adulthood. Among the renal patient population, 90% of even the most severely affected end-stage patients aged 10 to 19 years, those who are on dialysis or have had transplants, can expect to celebrate their 21st birthdays and beyond.[2]

Most pediatricians agree that at some point, patients with chronic health conditions should move from pediatric to adult medical facilities. It is the timing and method of transfer that remain open to debate. The American Academy of Pediatrics considers individuals from 0 to 21 years of age within its purview, while allowing that 'special circumstances' such as chronic illness or disability may make pediatric care optimal for some beyond the age of 21 years. However, healthy adolescents frequently undergo haphazard transitions, many coasting along for months or years with no medical provider of record after 'graduating' from their pediatricians. They are then thrust abruptly into the world of adult care only when a crisis, such as an accident, illness, or pregnancy, precipitates a sudden need.[9]

For the chronically ill adolescent, a lack of planning for transition can spell disaster. The problems related to transitioning for adolescents with special needs were highlighted in the *Consensus Statement on Health Care Transitions for Young Adults with Special Health Care Needs,* improvement recommendations published in December 2002 and adopted as policy by the American Academy of Pediatrics, the American Academy of Family Practice, and the American College of Physicians – American Society of Internal Medicine.[1] Given the parent/family-oriented focus of most pediatricians, this delivers a message to the young adult that he or she is not believed capable of independent care; is not expected to assume self-responsibility and will be taken care of indefinitely; and is very different from his or her peers who are, in a developmentally appropriate way, moving towards independence. It may even be interpreted as a sign that his or her medical prognosis is too poor to warrant planning for the future.[3] Others, like their healthy counterparts, drop out of the healthcare system altogether, with no provider replacing their pediatric services.[2]

Even when the message is clearly stated by parents and care-givers that growing up is inevitable and desirable, remaining in the pediatric environment for too long can serve as an impediment to the achievement of this goal. In light of the recent emphasis on family-centered care, pediatricians now by and large view their patients in the context of their parents. Medical decision-making and adherence have become responsibilities to be shared by parents and patient. Questions regarding financial arrangements, including insurance, and logistics such as

<table><tr><td>

Box 11-1   Barriers to Effective Transitioning[8]

- The overprotected *patient* has emotional and developmental immaturity
- The *family* may have difficulty ceding control for fear of dire medical consequences if their involvement lessens.
- The *pediatric care-giver* often has made a huge investment in his or her patients.
- Many *adult care-givers* do not have the same resources or patience as pediatricians to devote to individual patients.

</td><td>

Clinical Pearl

Transition to adult care should be a gradual process.
- Discussions should be held at regular intervals, starting in early adolescence.
- Lack of progress towards independence should be detected early and corrected.
- The goal is to transfer all patients by the age of 21 years, although many will be ready by age 18 years.

</td></tr></table>

making appointments and transportation to and from appointments are generally directed at the parents rather than the young person. School is considered the patient's main developmental task, rather than the more complex, young-adult task of balancing higher education or a job with the building of meaningful relationships independent of one's birth family.[8] While this is a developmentally appropriate approach for patients younger than the mid-teens, the pediatric team's expectation of parental involvement in and control over their children's lives flies in the face of the needs and desires of older teenagers and young adults. Indeed, the older adolescent's developmental priorities of moving towards independence, relating with peers, and becoming sexually mature should be expected as a matter of course to interfere with adherence to medical regimens (Box 11-1).[4]

Despite these barriers to success, and despite the lack of collected data tracking transition programs, a survey of literature from the field of adolescent medicine reveals elements that are generally agreed to be essential to effective transitioning (Box 11-2).[6]

With these general principles in mind, the following transitioning program has been designed specifically for use with pediatric renal patients.

OVERVIEW

Age 14–16 years

Adolescents should start to become more independent in making the decisions that affect their health. Sexual issues, in particular, begin to arise which may be complicated by chronic illness (Box 11-3).

Private discussions allow the adolescent to speak for him or herself. By the completion of this stage they should be able to:
- Know the names of their medications and know their purpose
- Administer medications to themselves
- Understand and follow fluid and dietary limitations
- Give relevant medical and surgical histories
- Recognize symptoms that indicate a need for immediate treatment
- Negotiate the process of seeking help when problems arise.

Age 17 years

Each year, patients who will be turning 18 in the next calendar year should be identified, and the team should discuss their progress toward transition. Concerns about a patient who is not on track to transition by age 18 years

Box 11-2   Essential Elements to Effective Transitioning

- Obtaining the consent and engaging the cooperation of the patient
- Enlisting the support of the family
- Having the support of all professionals on the medical team[7]
- Instituting a policy on timing of transfers
- Establishing a preparation and education program prior to transition
- Gathering information about available adult services

Box 11-3   Adolescents should be Interviewed Independent of their Parents to Discuss

- Drug use
- Alcohol use
- Cigarette use
- Risk-taking behavior
- Sexual activity
- Birth control
- Mental health status
- Any other issue the adolescent prefers to address privately

---

Box 11-4 Plan for Future Care Between Ages 17½ and 18 Years

- Vocational interests and plans for higher education or career
- Insurance coverage after age 18 years
- Recognition of the legal differences in medical care for those over age 18 years
- Proceeding to have a patient declared mentally incompetent, if necessary

---

can then be clarified and a plan devised for future care (Box 11-4).

Goals for transfer to adult care include potential medical providers and a timetable. A transition readiness checklist can help in uniformly evaluating each patient nearing age 18 and clarifying which, if any, issues are standing in the way of effective transfer to adult care. The team can then use this documentation to formulate a plan to address the patient's needs.

Clinical Pearl

Legal differences in medical care for those over age 18 years include:
- Signing in and out of hospital
- Signing informed consent for treatment
- Executing advance directives or living wills
- Recognizing the maintenance of confidentiality regarding medical care
- Deciding what information will be shared with family members, and under what circumstances

---

Age 18–21 years

The patient should be able to meet team members without family members present. Discussions about transfer should become more frequent and emphatic as the patient approaches the age of 21. When an adult-care medical provider has been identified and the patient has given consent, contact should be made with this provider, and the medical records forwarded. If appropriate, a social worker or advanced nurse practitioner may accompany the patient to his or her first visit with the new care-giver. This can reduce the stress associated with locating the center and meeting the new team (Box 11-5).

Contact between the patient and a designated member of the pediatric team may need to continue for a period of time following transfer. The purpose of such contact would be to troubleshoot potential problems and to encourage the patient to adhere to the new team's

---

Box 11-5 The Following Questions should be Asked During the First Appointment:

- How often should I see the physician/medical team?
- Will my appointment schedule have a major impact on my education or employment?
- How will I find out test results?
- How will I obtain prescriptions?
- Who do I call if I become ill between visits, during office hours and outside of office hours?
- Who do I contact if I have problems with transportation or insurance?
- If surgery becomes necessary, who will be consulted?

---

recommendations. The team member should assuage concerns that invariably arise due to differences in management or style, without offering medical opinions or giving contradictory advice. Ideally, the need for contact will gradually decrease. One problem that sometimes arises is patients who become 'homesick' for their old, familiar medical team and who wish to 'untransfer', despite its inappropriateness. If a patient or family contacts a pediatric team member expressing a strong wish to return to the pediatric facility, the social worker should offer to speak with them to discuss the issues that have led to this desire. The social worker can reinforce the need to transfer from the pediatric facility while still assisting with problem-solving within the patient's new situation. The social worker should advise the patient how to find a different adult-care facility by using the social work services at the current facility, if the situation is untenable.

Clinical Pearl

Ex-patients should not be readmitted to the pediatric facility after transfer, even for emergencies, but be redirected to the current adult-care provider.

By utilizing this protocol the transition to adult care should become a gradual, developmentally appropriate process, rather than a sudden and traumatic event.[5] Nevertheless, a few patients and families will remain anxious about changing care-givers and unwilling to engage in any dialogue about transfer or take concrete action toward achieving that end. Every attempt should be made to identify these 'reluctant' patients at an early stage in order to determine the reasons behind their concerns and fears and to devise a plan of intervention.

If all attempts at transfer fail, the nephrology team should meet to determine a timetable for involuntary

---

Box 11-6 Unilateral Transitioning of Patients Over the Age of 18 Years

- Provide the patient, in writing, with a list of appropriate adult-care facilities, including addresses, phone numbers, names of contact personnel, and directions.
- Send the patient a certified letter stating the date at which pediatric care will no longer be provided.
- Offer to transfer records to the new adult-care provider of the patient's choice (including a release of information form for the patient's signature along with a self-addressed, stamped envelope for return to the pediatric Nephrology division). The letter should be reviewed by the pediatric facility's counsel and signed by the Nephrology division chief.
- In the event the patient arrives at the pediatric facility for treatment following the stated deadline, he or she should be directed to the emergency room at the nearest adult hospital.
- Providing 'one last appointment' or writing new prescriptions after the deadline out of well-intentioned kindness or in order to avoid confrontation will reinforce the patient's attempts to maintain pediatric care, and is counter-productive.

---

transfer. This simple, legal, and ethical method for unilateral transitioning of patients over the age of 18 years has proved effective (Box 11-6).

TRANSITIONING THE PATIENT WITH ADDITIONAL SPECIAL NEEDS

The guidelines addressed above assume that patients will ultimately be able to achieve independence. However, some patients with cognitive limitations or serious mental illness may never reach this stage of development. In this event, the renal team should encourage and help families as the individual's 18th birthday approaches to obtain a medical power of attorney. This gives parents or other designated care-givers the legal right to make decisions regarding an adult patient's treatment.

Although the emotional benefits of transitioning to adult care may not be realized in all of these cases, there are still cogent medical indications for transfer. The transitioning protocol should still be followed with the family with the goal of transfer by age 21. Special consideration should be given to finding an adult-care facility with experience/expertise in taking care of patients who continue to depend on their parents or other care-givers.

TRANSITIONING THE TRANSPLANT PATIENT

Renal transplant patients have a unique perspective on change, mainly due to the more serious consequences that may result from inadequate care such as loss of the transplant.

Clinical Pearl

The trepidation that many patients feel about changing healthcare providers can, for transplant patients and their families, magnify into paralyzing fear.

Patients and families feel that because their pediatric nephrologist and other renal team members took care of them before, during, and after a transplant, the medical and psychosocial histories are well known and this shared experience can help to tailor treatment decisions.

Some of the fears expressed by transplant patients faced with imminent transfer, along with ways the renal team can acknowledge and allay these concerns, are:

- "Nobody will know me." Assure the patient that detailed records will be sent. Let the patient know that the new facility will be able to contact the pediatric team with questions, even after the transfer has taken place. Advise the patient that because he or she is the ultimate expert regarding their history, they will be able to educate the new care-givers. Compare the transition to leaving high school and starting college or a job. Explain that transitions occur throughout a person's life and are a normal part of growing up.
- "I don't know anybody there." References should be made available to the patient with the names and roles of all care-givers on the adult renal team. A site visit to the new facility prior to transfer, accompanied by a pediatric team member, may be offered if this fear is particularly severe.
- "How do I decide where to go? There are too many choices!" Guidance should be offered in helping the patient determine what they consider to be the most important features of a medical facility and care-giving team. Is proximity to home a top priority? Is automobile transportation available to the patient, or must the facility be accessible by public transportation? Does the facility accept the patient's insurance? Do the hours and days available for appointments match the configuration of the patient's schedule? Is a smaller program with shorter waits for physician visits and laboratory testing desirable, or is having the expertise of a program in a large, multidisciplinary facility more important? A meeting with the renal social worker can help to

---

Box 11-7 Provide Sufficient Information About Adult Programs

- Name of program
- Street address
- Specific location of transplant clinic
- Phone number to call for appointments
- Staff names and roles
- Days and times that transplant patients are seen
- Who to contact if patient becomes ill between appointments
- Where parking is located
- Cost of parking

Box 11-8 Moving to an Adult Care Center Has Many Advantages for those Over Age 18 Years

- Care by a nephrologist who has more experience with the unique medical needs of patients who have been on dialysis for long periods of time
- Access to a social worker who is familiar with vocational rehabilitation, work-related laws concerning disability, and government entitlements for adults

---

clarify these priorities, much as a student's meeting with the high-school guidance counselor helps to sort out post-graduation plans.

- "What if I get sick?" Patients need to feel confident that the care they will receive after transfer will be as good as the pediatric care they have been receiving. It is helpful for the pediatric team to be familiar with the strengths and weaknesses of local adult programs in order to provide honest information.

Clinical Pearl

A transitioning patient should be helped to recognize that while their pediatric care-givers are experts in pediatric care, adult-care teams specialize just as adeptly in providing care to those over 18 years old.

- "You're only transferring me because you don't like me/because you don't like my family/because I didn't do exactly what you asked me to do!" Assure the patient that transfer is no easier for the medical team than it is for the patient, but that the patient's best interest demands adult care when age-appropriate. It is not uncommon for young adults to personalize transition as a form of rejection. Recognizing and acknowledging this fear with sensitivity, while providing reassurance that transfer is the soundest course of action medically, is important for a successful transition.

Most concerns about transition stem from a fear of the unknown; therefore, providing ample information about adult programs is important (Box 11-7).

TRANSITION OF THE DIALYSIS PATIENT

Like transplant patients, many dialysis patients have a unique perspective on transferring care. For hemodialysis patients in particular, so many hours are spent at the dialysis center site and in the company of the center's personnel that having an agreeable experience three times a week becomes a focus of decision-making about transition. It is important for patients to be helped to realize that patient populations and patient:staff ratios at adult-care facilities will almost inevitably be larger than at pediatric units (Box 11-8).

Information on dialysis centers across the country can be found on the Medicare web site (http://www.medicare.gov). A meeting with the social worker can help the hemodialysis patient understand that no center is perfect, but that some facilities better match his or her particular priorities than others.

A site visit is recommended for all patients when a transfer is under consideration. If necessary, the pediatric social worker can accompany the patient and family to ease the transition. The following list of questions regarding dialysis care may help patients gather complete information regarding a new unit in order to make an informed choice for transfer:

- How often will I see the physician; social worker; nutritionist?
- Can I eat/drink in the unit?
- Are blankets/pillows available?
- Who do I call if I'm sick at home?
- What do I do if I don't like the shift I'm assigned?
- Can I change my schedule temporarily if I need to travel or have a special event to attend that conflict with my usual shift?
- Who can help if I have transportation problems?
- How often is lab work done?
- Are there TVs/VCRs available at the dialysis stations? Do I have to use/bring my own headphones?
- Is there a refrigerator for storing patient food/drinks?
- What happens if my fistula/graft/catheter stops working?
- Will I learn/be required to set up my own machine? Participate in any other aspects of treatment?

CONCLUSION

A comprehensive protocol for transitioning, if gradually introduced during the teenage years and utilized uniformly with all patients, offers the best chance of fostering successful transitions from pediatric to adult nephrology care.

REFERENCES

1. American Academy of Pediatrics, American Academy of Family Physicians, American College of Physicians – American Society of Internal Medicine. A consensus statement on health care transitions for young adults with special health care needs. Pediatrics 2002;110:1304–1306.
2. Blum RW. Introduction, improving transition for adolescents with special health care needs from pediatric to adult-centered health care. Pediatrics 2002;110:1301–1303.
3. Blum RW, Garell D, Hodgman CH, et al. Transition from child-centered to adult health-care systems for adolescents with chronic conditions. J Adolesc Health 1993;14:570–590.
4. Court JM. Outpatient-based transition services for youth. Pediatrician 1991;18:150–156.
5. Cystic Fibrosis Center, The Children's Hospital of Philadelphia. Protocol for transition to adult care program, 1994.
6. Rosen D. Between two worlds: bridging the cultures of child health and adult medicine. J Adolesc Health 1995;17:10–16.
7. Scal P. Transition for youth with chronic conditions: primary care physicians' approaches. Pediatrics 2002;110:1315–1321.
8. Schidlow DV, Fiel SB. Life beyond pediatrics: transition of chronically ill adolescents from pediatrics to adult health-care systems, Med Clin North Am 1990;74:1113–1120.
9. Viner R. Transition from paediatric to adult care: bridging the gaps or passing the buck? Arch Dis Child 1999;81:271–275.

PART II

CHAPTER 12

Evaluation of Hematuria

MADHURA PRADHAN, M.D. AND

BERNARD S. KAPLAN, M.B., B.Ch.

INTRODUCTION

The detection of even microscopic amounts of blood in the urine of a well child causes much consternation. This usually occurs when blood is found by the dipstick method during a routine examination. This discovery alarms the patient, parents, and physician, and often results in the performance of a large number of laboratory studies. The physician has to ensure that serious conditions are not overlooked, while at the same time avoiding unnecessary laboratory studies that are often expensive. In addition, he or she must be able to reassure the family and provide guidelines for additional studies in the event that there is a change in the child's course.[8] Macroscopic (gross) hematuria is even more frightening, and should be evaluated as soon as possible. Gross hematuria, in the absence of significant proteinuria and/or red blood cell casts, is an indication for a renal and bladder ultrasound examination to exclude a malignancy.

Clinical Pearl
- Hematuria is one of the most important signs of renal or bladder disease.
- Proteinuria, however, is a more important diagnostic and prognostic finding except in the case of calculi or malignancies.
- Hematuria is almost never a cause of anemia.

DEFINITIONS

Hematuria is the medical term for the presence of blood in the urine. Gross hematuria is visible to the naked eye, whereas microscopic hematuria is detected by a dipstick test and is confirmed by microscopic examination of the spun urine sediment.

Clinical Pearl
Microscopic hematuria, in practice is really dipstick hematuria.

95

Table 12-1   Urine Color in Hematuria

Color	Causes
Dark yellow Dark brown or black Red or pink urine	• Normal concentrated urine • Bile pigments • Homogentisic acid, thymol, melanin, tyrosinosis, methemoglobinemia, alkaptonuria • Alanine, cascara, resorcinol • Red blood cells, free hemoglobin, myoglobin, porphyrins • Benzene, chloroquine, deferoxamine, phenazopyridine, phenolphthalein • Beets, blackberries, rifampin, red dyes in food • Urates

The evaluation of a child with gross hematuria differs from that of one with microscopic hematuria. Gross hematuria of glomerular origin is usually described as brown, tea-colored or cola-colored urine. Gross hematuria from the lower urinary tract (bladder and urethra) usually leads to pink or red urine. The incidence of gross hematuria among children presenting to an emergency room is 1.3 per 1000.[7] Microscopic hematuria is defined as more than five red blood cells per high-power field (HPF). Microscopic hematuria is almost always a medical problem that may warrant referral to a nephrologist rather than to a urologist. Microscopic hematuria in two or more urine samples is found in 1–2% of children aged between 6 and 15 years.[4,15]

Clinical Pearl

Most children with isolated microhematuria do not have a treatable or serious cause for hematuria, and do not require an extensive evaluation.

The presence of hematuria must be confirmed by microscopy examination of spun sediment of urine, because other substances besides blood can produce red or brown urine or give a false-positive dipstick test for blood (Table 12-1).

DIAGNOSIS OF HEMATURIA

Significant microscopic hematuria should be diagnosed when at least three urinalyses show the presence of five or more red blood cells (RBCs) per HPF over a 2- to 3-week period. The urine dipstick is a sensitive screening test for the presence of blood in urine. The dipstick is impregnated with hydroperoxide and tetramethylbenzidine, and

the peroxidase-like activity of hemoglobin catalyzes a reaction which results in the formation of a blue-green color. The test detects intact RBCs, free hemoglobin, and myoglobin. It can detect as little as 150 µg/l of free hemoglobin, equivalent to approximately 5–20 intact RBC per mm^3 urine.[3] False-positive results occur in the presence of oxidizing agents such as household bleach that is used to clean urine collection containers. False-negative results occur in samples with high specific gravity or with high ascorbic acid concentrations.

Urine samples positive for blood on the dipstick test should always be examined microscopically, as microscopic evaluation provides information on the number of RBCs and other cells, casts, crystals, and bacteria. In the past, Addis counts were used in timed urine collections to quantify RBCs, but today these are of only historical significance.

The American Academy of Pediatrics recommends a screening urine analysis at school entry (ages 4–5 years) and once during adolescence (ages 11–21 years).[1]

LOCALIZATION OF HEMATURIA

Blood may originate from anywhere in the kidney – the glomeruli, renal tubules, and interstitium, or from the urinary tract collecting systems of the ureter, bladder, and urethra.[5] RBCs pass from the capillary lumen through the glomerular capillary via structural discontinuities in the capillary wall that usually cannot be detected even by electron microscopy. Proteinuria, RBC casts, and deformed RBCs in the urine usually accompany hematuria resulting from glomerular injury. The renal papillae may be damaged by microthrombi and/or anoxia in patients with a hemoglobinopathy or toxins.[11] Patients with renal parenchymal disease may have transient microscopic or gross hematuria during systemic infections, or after moderate exercise. This may be the result of renal hemodynamic responses to exercise or fever. It is important to differentiate between glomerular and non-glomerular causes of hematuria in order to limit the diagnostic possibilities and perform focused investigations.[12] This is done by taking a careful history and physical examination, together with urinalysis (Table 12-2). A history of trauma may be important in patients with bright-red urine.

DIFFERENTIAL DIAGNOSIS OF HEMATURIA

The various causes of hematuria in children are shown in Box 12-1.

Table 12-2 Distinguishing Features of Glomerular and Non-glomerular Hematuria

Feature	Glomerular Hematuria	Non-glomerular Hematuria
History		
Burning on micturition	No	Urethritis, cystitis
Systemic complaints	Edema, fever, pharyngitis, rash, arthralgias	Fever with urinary tract infections. Severe pain with calculi.
History of trauma	No	Yes
Family history	Deafness in Alport syndrome, renal failure	Usually negative. May be positive with calculi.
Physical Examination		
Hypertension	Often present	Unlikely
Edema	May be present	No
Abdominal mass	No	Important with Wilms' tumor, polycystic kidneys
Rash, arthritis	Lupus erythematosus, Henoch–Schönlein purpura	No
Urine Analysis		
Color	Brown, tea, cola	Bright red
Proteinuria	Often present	No
Dysmorphic RBCs	Yes	No
RBC casts	Yes	No
Crystals	No	May be informative

Benign Familial Hematuria (BFH)

BFH is defined by the familial occurrence of persistent hematuria without proteinuria, progression to renal failure or hearing loss. Many – but not all – of these individuals have thin glomerular basement membranes.

Clinical Pearl
- Benign familial hematuria and so-called thin basement membrane disease are confusing, over-lapping entities.
- Thin basement membranes can occur in normal individuals, in individuals with other causes of glomerular injury and in some patients with Alport syndrome.

Box 12-1 Causes of Hematuria in Children

Glomerular diseases
- IgA nephropathy, benign familial hematuria (BFH), Alport syndrome
- Acute post-streptococcal glomerulonephritis (PSGN), membranoproliferative glomerulonephritis
- Systemic lupus erythematosus, membranous nephropathy
- Rapidly progressive glomerulonephritis, Goodpasture's disease
- Henoch–Schönlein purpura, hemolytic-uremic syndrome

Infection
- Bacterial, viral (adenovirus), tuberculosis
- Hematologic
- Sickle cell disease, coagulopathies (von Willebrand's disease),
- Renal vein thrombosis, thrombocytopenia

Nephrolithiasis and hypercalciuria

Structural abnormalities
- Congenital anomalies, polycystic kidney disease, vascular anomalies (arteriovenous malformations, hemangiomas)

Trauma

Tumors

Medications
- Penicillin, aminoglycosides, anticonvulsants, diuretics, coumarin, aspirin
- Amitryptiline, cyclophosphamide, chlorpromazine, thorazine

BFH usually manifests with persistent microhematuria, occasionally with intermittent microhematuria, and rarely manifests with episodic gross hematuria. BFH may be autosomal recessive, autosomal dominant, or sporadic. The hematuria is usually detected in childhood by routine testing.

Thin Basement Membranes

Thin basement membranes (TBM) occur in 5.2–9.2% of the general population (Box 12-2). The finding of defects in type IV collagen in some patients indicates that individuals with BFH or TBM are carriers of an Alport syndrome mutation. A detailed family history of renal failure and deafness must be obtained. A urine analysis should be performed in the parents. BFH implies a favorable prognosis, but these children should be evaluated regularly for proteinuria, and for hearing loss or other extra-renal symptoms, as clinically indicated.

Glomerulonephritis

Acute Post-Infectious Glomerulonephritis (APIGN)

Children with APIGN usually present with an abrupt onset of gross hematuria and edema in the context of a history of antecedent pharyngitis or impetigo (see Chapter 16). A diagnosis of APIGN requires evidence of antecedent streptococcal infection (high ASO titer or positive Streptozyme® test and/or positive throat culture for β-hemolytic streptococcus) and low serum complement (C3) level. Proteinuria and red blood cells are detected by dipstick testing; laboratories often miss RBC casts. Therefore, a careful microscopic examination of urine is essential in patients with hematuria who have a combination of proteinuria, hypertension, or edema. Microhematuria can persist for as long as 2 years in patients with APIGN.

Henoch–Schönlein Purpura (HSP) Nephritis and IgA Nephropathy

Patients with immunoglobulin A (IgA) nephropathy typically present with recurrent gross hematuria, or are found to have microscopic hematuria during routine examinations (see Chapter 17). Hematuria and/or proteinuria may be detected prior to the appearance of the purpuric rash in some patients with HSP nephritis (see Chapter 18).

Rapidly Progressive Glomerulonephritis (RPGN)

This usually presents with gross hematuria, and occasionally with microscopic hematuria. It is usually associated with rapidly deteriorating renal function and warrants a renal biopsy. RPGN may be idiopathic or secondary to IgA nephropathy, Wegener granulomatosis, microscopic polyangiitis, Goodpasture syndrome, APIGN, and HSP nephritis.

Hereditary Nephritis

Alport syndrome or hereditary nephritis is caused by mutations in the gene encoding for the alpha 5 strand of type IV collagen. This results in an abnormal glomerular basement membrane. Alport syndrome usually presents in childhood with gross or microhematuria. Episodes of gross hematuria may follow upper respiratory infections (see Chapter 20).

Interstitial Nephritis

The numerous causes of acute interstitial nephritis are shown in Box 12-3. Typical symptoms are fatigue, malaise, and flank pain. Urine output may be either increased, decreased or normal. A urine analysis can be benign or may show hematuria, mild proteinuria, pyuria with white blood cell (WBC) casts and eosinophils. Interstitial nephritis does not present with isolated hematuria or with gross hematuria.

Infections

Urinary tract infections (UTIs) are an important cause of gross hematuria, but they rarely cause isolated microhematuria. Bacterial UTIs are associated with fever, dysuria, flank and/or abdominal pain and urinary symptoms of burning, frequency, or wetting. Adenoviral cystitis presents with dysuria and gross hematuria.

Hematologic Conditions

Patients with sickle cell disease or trait may have painless gross hematuria. The hematuria may be recurrent,

---

Box 12-2 Glomerular Basement Membrane Thickness in Children

- 1st to 9th year – 100 to 340 nm
- Over 9th year – 190 to 440 nm
- Thinner in female than male
- Local normal range should be established

Box 12-3 Common Causes of Acute Interstitial Nephritis

Medications:	Non-steroidal anti-inflammatory agents, antibiotics, rifampin
Infections:	Epstein–Barr virus (EBV), cytomegalovirus (CMV), bacterial associated, mycobacterial
Systemic:	Systemic lupus erythematosus
Idiopathic	

and usually originates from the left kidney. Some patients have asymptomatic microhematuria. Coagulopathies and thrombocytopenia are uncommon causes of gross hematuria. A coagulation abnormality should be looked for only if there is no other apparent cause of painless gross hematuria in a patient with a positive family history of bleeding and a history of bruising or bleeding from other sites.

Nephrolithiasis/Hypercalciuria

The presentation of nephrolithiasis is variable with combinations of renal colic, gross hematuria, asymptomatic microhematuria, or incidental findings on imaging studies (see Chapter 19).

Structural Abnormalities/Masses

Gross hematuria can occur with even minor trauma in patients with renal cysts or hydronephrosis caused by ureteropelvic junction obstruction.

Clinical Pearl

- Gross hematuria is often a presenting sign in Wilms' tumor.
- All patients with gross hematuria require an imaging study.

Vascular Anomalies

Renal vein thrombosis rarely presents with gross hematuria, but renal venous thrombosis is an important cause of bloody urine in the newborn period. Urinary tract arteriovenous malformations and hemangiomas rarely cause episodic gross hematuria. They are extremely difficult to diagnose, even with cystoscopy and renal angiography.

Loin Pain-Hematuria Syndrome[2]

Loin pain-hematuria syndrome is a descriptive diagnosis of recurrent episodes of loin pain accompanied by hematuria in which investigations do not reveal adequate pathology to account for the symptoms. The pain may be either unilateral or bilateral, and the hematuria may be either gross or microscopic. The pain often radiates across the abdomen or to the groin. It is most commonly seen in young women aged between 20 and 40 years, but it can occur in older children. All laboratory investigations and imaging studies are normal. The renal pathology is inconsistent and non-specific, showing mild abnormalities ranging from mesangial proliferation to interstitial fibrosis and microaneurysms. The diagnosis of loin pain-hematuria syndrome is made by exclusion, and patients do not have infection, malignancy, nephrolithiasis, hypercalciuria, and trauma. Moreover, their genitourinary system is normal. The differential diagnosis includes obstructive uropathy, UTI, calculi, tumors, glomerulonephritis, renal vein thrombosis, hypercalciuria,

and medullary sponge kidney. Renal angiography has shown a variety of abnormalities such as beading, tortuosity, cortical infarcts, and microaneurysms. An anatomical abnormality in which the left renal vein is compressed between the aorta and the superior mesenteric artery may be associated with loin pain ('nutcracker syndrome'). A significant number of patients show psychological or psychopathological features, and hence the evaluation should include detailed psychiatric history, the patient's perception of pain, and the psychosocial environment. The pain can be severe, leading to the use of addictive analgesics. Treatment is mainly symptomatic in the form of analgesic therapy. Autotransplantation or denervations of the kidney have been used as treatments, albeit with variable results.

Urologic Conditions

These are discussed in Chapters 26, 27, and 40. Meatal stenosis can be the cause of gross or microscopic hematuria, especially in the newborn period. Bladder polyps and ulceration are rare causes of hematuria in children.

Urethrorrhagia[16]

Boys who present with bloody spots in their underwear elicit a great deal of anxiety that can be allayed easily by knowing about urethrorrhagia. The mean age at presentation is about 10 years. Symptoms include terminal hematuria in 100% and dysuria in 29.6% of cases. Radiographic and laboratory evaluations are normal in all patients, except for microscopic hematuria in 57%. Cystourethroscopy shows bulbar urethral inflammation without strictures. Complete resolution occurs in half the cases at 6 months, in 71% at 1 year, and in 91.7% overall. The average duration of symptoms is 10 months (range from 2 weeks to 38 months), but the condition may persist for about 2 years. Treatment consists of watchful waiting. Routine radiographic, laboratory and cystoscopic evaluation are unnecessary for evaluating urethrorrhagia. Cystoscopy should be avoided because it can cause a urethral stricture.

Clinical Pearl

- Urethrorrhagia is a cause of painless terminal hematuria.
- It occurs in prepubertal and pubertal boys.
- It typically presents with bright red blood in the underpants.

Miscellaneous

Heavy exercise can lead to gross hematuria. Microhematuria can also occur with exercise, and so the urine should be rechecked after the patient has refrained from exercise for 48 hours. Microhematuria is often seen in young women with the onset of menstruation.

Munchausen Syndrome

This is a rare, difficult to prove, cause of hematuria. The source of the blood may be from self-inflicted finger pricks, or a parent may feign the hematuria.

EVALUATION OF GROSS HEMATURIA

Gross hematuria is an alarming symptom to the child and parents, and requires prompt evaluation (Box 12-4).

A urine analysis must be performed to confirm the presence of RBCs and to look for casts and crystals. Occasionally, *S. haematobium* is diagnosed by finding ovae in the urine of an immigrant child with unexplained gross hematuria.[9]

Clinical Pearl
- Painful gross hematuria is usually caused by infections, calculi, or urological conditions.
- Glomerular causes of hematuria are painless.

The most common glomerular causes of gross hematuria in children are acute post-streptococcal glomerulonephritis (APSG) and IgA nephropathy. A detailed history must be obtained to elicit the cause of hematuria. An antecedent sore throat, pyoderma, or impetigo proteinuria, edema, hypertension, and casts suggests glomerulonephritis. If the ASO titer and Streptozyme®

Box 12-4   Indications for Prompt Evaluation of Hematuria

- Potentially life-threatening causes of hematuria must be excluded in any child with any of the following: hypertension, edema, oliguria, significant proteinuria (>500 mg per 24 hours), or red blood cell casts
- These causes include acute post-infectious nephritis, Henoch–Schönlein purpura, hemolytic-uremic syndrome, membranoproliferative glomerulonephritis, IgA nephropathy, and focal segmental glomerulosclerosis
- The evaluation must include a complete blood count (hemolytic-uremic syndrome); throat culture, Streptozyme® panel and serum C3 concentration (acute post-streptococcal glomerulonephritis); and serum creatinine and potassium concentrations (to exclude renal insufficiency)
- While awaiting the results of these tests, the blood pressure and urine output must be monitored at frequent intervals

---

test, and serum C3 concentration are informative, the diagnosis is PSGN. If these are not informative, further investigations are warranted to rule out other causes of glomerulonephritis. IgA nephropathy can cause recurrent gross hematuria, and this may be preceded by an upper respiratory tract infection and even flank or abdominal pain.

Fever, dysuria, flank pain with or without voiding symptoms suggests a UTI. This is the most common cause of gross hematuria in children presenting to an emergency room. A computed tomography (CT) scan of the abdomen and pelvis must be obtained promptly with a history of abdominal trauma, and the child must be referred to a urologist. A family history of renal calculi or severe renal colic with gross hematuria suggests urinary calculi. Hypercalciuria can cause recurrent gross or microscopic hematuria in the absence of calculi on imaging studies.

Clinical Pearl
- If no obvious cause is found for gross hematuria by history, physical and preliminary studies, the differential diagnosis should include hypercalciuria, sickle cell trait or thin basement membrane disease.
- Cystoscopic examination in children rarely reveals a cause for hematuria.

If a cystoscopy is performed to lateralize the source of bleeding, it is best carried out during active bleeding. In young girls with recurrent gross hematuria it is important to enquire about a history of child abuse, or the insertion of a vaginal foreign body; the genital area must also be examined for signs of injury.

If no RBCs are seen in the urinalysis, but the dipstick test is positive for blood, then hemoglobinuria and myoglobinuria must be considered as causes. A stepwise approach to the evaluation of gross hematuria is shown in Figure 12-1.

EVALUATION OF MICROHEMATURIA

Isolated Microhematuria

Isolated microhematuria, without any abnormal findings on history or physical examination, is often found during routine urine screening. The urinalysis should be repeated two to three times over several months (without preceding exercise) before embarking on further investigations. If the microhematuria persists, a careful history should be obtained for use of medications, family history of hematuria, deafness, renal failure, urinary calculi; history of sickle cell disease or trait; and the parents' urines should be examined for hematuria.[13,14] If all the enquiries and the examination are negative, the

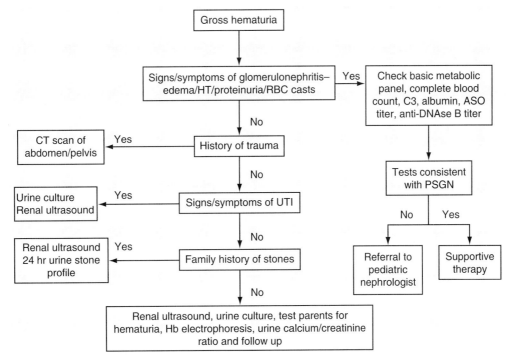

Figure 12-1   A stepwise approach to the evaluation of gross hematuria.

parents should be reassured and further investigations such as renal ultrasound and cystoscopic studies should be avoided.[6] The child can be re-evaluated yearly by urine analysis, and further studies can be carried out if anything evolves. Testing for microhematuria is being challenged even in adult medicine (Figure 12-2 and Box 12-5).[10]

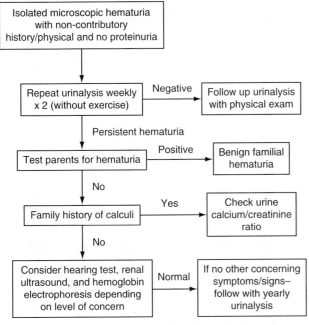

Figure 12-2   A stepwise approach to the evaluation of microscopic hematuria.

Clinical Pearl

- A renal ultrasound, voiding cystourethrogram, cystoscopy, and renal biopsy are not indicated in the evaluation of microscopic hematuria.
- Microhematuria in the otherwise healthy child is a minimal health threat, and is rarely indicative of serious illness.

Microhematuria with Abnormal Findings

Children with microhematuria and any abnormal finding on history, physical examination, or urine analysis should be investigated for kidney disease (Figure 12-3). Edema, hypertension, decreased urine output, rashes,

Box 12-5   Testing for Microhematuria in Adults

- Microhematuria is poorly predictive of cancers of the urinary tract
- Hemoglobin dipstick testing is not a reliable way of detecting early bladder cancer in patients at high risk
- Microhematuria is not reliable evidence of a stone in the ureter and may be misleading, as it is often present in other serious conditions that cause acute loin pain
- Testing for microhematuria is not helpful in evaluating men with lower urinary tract symptoms

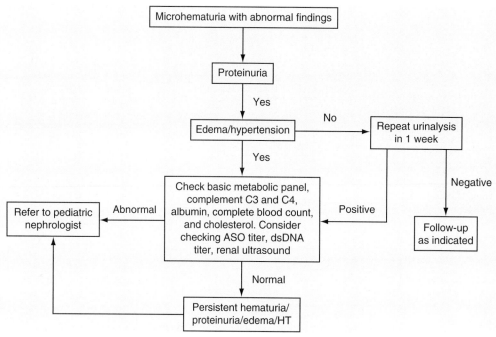

Figure 12-3 A stepwise approach to the evaluation of kidney disease.

arthralgias, or constitutional symptoms, loss of appetite, and/or weight loss are suggestive of intrinsic renal disease. Patients with any of these signs or symptoms should undergo laboratory tests that include a basic metabolic panel, complement levels, and a complete blood count. Additional tests that can be carried out are based on clinical suspicions, and include ASO titer, DNA-binding antibodies and serological tests for hepatitis. A child with hematuria and proteinuria who does not have edema or hypertension should have repeated urine analysis unless the proteinuria is greater than 2+ positive. If the abnormal urinary findings persist, then the above investigations should be carried out even in the absence of edema or hypertension. Persistent proteinuria should be quantified, and if the excretion is greater than 1 g per day the patient should be referred to a pediatric nephrologist for further evaluation.

REFERENCES

1. American Academy of Pediatrics: Committee on Practice and Ambulatory Medicine. Recommendations for preventive pediatric health care. Pediatrics 1995;96:373–374.

2. Burke JR, Hardie IR. Loin pain hematuria syndrome. Pediatric Nephrol 1996;10:216–218.

3. Diven SC, Travis LB. A practical primary care approach to hematuria in children. Pediatr Nephrol 2000;14:65–69.

4. Dodge WF, West EF, Smith EH, Bunce H. Proteinuria and hematuria in school children: epidemiology and early natural history. J Pediatr 1976;88:327.

5. Feld LG, Waz WR, Perez LM, Joseph DB. Hematuria. Pediatr Clin North Am 1997;44:1191–1210.

6. Feld LG, Meyers KEC, Kaplan BS, Stapleton FB. Limited evaluation of microscopic hematuria in pediatrics. Pediatrics 1998;102:E42.

7. Ingelfinger JR, Davis AE, Grupe WE. Frequency and etiology of gross hematuria in a general pediatric setting. Pediatrics 1977;59:557–561.

8. Lieu TA, Grasmeder M, Kaplan B. An approach to the evaluation and treatment of microscopic hematuria. Pediatr Clin North Am 1991;38:579–592.

9. Kaplan BS, Meyers KEC. Images in clinical medicine. *Schistosoma haematobium*. N Engl J Med 2000;343:1085.

10. Malmström PU. Time to abandon testing for microscopic haematuria in adults? Br Med J 2003;326:813–815.

11. Northway JD. Hematuria in children. J Pediatr 1971;78: 381–396.

12. Patel HP, Bissler JJ. Hematuria in children. Pediatric Urol 2001;48:1519–1537.

13. Stapleton FB, Roy S, Noe N, Jerkins G. Hypercalciuria in children with hematuria. N Engl J Med 1984;310:1345–1348.

14. Stapleton FB. Hematuria associated with hypercalciuria and hyperuricosuria: a practical approach. Pediatr Nephrol 1994;8:756–761.

15. Vehaskari VM, Rapola J, Koskimies O, et al. Microscopic hematuria in schoolchildren: epidemiology and clinico-pathologic evaluation. J Pediatr 1979;95:676–684.

16. Walker BR, Ellison ED, Snow BW, Cartwright PC. The natural history of idiopathic urethrorrhagia in boys. J Urol 2001;166:231–232.

CHAPTER 13

Proteinuria

MADHURA PRADHAN, M.D. AND

BERNARD S. KAPLAN, M.B., B.Ch.

INTRODUCTION

Proteinuria is one of the most important clinical markers of kidney disease, is associated with progressive renal disease, and is implicated as a risk factor for cardiovascular disease.[3,12] However, transient proteinuria is associated with several physiological conditions, and therefore it is important to differentiate between physiological and pathological proteinuria.[2]

Proteinuria is the excretion of abnormal amounts of protein in the urine. Protein excretion in normal children is less than 4 mg/m²/h, and in healthy adults is less than 150 mg in 24 hours (Table 13-1).

Not all the protein in the urine is derived from plasma: 50% is derived from plasma, and 50% is secreted from the kidney as Tamm–Horsfall protein. Albumin accounts for less than 30% of the total urinary protein in normal individuals.

Urinary Protein	mg/24 h	mg/m²/h	Protein:Creatinine (mg:mg)
Adults			
Normal	<150		<0.2
Nephrotic range	2000–3000		>2
Children			
Normal		<4	<0.5 (age <2 years)
		4–40	<0.2 (age >2 years)
Nephrotic range		>40	>2

Table 13-1 Urinary Protein Excretion

MECHANISMS OF PROTEINURIA

Protein excretion in urine depends on two processes: glomerular filtration, and tubular reabsorption. Proteinuria therefore can occur as a result of increased glomerular capillary wall permeability, or decreased tubular reabsorption, or both mechanisms. The permeability of the glomerular capillary wall is determined by the size of plasma proteins, the electrostatic charge of the capillary wall, and by hemodynamic factors such as glomerular plasma flow, capillary hydrostatic pressure and the ultrafiltration coefficient of the capillary wall. The slit pores between the interdigitating foot processes of glomerular visceral epithelial cells (podocytes) are called the slit diaphragm. The ultimate barrier to the passage of protein across the glomerular capillary wall is provided by these specialized cell adhesion structures. The capillary basement membrane and slit diaphragms impede the egress of molecules above a molecular weight of 40,000 daltons (Da). Therefore, only that fraction of the plasma albumin which has a molecular weight of 69,000 Da is filtered. This size-selectivity appears to correspond to 'pores' of predetermined dimensions that limit the passage of large solutes across the glomerular basement membrane. The glomerular capillary wall also contains heparan sulfate proteoglycans and sialoproteins that are negatively charged. These also impede the filtration of other negatively charged molecules such as albumin by electrostatic repulsion. However, the role of charge selectivity in the permeability of the glomerular capillary wall is questionable. The precise contributions of loss of size selectivity and charge selectivity to proteinuria are not known, and the subject is in a state of flux.[5] Hemodynamic changes in glomerular blood flow cause proteinuria by altering convection (the solute is carried across the membrane with a solvent) or diffusion (the solute moves across a concentration gradient) across the capillary wall. This is important in individuals with chronic renal failure because the filtration rates in remnant nephrons are increased, and this increases transglomerular protein loss by convection. Albumin infusions can result in increased proteinuria by increased diffusion.

Tubular proteinuria occurs when the tubules are unable to reabsorb normally filtered low molecular-weight proteins or albumin. This occurs in most types of renal disease, including the nephrotic syndrome. Tubular proteinuria also occurs in Fanconi syndrome, acute tubular necrosis, interstitial nephritis, and in multiple myeloma. Low molecular-weight proteins such as beta-2 microglobulins and lysozymes are detected by urine protein electrophoresis. Tubular proteinuria does not exceed 1–1.5 g in 24 hours.

The concept of selectivity of proteinuria was introduced in 1960 in an attempt to predict the response to treatment of patients with nephrotic syndrome. Patients with minimal change nephrotic syndrome have increased excretion of intermediate molecular weight proteins such as albumin, but do not excrete high molecular-weight proteins, such as immunoglobulin G (IgG). This is referred to as selective proteinuria, and is assessed by the selectivity index (SI) based on the comparison of the clearance of IgG and transferrin. Patients with a SI of 0.2 or higher are said to have non-selective proteinuria. Although this concept had limited clinical applications in the past, recent reports note decreased tubulointerstitial involvement and better outcomes in patients with selective proteinuria versus non-selective proteinuria.

DETECTION OF PROTEINURIA

Qualitative

Proteinuria is usually detected using the dipstick method. This mainly detects albumin and not low molecular-weight proteins. The concentration of urinary protein is measured by a colorimetric method (Table 13-2). Impregnated tetrabromophenol blue changes color when it reacts with amino groups. Tetrabromophenol blue is a pH indicator, and therefore false-positive results occur when the urine pH is above 7 (Box 13-1).

Clinical Pearl

Trace-positive proteinuria by the dipstick method does not imply abnormal proteinuria.

A urine sample is considered positive for protein if the dipstick registers ≥1+ in urine sample with a specific gravity of ≤1.015. If the specific gravity of the urine is >1.015, the dipstick must be ≥2+ to be considered positive. When the urine is very dilute (specific gravity <1.005), the dipstick can give a false-negative result. At least two out of three urine samples collected ≥1 week apart must be positive for a diagnosis of persistent proteinuria.

The sulfosalicylic acid, trichloroacetic acid, nitric acid, and sodium sulfate qualitative methods are also available

Table 13-2 Qualitative Evaluation of Proteinuria by Dipstick Test

Grade	Protein Concentration (mg/dl)
Trace	10–20
1+	30
2+	100
3+	300
4+	1000–2000

for the detection of proteinuria. The sulfosalicylic acid method detects all forms of protein, but gives false-positive results with radiographic contrast dyes, penicillins, cephalosporins, sulfonamides, and high uric acid concentrations.

Quantitative

Qualitative tests are convenient, but are often imprecise. Therefore timed urine collections are essential for establishing the presence and amount of proteinuria. A 24-hour urine collection is the best method. The individual discards the first voided sample in the morning and then collects every sample of urine, including the first specimen the following morning. The urine sample should be refrigerated until submission to the laboratory. Timed urine collections are often difficult to carry out accurately in a child. A 24-hour collection can be substituted by determining the protein:creatinine ratio in a random urine sample, preferably the first voided sample. The ratio of the urine protein (mg) to the urine creatinine (mg) ($U_{P:C}$) correlates with the 24-hour urine protein excretion.[1] The 24-hour urine protein excretion can be derived from the $U_{P:C}$ by the following formula: $0.63 \times U_{P:C}$ = urine protein excretion in g/m^2/day. Specimens should not be obtained after exercise because the upper limit of normal is higher in these specimens. The urine protein:creatinine ratio is not an accurate estimate of proteinuria in malnourished children because of decreased creatinine secretion, or in those with low levels of renal function because of increased creatinine secretion.

Microalbuminuria

Measurement of urinary albumin rather than total protein is recommended in adults and postpubertal children with diabetes for the diagnosis of chronic kidney disease (CKD).[4,9,10] First-morning spot collections are now considered optimum for children and adolescents to avoid the confounding effect of orthostatic proteinuria. Albuminuria is reported as milligrams of albumin per gram of creatinine. This is often referred to as microalbuminuria, as the test measures very small quantities of albumin, which are below the level of detection by dipstick test for total protein. A value of <30 mg protein per gram creatinine is normal, and 30 to 300 mg/g is consistent with microalbuminuria. It is recommended that children with diabetes of more than 5 years' duration have their urine checked for microalbuminuria. Values greater than the reference range should be confirmed in two of three tested samples. Microalbuminuria is considered to be an early sign of incipient diabetic nephropathy.

EPIDEMIOLOGY OF PROTEINURIA

The prevalence of proteinuria in children varies depending on the definition of proteinuria (degree of positivity on a dipstick), and the number of specimens examined.[6] Some 10% of school-aged children will have proteinuria, defined as 1+ on dipstick test, at some time. If the definition is a positive dipstick reading of ≥ 1+ in two out of four specimens, the prevalence falls to 2.5%. The prevalence of proteinuria increases with age, peaking in adolescence (age 13 years in girls and 16 years in boys), and declining thereafter.

ETIOLOGY

Asymptomatic proteinuria is common in children. It is important to recognize that although proteinuria is a hallmark of many kidney diseases, many physiologic/functional situations cause transient proteinuria. Causes of proteinuria in children are listed in Table 13-3.

DIFFERENTIAL DIAGNOSIS OF PROTEINURIA

Functional/Transient Proteinuria

Functional proteinuria is typically transient, and resolves when the inciting factor remits. It is generally ≤2+ on a dipstick. Febrile proteinuria occurs with the onset of fever and resolves within 10–14 days even if the fever defervesces earlier. Proteinuria associated with exercise generally abates within 48 hours of cessation of exercise. Proteinuria with fever, exercise, and heart failure is most likely the result of hemodynamic alterations in glomerular blood flow that causes increased diffusion of proteins across the glomerular basement membrane.

Orthostatic (Postural) Proteinuria

Orthostatic proteinuria is defined as abnormally high protein excretion only when the subject is in the

Table 13-3	Classification and Etiology of Proteinuria in Children
Transient proteinuria	• Fever, dehydration, exercise, cold exposure. Congestive heart failure, seizures, emotional stress, epinephrine administration, serum sickness
Isolated proteinuria	• Orthostatic proteinuria, persistent asymptomatic isolated proteinuria
Glomerular proteinuria	• Minimal change nephrotic syndrome • Focal segmental glomerulosclerosis • Post-infectious glomerulonephritis • Membranoproliferative glomerulonephritis • Membranous nephropathy • Immunoglobulin A nephropathy • Henoch–Schönlein purpura • Hemolytic uremic syndrome • Hereditary nephritis (Alport syndrome) • Systemic lupus erythematosus • Vasculitis (Wegener's granulomatosis, microscopic polyangiitis) • Diabetes mellitus • Sickle cell disease • HIV-associated nephropathy • Malaria • Hepatitis B and C • Bacterial endocarditis • Congenital nephrotic syndrome
Tubulointerstitial disease	• Reflux nephropathy, pyelonephritis • Interstitial nephritis, Fanconi syndrome • Medications and toxins – aminoglycosides, penicillins, heavy metals, lithium, gold salts • Ischemic tubular injury • Renal hypoplasia/dysplasia, polycystic kidney disease

upright position. It is the most common cause of asymptomatic proteinuria in children, and the prevalence is greatest in adolescents. Orthostatic proteinuria usually does not exceed 1 g/day; moreover, it can be fixed and reproducible on repeated measurements, or it can be intermittent and transient. Orthostatic proteinuria may be the result of altered renal hemodynamics with activation of the renin-angiotensin system in response to decreased effective circulating volume due to venous pooling in the legs when in the upright position. Circulating immune complexes have also been suggested as the cause of orthostatic proteinuria.

Orthostatic proteinuria is diagnosed by checking the first-morning urine sample for protein: a diagnosis of postural proteinuria is made if there is no protein in this sample. A timed split urine collection is a more definitive test: before going to bed, the child voids and discards the urine; the next first-morning urine is collected in a container marked 'recumbent' immediately on rising; all

urine produced during the day – including the last void of the day – is collected in another container labeled 'ambulatory'; the start and end times for both samples are recorded. Protein excretion in the recumbent specimen should be normal (<4 mg/m^2/h), whereas that in the ambulatory collection is two- to four-fold that found when in the recumbent collection.

Orthostatic proteinuria is benign, and long-term follow-up studies in young adults show a benign course. However, before reassuring the individual and family, the history, physical findings and laboratory evidence of renal disease must be excluded.

> **Clinical Pearl**
> • Only first-morning urine analysis should be performed in children with postural proteinuria at their yearly physical examinations.
> • The clinician should emphasize that a diagnosis of orthostatic proteinuria does not indemnify the individual from subsequent renal diseases due to other causes.

Persistent Asymptomatic Isolated Proteinuria (PAIP)

PAIP is said to be present when proteinuria is present persistently (in >80% of samples), including in recumbent specimens in an otherwise healthy child in whom clinical and laboratory work-up is normal. Renal biopsy studies in some children with PAIP have revealed glomerular abnormalities including focal sclerosis, immunoglobulin A (IgA) nephropathy, membranous nephropathy, and diffuse mesangial proliferation. There is also a concern that unremitting proteinuria itself can cause focal sclerosis. Hence this entity is viewed with caution and deserves close follow-up. The proteinuria should be quantified if possible and monitored every 6 to 12 months. A progressive increase in proteinuria beyond 1 g/day warrants a renal biopsy. However, the yield of a renal biopsy is poor in the presence of mild-moderate proteinuria (<1 g/day).

Glomerular Diseases

Proteinuria occurs in most glomerular diseases. Glomerular proteinuria can be in excess of 10 g/24 hours, especially in membranous nephropathy.

Nephrotic Syndrome

The nephrotic syndrome is defined by the presence of proteinuria, hypoalbuminemia, hypercholesterolemia, and edema. Minimal change disease is the most common type of primary nephrotic syndrome in children. Other causes are mesangioproliferative glomerulonephritis and focal segmental glomerulosclerosis. The urine protein excretion in nephrotic syndrome exceeds 40 mg/m²/h or 50–100 mg/kg/day (see also Chapter 20).

Focal Segmental Glomerulosclerosis (FSGS)

FSGS accounts for 30% of cases of idiopathic nephrotic syndrome in children. However, it can present in older children and adolescents as asymptomatic proteinuria. It is the most common glomerular cause of end-stage renal failure in children, and occurs frequently in African-Americans (see also Chapter 22).

Glomerulonephritis

Membranoproliferative Glomerulonephritis (MPGN)

MPGN is characterized by diffuse thickening of the glomerular capillary wall and increased mesangial cellularity. It is common in older children and adolescents and presents with nephrotic syndrome and hematuria. Complement levels are low. It should be considered in the differential diagnosis of proteinuria with associated hematuria, renal insufficiency, or low complement levels (see also Chapter 19).

Membranous Nephropathy

This is an uncommon cause of nephrotic syndrome in children, and can also present with asymptomatic proteinuria. It is characterized by diffusely thickened glomerular capillary walls without mesangial proliferation. The proteinuria in membranous nephropathy is often massive (see also Chapter 23).

IgA Nephropathy (IgA N)

IgA N can present with combinations of nephrotic syndrome, asymptomatic proteinuria, hematuria, recurrent gross hematuria, or acute nephritis. Isolated proteinuria is rarely seen in IgA N. The pathological lesion is characterized by mesangial proliferation and IgA deposits (see also Chapter 17).

Tubular Diseases

Tubular diseases causing proteinuria can be either congenital (dysplastic kidneys, polycystic kidneys, Fanconi syndrome) or acquired (acute tubular necrosis, interstitial nephritis secondary to drugs or infections). Tubular proteinuria generally does not exceed 1.5 g per day.

Miscellaneous Causes of Proteinuria in Children

Diffuse Mesangial Sclerosis

Diffuse mesangial sclerosis (DMS) presents in infants and toddlers with the nephrotic syndrome. DMS can be a sporadic condition, an autosomal recessively inherited disease, or a component of Denys–Drash syndrome (DDS). DDS consists of combinations of male pseudo-hermatophroditism, nephrotic syndrome, and Wilms' tumor. DMS can progress to end-stage renal disease in childhood and require renal transplantation. The presence of proteinuria in a young male child with undescended testes should alert the clinician to the possibility of DDS.

Fabry Disease

This X-linked disorder is caused by a deficiency of α-galactosidase A that leads to recurrent painful crises of the hands and feet, a characteristic skin rash, and corneal and lenticular opacities. Glycosphingolipid deposition in the kidneys can lead to progressive renal damage with proteinuria and chronic renal failure. Fabry disease can now be treated with infusions of rHα-galactosidase A.

Nail-patella Syndrome

This is a rare autosomal dominant disorder with nail dysplasia, bone abnormalities, and renal disease. The patellae are hypoplastic or absent, and renal involvement occurs in 30–40% of patients as proteinuria or nephrotic syndrome.

EVALUATION OF PROTEINURIA

The presence of proteinuria must be confirmed on at least three occasions before initiating its evaluation. The evaluation should be focused on finding the cause of the condition, using a stepwise approach to avoid unnecessary and invasive investigations.[7,8] The first step is to obtain a complete history and perform a careful physical examination, with emphasis on the detection of renal diseases (Table 13-4).

Table 13-4	History and Physical Examination in the Evaluation of Proteinuria
History	Systemic illnesses, fever preceding detection of proteinuria, urinary tract infections, family history of renal disease, deafness
Examination	Height and weight, blood pressure, edema, rash, abdominal mass, arthritis, absent lunae and absent patellae (nail patella syndrome), eye examination (SLE, hypertension, Fabry disease), ambiguous genitalia (Denys–Drash syndrome)

SLE = systemic lupus erythematosus.

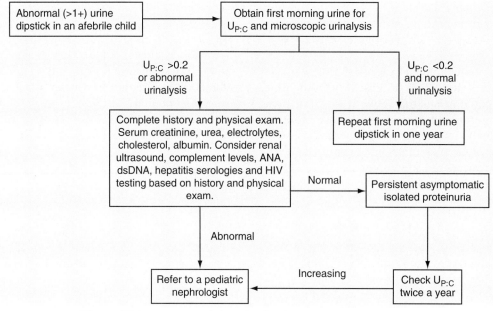

Figure 13-1   A suggested algorithm for the evaluation of proteinuria.

Laboratory investigations should begin with the first-morning urine analysis and urine protein:creatinine ratio, followed in stages by tests for renal function, serological tests, and imaging studies of the kidneys (Figure 13-1). If the first-morning urine protein:creatinine ratio is <0.2, then a diagnosis of orthostatic proteinuria is made and no further tests are necessary.

Additional investigations are based on the results of the studies listed in Table 13-5. If these are normal, and if there is significant and persistent proteinuria, then a renal biopsy may be indicated to rule out specific renal diseases (Box 13-2). A suggested algorithm for the evaluation of proteinuria is provided in Figure 13-1.

TREATMENT

The treatment of proteinuria is based on its cause. If no cause is found, then treatment to reduce the urinary protein excretion is often offered in the presence of significant (>1 g/day) proteinuria. Therapies to ameliorate proteinuria have gained much importance due to the impact of persistent proteinuria on progression of renal failure.[11] Angiotensin-converting enzyme inhibitors (ACE I) and angiotensin receptor blockers (ARB) are used to decrease proteinuria. However the long-term benefit of ACE I in children and adolescents with proteinuria remain

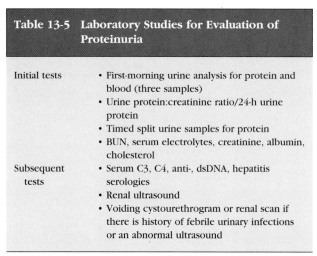

Table 13-5	Laboratory Studies for Evaluation of Proteinuria
Initial tests	• First-morning urine analysis for protein and blood (three samples) • Urine protein:creatinine ratio/24-h urine protein • Timed split urine samples for protein • BUN, serum electrolytes, creatinine, albumin, cholesterol
Subsequent tests	• Serum C3, C4, anti-, dsDNA, hepatitis serologies • Renal ultrasound • Voiding cystourethrogram or renal scan if there is history of febrile urinary infections or an abnormal ultrasound

BUN = blood urea nitrogen; dsDNA = double-stranded DNA.

Box 13-2   Indications for a Renal Biopsy in the Evaluation of Proteinuria

• Nephrotic range proteinuria
• Proteinuria with a family history of chronic glomerulonephritis or unexplained renal failure
• Proteinuria associated with hematuria and red blood cell casts, except with post-streptococcal glomerulonephritis
• Proteinuria with a low C3 level, except with post-streptococcal glomerulonephritis
• Proteinuria with hypertension or azotemia
• Persistent non-orthostatic proteinuria for more than 1 year

to be established. Although dietary protein restriction does not have a significant impact on the rate of progression of renal disease, it is reasonable to avoid excess dietary protein in children with proteinuric renal disease.

REFERENCES

1. Abitol C, Zilleruelo G, Freundlich M, Strauss J. Quantitation of proteinuria with urinary protein/creatinine ratios and random testing with dipsticks in nephrotic children. J Pediatr 1990;116:243-247.

2. Bergstein JM. A practical approach to proteinuria. Pediatr Nephrol 1999;13:697-700.

3. Cameron JS. Proteinuria and progression in human glomerular diseases. Am J Nephrol 1990;10:81-87.

4. National Kidney Foundation (K/DOQI). Clinical Practice Guidelines for Nutrition of Chronic Renal Failure. Evaluation, classification and stratification. Am J Kidney Dis 2002;39:S1-S266.

5. D'Amico G, Bazzi C. Pathophysiology of proteinuria. Kidney Int 2003;63:809-825.

6. Dodge WF, West EF, Smith EH, Bunce H. Proteinuria and hematuria in school children: epidemiology and early natural history. J Pediatr 1976;88:327.

7. Ettenger RB. The evaluation of the child with proteinuria. Pediatr Ann 1994;23:486-494.

8. Hogg RJ, Portman RJ, Milliner D, et al. Evaluation and management of proteinuria and nephrotic syndrome in children: recommendations from a pediatric nephrology panel established at the National Kidney Foundation Conference on Proteinuria, Albuminuria, Risk, Assessment, Detection and Elimination (PARADE). Pediatrics 2000;105:1242-1249.

9. Hogg RJ, Furth S, Lemley KV, et al. National Kidney Foundation's Kidney Disease Outcomes Quality Initiative Clinical Practice Guidelines for Chronic Kidney Disease in Children and Adolescents: Evaluation, Classification, and Stratification. Pediatrics 2003;111:1416-1421.

10. Keane WF, Eknoyan G. Proteinuria, albuminuria, risk, assessment, detection, elimination (PARADE): a position paper of the National Kidney Foundation. Am J Kidney Dis 1999;33:1004-1010.

11. Peterson JC, Adler S, Burkart JM. Blood pressure control, proteinuria and the progression of renal disease. Ann Intern Med 1995;125:754-762.

12. Remuzzi G, Ruggenenti P, Benigni A. Understanding the nature of renal disease progression. Kidney Int 1997;63:S10-S14.

Hypertension: Principles for the Practitioner

JONATHAN M. SOROF, M.D.

INTRODUCTION

Hypertension affects more than 50 million Americans, and is a leading cause of cardiovascular disease, end-stage renal disease, and cerebrovascular accidents. Hypertension and its complications also occur in children. Children are more likely to have secondary hypertension due to underlying cardiorenal disease. However, the changing epidemiology of pediatric hypertension has resulted in a relative increase in the prevalence of primary hypertension in the face of an epidemic of childhood obesity, inactivity, and poor dietary habits. In pediatric hypertension clinics, the typical patient is now an otherwise healthy adolescent often with combinations of cardiovascular risk factors of obesity, family history of hypertension, and an ethnic predisposition to hypertensive disease and/or type II diabetes mellitus.

> **Clinical Pearl**
>
> As a general rule, the younger the patient and the more severe the hypertension, the more likely it is that a secondary cause for the hypertension is present.

Very young children or children with marked blood pressure (BP) elevation always require comprehensive evaluation and management. However, the majority of hypertensive children are adolescents with mild to moderate hypertension. For these, the appropriate level of diagnostic evaluation, indications for pharmacological treatment, and the target BP values to aim for in response to treatment, have not been established. Thus, the practice of truly evidence-based medicine remains a challenge for physicians who care for hypertensive children. Nonetheless, as the prevalence of hypertension, often in association with obesity, increases, responsibility for the care of these children will fall increasingly to primary healthcare providers. This chapter summarizes current concepts in the diagnosis, evaluation, and management of hypertension in children, as well as the indications for subspecialty referral.

MEASUREMENT OF BP IN CHILDREN

Cuff Size

It is important to establish that the BP was measured by the correct technique. Factors that affect the accuracy and reliability of this measurement are anxiety, position of the arm, observer bias, type of equipment, and the size of the cuff. A larger than appropriate cuff size can give falsely low measurements, while a smaller one can give falsely high readings. This is of particular importance in children because of significant differences in arm sizes at various ages. Selection of the appropriate cuff size is even more difficult because of inconsistent recommendations for cuff selection. The 1987 Task Force on BP Control in Children recommended that the cuff bladder should be wide enough to cover three-quarters of the upper arm length, measured from the acromion to the olecranon process.[24] The most recent update to the Task Force recommended that the width of the bladder cuff should equal 40% of the mid-upper arm circumference.[25] When these two recommendations are compared, cuffs chosen based on upper arm length criteria are larger on average than those based on upper arm circumference. In many cases, perceptions on proper cuff selection among healthcare providers do not match either of the Task Force recommendations. Irrespective of the selection method, intra-arterial measurements often correlate poorly with those obtained by cuffs. The problem of the appropriate cuff size for indirect measurement of both systolic and diastolic BP is unresolved. Nevertheless, criteria for choosing a cuff must be used to measure BP. The most recent recommendations on the Task Force Report on High BP in Children and Adolescents are summarized in Box 14-1. The appropriate cuff size is shown in Figure 14-1. The bladder width is approximately 40% of the arm circumference midway between the olecranon and the acromion processes. Careful attention to this protocol allows consistency between patients and the best comparability with the Task Force normative BP data (Table 14-1).

Auscultatory and Oscillometric Methods

Auscultation and oscillometry are the main techniques for indirect measurement of BP. The 'gold standard' technique for BP measurement in children is auscultation with a sphygmomanometer containing a mercury column, using the stethoscope placed over the brachial artery pulse, proximal and medial to the antecubital fossa and below the bottom edge of the cuff (i.e., about 2 cm above the cubital fossa). An alternative to the mercury-based equipment is the aneroid sphygmomanometer. The auscultatory method relies on the detection of Korotkoff sounds for determining systolic and diastolic BP values. Systolic BP is determined by the onset of the 'tapping' Korotkoff sounds. The phase of the Korotkoff sounds that defines diastolic BP has been controversial (see Development of Normative Data). The American Heart Association has established the fifth Korotkoff sound (K5), or the disappearance of Korotkoff sounds, as the definition of diastolic pressure. Similarly, the Task Force Report now recommends using K5 to define diastolic BP in children of all ages, and the BP tables provided in the Task Force Report use K5 as the diastolic BP.

Oscillometric devices are increasingly used for determining BP. These devices are based on the correlation between the oscillation generated by pulses and the BP. At a minimum, the devices determine mean arterial pressure and may also estimate systolic pressure. Systolic and diastolic pressures are reported using algorithms that are proprietary to the companies that manufacture each device. Since reference standards in children are based on auscultatory measurements, oscillometric devices are generally calibrated to mirror the values obtained through auscultation. However, oscillometric devices do not necessarily yield values that approximate auscultatory readings, nor do oscillometric values from one device

Box 14-1	Recommendations for the Accurate Measurement of BP in Children

- Use the appropriate cuff size
- Measure BP in a controlled environment
- Allow 3–5 minutes of rest in the seated position
- The antecubital fossa must be supported at heart level
- Record BP at least twice on each occasion
- Use the average of each measurement to estimate BP

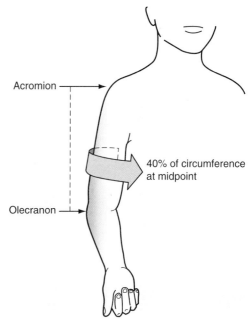

Figure 14-1   Diagram of proper placement of BP cuff. (From Update on the 1987 Task Force Report on High BP in Children and Adolescents: a working group report from the National High BP Education Program. National High BP Education Program Working Group on Hypertension Control in Children and Adolescents. Pediatrics 1996;98:649–658.[25])

Table 14-1 Blood Pressure Levels for the 90th and 95th Percentiles of Blood Pressure for Boys Aged 1–17 years by Percentiles of Height

Age (years)	BP percentile*	Systolic BP by percentile of height (mmHg)**							Diastolic BP by percentile of height (mmHg)**						
		5%	10%	25%	50%	75%	90%	95%	5%	10%	25%	50%	75%	90%	95%
1	90th	94	95	97	98	100	102	102	50	51	52	53	54	54	55
	95th	98	99	101	102	104	106	106	55	55	56	57	58	59	59
2	90th	98	99	100	102	104	105	106	55	55	56	57	58	59	59
	95th	101	102	104	106	108	109	110	59	59	60	61	62	63	63
3	90th	100	101	103	105	107	108	109	59	59	60	61	62	63	63
	95th	104	105	107	109	111	112	113	63	63	64	65	66	67	67
4	90th	102	103	105	107	109	110	111	62	62	63	64	65	66	66
	95th	106	107	109	111	113	114	115	66	67	67	68	69	70	71
5	90th	104	105	106	108	110	112	112	65	65	66	67	68	69	69
	95th	108	109	110	112	114	115	116	69	70	70	71	72	73	74
6	90th	105	106	108	110	111	113	114	67	68	69	70	70	71	72
	95th	109	110	112	114	115	117	117	72	72	73	74	75	76	76
7	90th	106	107	109	111	113	114	115	69	70	71	72	72	73	74
	95th	110	111	113	115	116	118	119	74	74	75	76	77	78	78
8	90th	107	108	110	112	114	115	116	71	71	72	73	74	75	75
	95th	111	112	114	116	118	119	120	75	76	76	77	78	79	80
9	90th	109	110	112	113	115	117	117	72	73	73	74	75	76	77
	95th	113	114	116	117	119	121	121	76	77	78	79	80	80	81
10	90th	110	112	113	115	117	118	119	73	74	74	75	76	77	78
	95th	114	115	117	119	121	122	123	77	78	79	80	80	81	82
11	90th	112	113	115	117	119	120	121	74	74	75	76	77	78	78
	95th	116	117	119	121	123	124	125	78	79	79	80	81	82	83
12	90th	115	116	117	119	121	123	123	75	75	76	77	78	78	79
	95th	119	120	121	123	125	126	127	79	79	80	81	82	83	83
13	90th	117	118	120	122	124	125	126	75	76	76	77	78	79	80
	95th	121	122	124	126	128	129	130	79	80	81	82	83	83	84
14	90th	120	121	123	125	126	128	128	76	76	77	78	79	80	80
	95th	124	125	127	128	130	132	132	80	81	81	82	83	84	85
15	90th	123	124	125	127	129	131	131	77	77	78	79	80	81	81
	95th	127	128	129	131	133	134	135	81	82	83	83	84	85	86
16	90th	125	126	128	130	132	133	134	79	79	80	81	82	82	83
	95th	129	130	132	134	136	137	138	83	83	84	85	86	87	87
17	90th	128	129	131	133	134	136	136	81	81	82	83	84	85	85
	95th	132	133	135	136	138	140	140	85	85	86	87	88	89	89

*Blood pressure percentile was determined by a single measurement.

**Height percentile was determined by standard growth curves.

From: National High Blood Pressure Education Program Working Group on Hypertension Control in Children and Adolescents. Update on the 1987 task force report on high blood pressure in children and adolescents: a working group report from the National High Blood Pressure Education Program. Pediatrics 1996;98:649–658.[25]

necessarily equal values obtained from another device made by other manufacturers. It is therefore important to understand that oscillometric BPs are not completely interchangeable with auscultatory values, and that there are no established reference standards for oscillometric BP values in children. Nonetheless, the ease of use, independence from potential user bias such as terminal digit preference (e.g., over-reporting of BP values ending in zero), and the movement to remove sources of mercury from hospital or clinic environments has led to the use of oscillometric monitors as the *de facto* standard for BP measurement in children. This is particularly true in newborns and young infants in whom auscultation is difficult, as well as in the intensive care units where frequent BP measurement is needed. However, when treatment decisions are to be made based on specific BP values, oscillometric measurements should be confirmed by standard auscultatory methods whenever possible.

Ambulatory BP Monitoring (ABPM)

ABPM is useful for the assessment of BP in children[16] (Box 14-2). ABPM measures BP multiple times during a predefined time period, and more accurately reflects the continuous nature of BP as a hemodynamic variable (Figure 14-2).

Techniques for ABPM include auscultatory, auscultatory with R-wave gating, and oscillometry. Auscultatory technology relies on the detection of Korotkoff sounds for determining systolic and diastolic BP values, similar to stethoscope and manual mercury manometer measurements. A microphone is placed under the BP cuff over the brachial artery, and this must remain in place throughout the monitoring period. While this potentially provides acceptable accuracy under controlled circumstances, ambient noise levels may interfere with detection of Korotkoff sounds and lead to erroneous values.

> ### Box 14-2 Advantages of Ambulatory BP Monitoring (ABPM)
>
> - It measures BP multiple times during a predefined time period, and more accurately reflects the continuous nature of BP as a hemodynamic variable
> - It measures BP in the normal environment while awake and during sleep
> - It takes into account transient stress-induced elevations in BP
> - It evaluates alterations in the 24-hour circadian patterns of BP
> - It can be used to assess the efficacy of antihypertensive medications over a 24-hour period

The inclusion of R-wave gating synchronizes the Korotkoff sounds with the electrocardiographic waveforms. Although this may increase accuracy, ambient noise may continue to be a problem. Adding electrocardiograph (ECG) leads and microphones, which may slip during monitoring, limits the use of these technologies in children. Oscillometry is used most frequently, and BP is measured using a similar technique to that in standard oscillometric BP equipment. The major technical limitation oscillometry is movement artifact. Nonetheless, using oscillometric monitors programmed to measure BP two to three times an hour for 24 hours is tolerated in children, with the most common complaint being sleep disruption. Wake and sleep periods are usually determined by patient diaries, which may be subject to recall inaccuracy but are preferable to arbitrary wake-sleep definitions.

The physician predetermines the timing and frequency of measurement of BP during ABPM. Multiple time intervals may be identified with a different frequency of BP

Figure 14-2 Normal ambulatory BP monitoring (ABPM) pattern in an 11-year-old female. The graph shows the systolic and diastolic BP tracing for the 24-hour monitoring period. BP (in mmHg) is shown on the vertical axis and time of day is shown on the horizontal axis. The solid horizontal lines within the graph show the age- and size-specific 95th percentile for both wake and sleep periods. The mean wake BP is below the 95th percentile by Task Force criteria, and the BP loads are close to zero.

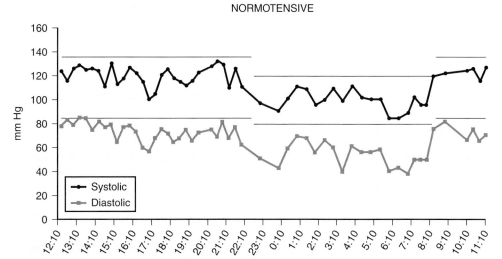

measurement for each interval. Typically, measurements are programmed for every 20 minutes during wake periods and every 30–60 minutes during the expected sleep periods. Assuming an 8-hour sleep period with every 30-minute BP measurements, 60 BP measurements should be made for each 24-hour period. However, errors during attempted measurements may reduce the number of successful readings. Error control within the monitors allows for a single additional attempt 3 minutes after a failed reading. From the raw data generated from the 24-hour ABPM, more specific analyses may be performed. The most basic is calculation of the mean BP values. Mean BP can be determined for the entire 24-hour period, or independently for wake and sleep periods. In addition to mean values, BP load can be calculated, which is the percentage of BP readings for a given time period that exceeds the 95th percentile of normal for the individual patient.

NORMATIVE BP VALUES IN CHILDREN

History of the Task Force on High BP in Children

Incorporation of BP measurement into routine pediatric examinations, and the publication of the Task Force national norms for BP in children[16,24,25] enabled the detection of significant asymptomatic secondary hypertension and also confirmed the suspicion that mild elevations in BP during childhood and adolescence were more common than previously recognized. The report of the Second Task Force for BP Control in Children and Adolescents provided additional data that described the distribution of BP values in over 70,000 normal children.[25] These reports provide the foundation for virtually all current research and clinical practice in the evaluation of pediatric hypertension.

Height percentile, gender, and age are now incorporated in calculating normative percentile values for BP in children (see Table 14-1). The addition of height percentiles recognizes the fact that the relative degree of maturity and/or physical stature of a child within a chronological year increment may have substantial effects on BP. In fact, the difference in the 95th percentile of BP between children at the 5th percentile of height compared to the 95th percentile is consistently 8–9 mmHg. This wide difference based on height has obvious practical clinical implications for the diagnosis of hypertension in children. Conversely, there are no normative standards that account for weight or body mass index (BMI) in children because increased BMI is considered to be a pathological state associated with increased cardiovascular risk. As such, pediatric patients get 'credit' for being taller, but not for being heavier.

Controversies in Determining Diastolic BP (DBP) in Children (K4 versus K5)

The reliability of the measurement of DBP is an important issue in the evaluation of BP in children. Whether to use the K4 (muffling of the Korotkoff sounds) or the K5 sound (disappearance of Korotkoff sounds) to define the auscultatory DBP is controversial. This affects the prevalence of DBP hypertension. Sinaiko et al. compared K4 with K5 in 19,274 children aged 10–15 years, and found that the K4–K5 difference was 5–10 mmHg in 20%, 11–20 mmHg in 11%, and greater than 21 mmHg in 3% of the children.[12,13] In this study, the choice of K4 or K5 to define DBP changed the prevalence for significant DBP hypertension by 2–3%. Biro et al. performed a cross-sectional analysis of BP from 2379 nine-year-old children in the National Heart, Lung, and Blood Institute Growth and Health Study (NGHS).[2] Of the 159 subjects potentially classified with elevated DBP, 60% would be classified differently depending on whether K4 or K5 was used to define elevated DBP. Thus, the choice of the onset of K4 or K5 for determining DBP in children may have important implications for comparing studies and determining the relative prevalence of systolic blood pressure (SBP) and diastolic blood pressure (DBP) hypertension. Nonetheless, the current standard for defining DBP in children is K5, and the BP tables provided in the Task Force Report use K5 to define the 90th and 95th percentile for DBP.

DEFINITION OF HYPERTENSION

Task Force Definition

The 2nd Task Force developed definitions based on the distribution of BP in healthy children, as well as clinical experience and consensus. Normal BP is defined as SBP and DBP less than the 90th percentile for age and sex. High-normal BP is defined as average SBP or DBP greater than or equal to the 90th percentile, but less than the 95th percentile. Hypertension is defined as average SBP or DBP greater than or equal to the 95th percentile for age and sex measured on at least three separate occasions. Elevated BP must be confirmed on repeated visits before characterizing an individual as having hypertension. This is because BP at the high levels tends to fall on subsequent measurement as the result of: (1) an accommodation effect; and (2) regression to the mean. A more precise characterization of an individual's BP level is an average of multiple BP measurements taken for weeks to months. According to the Task Report, with repeated measurement of BP, only about 1% of children and adolescents will be found to have hypertension.

Despite the importance of the Task Force normative data in furthering our understanding of the epidemiology of hypertension in children, the Task Force definition of hypertension has important conceptual limitations and weaknesses. The upper BP limit of normotension has been chosen somewhat arbitrarily as above the 95th percentile of the population distribution. This threshold limit of normality is statistical rather than functional and has not as yet been validated by association with outcomes. The widely quoted threshold of normality of 140/90 mmHg in adults is based on the association between BP values that exceed this threshold and subsequent morbidity and/or mortality. These associations are difficult to establish in children because morbid events such as stroke, myocardial infarction, and congestive heart failure are rare, except in the most severe cases of secondary hypertension. Hypertension defined by the Task Force criteria has not been found to be highly predictive of end-organ injury during childhood. As a result, there are few data to support early pharmacological treatment in children with borderline or moderate casual BP elevation. Furthermore, no longitudinal studies in children have investigated whether normalization of casual BP to less than the 95th percentile prevents or reverses end-organ injury.

Ambulatory BP Definition

The most important limitation of casual BP measurements relates to our conceptualization of BP as a hemodynamic variable. The percentile values traditionally used to define pediatric hypertension are generated from a single set of casual measurements in the school or from large population screenings. BP is not a static but a continuous variable that changes not only from year to year, but also from minute to minute. As a result, casual BP provides only a brief snapshot of the entire 24-hour circadian BP pattern. This circadian pattern may be altered in a number of ways that cannot be captured by intermittent daytime casual BP measurements, even when repeated on several occasions. In addition, some patients may repetitively manifest a transient, stress response when BP is measured in the presence of a medical professional ('White Coat hypertension'). This phenomenon may cause over-diagnosis of hypertension and lead to unnecessarily aggressive and costly diagnostic studies and treatment. The advantages of ABPM are listed in Box 14-2. Critical to the interpretation of ABPM data is the availability of normative data against which ABPM results may be compared. Task Force BP data are derived exclusively from awake casual BP measurements and therefore are of limited utility for interpretation of ABPM data. The largest multicenter study to date from Soergel et al. involved 1141 healthy children stratified by height to

---

> ### Box 14-3 Increasing Importance of Systolic Hypertension
>
> - Mild to moderate SBP elevation is associated with increased left ventricular mass
> - SBP is more closely linked to left ventricular morphology than DBP
> - Increased LVM is associated with SBP, even when SBP falls in the 'normal' range

establish the 50th, 90th and 95th percentile for 24-hour, day and night mean BP by ABPM.[14] These normative data provide better guidance in children for what constitutes not only daytime ambulatory hypertension, but also nighttime and 24-hour hypertension.

Systolic Versus Diastolic BP

In adults, the paradigm of essential hypertension has shifted to an emphasis on SBP because SBP hypertension in older patients is more common, is a marker for vascular disease, predicts cardiovascular morbidity and mortality and, when treated, results in decreased morbidity and mortality. In children and adolescents, data supporting a similar pattern of disease are emerging.[15,21] SBP hypertension is more common in children, whether examining an unselected sampling of patients by routine screening or a selected sampling of referred hypertensive patients. Evidence in children suggests that even mild to moderate BP elevation is associated with increased left ventricular mass (LVM), and that SBP appears to be more closely linked to left ventricular morphology than DBP. This association persists even when controlling for other variables such as age and body habitus. Among patients with hypertension by conventional definition, the reported prevalence of left ventricular hypertrophy (LVH) defined by pediatric standards ranges from 30 to 70%, and is more closely related to SBP than to DBP. Furthermore, increased LVM has been associated with SBP even in patients whose SBP falls within the 'normal' range. These data indicate that SBP hypertension in children should be considered to be of primary prognostic significance. This assertion has practical implications. The treatment of hypertension should be directed at the normalization of SBP, even when DBP is within the normal range. Trials of antihypertensive medications in children should incorporate SBP hypertension into the study inclusion criteria. Future pediatric studies should be aimed at demonstrating regression of LVM with effective treatment of both SBP and DBP elevation, and at prevention of cardiovascular morbidity by early initiation of such treatment.

PREVALENCE OF HYPERTENSION

The overall prevalence of pediatric hypertension is uncertain, but appears to be increasing. One of the earliest and largest studies was by Silverberg et al. in 1975, who performed BP screening on over 15,000 Canadian children.[11] BP was measured at a single visit with hypertension defined as BP greater than 140/90 mmHg. Using these criteria, the prevalence of hypertension was found to be 6.1% for SBP and 1.8% for DBP. Fixler et al. published the results of a similar screening program in the United States using the same definition of hypertension, but added two subsequent sets of BP measurements in the children found to be hypertensive on initial screening.[7] The overall prevalence of hypertension was lower after follow-up measurements, decreasing from approximately 9% initially to less than 2% by the third set of measurements.

The reliance on adult definitions rather than on currently accepted pediatric definitions from the Task Force data makes the validity of these earlier studies uncertain. By definition, the prevalence of hypertension in children should approximate 5% as the threshold for diagnosing hypertension is values that exceed the 95th percentile. However, the Task Force normative values are based on a single set of measurements. As recommended in the Task Force report, elevated BP must be confirmed on repeated visits before characterizing an individual as having hypertension. According to the Task Force estimates, with repeated measurement of BP using measurement techniques standardized for children, about 1% of children and adolescents will be found to have hypertension. A study by Sinaiko et al. in 1989 reported the prevalence of hypertension in approximately 15,000 school children using the age and gender-specific percentile values from the Task Force.[12] In contrast to the previous studies, the prevalence of hypertension after two sets of measurements on different visits was 0.3% for SBP and 0.8% for DBP. These low estimates must be balanced against the observation that the epidemiology of cardiovascular risk factors in children is changing for the worse. In the US, the prevalence of obesity among children has increased from 5 to 11% in national surveys from the 1960s to the 1990s.[8] Current estimates of the prevalence of obesity among school-aged children are even higher.[4] As the Task Force data were collected in the 1970s and 1980s, the current pediatric 95th percentile would almost certainly be higher than in previous decades. Recent studies place the prevalence of hypertension much higher than previously reported, particularly among ethnic minority adolescents.[9] Sorof et al. reported an estimated prevalence of hypertension of 9.5% after three sets of screenings in an urban public school system, in conjunction with a prevalence of obesity of 23%.[19] Thus, the current prevalence of pediatric hypertension, although still uncertain, is likely to be far greater than the 1% quoted in the most recent Task Force reports.

DIAGNOSTIC APPROACH TO HYPERTENSION

Differential Diagnosis

The complete differential diagnosis for persistent hypertension in children can be extensive. However, the more common causes of hypertension in children may be categorized into a few broad categories. As the potential cause of hypertension in children is often age-dependent, the differential diagnosis can be further narrowed simply by focusing on diagnoses consistent with the age of the patient (Table 14-2). As a general rule, the younger the patient and the more severe the hypertension, the more likely it is that a secondary cause for the hypertension is present. When the index of suspicion is very high for an underlying cause, an exhaustive evaluation may be necessary, and primary hypertension would be diagnosed by exclusion. However, an extensive and invasive battery of diagnostic studies is not always indicated or appropriate for every patient whether or not a secondary cause is suspected.

In hypertensive newborns and infants, an indwelling umbilical artery catheter during the perinatal period is virtually pathognomonic for a thromboembolic event via

Table 14-2   Causes of Pediatric Hypertension by Age Group

Age Group	Causes
Newborn/infants	Renal parenchymal infarct from umbilical artery catheter
	Prematurity with chronic lung disease
	Renal artery or vein thrombosis
	Coarctation of aorta
1 to 6 years	Renal parenchymal scarring from urinary tract infection
	Coarctation of aorta
	Renal artery stenosis
	Glomerular diseases (e.g., glomerulonephritis, nephrotic syndrome)
6 to 12 years	Glomerular diseases
	Renal parenchymal scarring from urinary tract infection
	Renal artery stenosis
	Primary hypertension
	Chronic renal failure
>12 years	Primary hypertension
	Glomerular diseases
	Chronic renal failure

the renal artery as the cause of hypertension. While basic renal function studies and a renal ultrasound would be indicated, further imaging studies in this age group are not useful as they are too insensitive to detect small infarcts caused by an indwelling umbilical catheter. Furthermore, the majority of these children will normalize their BP with age. Older children and adolescents with borderline or mild hypertension and known hypertension risk factors such as obesity may require minimal diagnostic evaluation prior to the diagnosis of primary hypertension. Thus, the extent to which a diagnostic evaluation should be aggressively pursued is highly dependent on the clinical context and on the clinical acumen of the treating physician.

Most hypertensive children have mild to moderate BP elevation and can be evaluated and treated on an outpatient basis. However, children with severe hypertension (defined as >20 mmHg above the 95th percentile) may require an inpatient evaluation. When symptomatic hypertension is present, as evidenced by severe headache, neurological changes, or congestive heart failure, an evaluation in the intensive care unit is prudent until the BP can be adequately controlled. A sub-specialist experienced in the evaluation of hypertensive children may best direct

a complete diagnostic evaluation. Figure 14-3 provides a very basic overview of how a focused diagnostic evaluation for hypertension might be directed based on: (1) clues from the history, physical examination, and preliminary evaluation; (2) suspected diagnoses based on those clues; and (3) diagnostic studies that might be considered based on the suspected diagnoses. Although other diagnoses are also possible and may ultimately need to be considered, the majority of hypertensive children will fall into one of these categories.

For all patients, a careful medical history and physical examination is critical. Whenever possible, documentation of previous BP values should be sought to determine whether the hypertension is acute or chronic. The medical history should include the neonatal history specifically regarding umbilical artery catheterization. A history of urinary tract infection(s) may suggest renal scarring secondary to reflux nephropathy and/or pyelonephritis. Symptoms suggestive of glomerulonephritis such as a recent history of pharyngitis, gross hematuria, edema, unusual rashes, or arthralgias may direct attention to a glomerular basis for the hypertension. The physical examination should include attention to demeanor, wet cold palms, and heart rate to determine

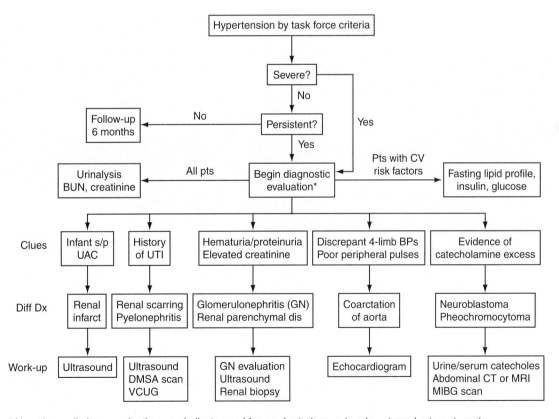

* Negative preliminary evaluation may indicate need for renal arteriogram to rule-out renal artery stenosis

Figure 14-3 Algorithm for the evaluation of an uncomplicated hypertensive patient. CV = cardiovascular; MIBG = meta-iodobenzylguanidine; Persistent = hypertension confirmed on at least three separate occasions; SEVERE = BP more than 20 mmHg above the 95th percentile; UAC = umbilical artery catheter; UTI = urinary tract infection; VCUG = voiding cystourethrogram.

Box 14-4 Syndromes Associated with Hypertension

Cushing's syndrome	Hyperthyroidism
Adrenal hyperplasia	Pheochromocytoma
Liddle's syndrome	Cohn's syndrome
Neurofibromatosis	Williams' syndrome

---

whether the patient has evidence of excessive anxiety. The neck should be examined to detect thyromegaly. The cardiovascular examination should include careful auscultation for murmurs, as well as palpation of femoral pulses and four-extremity BP measurement for possible coarctation of the aorta. The abdomen should be auscultated for bruits and palpated for masses. Rashes, arthritis, or peripheral edema would suggest a systemic disease with associated glomerulonephritis. Syndromes associated with hypertension are summarized in Box 14-4.

The least invasive and most cost-effective strategy for the evaluation of children with elevated BP is a staged diagnostic approach. The first step should be to follow the Task Force recommendation of three BP measurements on three different occasions at least 1 week apart. This recommendation is based in part on epidemiological studies showing that most children with elevated BP on an initial measurement will normalize with repeated measurements. In the absence of severe hypertension (i.e., >99th percentile or symptomatic), no further evaluation need be undertaken unless persistent hypertension is confirmed in clinic. Once a diagnosis of hypertension is confirmed by repeated BP measurements exceeding the 95th percentile, decisions must be made on further evaluation and treatment.

Most children and adolescents with BP levels at or just greater than the 95th percentile for their age and sex are overweight and have family histories of hypertension. For these, careful histories and physical examination are most important. They require few diagnostic tests other than a urinalysis and blood profiles to examine blood urea nitrogen and serum creatinine concentrations. An abnormal lipid profile is a cardiovascular risk factor that may be associated with hypertension in children. A lipid profile may provide useful information because many overweight children and adolescents with hypertension may have elevated triglycerides and low-density lipoprotein (LDL) cholesterol levels with low levels of high-density lipoprotein (HDL) cholesterol.

ABPM and 'White Coat Hypertension'

ABPM has increasingly become part of the initial evaluation at many pediatric centers, especially those with a large number of hypertension patient referrals. From the raw data generated from the 24-hour ABPM, detailed analyses may be performed to determine whether a patient is hypertensive in a non-medical setting. The most basic analysis is calculation of the mean BP values. Mean BP can be determined for the entire 24-hour period, or independently for wake and sleep periods. Hypertension may be defined as mean 24-hour BP exceeding the 95th percentile of mean ambulatory BP in children, or by separately comparing wake and sleep periods with normative values. Further analysis may include calculation of the BP load (percentage of BP readings for a given time period that exceeds the 95th percentile of normal for the individual patient). In hypertensive children, an elevated mean 24-hour SBP in combination with a SBP load greater than 50% was found to be associated with a prevalence of LVH of 47%, as compared to 10% when both criteria were not met.[18]

If both mean BP and BP load are in the normal range, 'White Coat hypertension' is diagnosed and no further diagnostic evaluation may be necessary at that time. In studies of adults with casual BP elevation, the reported prevalence of White Coat hypertension by ABPM is 20–60%. In the largest pediatric study to date, Sorof et al. found that the frequency of White Coat hypertension was 35% (40/115) for all patients, and 22% (11/51) for those with hypertension confirmed in the clinic prior to performing ABPM.[17,20] While these results suggest that the phenomenon of White Coat hypertension does occur commonly in children, it should be emphasized that it might not be an entirely benign condition, and in fact may represent a pre-hypertensive state. In adults, 37% of patients with White Coat hypertension developed persistent hypertension over a period of 6 months to 6.5 years.[26] There are currently no data available on the long-term follow-up of children with White Coat hypertension on initial assessment. Further research may determine whether early diagnosis of this condition in children allows early intervention to prevent the development of persistent hypertension and its sequelae.[6]

When hypertension is confirmed by ABPM, further evaluation should be tailored to the individual patient, depending on the patient's age, severity of hypertension, and associated risk factors (obesity, family history of hypertensions African-American ethnicity).[20] It is appropriate to consult with a physician experienced in childhood hypertension for children in whom further testing for underlying causes of hypertension is indicated to determine the type and extent of diagnostic testing necessary for a given child. Based on the determination of whether the hypertension is primary (essential) or secondary, specific targeted therapies may be appropriate.

Evaluation of Secondary Hypertension

Children and adolescents with DBP and SBP well above the 95th percentile frequently have an underlying cause of hypertension. The diagnostic evaluation may

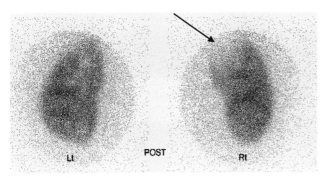

Figure 14-4   Dimercaptosuccinic acid (DMSA) renal scan showing renal scarring from pyelonephritis.

include various types of renal imaging studies, as secondary hypertension in children is most commonly due to underlying renal or renovascular pathology. A renal ultrasound may be useful as an initial non-invasive screening study to detect gross structural abnormalities and/or asymmetry between kidneys. When renal parenchymal injury causing unregulated overproduction of renin is suspected based on a previous history of urinary tract infections or by ultrasound abnormalities, a dimercaptosuccinic acid (DMSA) renal scan to detect focal functional defects consistent with renal scarring is often necessary (Figure 14-4). If a scar is detected, a voiding cystourethrogram to detect vesicoureteral reflux as the mechanism for scar formation is warranted. Among children with secondary hypertension, renal artery stenosis is relatively common, usually due to fibromuscular dysplasia (Figure 14-5). The only consistently reliable diagnostic study to diagnose renal artery stenosis is renal arteriography. Arteriography is often performed only after more non-invasive studies have failed to reveal the cause of hypertension. However, in patients with diseases that predispose to arteriopathy such as neurofibromatosis, arteriography is indicated early in the diagnostic evaluation. Sending a blood sample to centers capable of

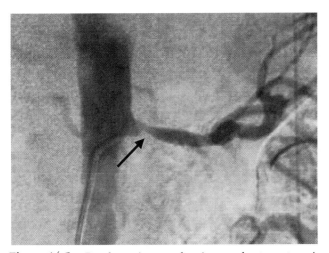

Figure 14-5   Renal arteriogram showing renal artery stenosis (arrow) secondary to fibromuscular dysplasia.

performing the genetic testing can now identify genetic types of hypertension, such as glucocorticoid-remediable aldosteronism.

Assessment for End-Organ Injury

Severe hypertension in children is associated with significant risk of short-term morbidity and mortality. In one of the earliest studies published in 1967, Still et al. described the morbidity and mortality of severe hypertension in children with 55 patients with DBP greater than 120 mmHg and cardiomegaly by examination or LVH by electrocardiography.[23] The presenting signs were papilledema in 36%, seizures in 22%, and facial palsy in 6%. The mortality rate was 56%. A more recent study systematically investigated 88 children with mild to moderate hypertension (either SBP or DBP greater than the 90th percentile) for evidence of target organ injury.[6] Retinopathy was found in 50% of patients, glomerular hyperfiltration in 49%, and LVH in 36%. These recent data suggest that target organ injury does occur in children with even moderate BP elevation.

Since morbid cardiovascular events are rare in the majority of hypertensive children, attention has focused on other markers of hypertensive injury such as increased left ventricular mass index (LVMI) and the presence of LVH. Studies of normal and hypertensive children have found that systolic BP and LVMI are positively associated across a wide range of BP values, with no clear BP threshold to predict pathologically increased LVMI. A recent multicenter study of LVH of 115 hypertensive children with a mean age of approximately 14 years found that the prevalence of LVH was 38% by pediatric criteria and 16% by adult criteria (consistent with severe LVH).[5] Thus, hypertensive sequelae in the form of cardiac remodeling appears to occur early in the course of disease well before the onset of clinical morbidity or mortality.

For these reasons, it can be argued that the assessment of a hypertensive child should include an echocardiogram to detect elevated LVMI and/or the presence of LVH. The protocol for measuring LVM, indexing to height, and determining the thresholds for defining LVH has been described.[18] If echocardiography reveals normal LVMI and ambulatory BP falls within the normal range, expectant care with a prolonged trial of non-pharmacological management may be recommended. Conversely, when ambulatory hypertension is confirmed and/or LVH is diagnosed, the echocardiographic findings may indicate the need for pharmacological therapy.

TREATMENT

One of the most difficult issues in the care of children with elevated casual BP is determining whether to initiate anti-hypertensive medication. Although the presence of elevated BP in children represents a cardiovascular risk factor, BP values of hypertensive children tend to normalize with repeated measurements over time without pharmacological treatment.[3] In addition, BP in children is inherently variable as evidenced by the greater than 75% prevalence of White Coat hypertension reported in children with persistent mild to moderate casual BP elevation.[26] These observations must be balanced against the accumulating body of evidence that children with cardiovascular risk factors suffer target organ injury relatively early in their disease course that may be reversible or preventable with appropriate intervention. The decisions regarding treatment are most difficult when the patient is an otherwise healthy adolescent with mild to moderate hypertension and some combination of the cardiovascular disease risk factors such as obesity, a family history of hypertension, and an ethnic predisposition to hypertensive disease.

Non-Pharmacological Treatment

Since the majority of children with primary hypertension are also overweight, the focus of non-pharmacological therapy in them has been on weight loss and exercise. The positive effect of weight loss on BP in children has been demonstrated in several uncontrolled interventional studies. The only controlled study was performed by Rocchini et al., who randomized overweight adolescents to three interventions over a 20-week period, namely diet alone, diet plus exercise, and control (no intervention). Changes in SBP from baseline in the diet plus exercise group, diet alone group, and control group were −16 mmHg, −10 mmHg, and +4 mmHg, respectively.[1,10] This study provides the most definitive evidence that weight loss – particularly in conjunction with exercise – can be beneficial in the treatment of obesity hypertension in children. However, the long-term benefits of weight loss on BP remain to be defined as it is unknown whether the decline of BP observed during acute weight loss is maintained.

Pharmacological Treatment

Although anti-hypertensive medications have been studied extensively in adults and used widely in children, until recently no anti-hypertensive medications had been approved for use in children under 12 years of age in the United States due to a lack of randomized controlled clinical trials. As a result, the pharmacological management of childhood hypertension had been based mainly on data from adult studies. To address this issue, the US Food and Drug Administration Modernization Act of 1997 offered extension of marketing exclusivity in return for approved clinical trials of medications with pediatric indication. This legislation has resulted in a significant increase in pediatric trials of anti-hypertensive medications. Recently completed or ongoing trials of anti-hypertensive medications have included virtually all classes of drugs, such as beta-blockers, calcium channel blockers, ACE inhibitors, and angiotensin II receptor blockers (ARB). At present, the results of only one of these studies on the combination drug bisoprolol fumarate/ hydrochlorothiazide (B/HT), consisting of a selective β-1 adrenoceptor blocking agent and hydrochlorothiazide (HCTZ), has been published. This randomized, double-blind, placebo-controlled trial in 94 randomized subjects showed that B/HT induced significant reductions compared to placebo for SBP (9.3 versus 4.9 mmHg; $p < 0.05$) and DBP (7.2 versus 2.7 mmHg; $p < 0.05$).[22] The preliminary results from other trials of drugs such as enalapril, lisinopril, losartan, and amlodipine have all shown efficacy for lowering BP with side-effect profiles comparable to placebo. Thus, there is good evidence that the same drugs that are effective in hypertensive adults are also effective in children.

The choice of drug as first-line therapy remains uncertain, and may depend on the etiology of the hypertension. Many causes of secondary hypertension in children are related to overproduction of renin and may thus be particularly responsive to the effects of ACE inhibitors or ARB medications. There are currently no data available to support a particular class of drug for the treatment of primary hypertension in children. Recent trials in hypertensive adults suggest superiority of ACE inhibitors over the conventional first-line therapies of beta-blockers and thiazides for the prevention of hypertension-related morbidity and mortality; the applicability of these studies to the treatment of children remains to be demonstrated. For the pharmacological treatment of pediatric hypertension, the choice of drug and the appropriate dosing of that drug is best left to the specialist in consultation with the primary care provider.

CONCLUSIONS

The prevalence and severity of hypertension is increasing in both children and adolescents. These observations suggest that the trend of decreasing cardiovascular disease in adults observed over the past 50 years may be reversed as the current population of hypertensive children and adolescents become adults.[4] Although significant progress has been made with regard to children with hypertension in the definition of hypertension, recognizing that the sequelae of hypertension begin in childhood, and in developing evidence-based guidelines for the pharmacological treatment of hypertension, much remains to be done. Hypertension in childhood should be considered a chronic medical condition that may require long-term treatment. If physicians who care for hypertensive children seek to promote health that extends beyond the traditional pediatric age range, early recognition and intervention for hypertension clearly must begin in childhood.

REFERENCES

1. Berenson GS, Shear CL, Chiang YK, et al. Combined low-dose medication and primary intervention over a 30-month period for sustained high BP in childhood. Am J Med Sci 1990;299:79–86.

2. Biro FM, Daniels SR, Similo SL, et al. Differential classification of BP by fourth and fifth Korotkoff phases in school-aged girls. The National Heart, Lung, and Blood Institute Growth and Health Study. Am J Hypertens 1996;9: 242–247.

3. Blumenthal S, Epps RP, Heavenrich R, et al. Report of the task force on BP control in children. Pediatrics 1977;59: 797–820.

4. Daniels SR. Is there an epidemic of cardiovascular disease on the horizon? J Pediatr 1999;134:665–666.

5. Daniels SR, Kimball TR, Morrison JA, et al. Indexing left ventricular mass to account for differences in body size in children and adolescents without cardiovascular disease. Am J Cardiol 1995;76:699–701.

6. Daniels SR, Meyer RA, Strife CF, et al. Distribution of target-organ abnormalities by race and sex in children with essential hypertension. J Hum Hypertens 1990;4:103–104.

7. Fixler DE, Laird WP, Fitzgerald V, et al. Hypertension screening in schools: results of the Dallas study. Pediatrics 1979;63:32–36.

8. Ogden CL, Troiano RP, Briefel RR, et al. Prevalence of over-weight among preschool children in the United States, 1971 through 1994. Pediatrics 1997;99:E1.

9. Rabinowitz A, Kushner H, Falkner B. Racial differences in BP among urban adolescents. J Adolesc Health 1993;14: 314–318.

10. Rocchini AP, Katch V, Anderson J, et al. BP in obese adolescents: effect of weight loss. Pediatrics 1988;82:16–23.

11. Silverberg DS, Nostrand CV, Juchli B, et al. Screening for hypertension in a high school population. Can Med Assoc J 1975;113:103–108.

12. Sinaiko AR, Gomez-Marin O, Prineas RJ. Prevalence of 'significant' hypertension in junior high school-aged children: the Children and Adolescent BP Program. J Pediatr 1989;114:664–669.

13. Sinaiko AR, Gomez-Marin O, Prineas RJ. Diastolic fourth and fifth phase BP in 10–15-year-old children. The Children and Adolescent BP Program. Am J Epidemiol 1990;132: 647–655.

14. Soergel M, Kirschstein M, Busch C, et al. Oscillometric twenty-four-hour ambulatory BP values in healthy children and adolescents: a multicenter trial including 1141 subjects. J Pediatr 1997;130:178–184.

15. Sorof JM. Systolic hypertension in children: benign or beware? Pediatr Nephrol 2001;16:517–525.

16. Sorof JM, Portman RJ. Ambulatory BP monitoring in the pediatric patient. J Pediatr 2000;136:578–586.

17. Sorof JM, Portman RJ. White Coat Hypertension in children with elevated casual BP. J Pediatr 2000;137:493–497.

18. Sorof JM, Cardwell G, Franco K, et al. Ambulatory BP and left ventricular mass index in hypertensive children. Hypertension 2002;39:903–908.

19. Sorof JM, Hanevold C, Portman RJ, Daniels SR. Left ventricular hypertrophy in hypertensive children: a report from the International Pediatric Hypertension Association. Am J Hypertens 2002;15:31A (abstract).

20. Sorof JM, Poffenbarger T, Franco K, et al. Evaluation of White Coat Hypertension in children: importance of the definitions of normal ambulatory BP and the severity of casual hypertension. Am J Hypertens 2001;14:855–860.

21. Sorof JM, Poffenbarger T, Franco K, et al. Isolated systolic hypertension, obesity, and hyperkinetic hemodynamic states in children. J Pediatr 2202;140:660–666.

22. Sorof JM, Cargo P, Graepel J, et al. β-Blocker/thiazide combination for treatment of hypertensive children: a randomized double-blind, placebo-controlled trial. Pediatr Nephrol 2002;17:345–350.

23. Still JL, Cottom D. Severe hypertension in childhood. Arch Dis Child 1967;42:34–39.

24. Task force on BP control in children: report of the second task force on BP control in children – 1987. Pediatrics 1987;79:1–25.

25. Update on the 1987 Task Force Report on High BP in Children and Adolescents: a working group report from the National High BP Education Program. National High BP Education Program Working Group on Hypertension Control in Children and Adolescents. Pediatrics 1996;98: 649–658.

26. Verdecchia P, Schillaci G, Borgioni C, et al. Identification of subjects with white-coat hypertension and persistently normal ambulatory BP. Blood Press Monit 1996;1:217–222.

CHAPTER 15

Rickets

ANN E. SALERNO, M.D.

LISA J. STATES, M.D. AND

BERNARD S. KAPLAN, M.B., B.Ch.

INTRODUCTION

Bones are dynamic structures with multiple physiologic activities. They are the major repositories for calcium and phosphorus, and have key roles in calcium metabolism and hematopoiesis. The kidney plays a major role in maintaining calcium and phosphorus balance in the bones. Therefore, renal disease can cause major perturbations in bones.

BONE MINERALIZATION

Rickets is caused by disorders that alter vitamin D metabolism, and is characterized by inadequate mineralization of growing bones. Bone development requires appropriate amounts of vitamins, minerals and, in particular, calcium and phosphorus, and the vitamin D hormones. Calcium and phosphorus are needed for the formation of hydroxyapatite crystals that are the mineral building blocks of bone. Bone mineralization occurs by intramembranous and enchondral ossification. In intramembranous ossification, bone is formed directly from bone cells. The cranial and facial bones form by intramembranous ossification. In enchondral ossification, calcified cartilage matrix is remodeled into bone. Enchondral ossification results in longitudinal growth of the bones, and occurs at the physis or epiphyseal cartilagenous growth plate. Tubular, flat, and cuboidal bones are formed by enchondral ossification. The mandible and clavicle develop by both mechanisms. The physis is composed of columns of cartilage cells organized into four parallel zones; these are the resting, proliferating, hypertrophic, and calcifying zones (Box 15-1). Bone remodeling with absorption of osteoid and calcium by

---

Box 15-1   Zones and Activities within the Physis

Resting zone	Little activity
Proliferating zone	Active cartilage cell division
Hypertrophic zone	Maturation
Calcifying zone (zone of provisional calcification)	Formation and mineralization of osteoid matrix

osteoclasts occurs in the adjacent metaphyseal region called the primary spongiosa.

The primary metabolic abnormality in rickets occurs at the zone of provisional calcification of the physis. Diminished calcification of cartilage cell columns, continued osteoid production by osteoblasts and diminished resorption of osteoid and calcium due to impaired osteoclast function results in a widened irregularly calcified physis. The contiguous metaphysis is also affected and manifests as enlargement of the wrists, knees, and rib ends (rachitic rosary). Metaphyseal broadening or 'cupping' results from changes related to stress at sites of ligament attachment, splaying of cartilage cells peripherally and microfracturing of the primary spongiosa by herniation of cartilage into this area. Softening of the bone results in bowing. Evaluation of the metaphyseal–physeal region is essential for the diagnosis of rickets because this is where the most specific abnormality occurs.

RADIOGRAPHIC APPEARANCES OF GROWING BONES

In a normal child, the first three zones of the physis are lucent and the zone of provisional calcification is similar in density to the mature mineralized bone. Abnormalities of mineralization affect the appearance of the zone of provisional calcification. As a result, radiographs of the physis of the growing child have a crucial role in the diagnosis and management of rickets. The plain radiograph is the primary imaging tool for the evaluation of suspected metabolic bone disease due to rickets. Currently, there is no role for computed tomography or nuclear bone scintigraphy in the evaluation of rachitic bone. Magnetic resonance imaging (MRI) is an ideal imaging modality for evaluating cartilaginous structures, but because subtle mineralization is not well seen, MRI has limited usefulness in the evaluation of rickets. In addition, sedation is necessary for most children aged less than 6 years. Ultrasound can be used to identify a metaphyseal fracture in rickets.

The degree of mineralization, the shape of the bone and the appearance of the physis should be noted. Hypomineralization of the skeleton (osteopenia) is a feature, but is not specific for rickets. Radiographically, osteoporosis and osteomalacia resemble osteopenia.

Clinical Pearl

The imaging findings of rickets – whether the cause is nutritional deficiency, medication, or diseases of the liver, kidneys, or gastrointestinal tract – are often indistinguishable.

Clinical Pearl

- Osteopenia is decreased bone mineralization.
- Osteoporosis is normal mineralization of diminished bone mass
- Osteomalacia is diminished mineralization of normal bone mass

---

Choosing the part of the body to image depends on the age of the child, because the rate of longitudinal growth and physiologic activity differs throughout the skeleton. A chest radiograph is useful for detecting abnormal mineralization in the neonate, infant, and young child. Abnormalities of the metaphyseal–physeal region can be seen in the proximal humeri and anterior rib ends. In most children, the wrists and knees are regions of rapid growth and show the most change. Bilateral views of these regions are recommended to help determine if abnormal findings are due to generalized metabolic disease or a unilateral process such as infection or trauma.

Accelerated or delayed bone-age is also a common manifestation of metabolic bone disease. Therefore, the radiograph of the left hand is useful because it not only provides a view of the physeal region of the distal radius and ulna, but also determines the patient's skeletal age. Similarly, in children less than 1 year of age, the knee radiograph evaluates the distal femoral and proximal tibial and fibular physes and also determines skeletal age.

Classic rachitic changes are present after the neonatal period. Radiographs of the long bones reveal widening and irregularity of all the physes as well as 'fraying' and broadening of the metaphyses. The fraying may resemble the appearance of a paintbrush, or be disordered and irregular. In addition, the bones are demineralized and the cortical outlines of the epiphyseal ossification centers become blurred or non-apparent. A chest radiograph shows irregularity of the proximal humeral metaphyses and enlargement and irregularity of the anterior rib ends. In the long bones there is loss of the metaphyseal collar, a straight-edged segment of 1–3 mm in length representing the newly ossified metaphysis.

In ongoing, untreated rickets, deformities due to softening of bone occur as a result of normal stress on the skeleton. Femoral and tibial bowing is most common and is typically seen in the newly crawling or walking child. Children with poor muscle tone may develop genu valgum (knock knees). Findings in the pelvis include coxa vara and protrusio acetabuli. The thorax may develop an hour-glass shape, and there may be postural molding and frontal bossing in the skull.

Radiographs are extremely useful for monitoring the response to therapy for rickets. Treatment with vitamin D results in calcium deposition in the zone of provisional calcification which, when newly repaired, appears as a dense metaphyseal band. These findings are seen

2–3 weeks after the initiation of therapy in children with nutritional rickets, and after 2–3 months in children with renal rickets. Deformities caused by bone softening may persist, even after successful treatment.

VITAMIN D METABOLISM AND CALCIUM HOMEOSTASIS

Vitamin D is essential for the maintenance of adequate levels of calcium and phosphorus in the bones by its actions on the intestine and kidney. In the gut, the vitamin is necessary for active absorption of dietary calcium, while in the renal tubules it stimulates reabsorption of calcium and inhibits reabsorption of phosphorus. Vitamin D deficiency can result from inadequate amounts of dietary vitamin D, inadequate exposure to sunlight, or from disorders affecting the intestine, kidneys, or liver. A lack of adequate calcium intake or metabolism causes abnormalities in bone mineralization.

Cholecalciferol (vitamin D_3) is produced endogenously in the skin by the conversion of 7-dehydrocholesterol to cholecalciferol (vitamin D_3) by ultraviolet radiation. Ergocalciferol (vitamin D_2) is obtained exogenously from the diet and absorbed in the gut. Both vitamin D_2 and D_3 are hydroxylated in the liver to 25-hydroxyvitamin D by the action of microsomal enzymes. 25-Hydroxyvitamin D is then converted in the kidney to 1,25-dihydroxyvitamin D by the enzyme 1-α-hydroxylase. 1,25-Dihydroxyvitamin D is the active form of vitamin D that binds to the vitamin D receptor and activates absorption of calcium and phosphorus from the intestine, and then mobilizes calcium and phosphorus from the bone into the blood. Elevated parathyroid hormone (PTH) levels, hypocalcemia, and hypophosphatemia increase the activity of 1-α-hydroxylase. Hyperparathyroidism also increases bone resorption and distal tubular reabsorption of calcium, thereby increasing the serum calcium concentration.

Clinical Pearl

An understanding of vitamin D metabolism and calcium homeostasis is essential in the evaluation and treatment of the child with rickets.

DIFFERENTIAL DIAGNOSIS OF RICKETS

Once the radiological features of rickets are documented, the etiology must be determined so that the appropriate therapy can be initiated to allow timely bone repair and growth.

Clinical Pearl

Rickets can be caused by nutritional deficiencies, renal disease, hepatic disease and primary bone disorders.

Nutritional Rickets

Inadequate dietary intake of vitamin D is the most common cause of nutritional rickets. Dark-skinned infants who are primarily or exclusively breast-fed are most at risk due to lack of sun exposure and production of endogenous vitamin D as well as insufficient dietary vitamin D. Other groups at risk are children on strict vegan diets that exclude dairy products. Children with malabsorption syndromes such as short gut syndrome, celiac disease, or cystic fibrosis have malabsorption of fat-soluble vitamin D.[12] Many antacids, by decreasing dietary phosphate absorption, can cause rickets. The incidence of rickets has recently increased,[13] this being partly due to an increase in breast-feeding without appropriate vitamin supplementation. In addition, recent efforts to prevent skin cancer such as protective clothing, avoidance of direct sunlight and regular use of sunscreens decrease endogenous vitamin D synthesis in the skin (Box 15-2).

Decreased vitamin D concentration prevents adequate calcium absorption from the intestine, and as a result the serum calcium concentration decreases. In response, PTH levels increase to restore serum calcium. PTH causes increased urinary losses of phosphorus and calcium loss from the bone. Consequently, phosphorus levels decline and the bone matrix breaks down. Alkaline phosphatase activity increases.[12]

The clinical presentation of nutritional rickets in children is variable. This condition most commonly comes to medical attention between 6 and 18 months of age with a failure to thrive and/or skeletal abnormalities, such as bowing of the legs, splaying of the wrists, costochondral beading or fracture. Some may present with developmental delay, hypocalcemia, tetany, weakness, or seizure.[13] Others are diagnosed incidentally by a radiographic finding.

The treatment of nutritional rickets is vitamin D supplementation. Oral ergocalciferol (vitamin D_2) is recommended at a dose of 2000–5000 IU daily for

Box 15-2 Nutritional Causes of Rickets

Vitamin D deficiency	Nutritional deficiency – breast milk
	Decreased sunlight
Malabsorptive disorders	Short gut syndrome, celiac disease, cystic fibrosis
Phosphate depletion	Antacids
	Prematurity
Calcium deficiency	Neonatal hyperalimentation
	Children in Kwa-Zulu, South Africa

6–12 weeks, followed by a maintenance dose of 400 IU daily after bone healing is complete.[19] A large single dose of vitamin D (15,000 μg; 600,000 IU) can also be given.[4] In 4 to 6 weeks, radiographs should be repeated to document bone healing. If bone healing is not complete after several months, other causes of rickets must be looked for.

The recommended daily requirement of vitamin D for the prevention of rickets in infants, children, and adolescents was previously 400 IU (10 μg), but it is now 200 IU.[9] The vitamin D content of human milk is approximately 25 IU/l. Infant formulas contain a minimum of 40 IU per 100 kcal, and a maximum of 100 IU per kcal. Therefore, infants must consume at least 500 ml of formula to receive the recommended 200 IU of vitamin D per day. The AAP recommends that all breast-fed infants who consume less than 500 ml of milk should receive vitamin D supplementation. In addition, all older children or adolescents who do not get regular sun exposure, do not drink at least 500 ml of vitamin D-fortified milk, or do not take a multivitamin preparation should also receive vitamin D supplementation of at least 200 IU daily.[9] The outcome of nutritional rickets is good. Bone healing starts only days after treatment is initiated and progresses over several months. Bony abnormalities may persist for several months or years, and in extreme cases may be permanent.

Congenital Rickets

In-utero causes must be considered when rickets develops in a term infant aged less than 6 months. These include maternal vitamin D deficiency,[17] poorly controlled hyperparathyroidism,[14] renal insufficiency,[1] administration of phosphate enemas during pregnancy, or infants born to mothers who are on strict vegan diets. Nutritional rickets in an otherwise normal infant usually does not become clinically apparent before 6 months of age due to maternally derived prenatal stores of vitamin D. Early presentation of rickets may also occur in term infants with proximal renal tubular acidosis or neonatal obstructive jaundice. Primary hyperparathyroidism[14] and hypophosphatasia[5] can be confused with rickets in this age group.

Prematurity

The increasing number of viable, premature (<32 weeks' gestation), low birth weight (<1500 g) infants has led to an increase in neonatal rickets.[16,20] These infants, who receive total parenteral nutrition (TPN), often have inadequate intake of calcium and phosphorus, and require more calcium than in standard TPN solutions. The term 'osteopenia of prematurity' has been used to categorize these patients, in whom a hypomineralized skeleton is often the only finding of rickets. An early finding of rachitic change is rarefaction

or lucency of the metaphyses and metadiaphyseal regions. The typical metaphyseal findings of irregularity and broadening are not present because these neonates are not weight-bearing and do not grow at a normal rate. After 8 weeks of age, the humeri, knees, wrists, and proximal femurs may show metaphyseal irregularity and growth plate widening. Findings may be seen earlier in a very small or early gestational-age premature infant. Ongoing rickets manifests as acute, and healing fractures most commonly in the ribs and forearms.

RENAL CAUSES OF RICKETS

Hypophosphatemic Disorders

X-linked Hypophosphatemic (XLH) Rickets (Vitamin D-resistant Rickets)

XLH rickets is an X-linked dominant disorder (Box 15-3). It is caused by decreased renal tubular phosphate reabsorption as well as a dysregulation of 1-α-hydroxylase in the proximal convoluted tubule. This results in inappropriately normal or low levels of 1,25-dihydroxyvitamin D for the degree of hypophosphatemia. XLH rickets is the most common inherited hypophosphatemic disorder, and accounts for 80% of familial phosphate wasting.[11] There is complete penetrance of the renal tubular abnormality, with variable clinical expression. Males, females, children, and adults can be affected, although males are usually more severely affected than females. Patients with XLH rickets usually come to medical attention around 18 months of age with progressive

> **Clinical Pearl**
>
> Hypophosphatemic disorders cause the same radiological features of calcium-deficient rickets; however, they are not associated with secondary hyperparathyroidism or increased bone resorption.

Box 15-3 Renal Causes of Rickets

Hypophosphatemic disorders
- X-linked hypophosphatemic rickets (vitamin D-resistant rickets)
- Vitamin D-dependent rickets: types 1 and 2
- Autosomal dominant hypophosphatemic rickets (ADHR)
- Hereditary hypophosphatemic rickets with hypercalciuria (HHRH)
- Fanconi syndrome
- X-linked recessive nephrolithiasis (XRN)[15]
- Tumor induced osteomalacia (TIO)/osteogenic osteomalacia

Chronic renal failure: renal osteodystrophy
Hepatic cause

femoral or tibial bowing. They typically have radiological findings of rickets and osteomalacia, severe skeletal abnormalities, and growth retardation. They may also have bone pain, late dentition, dental abscesses, deafness, craniosynostosis, and Chiari malformation. It is uncommon, however, for them to have the muscle weakness or pain that is associated with acquired hypophosphatemia. With time, patients with XLH rickets – especially those that are poorly controlled – may develop nephrocalcinosis, renal tubular acidosis, end-stage renal failure, hypertension, and hyperparathyroidism.

Serum phosphorus levels are usually less than 2.5 mg/dl (0.8 mmol/l), but serum calcium, PTH and 25-hydroxyvitamin D levels are normal. Alkaline phosphatase activity is elevated. 1,25-Dihydroxyvitamin D (calcitriol) levels are low or inappropriately normal. Stimulators of 1,25-dihydroxyvitamin D synthesis such as low phosphate diets and PTH fail to cause an increase in calcitriol in patients with XLH rickets.[11] Bone biopsies show low-turnover osteomalacia without osteopenia. The candidate gene for this disorder is the *PHEX* gene, or phosphate-regulating gene with homologies to endopeptidases on the X chromosome, [Xp22.1-p21].[8] PHEX encodes for a metalloprotease. The substrate for this enzyme has yet to be identified, and therefore the exact mechanism of this defect is unclear.[11] Interestingly, *PHEX* is not expressed in the kidney. Animal studies have suggested that the defect causing XLH rickets involves an intermediary circulating factor that is involved in mechanisms of cellular transport of phosphate as well as in osteoblast function, and 1-α-hydroxylase activity.

Two different radiographic patterns – type A and type B – are seen in this disorder. In type A, there are rachitic changes in the knees that are out of proportion to those in the wrists; this finding does not occur in any other type of rickets. In type B, there is a modeling defect with short, squat long bones and coarse bone trabeculation of the axial skeleton. This finding is seen predominantly in males, possibly as a reflection of the X-linked inheritance.

The treatment of XLH rickets is not curative, and is associated with long-term complications. The goals of treatment are growth, improvement in bone disease and bowing defects, and in activity limitations. Medical therapy includes frequent and regular oral phosphate salts as well as calcitriol supplements. In infants aged less than 2 years, 250–375 mg of elemental phosphorus given in two to three divided doses and calcitriol 0.25 μg once or twice daily is recommended.[3] Doses should be increased as needed for each individual child under the direction of a pediatric nephrologist.

Monitoring by laboratory studies and radiography is essential to assure appropriate therapy and to minimize side effects. Serum calcium and PTH levels, and urinary calcium and creatinine excretion, should be measured at regular intervals to assess adequate therapy. Serum alkaline phosphatase activity will remain abnormal until adulthood and is not useful in monitoring therapy. Serum phosphorus levels fluctuate throughout the day, and are not always reflective of bone health and parathyroid activity; therefore they should not be used to dictate dose changes. In young infants, laboratory studies should be performed 2 weeks after the initiation of treatment, and then every 3 months thereafter. The goal is to maintain normal serum calcium levels and urinary calcium excretion, without causing secondary hyperparathyroidism.[3] Small incremental changes should be made in doses, and followed by laboratory studies 1 month later. Once appropriate doses are achieved and growth is stable, children should be followed every 4–6 months for the first year and then annually thereafter, depending on the patient's adherence with the regimen. Children should be monitored more frequently again just before the pubertal growth spurt through the duration of puberty until growth ceases. Every 1–2 years, a renal ultrasound investigation should be performed to screen for the development of nephrocalcinosis, and radiographs of the knees should be performed to assess any need for changes in medication dosage.

This regimen has been shown to improve growth, bone density, and deformations. Although controversy persists in the literature regarding the effect of therapy on final adult height, most agree that medical therapy – especially in the first 2 years of life – results in improved outcomes.[3] Therefore, children of affected families who show abnormal serum and urine phosphorus levels and serum alkaline phosphatase activity should be screened in early infancy. Fewer osteotomies to correct bowing defects have been necessary in patients with XLH rickets since calcitriol treatment became widely available.[3]

Nephrocalcinosis can develop as a result of therapy and cause a decline in renal function over time. It has been suggested that nephrocalcinosis is a direct consequence of therapy, as patients who are poorly adherent to phosphate therapy have a decreased incidence of the condition.[22] The pathogenesis of nephrocalcinosis is unclear, and even after adequate treatment some patients still have hypomineralized periosteocytic lesions in bone that have been attributed to an intrinsic osteoblast defect in this condition. Short-term studies suggest that growth hormone therapy, particularly for very short patients, may improve height velocity and final height.[2,21,24]

Vitamin D-dependent Rickets: Types 1 and 2
Vitamin D-Dependent Rickets Type I [VDDR 1]:
1-α-Hydroxylase Deficiency

This condition, which is also known as pseudodeficiency rickets, is an autosomal recessive disorder. It is caused by a mutation in the 1-α-hydroxylase gene that causes impaired 1-α-hydroxylation of 25-hydroxyvitamin D in the renal proximal tubule. The defect is located on chromosome 12q13.3. Infants often present in the first few months of life with muscle weakness, tetany, seizures, and rickets. Serum calcium levels are low, while PTH levels are high and 1,25-dihydroxyvitamin D levels are either low or absent. Serum levels of 25-hydroxyvitamin D are normal or slightly high. The radiographic findings are indistinguishable from those of other forms of rickets. Life-long treatment with 1-α-hydroxyvitamin D (80–100 ng/kg/day) or with 1,25-dihydroxyvitamin D (8–400 ng/kg/day) at physiological doses causes normalization of laboratory values and healing of rickets.[23] Laboratory studies and growth must be monitored closely, however.

Vitamin D-dependent Rickets Type 2: Hereditary Vitamin D-resistant Rickets (HVDRR)

This condition is caused by the autosomal recessive inheritance of a mutation in the vitamin D receptor (VDR) gene (12q12-q14).[6] The defective gene product causes end-organ resistance to active 1,25-dihydroxyvitamin D. These patients are often of Middle Eastern origin. Hypocalcemic symptoms manifest during the first few months of life, and affected children may also have enamel hypoplasia and oligodentia.[12] Laboratory evaluation is characterized by low serum calcium and phosphorus levels, with secondary hyperparathyroidism and elevated 25-hydroxyvitamin D and 1,25-dihydroxyvitamin D levels. Over 50% of the cases are associated with alopecia. Mutations in the hairless gene (HR) cause this phenotype in mouse and humans. These patients require pharmacological doses of vitamin D metabolites, as well as periodic laboratory studies and radiographs to assure appropriate therapy. Some severely affected individuals require intravenous 1,25-dihydroxyvitamin D to overcome the intestinal resistance to large oral doses.[23]

Autosomal Dominant Hypophosphatemic Rickets (ADHR)

This condition may present in childhood or later in adulthood. Although in children it phenotypically resembles XLH rickets, evidence of male-to-male transmission and the phenotypic variability of ADHR distinguishes this disorder from XLH rickets. In addition, the renal phosphate wasting resolves post puberty. The defect has been associated with mutations in fibroblast growth factor (FGF)-23 on chromosome 12p13, although the mechanism of rickets is unclear.[11] As in XLH rickets, the serum phosphorus level is low, urine phosphorus is high, and levels of 1,25-dihydroxyvitamin D are inappropriately low or normal. Patients who present with adult-onset ADHR have osteomalacia with bone pain, weakness, and fractures. Adults do not present with the bony deformities typical of children with this disorder. Dental abscesses are also a feature. Treatment includes phosphate supplements and 1,25-dihydroxyvitamin D.

Hereditary Hypophosphatemic Rickets with Hypercalciuria (HHRH)

This condition is very rare, with only two families with the disorder having been reported. It appears to have autosomal recessive inheritance, although the genetic defect has not been defined. A defect in proximal tubule phosphate reabsorption causes renal phosphate wasting. There is an appropriate increase in 1,25-dihydroxyvitamin D production and thus, increased intestinal absorption of calcium and phosphate, hypercalciuria, and PTH suppression.[11] Chronic hypophosphatemia results in decreased bone mineralization, bone pain, rickets, muscle weakness, and short stature. Calcium levels are usually normal, phosphorus levels are low, and 1,25-dihydroxyvitamin D levels are increased. These patients are treated with daily oral phosphate alone, which corrects laboratory values and clinical features of rickets.

Fanconi Syndrome

This condition is due to a defect in the proximal tubule cells that causes wasting of phosphate, amino acids, glucose, and bicarbonate in the urine. In addition, 1-α-hydroxylation of 25-hydroxyvitamin D in the proximal tubule cells is impaired. As a result, affected children have type II renal tubular acidosis, hypophosphatemia, glycosuria, aminoaciduria, rickets, and growth failure. There may also be associated low molecular-weight proteinuria, polyuria and dehydration, hyponatremia or hypokalemia. Fanconi syndrome may be either idiopathic, or associated with metabolic disorders, recovery from acute renal failure or exogenous medications or toxins. Metabolic disorders associated with Fanconi syndrome include cystinosis, galactosemia, tyrosinemia, hereditary fructose intolerance, as well as mitochondrial disorders. Medications that have been associated with this disorder include azathioprine, cisplatin, gentamicin, ifosfamide, ranitidine, streptozotocin, and valproate, as well as Chinese herbal medicines. Exogenous toxins, such as aminoglycosides, glue sniffing (toluene), Lysol®, and lead and cadmium poisoning are also causes of Fanconi syndrome. Treatment of the rickets caused by Fanconi syndrome involves treatment of the underlying disorder or discontinuation of the offending agent, and maintenance of a normal serum phosphate with phosphate supplementation.

X-Linked Recessive Nephrolithiasis (XRN)

This is an unusual form of the renal Fanconi syndrome with low molecular-weight proteinuria, hypercalciuria with nephrocalcinosis and nephrolithiasis, hypophosphatemic rickets and renal failure. It is caused by mutations affecting a chloride channel expressed throughout renal tubule (CLCN5).[15] The locus is on Xp11.

Osteogenic Osteomalacia (Oncogenous Rickets)

This condition is caused by benign primitive mesenchymal tumors that secrete factors which inhibit proximal renal tubular phosphate reabsorption and impair synthesis of calcitriol. This results in hypophosphatemia that causes rickets or osteomalacia. Surgical removal of these tumors reverses the metabolic and bone abnormalities.

Chronic Renal Failure – Renal Osteodystrophy

Renal osteodystrophy is a syndrome of osteomalacia, rickets, and secondary hyperparathyroidism that develops in children with chronic renal disease (see Chapter 32). Glomerular and tubular dysfunction contributes to the development of this metabolic bone disease. Impaired glomerular function results in phosphorus retention with subsequent hypocalcemia. Tubular injury results in impaired synthesis of 1,25-dihydroxyvitamin D and hypocalcemia. Hyperparathyroidism develops in response to diminished serum calcium concentrations, and causes a variety of manifestations including demineralization of bones. This results in osteomalacia that may be exacerbated by chronic metabolic acidosis, aluminum toxicity, or total parenteral nutrition.[18] The classic features of secondary hyperparathyroidism are subperiosteal resorption, endosteal resorption and osteopenia. Subperiosteal resorption is best seen in the middle phalanges of the fingers, upper medial proximal tibias, medial femoral neck, distal clavicles, distal radius, and ulna, and lamina dura of teeth. The outer cortex has a hazy, ill-defined appearance. Endosteal resorption results in a lacy pattern of the inner cortex, referred to as cortical tunneling. Acro-osteolysis may also occur. Osteomalacia can appear as diminished density, or coarsening of the residual mineralized matrix and trabeculae. An additional feature of hyperparathyroidism is the development of cysts and brown tumors due to hemorrhage in fibrous tissue that has replaced the resorbed bone matrix. Children with renal osteodystrophy are at risk for developing slipped capital femoral epiphysis at a younger age than this is seen in the general population.[10] The therapy of renal osteodystrophy is with supplementation with 1,25-dihydroxyvitamin D and calcium, as well as dietary phosphorus restriction and phosphate binders (see Chapter 34).

Hepatic Causes of Rickets

Hepatic Osteodystrophy

Hepatic osteodystrophy occurs in chronic hepatic disorders in which cholestasis results in decreased bile salt secretion and malabsorption of fat-soluble vitamin D. It is characterized by the typical radiographic findings of rickets, hypocalcemia, elevated alkaline phosphatase activity, and decreased levels of 25-hydroxyvitamin D.

PTH levels are normal. These patients require very high doses of vitamin D to overcome malabsorption: 4000–10,000 IU (100–250 µg) of vitamin D_2, 50 µg of 25-hydroxyvitamin D, or 0.2 µg/kg of 1,25-dihydroxyvitamin D should be given daily with calcium supplementation.[4]

Medications

Altered metabolism of 25-hydroxyvitamin D has been observed in patients taking certain anti-epileptic medications and anti-tuberculous therapy. For example, phenobarbital, primidone, phenytoin, and rifampin accelerate hepatic inactivation of 25-hydroxyvitamin D.[23] Phenytoin causes target end-organ resistance to 1,25-dihydroxyvitamin D, and isoniazid decreases the 25-hydroxylation of vitamin D.[23] If the offending medication cannot be discontinued, vitamin D supplementation in large doses (4000–40,000 IU daily) should be given, together with frequent monitoring of serum calcium levels and radiography.[19]

Osteopetrosis with Rickets

Osteopetrosis is a rare, autosomal recessive disorder characterized by abnormal osteoclast function resulting in failure of resorption of bone. As a result, the bones throughout the skeleton are extremely dense. In some of these patients, despite a positive calcium balance, the calcium phosphorus product in the extracellular fluid is insufficient and rickets develops.[7] There may be widening of the physes, osteopenia, pseudofractures, and widening and cupping of the metaphyses.

DISORDERS THAT CAN BE CONFUSED WITH RICKETS

Primary hyperparathyroidism, hypophosphatasia, osteogenesis imperfecta, non-accidental trauma, and some of the metaphyseal dysplasias may be confused with rickets in children. Close attention to the radiographic findings can be helpful in making the proper diagnosis.

Primary Hyperparathyroidism

This rare disorder in children is usually diagnosed within the first 3 months of life. Radiographs demonstrate osteopenia, subperiosteal bone resorption, and pathologic fractures. Focal lytic lesions may be present. Metaphyseal changes are not a feature of this disorder.

Hypophosphatasia

This uncommon inherited disorder is the result of deficiency of alkaline phosphatase that results in the accumulation of inorganic pyrophosphate.[5] Excess inorganic pyrophosphate results in undermineralized bone with incomplete ossification of cartilage and metaphyseal regions. Calcium accumulation by mature chondrocytes does not occur, causing hypercalcemia and rickets.[4] Hypercalcemia may cause soft tissue calcification and nephrocalcinosis. Radiographs reveal short, irregular long bones with poor ossification. Bowed long bones and fractures are often present. Focal, round, lytic areas in the metaphyses due to clusters of unmineralized osteoid distinguish this disorder from rickets.

Hyperphosphatasia

This autosomal recessive disorder is characterized by extremely elevated levels of bone alkaline phosphatase, normal serum levels of calcium and phosphorus, and growth failure. Osteoid proliferation in the subperiosteal bone results in separation of the periosteum from the bone cortex. This leads to bowing and thickening of the diaphysis and osteopenia. Children present at around 2-3 years of age. The skull is large and the cranium is thickened and may be deformed. The bony texture on radiographs is variable, with dense areas interspersed with radiolucent areas and generalized demineralization. The long bones contain pseudocysts showing a dense bony halo.[4]

Osteogenesis Imperfecta (OI)

This condition is caused by a defect in type II collagen that results in brittle bones. It may present with bowing and fractures. The bones are demineralized, but have normal metaphyses. Broad or gracile long bones and wormian bones in the skull are features of OI that are not seen in rickets. Alkaline phosphatase activity is elevated.

Metaphyseal Chondrodysplasia (Primary Chondrodystrophy)

This type of short-limbed dwarfism is characterized by bowing of the legs, short stature and waddling gait in the absence of abnormalities of serum levels of calcium, phosphorus, alkaline phosphatase or vitamin D metabolites. There are several types, with varying degrees of dysmorphism. The metaphyseal findings of irregularity and flaring with widening of the growth plates resemble rickets. The intact metaphyseal collar distinguishes this from rickets. A full skeletal survey in these patients may show additional findings that are not seen in rickets. There is no effective treatment.

REFERENCES

1. Al-Senan K, Al-Alaiyan S, Al-Abbad A, et al. Imaging casebook: congenital rickets secondary to untreated maternal renal failure. J Perinatol 2001;21:473-475.

2. Baroncelli GI, Bertelloni S, Ceccarelli C, et al. Effect of growth hormone treatment on final height, phosphate metabolism, and bone mineral density in children with X-linked hypophosphatemic rickets. J Pediatr 2001;138:236-243.

3. Carpenter TO. New perspectives on the biology and treatment of X-linked hypophosphatemic rickets. Pediatr Clin North Am 1997;44:444-466.

4. Chesney R. Metabolic bone disease. In: Behrman RE, Kliegman RM (eds), *Nelson Textbook of Pediatrics*, 16th edn. WB Saunders Company, 2000.

5. Currarino GD, Neuhauser EBD, Reyersbach GC, et al. Hypophosphatasia. Am J Roentgenol 1957;78:392-419.

6. Demay M. Inherited defects of vitamin D metabolism. In: Holick MF (ed), *Vitamin D Physiology, Molecular Biology and Clinical Applications*. Nutrition and Health Series (ed. Bendich A). Humana Press, Totowa, NJ, 1999.

7. Di Rocco M., Buoncompagni A, Loy A, et al. Osteopetrorickets: case report. Eur J Pediatr 2000;159:579-581.

8. Drezner MK. PHEX gene and hypophosphatemia. Kidney Int 2000;57:9-18.

9. Gartner LM, Greer FR, et al. New guidelines for vitamin D Intake. Pediatrics 2003;111:908-910.

10. Goldman HB, Lane JM, Salvata E. Slipped capital femoral epiphyses complicating renal dystrophy: a report of three cases. Radiology 1978;126:333-339.

11. Jan De Beur SM, Levine MA. Molecular pathogenesis of hypophosphatemic rickets. J Clin Endocrinol Metab 2002;87:2467-2473.

12. Joiner TA, Foster C, Shope T. The many faces of vitamin D deficiency rickets. Pediatr Rev 2000;21:296-302.

13. Kreiter SR, Schwartz RP, Kirkman HN, et al. Nutritional rickets in African American breast-fed infants. J Pediatr 2000;137:153-157.

14. Landing BH, Kamoshita S. Congenital hyperparathyroidism secondary to maternal hypoparathyroidism. J Pediatr 1970;77:842-847.

15. Langlois V, Bernard C, Scheinman SJ, et al. Clinical features of X-linked nephrolithiasis in childhood. Pediatr Nephrol 1998;12:625-629.

16. Lyon AJ, McIntosh N, Wheeler K, et al. Radiological rickets in extremely low birthweight infants. Pediatr Radiol 1987;17:56-58.

17. Moncrieff H, Fadahunsi T. Congenital rickets due to maternal vitamin D deficiency. Arch Dis Child 1974;49:810-811.

18. Norman ME. Vitamin D in bone disease. Pediatr Clin North Am 1982;229:947-971.

19. Ozauh PO. Planning the treatment of a patient who has rickets. Pediatr Rev 2000;21:286.

20. Roberts L, Badger V. Osteomalacia of very-low-birth-weight infants. J Pediatr Orthop 1984;4:593-598.

21. Saggese G, Baroncelli G, Bertelloni S. Long-term growth hormone treatment in children with renal hypophosphatemic

rickets: effects on growth, mineral metabolism and bone density. J Pediatr 1995;127:395–402.

22. Taylor A, Sherman NH, Norman ME. Nephrocalcinosis in X-linked hypophosphatemia: effect of treatment versus disease. Pediatr Nephrol 1995;9:173–175.

23. Thomas MK, Demay MB. Vitamin D deficiency and disorders of vitamin D metabolism. Endocrinol Metab Clin North Am 2000;29:611–627.

24. Wilson DM, Lee PDH, Morris AH. Growth hormone therapy in hypophosphatemic rickets. Am J Dis Child 1991;145: 1165.

CHAPTER 16

Acute Post-Infectious Glomerulonephritis

PETER D. THOMSON, M.B., B.Ch., F.C.Paed. (SA),

BERNARD S. KAPLAN, M.B., B.Ch., AND

KEVIN E.C. MEYERS, M.B., B.Ch.

> **Clinical Pearl**
>
> *"When the patient dies the kidneys go to the pathologist, but while he lives the urine is ours. The examination of the urine is the most essential part of the physical examination of any patient."* Thomas Addis, 1948[1]

INTRODUCTION

Acute post-streptococcal glomerulonephritis (APSGN) is characterized by sudden onset of combinations of painless gross hematuria, periorbital puffiness, and hypertension with red blood cell casts, evidence of antecedent streptococcal infection and interstitium concentrations.[7] APSGN is the most common cause of acute nephritis in children in developing countries, and continues to occur at a lower prevalence rate, with occasional epidemics, in developed countries. APSGN must be confirmed or excluded before less common causes of acute post-infectious glomerulonephritis in children are considered.

ETIOLOGY

APSGN is caused by β-hemolytic *Streptococcus*, Lancefield Group A. The capsular M-protein defines whether the bacterial strain is rheumatogenic or nephritogenic. Nephritogenic strains are divided into pharyngitis-associated serotypes (1, 3, 4, 12 and 49) and skin infection-associated serotypes (2,49, 55, 57, and 60).[15]

> **Clinical Pearl**
>
> Recurrences of rheumatic fever are common, whereas APSGN rarely reoccurs despite skin infection with associated streptococcal serotypes.

PATHOGENESIS

APSGN is an immunologically mediated disease with antigen–antibody reactions in the circulation or *in situ* in glomeruli.[15,20] These antigen–antibody reactions result in the activation of the complement cascade through the alternative pathway. Complement activation precedes the clinical onset of APSGN. Markedly reduced serum concentrations of C3 and moderately reduced levels of C5 and properdin characterize the hypocomplementemia of APSGN. In addition, the classical complement pathway is frequently activated in patients with APSGN early in the course.[25] Chemotaxis (C5a) and platelet-derived inflammatory mediators are generated. Cellular immunity also has a role. Cytokines participate and amplify the damage.

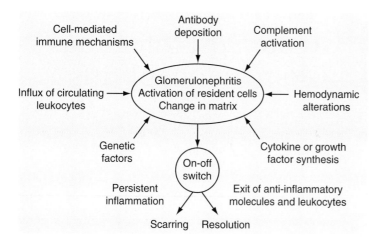

Figure 16-1   Mechanisms of glomerulonephritis. A number of pathogenic mechanisms have been implicated in the induction, resolution and progression of glomerular inflammation. Mechanisms leading to resolution or scarring are not fully elucidated. Their clarification will lead to more specific targeted efficacious therapy. (Reprinted with permission from Hricik DE, Ching-Park M, Sedor JR. Glomerulonephritis. N Engl J Med 1998; 339:889. Copyright © 1998 Massachusetts Medical Society. All rights reserved.)

The major mechanism for resolution of the inflammatory hypercellularity that results from this response is by apoptosis. At least three potential nephritogenic streptococcal antigens are proposed: pre-absorbing antigen; nephritis strain-associated protein (probably streptokinase C); and streptococcal pyrogenic exotoxin B. The latter also activates C3 via the alternative complement pathway. Both streptococcal M proteins and pyrogenic exotoxins can act as superantigens.[5] This can result in T-cell expansion and polyclonal B-cell activation with production of auto-antibodies (Figure 16-1). Streptococcal neuraminidase may be responsible for anti-IgG generation, and may play a role in facilitating the infiltration of the kidney by peripheral blood leukocytes.[6,16]

PATHOLOGY

In APSGN the kidneys are enlarged, with all glomeruli being equally affected by an acute generalized glomerulonephritis. The glomeruli are enlarged with diffuse mesangial cell proliferation and mesangial expansion. Polymorphonuclear neutrophil exudation is more apparent early in the course of the disease. The capillary loops are compressed, but the tubules are mainly unaffected, except for the presence of red blood cell casts. The interstitium is largely spared, although there can be cellular infiltrates. Immunofluorescence studies show fine granular deposits of IgG and C3 along the capillary walls. In some cases, C3 may be present without IgG. The typical electron microscopic findings are subepithelial 'humps', although there may also be intramembranous and even subendothelial deposits early in the course. Glomerular crescents rarely occur in patients with APSGN.

PATHOPHYSIOLOGY

The glomerular filtration rate (GFR) and effective renal plasma flow (ERPF) are decreased during the acute phase

of APSGN, there being a greater reduction in GFR than in ERPF. The resulting renal hyperperfusion normalizes within a year of onset of the disease.[11] There is positive salt and water balance in APSGN (Figure 16-2). Plasma renin activity (PRA) is normal in APSGN, and does not increase after a furosemide challenge.[19] Echocardiographic changes in the acute phase of APSGN show greater left ventricular (LV) internal end-diastolic diameter (LVIDd) (p = 0.022), interventricular septum thickness (IVSd) (p = 0.038), LV mass (LVM) (p = 0.0001), longer early diastolic flow deceleration time (DT) (p = 0.0001), and higher numbers of cases with mitral regurgitation (MR) (p = 0.0001) and pericardial effusion (p = 0.0001) in comparison with the controls. Six to eight weeks later, there is a significant improvement, but the LV posterior wall thickness, IVSd, LV end-diastolic volume, LVM and DT remain greater than in controls. These parameters were influenced by reduced GFR and edema.[13]

CLINICAL FEATURES

Approximately 90% of APSGN cases occur in young children after streptococcal pharyngeal or skin infections. The latency period from infection to presentation is 7–14 days for pharyngeal and 14–21 days for post-impetigo disease. The diagnosis is made in a patient with abnormal urinalysis,[8] evidence of recent streptococcal infection, a positive ASO-titer or anti-DNase B titer, and hypocomplementemia. The disease is usually self-limited, and generally requires only supportive therapy. Resolution occurs over a period of weeks to months. There are usually no permanent sequelae in children. Adults may have a higher incidence of hypertension and chronic renal failure as a result of APSGN (Box 16-1).

The peak incidence of APSGN is in children aged 5 to 15 years. However, APSGN can occur in anyone aged over 2 years. There are a number of possible clinical presentations. The classic presentation is with an acute nephritic syndrome that consists of combinations of gross

Figure 16-2 Fluid and salt balance differences in the acute nephritic and nephrotic syndromes. In health, the intravascular volume (V) is approximately 80 ml/kg and the extracellular fluid (ECF) volume is 200 ml/kg. In the nephrotic state, loss of albumin leads to a fall in intravascular oncotic pressure, resulting in movement of water into the tissues with a consequent contraction of intravascular volume (1) and edema (E). The accumulation of water leads to an expansion of the ECF with consequent weight gain. In the nephritic state, there is an expansion of the intravascular compartment (2) because of water overload as a consequence of a reduction in the glomerular filtration rate. The expansion of the ECF results in tissue edema and hypertension, necessitating treatment with diuretics. (Modified and used with permission from Milford DV. Glomerulonephritis in children. Br J Hosp Med 1995;54(2-3):87–91.)

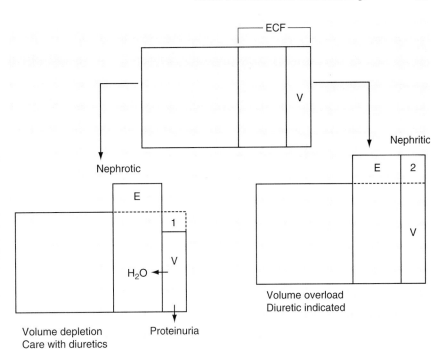

hematuria with red blood cell casts and proteinuria, oligoanuria, hypertension, edema and azotemia. However, the clinical presentation varies from full-blown acute nephritis to predominant nephrotic syndrome to microscopic hematuria with few or only subtle signs. Some patients, with or without abnormal urine, may present with severe hypertension and encephalopathy. Subclinical manifestations are five times more frequent than clinical disease, particularly during epidemics.[21]

The major symptoms are peri-orbital and macroscopic hematuria described as cola- or tea-colored. A third of patients complain of cough, sore throat, fever, and headaches. Nausea, vomiting, anorexia and abdominal pain are less frequent. Oliguria, seizures, and symptoms of congestive cardiac failure occur in less than 20% of

patients. Physical findings include combinations of edema, hypertension, and macroscopic hematuria.

Clinical Pearl

A clinician must examine a fresh urine specimen by microscopy, and not rely on results from a laboratory, where the report seldom mentions red blood cell casts or the presence of dysmorphic red cells.[24]

LABORATORY STUDIES

The urinalysis is positive blood on dipstick. Protein excretion ranges from 1+ positive on the dipstick to many grams per day. Red blood cells, red blood casts, hyaline and granular casts and dysmorphic red blood cells are seen by microscopic examination of the urine sediment. Dysmorphic red blood cells are identified by their small variable size and club-like protrusions that resemble 'mouse ears.'

Abnormal hematological findings include a leukocytosis, thrombocytosis, and anemia in about one-third of cases. The serum creatinine and blood urea nitrogen (BUN) levels are often – but not always – increased. Some patients have combinations of hypoalbuminemia and/or hyponatremia. Hyperkalemia occurs mainly in anuric patients, and these are at greater risk for the development of a major medical emergency in APSGN (Box 16-2).

The ASO titer and anti-DNase B are often elevated unless the patient has been treated with antibiotics.

Box 16-1   Clinical Presentations of Acute Post-Streptococcal Glomerulonephritis (APSGN)

Typical (>90% of cases)	Acute nephritic syndrome with hematuria, edema, and hypertension with/without oliguria.
Rare	Nephrotic syndrome
	Severe acute renal failure with rapidly progressive glomerulonephritis (RPGN)
	Hypertensive encephalopathy with normal urinalysis

Box 16-2 Medical Emergencies in APSGN

- Hyperkalemia
- Hypertensive encephalopathy
- Congestive heart failure

Serum concentrations of C3 are almost always depressed, and C4 is low normal in about 25% of the cases.

Scarlet fever – a major association of APSGN in the past – is rarely associated with APSGN except during epidemics. Pharyngitis-induced APSGN occurs in temperate climates, and is more common in males and children of school-going age. The latent period is shorter than pyoderma-induced APSGN. Pyoderma-induced APSGN occurs in tropical climates, affects the sexes equally, at a younger age, and complicates scabies.[21] These associations are not absolute. The diagnosis of impetigo can be missed in older children whose skin infections may have healed by the time they present with APSGN. APSGN may present in association with other conditions and in a number of unusual ways (Box 16-3). There are several uncommon associations of APSGN, but any patient is at risk for the development of APSGN regardless of the underlying renal disease.

DIAGNOSIS

The ASO titer is a screening test for APSGN. These titers do not rise significantly when antibiotics are used to treat pharyngitis, and are not reliable with post-impetigo glomerulonephritis. Therefore, the anti-DNase B and anti-hyaluronidase titers (Streptozyme test®) should be measured. The anti-DNase B and anti-hyaluronidase titers are more reliable for diagnosing impetigo-induced APSGN. The serum C3 concentration should be measured early in the course of the disease because it usually normalizes 4–8 weeks after onset. It is not necessary to measure serum C4 to diagnose APSGN (Box 16-4).

Box 16-3 Unusual Associations of APSGN

- Acute rheumatic fever
- Henoch–Schönlein purpura
- Thrombocytopenic purpura
- Hemolytic uremic syndrome
- Cerebral vasculitis

Box 16-4 Diagnostic Criteria for APSGN

- Clinical features of acute glomerulonephritis
- Dysmorphic red cells/red cell casts on urine microscopy
- Evidence for recent streptococcal infection:
  - Positive throat culture for β-hemolytic *Streptococcus*; and/or
  - Increased ASO and/or anti-DNase B titers
- Decreased serum C3 concentration
- Normalization of serum C3 concentration within 4–8 weeks after presentation

---

DIFFERENTIAL DIAGNOSIS

The differential diagnosis of APIGN is summarized in Table 16-1. Glomerulonephritides with a predominantly nephritic presentation includes APSGN, IgA nephropathy, Henoch–Schönlein nephritis, and Alport hereditary nephritis. The differential diagnosis of conditions with predominantly nephrotic syndrome presentation includes membranoproliferative glomerulonephritis (MPGN), focal segmental glomerulosclerosis, hepatitis B membranous nephropathy, mesangial proliferative glomerulonephritis, and lupus nephritis. Each of these conditions is discussed in more detail in other chapters of this book.

Clinical Pearl

A renal biopsy is indicated to exclude MPGN if:
- Proteinuria >1 g per day persists for more than 4 weeks
- Or, if the serum C3 does not normalize in 6 weeks
- Or, if renal dysfunction persists for more than 2 weeks

COMPLICATIONS

Hypertension is mainly, but not entirely, the result of intravascular volume expansion. Therefore, some children with minimal signs of volume overload may also have severe hypertension. Some patients may present with pulmonary edema, minimal urinary sediment changes, and variable increases in blood pressure. Central nervous system complications usually occur in the context of salt and water retention with severe hypertension. Rapid changes in blood pressure, as a result of dysregulation of the blood–brain barrier may cause posterior leukoencephalopathy and cerebral edema.[9] This may result in encephalopathy with headaches, confusion and even

Table 16-1   Causes of Post-Infectious Glomerulonephritis

Organism	Syndrome	Pathology
Viral		
Hepatitis B	Nephrotic-nephritic	Membranous; MPGN; polyarteritis nodosa
Hepatitis C	Nephritic-nephrotic	MPGN; membranous; IgA nephropathy
HIV	Nephrotic	FSGS, interstitial nephritis
Bacterial		
Post-streptococcal	Nephritic; rarely rapidly progressive GN	Acute exudative GN; crescentic GN
Infective endocarditis	Nephritic-nephrotic	MPGN; focal proliferative GN
Staph. aureus, Staph. viridans		

FSGS = focal segmental glomerulosclerosis; GN = glomerulonephritis; MPGN = membranoproliferative glomerulonephritis.

seizures that may be prevented by prompt control of hypertension.[10] Although T2-weighted magnetic resonance images characteristically show diffuse hyperintensity that selectively involves the parieto-occipital white matter, the gray matter occasionally may also be involved. These findings are sometimes confused with the findings of a vasculitis, but can be rapidly reversed with control of the hypertension. However, cerebral vasculitis does occur in rare cases of APSGN.[14]

TREATMENT

The decreasing incidence of APSGN may be due to widespread use of antibiotics, improvement in socio-economic or healthcare status, and urbanization. The standard 10-day course of penicillin therapy may not be the best therapeutic choice for treatment of streptococcal pharyngitis, and shorter courses of a cephalosporin may be preferable.[17] Penicillin eradicates the causative organism but is not used for prophylaxis. Bed rest is seldom required unless there is cardiac failure. The patient must be weighed at least once a day, blood pressures must be recorded frequently, and salt, potassium and fluids are restricted if there is oliguria. Protein is only restricted when the BUN is elevated and should not be reduced below 0.3 g/kg/day. A diet high in carbohydrates is provided for energy. Patients with APSGN seldom require dialysis unless there is severe acute renal failure. An urgent biopsy is indicated if a rapidly progressive glomerulonephritis (RPGN) with crescents is suspected.

Furosemide is used to manage hypertension and fluid overload. The initial dose is 0.5 mg/kg/dose, but if increased dosage is used with subsequent dosages, none of them should exceed 5 mg/kg/dose. Although this diuretic may reduce the length of hospital stay, there is the danger of sudden intravascular volume depletion. Nifedipine can be given in a dose of 0.1 to 0.3 mg/kg/dose orally

2 to 8 hourly as required for severe hypertension. It is prudent to start with the lowest dose. If hypertension appears to be established, a longer-acting calcium channel blocker such as amlodipine (2.5–10 mg daily or in two divided doses) or a β-blocker, such as atenolol can be given. A peripheral α-blocker (vasodilator) such as prazosin or doxazosin can be given if the hypertension is severe or difficult to control. ACE inhibitors can be given to patients who are nephrotic (Ramipril®; 0.3 mg/kg/day in two divided doses). It is important to monitor the serum potassium level when ACE inhibitors are used in patients with reduced renal function. There is usually no indication for corticosteroids or other immunosuppressives. If the patient has RPGN, methylprednisolone should be given as a single intravenous dose of 500 mg/m^2/day for 3 days. Oral prednisone can then be given at 2 mg/kg/day and tapered as clinically indicated (Box 16-5).

PROGNOSIS

Most patients with APSGN recover within 6 weeks, with return of renal function.[18] Some continue to have microscopic hematuria for as long as 5 years, but despite this the majority show progressive healing and a good long-term prognosis.[12,24] In the recovery phase, orthostatic proteinuria is common, and therefore an early

Box 16-5   Indications for Admission of APSGN to Hospital

- Hyperkalemia
- Hypertension
- Seizures
- Oliguria
- Congestive heart failure

morning urine protein:creatinine ratio is the best way to assess significant proteinuria. Recurrent episodes of APSGN are extremely uncommon.[23] Patients with crescentic RPGN have a potential to scar formation, and therefore a biopsy may be required in the first 2 weeks so that aggressive immunosuppressive therapy can be started.[4] The prognosis of acute APSGN is generally excellent, and few patients in developed countries progress to end-stage renal failure. A minority of patients develops progressive scarring after many years.[2] For example, APSGN is the second most frequent reason for renal transplantation in black South African children.[22] Fewer than 5% of patients studied for 5 to 17 years after recovery have hypertension and proteinuria. However, although the serum creatinine concentrations are usually normal in long-term studies, there may be reduced renal functional reserve.[3] Rapidly progressive glomerulonephritis with glomerular crescents is associated with a greater likelihood of progression to end-stage renal failure.

REFERENCES

1. Addis T. *Glomerulonephritis. Diagnosis and Treatment*. MacMillan, New York, 1948, p. 2.

2. Baldwin DS, Gluck MC, Schacht RG, et al. The long-term course of poststreptococcal glomerulonephritis. Ann Intern Med 1974;80:342-358.

3. Cleper R, Davidovitz M, Halevi R, Eisenstein B. Renal functional reserve after acute poststreptococcal glomerulonephritis. Pediatr Nephrol 1997;11:473-476.

4. Cole BR, Salinas-Madrigal L. Acute proliferative glomerulonephritis and crescentic glomerulonephritis. In: Barratt TM, et al. (eds), *Pediatric Nephrology*, 4th edn. Lippincott, Williams & Wilkins, Baltimore, 1999, pp. 669-689.

5. Couser WG, Johnson RJ. Postinfectious glomerulonephritis. In: Neilson EG, Couser WG (eds), *Immunologic Renal Diseases*. Lippincott-Raven, Philadelphia, 1997, pp. 915-943.

6. Cu GA, Mezzano S, Bannan JD, et al. Immunohistochemical and serological evidence for the role of streptococcal proteinase in acute post-streptococcal glomerulonephritis. Kidney Int. 1998;54:819-826.

7. Falk RJ, Jennette JC, Nachman PH. Primary glomerular disease. In: Brenner BM (ed), *Brenner and Rector's: The Kidney*, 6th edn. WB Saunders, Philadelphia, 2000, vol. 2, pp. 1263-1349.

8. Fogazzi GB, Ponticelli C, Ritz E. *The Urinary Sediment: An Integrated View*, 2nd edn. Oxford University Press, New York, 1999, pp. 30-31.

9. Froehlich T, Sandifer S, Varma PK, Testa F. Two cases of hypertension-induced reversible posterior leukoencephalopathy syndrome secondary to glomerulonephritis. Curr Opin Pediatr 1999;11:512-516.

10. Garg RK. Posterior leukoencephalopathy syndrome. Postgrad Med J 2001;77:24-28.

11. Herthelius M, Berg U. Renal function during and after childhood acute poststreptococcal glomerulonephritis. Pediatr Nephrol 1999;13:907-911.

12. Hinglais N, Garcia-Torres R, Kleinknecht D. Long-term prognosis in acute glomerulonephritis. Am J Med 1974; 56:52-60.

13. Jankauskiene A, Jakutovic M, Cerniauskiene V, et al. Echocardiographic findings in children ill with acute postinfectious glomerulonephritis. Eur J Pediatr 2003;162: 500-505.

14. Kaplan RA, Zwick DL, Hellerstein S, et al. Cerebral vasculitis in acute post-streptococcal glomerulonephritis. Pediatr Nephrol 1993;7:194-195.

15. Khandke KM, Fairwell T, Manjula BN. Difference in the structural features of streptococcal M proteins from nephritogenic and rheumatogenic serotypes. J Exp Med 1987;166:151-162.

16. Marin C, Mosquera J, Rodríguez-Iturbe B. Histological evidence of neuraminidase activity in acute nephritis: desialized leukocytes infiltrate the kidney in acute post-streptococcal glomerulonephritis. Clin Nephrol 1997;47: 217-221.

17. Pichichero ME, Casey JR, Mayes T, et al. Penicillin failure in streptococcal tonsillopharyngitis: causes and remedies. Pediatr Infect Dis J 2000;19:917-923.

18. Popovic-Rolovic M, Kostic M, Antic-Peco A, et al. Medium- and long-term prognosis of patients with acute poststreptococcal glomerulonephritis. Nephron 1991;58:393-399.

19. Powell HR, McCredie DA, Rotenberg E. Response to furosemide in acute renal failure: dissociation of renin and diuretic responses. Clin Nephrol 1980;14:55-59.

20. Rodriguez-Iturbe B. Postinfectious glomerulonephritis. Am J Kidney Dis 2000;35:XLVI-XLVIII.

21. Sarkissian A, Papazzian M, Azatian G, et al. An epidemic of acute postinfectious glomerulonephritis in Armenia. Arch Dis Child 1997;77:342-344.

22. Thomson PD. Renal problems in black South African children. Pediatr Nephrol 1997;11:508-512.

23. Watanabe T, Yoshizawa N. Recurrence of acute post-streptococcal glomerulonephritis. Pediatr Nephrol 2001;16:598-600.

24. White RHR. The investigation of haematuria. Arch Dis Child 1989;64:159-165.

25. Wyatt RJ, Forristal J, West CD, et al. Complement profiles in acute post-streptococcal glomerulonephritis. Pediatr Nephrol 1988;2:219-223.

CHAPTER *17*

IgA Nephropathy

BERNARD S. KAPLAN, M.B., B.Ch.

INTRODUCTION

Primary immunoglobulin A nephropathy (IgA N) is an immune-complex-mediated glomerulonephritis which is characterized by glomerular mesangial IgA deposits and several different histopathologic lesions that usually cause microscopic hematuria or recurrent macroscopic hematuria. Primary IgA N is an important cause of chronic renal disease and end-stage renal failure (ESRF). The diagnosis requires a kidney biopsy, and the biopsy must be studied by immunofluorescence techniques. It is important to bear in mind the highly variable nature of IgA N.

Clinical Pearl

IgA nephropathy (IgA N) was first described by Berger and Hinglais in 1968.
It may be the most common type of primary glomerulo-nephritis in the world.
Henoch–Schönlein purpura nephritis may be the systemic form of the primary IgA N.

EPIDEMIOLOGY

IgA N is uncommon under the age of 3 years, but all ages are affected. Males are affected more often than females; IgA N occurs more often in whites and Asians than in blacks. The incidence of IgA N in the pediatric age group is unknown. IgA N aggregates in some families.[7] IgA nephropathy is the most common form of primary glomerulonephritis in children and adults in Japan. Almost 70% of patients have microscopic hematuria or asymptomatic proteinuria. The prevalence of the disease varies widely from one country to another, and may comprise between 2% to 40% of all primary glomerular diseases. Prevalence rates also vary within the United States, where the overall rates are 2–10% compared with 38% in New Mexico Native Americans.[8] Differences within and among countries may be due to kidney biopsy criteria, environmental and genetic factors (Boxes 17-1 and 17-2).

ETIOLOGY OF IgA N

The cause/causes of IgA N are unknown, and no causative infectious agent has been found. There is an inconstant association with certain human lymphocyte antigens (HLA). The ethnic variation in prevalence,

---

Box 17-1 Incidence of IgA N in Japan[10]

- 4.5 cases each year per 100,000 children aged between 6 and 15 years
- 20 cases detected in 17 years

Box 17-2 IgA N is a Variable Disease

- Variable incidence
- Variable clinical presentation
- Variable indications for kidney biopsy
- Variable renal histopathology
- Variable treatment
- Variable outcomes

familial clustering, and subclinical renal abnormalities among relatives of IgA N cases, suggest a genetic component. Among 30 multiplex IgA N kindreds, 60% had linkage of IgA N to 6q22-23; the mode of transmission is autosomal dominant with incomplete penetrance.[7]

Clinical Pearl

Some 35% of IgA N patients have biopsy-proven recurrence after transplant.
Younger patients are more prone to the risk of recurrence.
Recurrence did not affect the ten-year graft survival.[10]
IgA deposits in a donor kidney disappear when it is transplanted into a recipient with end-stage renal disease.

PATHOGENESIS

The glomerular deposits of IgA consist of the IgA1 subclass that is produced in plasma cells in the gastrointestinal tract, respiratory tract, bone marrow, lymph nodes, and spleen. No antigens have been identified. Mucosal immunity is decreased in patients with IgA N,[2] and in some patients there is increased production of IgA1 in the bone marrow.[4] An abnormality in the IgA molecule may be required for IgA N to occur, because increased production of IgA is not sufficient to produce the disease.[1] The galactosylation of serum IgA1 and in IgA1 eluted from nephrectomy specimens of patients with IgA N is defective. Mesangial cells have a receptor for IgA1 that may be specific for undergalactosylated IgA1, and incubation of IgA1 from normal individuals with β-galactosidase increases its binding to human mesangial cells.[3]

The deposition of IgA1 in the kidney triggers the production of cytokines and growth factors (including transforming growth factor β1; TGF-β1) by mesangial and inflammatory cells, and this leads to mesangial cell proliferation and extracellular matrix deposition. The activation of TGF-β1 may be one of the common pathways that results in glomerulosclerosis, interstitial fibrosis, and tubular atrophy.[15]

PATHOLOGY

The light microscopy findings of IgA N are not specific. The most common alteration is focal or diffuse cellular and matrix expansion of the mesangium. Additional alterations include diffuse endocapillary proliferation, focal segmental sclerosis, segmental necrosis, and epithelial crescents. Immunofluorescence studies that show predominant deposition of IgA are required to establish a definitive diagnosis of IgA N. The IgA deposits are mainly in the mesangium, with focal perimesangial or subendothelial extensions. IgM, IgG, C3, lambda light chain, and kappa light chain may also be detected. Electron-dense deposits are also seen mainly in mesangium.

Tubulointerstitial changes may include interstitial fibrosis, tubular atrophy, interstitial or inflammation, and vascular sclerosis. Red blood cell casts and proteinaceous casts may be seen in the tubules.

There are no specific guidelines for a kidney biopsy in an asymptomatic patient with IgA N. However, a biopsy is indicated in all patients with combinations of unexplained macroscopic hematuria with red blood cell casts, proteinuria in excess of 1 g per 24 hours, clinical features of the nephrotic syndrome, and azotemia. The indications for performing a biopsy on a patient with microscopic hematuria with or without red blood cell casts vary among pediatric nephrologists within and among centers and countries. The indications for carrying out a biopsy on a patient with proteinuria of <1 g per 24 hours also vary considerably.

CLINICAL FEATURES

The clinical presentation of IgA N is variable (Box 17-3), and depends to a large degree on the level of suspicion of the nephrologists and the criteria for performing a kidney biopsy. In Japan, almost 70% of patients with IgA N have microscopic hematuria or asymptomatic proteinuria.[14] IgA N is first suspected in patients with gross

Box 17-3 Variable Clinical Manifestations of IgA N

- Microscopic hematuria
- Macroscopic hematuria
- Recurrent episodes of macroscopic hematuria
- Macroscopic hematuria with nephrotic syndrome
- Acute renal failure
- 'Malignant' IgA nephropathy with loin pain
- Chronic renal failure

hematuria and red blood cell casts. However, many patients have no obvious symptoms, and IgA N is suspected only after the finding of a positive dipstick test for blood during routine screening of the urine. Nonetheless, IgA N can present in several different ways.

Recurrent episodes of macroscopic hematuria may be triggered by an upper respiratory tract infection. Progression to ESRF within 4 years was reported in patients who presented with macroscopic hematuria, loin pain, persistent microscopic hematuria, and crescents in renal biopsies. The term 'malignant' IgA nephropathy was used to characterize this subset of patients.[5] Some asymptomatic patients present with microscopic hematuria and variable amounts of proteinuria.

Up to 20% of patients with IgA N can present with chronic renal failure, many without a clear history of previous renal disease.

LABORATORY INVESTIGATIONS

The urine must be tested with a dipstick for protein and blood. Examination of the spun urinary sediment for red blood cells and red blood cell casts is essential. The excretion of protein must be quantified by an early morning specimen of urine, or in a 24-hour urine collection. The serum creatinine and cholesterol concentrations may be either normal or elevated, while the serum albumin concentration may be decreased. The hemogram shows no particular changes. Serum complement levels are normal. Although the serum IgA and fibronectin concentrations may be elevated, little useful information is gained by measuring them.

OUTCOME

There are many difficulties in interpreting the published results of long-term outcomes of patients with IgA N (Box 17-4). IgA nephropathy is characterized by a variable course that ranges from a benign to rapidly progressive renal failure to chronic progressive renal failure. The reported incidence of end-stage renal disease in adult patients with IgA N varies from 15% to 40%, but this condition may appear up to 20 years after the initial diagnosis of the IgA N. In the United States, predicted kidney survival from the time of apparent onset was 94% at 5 years, 87% at 15 years, and 70% at 20 years. Unfortunately, follow-up data were available in only 40 of 103 patients more than 10 years from the time of diagnosis.[11]

Despite certain caveats, poor prognostic features for renal survival are hypertension, elevated serum creatinine at the time of diagnosis, severity of renal histological findings, persistent proteinuria of >1 g per 24 hours,

Box 17-4 Difficulties in the Interpretation of Long-Term Follow-up Data for IgA N

- Ascertainment of initial cases
- Indications for kidney biopsy
- Loss of cases for follow-up

and black race.[11] Age at clinical onset, gender, and ACE I polymorphisms are not associated with a poor outcome. Patients with familial IgA N have a worse outcome.[7]

Clinical Pearl

- Prognostic indicators are weak on a case-by-case basis for most patients.
- Overall prognosis may be better than suggested in the literature because patients with mild asymptomatic hematuria are often not biopsied and are frequently not included in published articles.

TREATMENT

There is no accepted treatment of IgA N, and most of the proposed regimens are controversial.[12] Reports of a favorable effect of tonsillectomy on long-term renal survival in patients with IgA N need to be substantiated before this can be recommended for all patients with this disease.[13] An attempt to produce evidence-based recommendations offers the following approaches to treatment.[6]

1. Patients with proteinuria over 3 g per day, mild glomerular changes, and preserved renal function (creatinine clearance >70 ml/min) should be treated with prednisone. Steroids reduce proteinuria (grade B recommendation) and stabilize kidney function (grade C). The combination of cyclophosphamide, dipyridamole and warfarin should not be used (grade A), nor should cyclosporine A (grade B).
2. Patients with progressive disease (creatinine clearance <0 ml/min) should be treated with fish oil (grade B). Use of fish oil is not supported by another evidence-based survey.[9]
3. Patients with proteinuria and hematuria and recurrent tonsillitis may benefit from a tonsillectomy (grade D).
4. Patients with hypertension should be treated with an angiotensin-converting enzyme (ACE) inhibitor (grade B).

It may be prudent to treat patients with active glomerular disease (macroscopic hematuria with proteinuria, azotemia and histological findings of diffuse proliferative glomerulonephritis) with corticosteroids and an ACE inhibitor. Advice should also be given about strategies for renal protection (see Chapter 33).

From about 5 years after renal transplantation, IgA N recurs in 20–60% of renal grafts, regardless of the source of the kidney. This is not, however, a contraindication to kidney transplantation.

DIFFERENTIAL DIAGNOSIS

The differential diagnosis of IgA N can be divided into clinical diagnoses and histopathological diagnoses. Clinical conditions that can present with microscopic hematuria, and which must be distinguished from IgA N, are thin glomerular basement membrane disease, Alport hereditary nephritis, and membranoproliferative glomerulonephritis. The renal biopsy findings can easily differentiate IgA N from these other conditions because of the presence of IgA in the mesangium.

However, mesangial IgA is seen in Henoch–Schönlein purpura nephritis. Secondary causes of mesangial IgA deposition are uncommon in children.

REFERENCES

1. Allen AC, Bailey EM, Brenchley PE, et al. Mesangial IgA1 in IgA nephropathy exhibits aberrant O-glycosylation: observations in three patients. Kidney Int 2001;60:969–973.

2. Bene MC, Faure GC. Mesangial IgA in IgA nephropathy arises from the mucosa. Am J Kidney Dis 1988;12:406–409.

3. Julian BA, Tomana M, Novak J, et al. Progress in the pathogenesis of IgA nephropathy. Adv Nephrol Necker Hosp 1999;29:53–72.

4. Layward L, Allen AC, Hattersley JM, et al. Elevation of IgA in IgA nephropathy is localized in the serum and not saliva and is restricted to the IgA1 subclass. Nephrol Dial Transplant 1993;8:25–28.

5. Nicholls K, Walker RG, Dowling JP, et al. 'Malignant' IgA nephropathy. Am J Kidney Dis 1985;5:42–46.

6. Nolin L, Courteau M. Management of IgA nephropathy: evidence-based recommendations. Kidney Int Suppl 1999;70:S56–S62.

7. Schena FP, Cerullo G, Rossini M, et al. Increased risk of end-stage renal disease in familial IgA nephropathy. J Am Soc Nephrol 2002;13:453–460.

8. Smith SM, Tung KS. Incidence of IgA-related nephritides in American Indians in New Mexico. Hum Pathol 1985;16: 181–184.

9. Strippoli GF, Manno C, Schena FP. An 'evidence-based' survey of therapeutic options for IgA nephropathy: assessment and criticism. Am J Kidney Dis 2003;41:1129–1139.

10. Utsunomiya Y, Koda T, Kado T, et al. Incidence of pediatric IgA nephropathy. Pediatr Nephrol 2003;18:511–515.

11. Wyatt RJ, Kritchevsky SB, Woodford SY, et al. IgA nephropathy: long-term prognosis for pediatric patients. J Pediatr 1995;127:913–919.

12. Wyatt RJ, Hogg RJ. Evidence-based assessment of treatment options for children with IgA nephropathies. Pediatr Nephrol 2001;16:156–167.

13. Xie Y, Nishi S, Ueno M, et al. The efficacy of tonsillectomy on long-term renal survival in patients with IgA nephropathy. Kidney Int 2003;63:1861–1867.

14. Yoshikawa N, Tanaka R, Iijima K. Pathophysiology and treatment of IgA nephropathy in children. Pediatr Nephrol 2001;16:446–457.

15. Yoshioka K, Takemura T, Murakami K, et al. Transforming growth factor-beta protein and mRNA in glomeruli in normal and diseased human kidneys. Lab Invest 1993;68: 154–163.

SUGGESTED READING

Donadio JV, Grande JP. IgA nephropathy. N Engl J Med 2002;5347:738–748.

CHAPTER 18

Henoch–Schönlein Purpura Nephritis

BERNARD S. KAPLAN, M.B., B.Ch.

Clinical Pearl

- Henoch–Schönlein purpura nephritis and IgA nephropathy are related diseases.
- Both can occur consecutively in the same patient.
- Both can occur simultaneously in identical twins.
- Henoch–Schönlein purpura nephritis and IgA nephropathy have identical pathological and biological abnormalities.
- Clinically silent, but histologically detectable IgA deposits, are found in skin and gastrointestinal biopsies of IgA nephropathy patients.

INTRODUCTION

Some 200 years ago, William Heberden described a 5-year-old boy with a skin rash, macroscopic hematuria, abdominal pain, bloody stools, arthralgia, and edema. Forty-six years later, Schönlein called this condition *purpura rubra.* Henoch later added abdominal colic, bloody diarrhea, and hemorrhagic nephritis to the features of the syndrome.[13]

Henoch–Schönlein purpura (HSP) is defined as a vasculitis with predominantly IgA deposits in the walls of small vessels in the skin, gastrointestinal tract, and kidney, associated with arthralgias or arthritis.[6,7,13,18] The leukocytoclastic vasculitis of HSP with inflammation and necrosis of small vessels is the most common type of systemic vasculitis in children. HSP is also known as anaphylactoid purpura, leukocytoclastic vasculitis, allergic vasculitis, and rarely, as rheumatoid purpura. It is generally a benign, self-limited disorder that follows an intercurrent illness, usually of the upper respiratory tract. The spectrum of the clinical expression of HSP may vary from a minimal petechial rash to severe gastrointestinal, renal, neurological, pulmonary, and joint disease (Box 18-1). Most children have self-limited disease. Systemic involvement or serious sequelae are infrequent on long-term follow-up.[31]

EPIDEMIOLOGY

The peak incidence of HSP occurs in the first and second decades of life, with 90% of patients aged less than 10 years. The male to female ratio is 2:1. HSP is uncommon in blacks. The incidence in children varies

Box 18-1 The Dominant Features of HSP in 100 Cases[29]	
Cutaneous purpura	100%
Arthritis	82%
Abdominal pain	63%
Gastrointestinal bleeding	33%
Nephritis	40%

Box 18-2   Possible Causes of HSP

Infections:	Parvovirus B19, hepatitis B virus, hepatitis C virus, human immunodeficiency virus, *Streptococcus* species, *Salmonella* species, *Shigella* species, *Staphylococcus aureus*
Medications:	Antibiotics, angiotensin-converting enzyme (ACE) inhibitors, angiotensin II receptor antagonists, non-steroidal anti-inflammatory agents
Toxins:	Vaccinations, insect bites, food allergy

from country to country and among different populations within a country,[12] and is highest in the fall and winter.

ETIOLOGY

Although there is often a history of a recent or simultaneous upper respiratory tract infection, no consistent causative organism is found. Virtually every known pathogen has been implicated, usually circumstantially, as a trigger for HSP (Box 18-2).

PATHOGENESIS OF HSP NEPHRITIS[6,7]

The pathogenesis of HSP nephritis (HSP N) is similar to that of IgA nephropathy (Box 18-3). No major biological differences are found between the two illnesses, except for a larger size of circulating IgA-containing complexes (IgA-CC) and a greater incidence of elevated plasma IgE concentrations in HSP N. A role for more potent activation of the leukocytes by IgA-CC and/or

Box 18-3   Immunologic Abnormalities in HSPN

- Increased serum IgA1 concentrations
- Increased IgA1-containing circulating immune complexes
- Positive IgA-rheumatoid factor
- Polymeric IgA1 deposited in the mesangium
- Abnormal hinge region of IgA1 molecule
- Decreased IgA1 galactosylation correlates with nephritis
- Abnormal O-glycosylation of mesangial IgA1 in IgA N

circulating chemokines in HSP N may occur because tissue infiltration by leukocytes is a major feature of HSP N vasculitis. Deposits of abnormal IgA1 in the mesangium trigger many mediators of inflammation that modulate the disease activity including the alternate complement pathway, interleukin (IL)-1, IL-6, platelet-derived growth factor, tumor necrosis factor, free-oxygen radicals, vascular cell adhesion molecule-1, and membrane attack complex (C5b-9).

PATHOLOGY[9]

Renal Pathology

HSP is characterized by predominant deposits of IgA in the mesangium. The major histopathologic changes are an endocapillary glomerulonephritis, but the findings on renal biopsy vary among patients, and also within and among glomeruli. The classical features of HSP N include neutrophil infiltration in glomeruli, nuclear fragmentation (karyorrhexis), and areas of necrosis. Necrotizing glomerular lesions, diffuse endocapillary proliferation, and fibrin deposits are seen in HSP N more often than in IgA N, and glomerular crescents occur in more than 50% of cases. Immunofluorescence microscopy demonstrates mesangial deposits of IgA, polymeric IgA1, and inconsistent staining for IgA in glomerular capillary walls. Glomerular fibrin deposits are frequently seen, but detection of glomerular deposits of IgG, IgM, C3, and alternative complement pathway components is more variable.

Ultrastructural findings include mesangial electron-dense deposits, subepithelial and subendothelial deposits.

Skin Pathology

Capillaries and venules of the dermis are affected by a leukocytoclastic vasculitis with vessel wall necrosis and perivascular accumulation of polymorphonuclear leukocytes and mononuclear cells. Immunofluorescence microscopy is positive for IgA, C3c, and fibrin/fibrinogen in small vessels and connective tissue in the purpuric lesions.[9,10,13]

CLINICAL FEATURES

The prevalence of each of the clinical features depends on the center from which they are reported. Initial signs of HSP N reported from pediatric nephrology centers[16] were hematuria and proteinuria in 50%, acute nephritic syndrome in 8%, nephrotic syndrome in 13%, and nephritic/nephrotic syndrome in 29% of patients.

Rash

By definition, the rash occurs in 100% of children with HSP N. These lesions start as red macules that pass through an urticarial phase to become purpuric papules. The urticaria is typically non-blanching. In some cases, purpuric papules – usually on the ankles – enlarge and become confluent areas that may break down to form necrotic ulcers. The rash is symmetrical and starts on the lower extremities, but it can occur on many parts of the body including the buttocks, abdomen, elbows, genitalia, face, and ears. Discrete areas of edema can occur over the forehead, feet, hands, and scalp. The rash may last for days to weeks and may recur, in some cases, once or many times, even 10 years after the first episode.

Joints

Joint involvement varies from mild arthralgia to severe, debilitating arthritis with swelling and redness. Larger joints such as ankles, knees, and wrists are usually affected. Swelling of the feet may be so severe that the patient is incapable of walking.

Gastrointestinal

Gastrointestinal involvement occurs in two-thirds of children with HSP, and usually manifests with colicky abdominal pain associated with combinations of nausea, vomiting, bloody stool, and upper gastrointestinal bleeding.[19] Abdominal symptoms precede the appearance of the rash in as many as 36% of patients. The abdominal symptoms may mimic an acute surgical abdomen and result in unnecessary laparotomy.[3] However, major complications of abdominal involvement develop in up to 14% of patients. Intussusception is the most common, most serious, and often the most difficult to diagnose gastrointestinal problem. The investigation of choice is ultrasonography. Infrequent complications are bowel

Box 18-4 Patterns of Renal Involvement in HSP N

- Microscopic hematuria
- Microscopic hematuria with minimal proteinuria
- Macroscopic hematuria – single or multiple episodes
- Acute nephritis – single or multiple episodes
- Acute nephritis with nephrotic syndrome
- Acute renal failure[20]
- Acute hypertension without apparent renal disease[8]
- Chronic renal failure

ischemia, infarction, perforation, fistula formation, late ileal stricture, acute appendicitis, pancreatitis, gallbladder hydrops, and pseudomembranous colitis. Occasionally there can be massive upper or lower gastrointestinal hemorrhage, but bleeding tends to be self-limiting with frank blood or melena in half the patents.

Renal Disease

Renal involvement varies from trivial microscopic hematuria to acute renal failure (Box 18-4).[1] Nephritis occurs in up to 40% of patients, and fewer than 10% are under 2 years of age. In 90% of patients the renal manifestations occur within the first month of onset of HSP, rarely manifest before the other features of the syndrome, and may be delayed for weeks after the onset of the other components.

Scrotum and Testis

Involvement of the scrotum and testis occurs in 30% of cases. This may mimic torsion of the testis and *very* rarely be a cause of torsion.[5]

LABORATORY STUDIES

The diagnosis of leukocytoclastic vasculitis is confirmed, if in doubt, by a skin biopsy. Depending on the patient's history, a complete blood cell count, serum chemistries, blood urea nitrogen (BUN), serum creatinine and albumin, blood cultures, cryoglobulins, rheumatoid factor, antinuclear antibody, autoantibodies to neutrophilic cytoplasmic antigens and serum complement values may be checked. The urine must be tested by dipstick, and the spun sediment must be examined by microscopy for red blood cell casts and red blood cells if the test is positive for blood. The urine protein excretion must be quantified if the dipstick shows more than 1+ protein. In general, the indication for a kidney biopsy is a 24-hour urine protein excretion of >1.0–1.5 g.

Every patient with severe abdominal pain must be examined, at a minimum, by ultrasonography to rule out an intussusception.

Clinical Pearl

- The platelet count is normal or increased in HSP.[11]
- The serum albumin concentration may be decreased as a result of nephrotic syndrome or protein-losing enteropathy.[27]

DIFFERENTIAL DIAGNOSIS

Systemic lupus erythematosus (SLE) should be considered, although it is usually not difficult to differentiate HSP N from SLE. The renal histopathologic findings are similar in HSP N and IgA N. Although pulmonary involvement rarely occurs in HSP, a diagnosis of Wegener granulomatosis must be considered in patients with pulmonary changes (Box 18-5) or atypical vasculitic skin eruptions. A differential diagnosis of purpuric rashes is listed in Box 18-6. Consideration of these is especially important in atypical cases of HSP N. Acute infantile hemorrhagic edema is a cutaneous leukocytoclastic vasculitis characterized by the symptom triad of fever, large purpuric skin lesions, and edema. The clinical picture has a violent onset, a short benign course, and spontaneous complete recovery.[2] Patients with meningococcemia can have a purpuric rash, with renal, lung, gastrointestinal and central nervous system impairment.[25] Hypersensitivity vasculitis and HSP are similar, but separable, clinical syndromes.[22] Major differences are the occurrence of low serum C3 concentrations and histopathologic findings of membranoproliferative glomerulonephritis in hypersensitivity vasculitis (Box 18-7). Unusual variants of post-streptococcal glomerulonephritis may present with a clinical picture that mimics many of the features of HSP.[17]

TREATMENT

General measures include maintaining hydration, correcting electrolyte abnormalities, treating hypertension, and providing analgesia for abdominal pain and arthralgias. Any assessment of studies on the treatment of the nephritis must take into account a number of difficulties: there are no prospective, randomized, controlled studies on the treatment of HSP N; there is a great deal of ascertainment bias; and there is a high rate of spontaneous remission in up to 50% of patients.[4] Despite these important caveats and reservations, several studies show that corticosteroids, immunosuppressive agents, and anticoagulants, either alone or in combination, may improve the renal outcome in patients with severe HSPN.[14,15,23,24,32]

Clinical Pearl

- Patients with normal kidney function need only supportive treatment
- There are no studies on the use of ACE inhibitors and/or angiotensin II receptor blockers in HSP N
- There are no clear guidelines on treatment of progressive renal disease in HSP N

No treatment protocol is universally effective, but early initiation of therapy appears to improve the renal outcome. The optimal duration of therapy is unknown, but it is suggested that immunosuppressive treatment should be given for at least 3 months. Plasma exchange may be indicated for patients who develop very severe nephritis, but there are no controlled studies and the effects may be transient.[30]

OUTCOME

The prognosis varies according to the clinical presentation (Table 18-1).[16] The severity of interstitial fibrosis,

---

Box 18-6 Differential Diagnosis of Purpuric Rashes

- Henoch–Schönlein purpura
- Meningococcemia
- Septicemia
- Purpura fulminans
- Acute infantile hemorrhagic edema

Box 18-5 Pulmonary Renal Syndromes[33]

- Systemic lupus erythematosus
- Wegener granulomatosis
- Goodpasture disease
- Henoch–Schönlein purpura
- *Strep. pneumoniae*-associated hemolytic uremic syndrome

Box 18-7 Features of Hypocomplementemic Urticarial Vasculitis (Hypersensitivity Vasculitis)[22]

- Polyarthritis
- Hypocomplementemia
- Purpuric rash
- Hematuria and proteinuria
- Membranoproliferative glomerulonephritis

Table 18-1 Outcome According to Initial Clinical Presentation[16]

Clinical Presentation	Chronic Renal Failure (%)
Hematuria and/or minimal proteinuria	<5
Non-nephrotic proteinuria/acute nephritis	15
Nephrotic syndrome	40
Nephritic/nephrotic syndrome	50

percentage of sclerotic glomeruli, and presence of glomeruli with fibrinoid necrosis are associated with a poor renal prognosis.[26] HSP can recur after renal transplantation, even in the absence of clinical signs and symptoms, and lead to graft loss in 11% to 35% of patients at 5 years after transplantation.[21] Patients with severe renal symptoms at onset require long-term follow-up during adulthood, and all women who had even mild renal symptoms at onset of HSP N should be carefully observed during and after pregnancy.[28]

Clinical Pearl

The severity of clinical presentation and initial findings on renal biopsy correlate well with outcome, but have poor predictive value in individuals.[16]

REFERENCES

1. Andreoli SP. Renal manifestations of systemic diseases. Semin Nephrol 1998;18:270-279.

2. Caksen H, Odabas D, Kosem M, et al. Report of eight infants with acute infantile hemorrhagic edema and review of the literature. J Dermatol 2002;29:290-295.

3. Choong CK, Beasley SW. Intra-abdominal manifestations of Henoch-Schönlein purpura. J Paediatr Child Health 1998; 34:405-409.

4. Coppo R, Mazzuco G, Cagnoli L, et al. Long-term prognosis of Henoch-Schönlein nephritis in adults and children. Italian Group of Renal Immunopathology Collaborative Study on Henoch-Schönlein purpura. Nephrol Dial Transplant 1997;12:2277-2283.

5. Crosse JE, Soderdahl DW, Schamber DT. "Acute scrotum" in Henoch-Schönlein syndrome. Urology 1976;7:66-67.

6. Davin JC, Weening JJ. Henoch-Schönlein purpura nephritis: an update. Eur J Pediatr 2001;160:689-695.

7. Davin JC, ten Berge IJ, Weening JJ. What is the difference between IgA nephropathy and Henoch-Schönlein purpura nephritis? Kidney Int 2001;59:823-834.

8. Drummond PM, Moghal NE, Coulthard MG. Hypertension in Henoch-Schönlein purpura with minimal urinary findings. Arch Dis Child 2001;84:163-165.

9. Emancipator SN. Primary and secondary forms of IgA nephritis and Schönlein-Henoch syndrome. In: Heptinshall RH (ed), Pathology of The Kidney, 5th edn. Lippincott Williams & Wilkins, Philadelphia, 1998, pp. 389-476.

10. Emancipator SN. IgA nephropathy: morphologic expression and pathogenesis. Am J Kidney Dis 1994;23: 451-462.

11. Evans-Jones LG, Clough JV. Thrombocytosis in Henoch-Schönlein syndrome. Clin Lab Haematol 1990;12:137-139.

12. Farley TA, Gillespie S, Rasoulpour M, et al. Epidemiology of a cluster of Henoch-Schonlein purpura. Am J Dis Child 1989;143:798-803.

13. Fervenza FC. Henoch-Schönlein purpura nephritis. Int J Dermatol 2003;42:170-177.

14. Flynn JT, Smoyer WE, Bunchman TE, et al. Treatment of Henoch-Schönlein purpura glomerulonephritis in children with high-dose corticosteroids plus oral cyclophosphamide. Am J Nephrol 2001;21:128-133.

15. Foster BJ, Bernard C, Drummond KN, et al. Effective therapy for severe Henoch-Schönlein purpura nephritis with prednisone and azathioprine: a clinical and histopathologic study. J Pediatr 2000;136:370-375.

16. Goldstein AR, White RH, Akuse R, et al. Long-term follow-up of childhood Henoch-Schönlein nephritis. Lancet 1992;339:280-282.

17. Goodyer PR, de Chadarevian JP, Kaplan BS. Acute post-streptococcal glomerulonephritis mimicking Henoch-Schönlein purpura. J Pediatr 1978;93:412-415.

18. Jennette JC, Falk RJ, Andrassy K, et al. Nomenclature of systemic vasculitides. Proposal of an international consensus conference. Arthritis Rheum 1994;37:187-192.

19. Harvey JG, Colditz PB. Henoch-Schönlein purpura – a surgical review. Aust Paediatr J 1984;20:13-16.

20. Kobayashi Y, Omori S, Kamimaki I, et al. Acute reversible renal failure with macroscopic hematuria in Henoch-Schönlein purpura. Pediatr Nephrol 2001;16:742-744.

21. Meulders Q, Pirson Y, Cosyns JP, et al. Course of Henoch-Schönlein nephritis after renal transplantation. Report on ten patients and review of the literature. Transplantation 1994;58:1179-1186.

22. Michel BA, Hunder GG, Bloch DA. Hypersensitivity vasculitis and Henoch-Schönlein purpura: a comparison between the 2 disorders. J Rheumatol 1992;19:721-728.

23. Niaudet P, Habib R. Methylprednisolone pulse therapy in the treatment of severe forms of Schönlein-Henoch purpura nephritis. Pediatr Nephrol 1998;12:238-243.

24. Öner A, Tinaztepe K, Erdogan Ö. The effect of triple therapy on rapidly progressive type of Henoch-Schönlein nephritis. Pediatr Nephrol 1995;9:6-10.

25. Pathan N, Faust SN, Levin M. Pathophysiology of meningococcal meningitis and septicaemia. Arch Dis Child 2003; 88:601-607.

26. Pillebout E, Thervet E, Hill G, et al. Henoch-Schönlein purpura in adults: outcome and prognostic factors. Am Soc Nephrol 2002;13:1271-1278.

27. Reif S, Jain A, Santiago J, et al. Protein losing enteropathy as a manifestation of Henoch-Schönlein purpura. Acta Paediatr Scand 1991;80:482-485.

28. Ronkainen J, Nuutinen M, Koskimies O. The adult kidney 24 years after childhood Henoch-Schönlein purpura: a retrospective cohort study. Lancet 2002;360:666-670.

29. Saulsbury FT. Henoch-Schönlein purpura in children. Report of 100 patients and review of the literature. Medicine (Baltimore) 1999;78:395-409.

30. Scharer K, Krmar R, Querfeld W, et al. Clinical outcome of Schönlein-Henoch purpura nephritis in children. Pediatr Nephrol 1999;13:816-823.

31. Szer IS. Henoch-Schönlein purpura. Curr Opin Rheumatol 1994;6:25-31.

32. Tanaka H, Suzuki K, Nakahata T, et al. Early treatment with oral immunosuppressants in severe proteinuric purpura nephritis. Pediatr Nephrol 2003;18:347-350.

33. von Vigier RO, Trummler SA, Laux-End R, et al. Pulmonary renal syndrome in childhood: a report of twenty-one cases and a review of the literature. Pediatr Pulmonol 2000;29:382-388.

CHAPTER 10

Membranoproliferative Glomerulonephritis

MICHAEL C. BRAUN, M.D. AND

C. FREDERIC STRIFE, M.D.

Clinical Pearl

Membranoproliferative glomerulonephritis (MPGN) is an uncommon form of renal disease.

INTRODUCTION

In the older literature, membranoproliferative glomerulonephritis (MPGN) is also referred to as mesangiocapillary glomerulonephritis (MCGN) or chronic lobular nephritis; however, these terms have now fallen out of favor. Like most forms of glomerulonephritis, MPGN is a pathologic diagnosis. The histologic criteria that characterize MPGN are expansion of the mesangial matrix, varying degrees of mesangial proliferation, a lobular appearance of the glomerular tufts, and distinct alterations of the glomerular basement membrane (GBM). Based largely on ultrastructural (electron microscopic) features, three types of MPGN have been defined.[22] Type I, the most common form, is characterized by the presence of an intact GBM with abundant subendothelial deposits. Type II, also referred to as 'dense deposit disease,' is defined by a thickened GBM with frequent intramembranous deposits. Lastly, type III is characterized by complex subendothelial and subepithelial deposits and a fragmented, disrupted, GBM. Although a substantial body of literature has emerged to support the classification of type III MPGN as a distinct pathologic disorder, this is not universally accepted. Some still regard type III solely as a variant of type I, and this is particularly evident in the adult literature, where most large case series of MPGN patients do not distinguish between type I and type III MPGN. Currently, none of the national renal or transplant databases separate type I from type III MPGN. In the 1970s it became apparent that some patients with chronic infectious diseases or malignancies developed glomerular pathology similar to MPGN. The classification system was then further refined by the addition of secondary as opposed to primary or idiopathic MPGN (Box 19-1).

EPIDEMIOLOGY

The incidence of MPGN is difficult to ascertain. One retrospective study of primary renal biopsies in the Italian city of Turin estimated the incidence of MPGN at

---

Box 19-1 Classification System of Membranoproliferative Glomerulonephritis (MPGN)

Idiopathic MPGN
    Type I
        Familial
    Type II
    Type III
        Familial
Secondary MPGN

0.75 cases per million children.[6] Large pediatric tertiary referral centers in the United States typically report one to two new cases of MPGN per year. Based on data from centers in Japan and Europe, there is some suggestion that the incidence of MPGN has been declining over the past decade. This issue remains unresolved. The most recent North American Pediatric Renal Transplant Cooperative Study (NAPRTCS) report indicates that MPGN is the primary etiology for approximately 3% of all pediatric patients with chronic renal insufficiency or end-stage renal disease (ESRD); 204 patients in total.[14] The relative frequency of the types of MPGN varies according to the reporting center.[3,10,17] Type I is the most common, accounting for roughly 55% of reported cases (range 36 to 78%), followed by type III with 25% (range 14 to 41%); type II is the least common at 20% (range 5 to 34%). MPGN occurs most commonly in older children and adolescents, with a mean age of onset of 9 years. The condition has, however, been reported in a child as young as 18 months. Males and females appear to be equally affected. In the United States, MPGN has been reported most frequently in the white population, although it has been seen in all ethnic groups. Some reports from Asia, Africa, and South America indicate a higher frequency of MPGN than is seen in the United States.

SECONDARY MPGN AND GENETIC ASSOCIATIONS

The incidence of secondary MPGN is unknown. With the exception of hepatitis-associated MPGN, most secondary forms of MPGN are rare and reports consist of single cases (Table 19-1). The most common form of secondary MPGN in adults is chronic hepatitis C

Table 19-1 Secondary Forms of Membranoproliferative Glomerulonephritis (MPGN). Frequently Reported Causes of Secondary MPGN are in Bold, the Remaining are Largely Single Case Reports of Associated but Not Proven Causes of Secondary MPGN.

Malignancy
B-cell lymphoma
Castleman's syndrome
Chronic lymphocytic leukemia
Gastric adenocarcinoma
Hydatidiform mole
Mixed-germ cell ovarian tumor
Monoclonal gammopathy
Transitional cell carcinoma of the bladder
Multiple myeloma
Non-Hodgkin's lymphoma
POEMS syndrome
Pulmonary carcinoid tumor
Reactive hemophagocytic syndrome
Small cell lung carcinoma
Wilms' tumor

Infectious
Coagulase-negative *Staphylococcus*
Candida albicans
Epstein–Barr virus
Hepatitis A
Hepatitis B
Hepatitis C
Hepatitis G
HTLV-1
HIV
Malaria
Meningococcus
Mycoplasma pneumoniae
Hantavirus
Q fever
Schistosoma mansoni
Tuberculosis

Immunologic
Complement deficiencies (Factor H)
Cryoglobulinemia
Hypogammaglobulinemia
Hyper-IgE syndrome
Sarcoidosis
Sjögren's syndrome
SLE
Hypocomplementemic urticarial vasculitis

Miscellaneous
Alpha-1 anti-trypsin deficiency
ADPKD
Crow–Fukase syndrome
Cushing's syndrome
Down's syndrome
Gaucher's disease
Gonadal dysgenesis
Hemolytic uremic syndrome
Heroin abuse
Partial lipodystrophy
Prader–Willi syndrome
Sherwood–Proesman syndrome
Sickle cell disease
Takayasu's arteritis
Turner's syndrome
Ulcerative colitis
Wiscott–Aldrich syndrome

ADPKD = autosomal dominant polycystic kidney disease; SLE = systemic lupus erythematosus.

infection; this association is seen much less frequently in the pediatric population. A retrospective study of children previously diagnosed with idiopathic MPGN failed to identify a single unrecognized case attributable to chronic viral hepatitis.[15] It is likely that the long latency period of hepatitis infections, combined with the relatively low incidence of these diseases in the pediatric population, accounts for the infrequency of hepatitis-associated MPGN. Other forms of chronic infectious antigenemia-associated MPGN are also rare in the United States. This is not the case in countries where malaria, schistosomiasis, and hepatitis are endemic. Malignancy-associated MPGN is uncommon in the pediatric population; indeed, the most frequent MPGN-associated malignancy, chronic lymphocytic leukemia (CLL) is rare in children.

There are reports of familial transmission of type I and type III MPGN, although specific chromosomal loci have not yet been identified. Familial clustering of type II MPGN has not been reported. There is one report of type I MPGN occurring in one sibling and type III in another, suggesting that there may be genetic susceptibility factors common to both diseases. This is supported by the finding of an increased frequency of the extended haplotype, HLA-B8, DR3, SCO1, GLO2 in 13% of patients with type I or type II compared to 1% of normal controls. There is also a higher frequency of inherited complement deficiencies in patients with type I and type III MPGN (22.7%) compared to healthy controls (6.7%).[5] These deficiency states include components of the classical pathway, C1q and C2, the alternative pathway protein Factor B, and terminal pathway components: C6, C7 and C9. Interestingly, an absolute deficiency in any of these proteins was not identified.

PRESENTATION AND CLINICAL FEATURES

MPGN is somewhat unique among forms of glomerulonephritis in that its clinical presentation is variable.[3,10,17,22] This can range from asymptomatic microscopic hematuria and/or proteinuria to acute nephritis with gross hematuria, nephrotic syndrome, or rapidly progressive glomerulonephritis (RPGN). The Japanese experience with urinary screening suggests that most patients with MPGN have a period of 'silent' disease. Iitaka et al. reported that of 41 children diagnosed with MPGN over a 20-year period, 33 (81%) were identified solely on the basis of isolated microscopic hematuria or proteinuria.[10] The absence of universal urinary screening in this country may account in part for the variability of presentation. Given the relative rarity of MPGN and its range of clinical presentations, MPGN is frequently not considered as a primary diagnosis.

Type I MPGN presents most commonly as asymptomatic microscopic hematuria and/or proteinuria. This is seen in roughly 50% of patients. The child is otherwise clinically well with normal renal function, serum albumin, and blood pressure. Nephrotic syndrome is seen in approximately 30% of type I patients. It is often associated with either microscopic or gross hematuria. Presentation with acute nephritis, marked by red cell casts and dark cola-colored urine, is seen in 25–30% of type I patients. Renal insufficiency is uncommon, and serum albumin concentrations are typically mildly depressed. Hypertension is also frequently seen. One feature that distinguishes MPGN type I at presentation is a history of prior systemic complaints. These are seen in about 25% of patients and include weight loss, decreased levels of activity, and easy fatigueability. These findings are uncommon in type II and almost never seen in type III.

Fewer than 25% of patients with type II MPGN present with isolated microscopic hematuria and/or proteinuria. Nephrotic syndrome is seen in over 50% of patients. Presentation with acute nephritis or gross hematuria is also more common in type II than in type I or III. Systemic hypertension is seen in about 50% of patients, and serum creatinine concentrations are greater than 1.2 mg/dl at presentation in 15% of patients with type II MPGN.

Type III MPGN presents most commonly as asymptomatic microscopic hematuria and/or proteinuria (67%). Nephrotic syndrome or acute nephritis is seen in less than 33% of patients. Renal function in most cases of type III is normal. In distinction to type I and type II, hypertension is rare and is noted in less than 10% of cases. Prior constitutional symptoms are exceedingly unusual.

Although uncommon, MPGN can present as RPGN. Serum C3 levels tend to be profoundly depressed, and rapid deterioration of renal function is accompanied by azotemia, oliguria, and accelerated hypertension. This is seen most commonly in type II MPGN, but it has also been reported in type I and III.

LABORATORY EVALUATION

While there are subtle differences in presentation between the different types of MPGN, it is difficult to clearly distinguish one type of MPGN from another based solely on clinical features. Analysis of abnormalities of serum complement proteins is particularly useful in this regard as abnormalities of the complement system are frequently associated with MPGN.[21] A low C3 level is seen is approximately 80% of patients with MPGN, regardless of type. The diagnostic evaluation of hypocomplementemic nephritis is shown in Figure 19-1. Measurement of C3, C4, and C5 are useful to the clinician

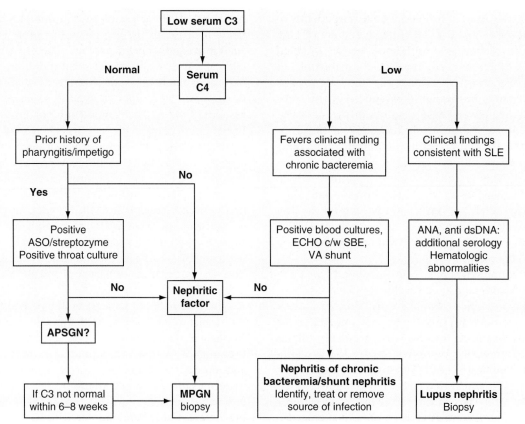

Figure 19-1 The diagnostic approach to a patient with hypocomplementemic nephritis. ANA = antinuclear antibodies; APSGN = acute post-streptococcal glomerulonephritis; MPGN = membrano-proliferative glomerulonephritis; SBE = subacute bacterial endocarditis; SLE = systemic lupus erythematosus; VA = ventriculo-atrial.

in identifying patients with MPGN as well as distinguishing the different types of MPGN serologically (Table 19-2).[20] It should be remembered that up to 20% of patients with MPGN have normal C3 levels at the time of presentation.

Type I MPGN is associated with low C3 levels (80% at presentation) and low C4 levels in about 40% of patients. C5 concentrations are typically normal, and there is little evidence of terminal pathway activation. Type II MPGN can be distinguished from type I in that C4 levels are universally normal. C3 levels are depressed

in approximately 75% of patients, whereas C5 levels are normal. Typically there is no suppression of terminal pathway components. In type III, the C3 levels tend to be profoundly depressed in over 80% of patients. The suppression of C3 seems to be greater and of longer duration than that seen in type I patients. C4 levels are frequently normal, although suppression of C4 can be seen in some patients. The primary hallmark of MPGN type III is a depressed C5 level, seen in 50% of patients. Depression of terminal components C6, C7, or C9 can be seen in up to 75% of type III patients.[21]

MPGN is also frequently associated with the presence of a complement-activating nephritic factor.[23] Nephritic factors are autoantibodies, typically IgG but occasionally IgM, which act to stabilize complement-activating convertases of either the classical or alternative pathways. Three nephritic factors have been characterized (Table 19-3).

NF_a (also referred to as $C3_{nef}$) stabilizes the alternative pathway convertase, C3bBb, and rapidly cleaves C3 *in vitro*. It is commonly seen only in type II MPGN. NF_c (also referred to as $C4_{nef}$) stabilizes the classical pathway convertase C4bC2b. NF_c is seen primarily in type I MPGN, and rarely in type III. NF_t, the nephritic factor of the terminal pathway, stabilizes the C5 convertase, $(C3b)_2BbP$,

Table 19-2	Patterns of Hypocomplementemia by MPGN Type		
	C3	**C4**	**C5**
Type I MPGN	Low	Low	Rarely low
Type II MPGN	Low	Normal	Normal
Type III MPGN	Low	Rarely low	Low
SLE	Low	Low	Rarely low
APSGN	Low	Rarely low	Low

APSGN = acute post-streptococcal glomerulonephritis; SLE = systemic lupus erythematosus.

Table 19-3 Nephritic Factors and Associated Type of MPGN

	Type I	Type II	Type III
NF_a	Not present	Common	Not present
NF_c	Common	Not present	Rare
NF_t	Rare	Not present	Common

Table 19-4 Immunofluorescent Findings by MPGN Type

	Type I	Type II	Type III
IgG	Capillary loop (Fringe) Co-localization	Absent	Faint No co-localization
C3	Fringe	Capillary loop Mesangium Bowman's capsule	Capillary Mesangium
C4	Fringe Co-localization	Absent	Absent

activating the terminal pathway. *In vitro*, NF_t is distinguished from NF_a by its slow cleavage C3; this is maximal at 4 hours compared to 20 minutes with NF_a. NF_t is seen primarily in type III MPGN, although it has occasionally been reported in association with type I MPGN. The serologic detection of nephritic factors is quite useful in distinguishing among the types of MPGN; however, assays for NF_c and NF_t are performed primarily by research laboratories and are not widely utilized clinically. In addition to complement activation and consumption, depressed C3 levels in patients with MPGN have been associated with reduced C3 production. This is mediated primarily by feedback inhibition of hepatic C3 synthesis by C3 cleavage fragments.

PATHOLOGY

It is difficult to distinguish the types of MPGN solely by light microscopy. All types of MPGN have an increase in glomerular cellularity with mesangial proliferation. Subtle differences in degrees of mesangial proliferation are seen, with proliferation being most dramatic in type I followed by types II and III. Focal mesangial proliferation is most commonly seen in type III. Using silver stain, the capillary walls are seen to be thickened, with a significant reduction in open capillary lumens. In type I MPGN, double contours of the capillary walls may be noted, resulting in a 'tram-track' appearance. Tram-tracking is less commonly noted in type II and type III.

Patterns of immunofluorescence staining can distinguish between the three types of MPGN (Table 19-4). In type I MPGN, C3 staining is typically seen in the periphery of the glomerular capillary loops in a 'fringe' pattern. Staining with C4 and IgG is frequently strongly positive and co-localizes in the capillary loops with C3. Type II can be distinguished by the lack of IgG and C4 staining. C3 staining is very strong, and localizes to the mesangium, as well as to the glomerular capillary loops. Ring-like staining is frequently seen along the GBM. C3 staining of Bowman's capsule is often also noted. In type III MPGN, C4 deposits are rarely seen. When noted, IgG is typically faint and seen only in a mesangial pattern. C3 is present in a mesangial and capillary loop distribution and does not co-localize with either IgG or C4. Staining for IgA or IgM is typically negative in all types of MPGN.

Ultimately, ultrastructural studies of the renal biopsy are required to diagnose the specific type of MPGN. The hallmark of type I is presence of an intact GBM with frequent subendothelial deposits. Subepithelial deposits can also be seen. Typically, there is marked mesangial proliferation extending around the glomerular capillaries and resulting in mesangial interposition. Type II MPGN can be identified by the presence of intramembranous deposits (dense deposits) in the lamina densa of the GBM. These deposits are discontinuous and may also be seen in the perimesangial region. The GBM lesions seen in type III are complex. Both subendothelial and subepithelial deposits can be seen, and the GBM appears to be thickened. It is often difficult to distinguish type I and type III deposits using standard electron microscopic techniques. However, with silver methenamine staining the GBM in type III is noted to be discontinuous, with a fragmented and laminated appearance; this is distinct from the intact GBM seen in type I MPGN (Table 19-5).

PATHOGENESIS

Idiopathic MPGN type I is thought to be mediated by immune complex formation. This hypothesis is based on evidence of activation of the classical pathway with low serum C4 and C3, and abundant IgG deposits in the kidney that co-localize with C3 and C4. Circulating immune complexes can frequently be detected in the serum of patients with type I. The association of type I with disorders producing either chronic antigenemia or abnormal immunoglobulin production strongly favors an immune complex-based mechanism of glomerular injury. It is thought that the deposition of these immune complexes in the subendothelial space induces mesangial proliferation and increased production of mesangial matrix components.

Table 19-5 Common Electron Microscopy Findings by MPGN Type

	Type I	Type II	Type III
GBM	Intact	Intact	Disrupted/thickened[*]
Intramembranous deposits	Absent	Abundant	Absent
Subendothelial deposits	Frequent	Absent	Common, variable
Subepithelial deposits	Variable	Absent	Common, variable

[*]The disrupted, laminated, appearance of the GBM in type III is best seen by silver methenamine staining.

Although the pathogenesis of type II is unknown, an emerging body of data suggests that chronic complement activation plays a primary role in the initiation of glomerular injury. Deficiency in Factor H – a complement regulatory protein that inactivates C3 convertase – is associated with the development of MPGN in humans and in animals. Humans with homozygous Factor H deficiency have an increased frequency of glomerulonephritis, including MPGN. Marder's disease – a mutation in Factor H that prevents Factor H binding to C3 convertase – is also associated with the development of MPGN. Animals with either naturally occurring Factor H deficiency (pigs) or targeted deletions in Factor H (mice) develop a spontaneous glomerulonephritis that is similar to MPGN.[16] In this model, glomerular injury is entirely complement-dependent. Mice deficient in Factor H when crossed with mice lacking Factor B, and thus unable to form C3 convertase, are protected from the development of nephritis. The lack of IgG deposits in humans with MPGN type II and the absence of classical pathway activation suggest that, as opposed to type I, type II is not an immune complex disease. The association of complement activation and MPGN is seen in patients with partial lipodystrophy.[11] These patients have a very high frequency of circulating NF_a and MPGN type II. It has been hypothesized that the concordance of lipodystrophy and MPGN in these patients is due to the high levels of Factor D produced by adipocytes. The pathogenic mechanisms by which this results in the destruction of adipocytes and in the development of MPGN are uncertain.

Less is known regarding the pathogenesis of type III. There are no known animal models of type III, and no specific complement-deficiency states are linked with type III. The absence of IgG deposits and normal C4 levels suggest that, like type II MPGN, type III is not a primary immune complex disease. West et al. have reported in a series of studies that there is a strong correlation between hypocomplementemia and the presence of perimesangial and subendothelial deposits in these patients.[24] They have hypothesized that the development of the ultrastructural changes seen in type III are dependent on the presence of circulating NF_t, and that

NF_t may play a primary pathogenic role in the development of this disease. However, a number of reports have failed to demonstrate any relationship between the presence of NF_t and either disease severity and/or renal survival.

NATURAL HISTORY

In the absence of therapy, the natural history of type I and type II MPGN is one of inexorable deterioration of renal function and progression to ESRD. There are no natural history studies of MPGN type III. Based on reports by Habib and Cameron, the outcome of type I and type II are similar, with 50% progressing to ESRD by 10 years, and 90% by 20 years.[4,9] It is important to note that in these studies no distinction was made between type I and type III MPGN. Cameron et al. noted a slower progression in children with type I MPGN compared to adults.[4] Regardless of type, the presence of nephrotic syndrome, renal insufficiency, or glomerular crescents has a negative impact on disease progression. Spontaneous remission of proteinuria and improvement in renal function has been noted in some cases of MPGN, although these are clearly the exception.

TREATMENT

Prior to any discussion of therapeutic options in the treatment of MPGN, there are a number of factors that are important to consider. First, given the rarity of this disease, a limited number of controlled therapeutic trials have been conducted. These studies typically contain few patients; in fact, the largest controlled study of the treatment of MPGN contained only 80 patients of all types. Second, most uncontrolled series contain patients accrued over years, if not decades. The improvement in care of patients with chronic renal insufficiency, combined with the fact that many patients have received additional therapies, presents a major confounding factor in data analysis. The largest published case series on the use of high-dose, alternate-day steroids contains slightly more than 85 patients enrolled over almost four decades. Many patients – particularly those from the 1960s to the late 1970s – received other forms of immunomodulatory therapy in addition to alternate-day steroids. Third, a number of trials have limited follow-up periods. In a disease where the mean time to renal failure is 10 years, it is difficult to evaluate the impact on long-term survival of any therapy when the follow-up time is limited. This is particularly relevant in regard to the studies on the use of anti-platelet therapies published during the 1980s and early 1990s. Fourth, it is important to recognize that many patients with MPGN have significant periods of silent disease. The duration of disease prior to entry time into the clinical trials is of critical importance; the time of diagnosis by biopsy may have been preceded by years of glomerular injury. The universally good outcome reported in the Japanese literature may in part be due to the early and aggressive treatment of individuals detected by asymptomatic urinary screening. Finally, the utility of renal survival analysis as a method of determining response to therapy has been questioned. Given the chronicity of these uncommon disorders, and the complexity of data analysis over many years of patient follow-up, the comparison of single-center experiences in relation to historical controls must be viewed with caution. For a complete discussion of this question, the reader is referred to an excellent analysis of the problem by Donadio et al.[8] With these caveats in mind, two basic approaches to treatment of MPGN have been advocated: corticosteroids and anti-platelet therapy.

Corticosteroids

The use of long-term high-dose, alternate-day steroids (2 mg/kg q.o.d. with a maximum of 80 mg per day) for a minimum of 2 years has been advocated by the Cincinnati group. Based on a series of uncontrolled reports spanning almost 30 years, they have reported encouraging results.[12] Renal survival for all types of MPGN was 84% at 10 years and 54% at 20 years – a significant improvement compared to historical controls. Most, if not all, patients had residual proteinuria, but serial follow-up biopsies confirmed improvement in many instances. Recent reports from this center indicate that patients with type I appear to respond more favorably to therapy than patients with type III, with 80% of type I patients having an estimated glomerular filtration rate (GFR) greater than 75 ml/min/1.73 m² compared to 70% of patients with type III at 10 years of follow-up.[3] Type III patients also had significantly more residual proteinuria and hematuria. The response of type II patients to the alternate-day prednisone regimen has been less encouraging. These reports have been criticized for their reliance on historical controls, and use of additional therapies in a number of patients in the early years of the study (1960s to 1970).

The largest and only randomized, placebo-controlled, trial of prednisone in the treatment of MPGN, the ISKDC (International Study of Kidney Disease in Children) study, supports the use of corticosteroids in these patients.[19] In this study, 80 patients with biopsy-proven MPGN and heavy proteinuria were randomized to either prednisone (40 mg/kg q.o.d.) or placebo (lactose). Seventeen patients with type III were enrolled and, due to limited statistical power, they were combined with the type I patients for analysis. The patients were followed for 5 years. Treatment failure was defined as either an increase in serum creatinine greater than 30% above baseline, or an absolute increase of >0.4 mg/dl. At the time of last follow-up, 33% of patients treated with prednisone had met the criteria for treatment failure compared to 55% of patients in the placebo group (p = 0.071). While this did not meet statistical significance, subset analysis of the combined type I and type III groups indicated a clear advantage with prednisone therapy (p = 0.035). A number of patients in the prednisone treatment group had to be withdrawn, or had their prednisone dose decreased, due to severe hypertension. This study has been criticized for a significant difference in duration of disease prior to enrollment in the treatment versus the placebo groups (8.9 months versus 18.1 months), which may have biased the data toward steroid responsiveness. Furthermore, others have suggested that a greater response to therapy would have been seen if higher doses of prednisone had been used. A smaller randomized trial reported by Mota-Hernandez et al. of eight patients with type I treated with high-dose, alternate-day steroids and 10 placebo control patients supported these findings.[13] At the last follow-up (mean of 6 years), all of the patients treated with prednisone had either stable or improved renal function, while 40% of placebo-treated patients had progressed to ESRD. A number of additional smaller studies have supported the use of alternate-day, high-dose prednisone.

Concern over the potential side effects of long-term steroid therapy in these patients, including hypertension, growth failure, and cataracts, has led a number of investigators to modify the Cincinnati protocol. This approach has been based on the observation that patients who present without nephrotic syndrome have a slower progression to ESRD, and thus may either not benefit from corticosteroid therapy or respond to lower doses of prednisone. Several studies have recommended that only patients with nephrotic range proteinuria be treated with high-dose steroids, including pulse solumedrol.[18] This issue remains unresolved, as Japanese investigators have shown significantly better outcomes in patients treated with high-dose prednisone, regardless of presentation.[10] It is also clear from historical studies that the absence of nephrotic syndrome does not preclude progression to ESRD.

Anti-Platelet Therapy

Based on early reports using dipyridamole and cyclophosphamide demonstrating improvement in renal function and proteinuria in patients with MPGN, a number of controlled trials on the use of these agents were undertaken. Significant improvement in proteinuria and stabilization of renal function were initially confirmed in a randomized, placebo-controlled trial employing aspirin and dipyramidole.[7] However, in a subsequent report of long-term follow-up in these patients the early differences in response to therapy were not validated.[8] A study of 18 MPGN patients using aspirin and dipyridamole reported an improvement in proteinuria in the treatment group, but failed to demonstrate any improvement in renal function in response to therapy.[25] The follow-up time was limited to 36 months, however. A number of other studies have failed to confirm benefits from anti-platelet therapy. Overall, the studies advocating the use of anti-platelet therapy, while encouraging, are limited due to small patient numbers, limited response to therapy, short periods of follow-up, and a high incidence of hemorrhagic complications.

Other Therapies

While there are isolated reports advocating the use of other therapies for the treatment of MPGN, including non-steroidal anti-inflammatory drugs (NSAIDs), cyclosporine, enalapril, and cyclophosphamide, few additional data are available to support the widespread use of these therapies. It is hoped that as our understanding of the pathogenic mechanisms of these diseases improves, targeted therapy directed at inhibition of complement activation or antibody formation will improve the outcome of these patients.

Renal Transplantation

As many patients will progress to ESRD despite medical therapy, disease recurrence in renal allografts is a significant issue for patients with MPGN.[1,2] The risk of recurrence appears to be highest in patients with type II MPGN, followed by type I. With only two case reports in the literature, the frequency of type III recurrence is unknown. Changes in immunosuppression had little impact on graft survival once the disease had recurred. Of concern was the finding that if the disease recurred in the primary allograft, the risk of disease recurrence in a subsequent graft was 80% (see Chapter 36).

REFERENCES

1. Andresdottir MB, Assmann KJ, Hoitsma AJ, et al. Recurrence of type I membranoproliferative glomerulonephritis after renal transplantation: analysis of the incidence, risk factors, and impact on graft survival. Transplantation 1997;63:1628–1633.

2. Andresdottir MB, Assmann KJ, Hoitsma AJ, et al. Renal transplantation in patients with dense deposit disease: morphological characteristics of recurrent disease and clinical outcome. Nephrol Dial Transplant 1999;14:1723–1731.

3. Braun MC, West CD, Strife CF. Differences between membranoproliferative glomerulonephritis types I and III in long-term response to an alternate-day prednisone regimen. Am J Kidney Dis 1999;34:1022–1032.

4. Cameron JS, Turner DR, Heaton J, et al. Idiopathic mesangiocapillary glomerulonephritis. Comparison of types I and II in children and adults and long-term prognosis. Am J Med 1983;74:175–192.

5. Coleman TH, Forristal J, Kosaka T, et al. Inherited complement component deficiencies in membranoproliferative glomerulonephritis. Kidney Int 1983;24:681–690.

6. Coppo R, Gianoglio B, Porcellini MG, et al. Frequency of renal diseases and clinical indications for renal biopsy in children (report of the Italian National Registry of Renal Biopsies in Children). Group of Renal Immunopathology of the Italian Society of Pediatric Nephrology and Group of Renal Immunopathology of the Italian Society of Nephrology. Nephrol Dial Transplant 1998;13:293–297.

7. Donadio JV, Jr, Anderson CF, Mitchell JC, III, et al. Membranoproliferative glomerulonephritis. A prospective clinical trial of platelet-inhibitor therapy. N Engl J Med 1984;310:1421–1426.

8. Donadio JV, Jr, Offord KP. Reassessment of treatment results in membranoproliferative glomerulonephritis, with emphasis on life-table analysis. Am J Kidney Dis 1989;14:445–451.

9. Habib R, Kleinknecht C, Gubler MC, et al. Idiopathic membranoproliferative glomerulonephritis in children. Report of 105 cases. Clin Nephrol 1973;1:194–214.

10. Iitaka K, Ishidate T, Hojo M, et al. Idiopathic membranoproliferative glomerulonephritis in Japanese children. Pediatr Nephrol 1995;9:272–277.

11. Levy Y, George J, Yona E, et al. Partial lipodystrophy, mesangiocapillary glomerulonephritis, and complement dysregulation. An autoimmune phenomenon. Immunol Res 1998;18:55–60.

12. McEnery PT. Membranoproliferative glomerulonephritis: the Cincinnati experience – cumulative renal survival from 1957 to 1989. J Pediatr 1990;116:S109–S114.

13. Mota-Hernandez F, Gordillo-Paniagua G, Munoz-Arizpe R, et al. Prednisone versus placebo in membranoproliferative glomerulonephritis: long-term clinicopathological correlations. Int J Pediatr Nephrol 1985;6:25–28.

14. Neu AM, Ho PL, McDonald RA, et al. Chronic dialysis in children and adolescents. The 2001 NAPRTCS Annual Report. Pediatr Nephrol 2002;17:656–663.

15. Nowicki MJ, Welch TR, Ahmad N, et al. Absence of hepatitis B and C viruses in pediatric idiopathic membranoproliferative glomerulonephritis. Pediatr Nephrol 1995;9:16–18.

16. Pickering MC, Cook HT, Warren J, et al. Uncontrolled C3 activation causes membranoproliferative glomerulonephritis in mice deficient in complement factor H. Nature Genet 2002;31:424–428.

17. Schwertz R, de Jong R, Gretz N, et al. Outcome of idiopathic membranoproliferative glomerulonephritis in children. Arbeitsgemeinschaft Padiatrische Nephrologie. Acta Paediatr 1996;85:308–312.

18. Somers M, Kertesz S, Rosen S, et al. Non-nephrotic children with membranoproliferative glomerulonephritis: are steroids indicated? Pediatr Nephrol 1995;9:140–144.

19. Tarshish P, Bernstein J, Tobin JN, et al. Treatment of mesangiocapillary glomerulonephritis with alternate-day prednisone – a report of the International Study of Kidney Disease in Children. Pediatr Nephrol 1992;6:123–130.

20. Varade WS, Forristal J, West CD. Patterns of complement activation in idiopathic membranoproliferative glomerulonephritis, types I, II, and III. Am J Kidney Dis 1990;16:196–206.

21. West CD. The complement profile in clinical medicine. Inherited and acquired conditions lowering the serum concentrations of complement component and control proteins. Complement Inflamm 1989;6:49–64.

22. West CD. Idiopathic membranoproliferative glomerulonephritis in childhood. Pediatr Nephrol 1992;6:96–103.

23. West CD. Nephritic factors predispose to chronic glomerulonephritis. Am J Kidney Dis 1994;24:956–963.

24. West CD, McAdams AJ. Membranoproliferative glomerulonephritis type III: association of glomerular deposits with circulating nephritic factor-stabilized convertase. Am J Kidney Dis 1998;32:56–63.

25. Zauner I, Bohler J, Braun N, et al. Effect of aspirin and dipyridamole on proteinuria in idiopathic membranoproliferative glomerulonephritis: a multicentre prospective clinical trial. Collaborative Glomerulonephritis Therapy Study Group (CGTS). Nephrol Dial Transplant 1994;9:619–622.

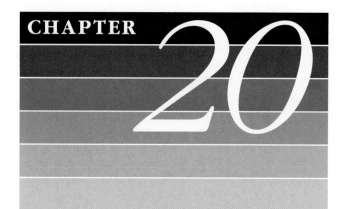

Hereditary Nephropathies

BERNARD S. KAPLAN, M.B., B.Ch.

> **Clinical Pearl**
>
> A renal syndrome may be the result of environmental cause(s) or genetic cause(s).

INTRODUCTION

Whenever a physician sees a patient with a renal syndrome, it is important to be aware of the following principles:

- Almost every renal syndrome can be the result of environmental causes or genetic causes. Nephritis can be caused by β-hemolytic *Streptococcus* and by mutations that give rise to Alport syndrome. Environmental causes of the nephrotic syndrome include hepatitis B and mercury, while genetic causes include mutations in the nephrin and podocin genes that result in congenital nephrotic syndrome and focal segmental glomerulosclerosis (FSGS), respectively. Shiga toxin-producing *E. coli* 0157: H is the most common environmental cause of the hemolytic uremic syndrome, and there are many other causes such as *S. pneumoniae,* and calcineurin inhibitors; however, an almost identical condition, atypical HUS, is caused by a mutation in Factor H on chromosome 1. Tubulointerstitial nephritis can be caused by antibiotics, viral infections, and numerous other agents, and by several mutations that result in nephronophthisis.

- Many renal syndromes are the result of more than one genetic or environmental cause. The same environmental agent can cause different renal syndromes. For example, *Treponema pallidum* can cause early-onset nephritis and later-onset membranous nephrotic syndrome. Mutations that result in Biedl–Bardet syndrome can cause combinations of small kidneys, obstructive uropathy, a glomerular disorder, and tubulointerstitial disease.

- It is important for treatment, counseling, and prognosis to determine whether the etiology of the syndrome is the result of an environmental insult or genetic mutation. HUS caused by *E. coli* 0157: H is treated differently and has a different outcome to HUS caused by a mutation in Factor H.

- A renal disease with a specific phenotype can be autosomal recessive, autosomal dominant, or X-linked. Alport syndrome and hypophosphatemic rickets are examples of inherited nephropathies with similar phenotypes caused by X-linked, recessive, and dominant modes of inheritance.

- A family history is important because many conditions once thought to be idiopathic or acquired may also be inherited. FSGS is an example of a glomerulopathy that can be idiopathic, or secondary to an acquired cause such as human immunodeficiency virus (HIV), or it can be inherited as autosomal recessive and autosomal dominant traits with mutations on different chromosomes.
- Some of the hereditary nephropathies, for example FSGS, affect only the kidney. Others, such as Biedl–Bardet syndrome, may affect other organs (retinitis pigmentosa, post-axial polydactyly) in addition to the kidneys.
- In many conditions there may be incomplete penetrance, such as polycystic kidney disease (PKD). A variable spectrum of involvement is common in PKD, but even more dramatic in tuberous sclerosis. For example, the kidneys in tuberous sclerosis may be affected by simple cyst, angiomyolipomas, polycystic disease, and renal cell tumors.
- In some genetic syndromes, such as Denys–Drash syndrome and Frasier syndrome, the condition is the result of a germline mutation, and is rarely inherited.
- Specific tests in presymptomatic individuals who are suspected of having a genetic condition must be undertaken with caution. It is important to ask whether presymptomatic diagnosis of a condition whose outcome cannot be affected by early diagnosis will benefit the individual, or have negative financial or psychological consequences.

In all patients with renal diseases, the clinical history and physical examination must be thorough, renal disease must be considered in patients with syndromes, and a careful family history must be obtained in all patients with renal disease (Table 20-1). The cystic kidney diseases and the renal dysplasia syndromes are described in Chapters 28 and 29, respectively.

Table 20-1 Inherited Nephropathies May Present with Discrete Renal Syndromes or Combinations of These Syndromes

Syndrome	Nephropathy
The nephrotic syndrome	Hypertension
The nephritic syndrome	Hematuria
Hemolytic uremic syndrome	Chronic renal failure
Fanconi syndrome	Rickets
Failure to thrive	Polydipsia, polyuria, and dehydration
Metabolic acidosis	Metabolic alkalosis
Vesicoureteric reflux	Cystic kidneys

NEPHROTIC SYNDROME

The nephrotic syndrome can be inherited as an entity that only affects the kidneys:
- Congenital nephrotic syndrome of the Finnish type (CNF)
- FSGS

Alternately, the nephrotic syndrome can be inherited as a part of a malformation syndrome:
- Denys–Drash syndrome
- Galloway–Mowat syndrome
- Nail-patella syndrome

The CNF *typically* presents with nephrotic syndrome at birth. Diffuse mesangial sclerosis (DMS),[15] Denys–Drash syndrome,[12] and Galloway–Mowat syndrome[2] rarely present with nephrotic syndrome during the neonatal period.

Congenital Nephrotic Syndrome of the Finnish Type (CNF)

Inheritance of CNF (also known as NPHS1) is autosomal recessive, with a mutation on 19q12-q13.1. The mutated gene codes for a cell-surface podocyte protein called nephrin. Two mutations, Fin-major and Fin-minor, occur in over 90% of Finnish patients.[10] CNF occurs in all population groups, but the highest prevalence is in Finland, with an incidence of 12.2 per 100,000 newborns. There is minor intrafamilial and interfamilial variability in the severity and age of onset of nephrotic syndrome. Proteinuria is detected within the first week of life in 71% of cases, and by 2 months in all affected infants. The placenta is large, with a mean placenta:neonatal weight ratio of 0.43 (normal ratio of 0.18). The babies are often premature and small for gestational age. Maternal serum and amniotic fluid alpha-fetoprotein levels are elevated, and amniotic fluid concentrations of albumin may be increased. The kidneys are echodense and are symmetrically enlarged on ultrasonography. Proximal tubules are dilated in 74% of cases, and the glomeruli initially appear normal. Later changes are interstitial fibrosis, lymphocytic and plasma cell infiltration, periglomerular fibrosis, and glomerular sclerosis. Ultrastructural studies show epithelial cell foot process effacement (Box 20-1).[10]

There are no typical dysmorphic features, but large anterior fontanels, limb deformations, pyloric stenosis, and pulmonic stenosis may occur. Affected babies have nephrotic syndrome complicated by failure to thrive, recurrent infections, and chronic renal failure (CRF). Early onset of hypertension and renal failure are uncommon. Renal vein thrombosis may occur *in utero* and postpartum. The nephrotic syndrome is resistant to treatment. Aggressive feeding by nasogastric or gastrostomy tubes may ensure weight gain. Massive edema is treated

---

Box 20-1 Finnish-Type Congenital Nephrotic Syndrome (CNF)

Alternate name	NPHS1
Gene product	Nephrin
Inheritance	Autosomal recessive
Mutation	Chromosome 19q12-q13.1
Onset	Birth to 3 months
Clinical features	Nephrotic syndrome
Specific treatment	Renal transplantation

Box 20-3 Denys–Drash Syndrome

Combinations of:
- Ambiguous genitalia – hypospadias, undescended testes[12]
- Early-onset nephrotic syndrome
- Diffuse mesangial sclerosis
- Wilms' tumor
- Zinc finger mutation on chromosome 11p
- Most patients die by 4 years of age unless transplanted

---

with intravenous albumin, and furosemide is added if the patient is not volume-depleted. Hypothyroidism is treated with thyroxin. Bilateral nephrectomy and dialysis are indicated if edema, volume depletion, and inanition cannot be controlled. The results of living-related renal transplantation are encouraging. CNF does not recur after transplantation, but a unique post-transplantation glomerular lesion resembling transplant glomerulopathy occurs in one-quarter of the patients and is resistant to treatment.[11]

Diffuse Mesangial Sclerosis (DMS)

Most patients with DMS present with nephrotic syndrome and CRF between 3 and 6 months of life and are hypertensive; they can also present at birth and in the neonatal period (Box 20-2).[15] There are no dysmorphic features unless the patient has Denys–Drash syndrome or Galloway–Mowat syndrome. The kidneys are enlarged and echodense. The renal lesion consists of mesangial sclerosis, collapsed tufts, embedded mesangial cells, thick glomerular basement membranes (GBM), and tubulointerstitial lesions. There is no specific treatment. Hypertension is treated with angiotensin-converting enzyme inhibitors, but often requires several additional agents. Treatment of DMS includes optimal calories, peritoneal dialysis, and transplantation. DMS does not recur after transplantation. It is important to determine whether there is a mutation in the *WT-1* gene on chromosome 11p in order to rule out Denys–Drash syndrome. If that cannot be done, renal ultrasound examinations may be

---

Box 20-2 Conditions Indicating the Presence of Diffuse Mesangial Sclerosis (DMS)

- Sporadic DMS
- Autosomal recessive inheritance
- Denys–Drash syndrome
- Galloway–Mowat syndrome

---

warranted every few months to monitor for Wilms' tumor, or both kidneys must be removed (Box 20-3).

Galloway–Mowat Syndrome

There is abnormal CNS development with microcephaly, wide sulci, abnormal gyral patterns, developmental retardation, and seizures.[2] The nephrotic syndrome presents before the age of three years, and is unresponsive to treatment. Inheritance is autosomal recessive. Death usually occurs before 6 months of age. There are various renal abnormalities that include FSGS, DMS, and even minimal changes.

Steroid-Responsive Nephrotic Syndrome

Patients in some families with steroid-responsive nephrotic syndrome have autosomal recessive inheritance with a median age of onset of 3.4 years. Some familial cases link to chromosome 2p.[14]

Focal Segmental Glomerulosclerosis (FSGS)[13]

Autosomal Recessive Disease

There is early onset of nephrotic syndrome, resistance to corticosteroid therapy, and rapid progression to end-stage kidney failure. Most affected children have FSGS on renal biopsy, but some have minimal change disease. The gene for this podocytopathy maps to chromosome 1q25-31, and the responsible gene, *NPHS2*, encodes podocin, a membrane protein. NPHS2 mutations also occur in 20–30% of children with *sporadic* steroid-resistant nephrotic syndrome.

Autosomal Dominant Disease

Autosomal dominant forms of FSGS present later and are more slowly progressive than recessive forms. There are two loci that are responsible for a fraction of the cases of dominant FSGS. Mutations in α-actinin-4 gene (*ACTN4*) cause a slowly progressive disease with dominant inheritance, minimal proteinuria, and renal insufficiency.

Table 20-2   Genetic Causes of Focal Segmental Glomerulosclerosis (FSGS)

FSGS Syndromes	Locus	Gene	Product	Inheritance
SRNS 1	1q25-q31	NPHS2	Podocin	Autosomal recessive
Dominant FSGS	19q13	ACTN4	α-actinin-4	Autosomal dominant
Dominant FSGS	11q21-q22			Autosomal dominant
Frasier syndrome	11p13	WT1	WT1	Autosomal dominant

SRNS = steroid-resistant nephrotic syndrome.

The penetrance of *ACTN4*-associated disease is high; some individuals in these families have disease-associated mutations, but no proteinuria or renal insufficiency. Most families with autosomal dominant FSGS do not map to *ACTN4*. One family mapped to chromosome 11q, but a mutation has not been found in the remainder.

Frasier Syndrome (FS)

FS is a rare disease of male pseudohermaphroditism and progressive glomerulopathy. Patients with normal female external genitalia, streak gonads, and XY karyotype frequently develop a gonadoblastoma. Renal symptoms in children are proteinuria and nephrotic syndrome with FSGS, and progression to end-stage renal failure in adolescence or early adulthood. Unlike Denys–Drash syndrome, they do not have Wilms' tumor. FS is caused by mutations in the donor splice site in intron 9 of *WT-1* (Table 20-2).[1]

Nail-Patella Syndrome (NPS)[17]

Inheritance of NPS is autosomal dominant. There is variable expression of dysplastic nails with absent lunae, absent or hypoplastic patellae, iliac horns, and elbow abnormalities (antecubital pterygium). There may be no renal manifestations; or there may be proteinuria and in some cases, nephrotic syndrome. The GBMs are abnormal. Fewer than 10% of NPS patients develop renal failure,[6] and the overall risk of having renal disease is less than 25%. Neurological and vasomotor symptoms, and gastrointestinal symptoms are also part of the NPS phenotype. The mutation is on chromosome 9q34.1 and the responsible gene is the lmx1b transcription factor (Box 20-4).

GLOMERULONEPHRITIS

Glomerulonephritis is defined by the occurrence of gross hematuria, proteinuria, red blood cell casts, oligoanuria, hypertension, and azotemia in various combinations. Acute post-streptococcal infection is the most frequent cause of acquired acute glomerulonephritis. A similar syndrome can also be seen in IgA nephropathy, ANCA-positive vasculitis/pauci immune glomerulonephritis, membranoproliferative glomerulonephritis, and lupus nephritis. Each of these conditions can be differentiated by specific tests and biopsy findings. However, it is important to note that Alport syndrome (hereditary nephritis) can present with a similar constellation of renal manifestations. Furthermore, IgA nephropathy,[4] MPGN and lupus nephritis may also be inherited in some cases.

Alport Syndrome (AS)[5]

Alport syndrome is a progressive, genetically heterogeneous nephropathy associated with deafness and/or ocular lesions. The renal disease in X-linked AS is worse in males than females, and typically progresses to end-stage renal failure by the second decade of life. Renal manifestations range from microscopic hematuria with red blood cell casts to macroscopic hematuria, variable proteinuria, and azotemia. Most patients have sensorineural deafness. Ocular findings include corneal abrasions, anterior lenticonus, and retinal flecks in the macular and mid-peripheral retina. The classical histopathologic changes in AS are laminated and basket-weave appearances of the GBMs. Carriers of X-linked disease have combinations of thinning and lamellation, while carriers of autosomal recessive disease have more widespread and more uniform thinning of the membrane and less lamellation. There is progressive glomerular sclerosis and tubulointerstitial damage. The Goodpasture antigen is identified with type IV collagen and is not detected in males, but may be present in affected females. Fewer than 5% of patients with AS develop anti-GBM nephritis in the allograft after

---

Box 20-4   Features of Nail-Patella Syndrome (NPS)

Skeletal features
- Absent or hypoplastic patellae, patella dislocations, elbow abnormalities, talipes, and iliac horns

Kidney involvement
- Proteinuria, chronic renal failure

Eyes
- Glaucoma

renal transplantation. IgG from patients with Goodpasture syndrome binds *in vitro* to normal GBM, but may not bind to the GBM of some patients with Alport syndrome. The mutation for the *COL4A5* gene in X-linked AS is mapped to Xq22-q23. A molecular diagnosis of AS is difficult because there is a wide phenotypic spectrum of collagen IV disorders with several underlying loci and mutational heterogeneity, especially in small families and sporadic cases. Therefore, a formal genetic analysis may not suggest what gene to study and what genotype to expect (homozygous/genetic compound versus heterozygous).

AS is usually the result of X-linked inheritance, but there are also patients with autosomal recessive and autosomal dominant inheritance of AS. There are at least two other syndromes with similar renal manifestations to AS but with additional features: the leiomyomatosis-nephropathy syndrome, and hereditary nephritis with giant platelets (Table 20-3).

Leiomyomatosis-Nephropathy Syndrome[8]

Patients with the leiomyomatosis-nephropathy syndrome have features of AS. This syndrome is the result of a contiguous gene syndrome due to deletions that disrupt the *COL4A5* and *COL4A6* genes.

Hereditary Nephritis with Giant Platelets[16]

Epstein syndrome is an autosomal dominant disease characterized by nephritis, mild hearing loss, and thrombocytopenia with giant platelets. The renal and hearing abnormalities are indistinguishable from those in an Alport-like variant that has been called Fechtner syndrome. Various combinations of nephritis, sensorineural deafness, congenital cataracts, macrothrombocytopenia, and Dohle-like leukocyte inclusions characterize the Fechtner syndrome. Renal disease ranges from microscopic hematuria to end-stage renal failure. Epstein syndrome with macrothrombocytopenia is similar to that described in Fechtner syndrome, May–Hegglin anomaly, and Sebastian syndrome. These latter three platelet disorders are caused by mutations in the non-muscle heavy chain myosin IIA (MYH9). In Epstein syndrome, however, there are no inclusion bodies in the leukocytes. The clinical features of these syndromes and the chromosomal localization of the respective gene in the same region as MYH9 suggest that they are allelic with the other giant platelet disorders associated with mutations of non-muscle myosin IIA on chromosome 22q.

Benign Familial Hematuria (BFH)

This is a heterozygous condition, usually with persistent microhematuria and occasionally intermittent microhematuria. There are rare episodes of macroscopic hematuria. BFH with normal renal function cannot be differentiated clinically from the initial stages of Alport syndrome. In some cases there are mutations of either *COL4A3* or *COL4A4*. BFH patients can be carriers of autosomal recessive Alport syndrome. There is thinning of the GBM. There may also be autosomal dominant inheritance.

Thin Glomerular Basement Membrane Disease (TBMD)[7]

This is where things can get really difficult. For example, is TBMD really a specific disease, a normal variant, or a manifestation of many different conditions? Isolated microscopic hematuria in childhood of glomerular origin may occur in Alport syndrome, IgA nephropathy and benign familial hematuria. In a series of 322 children with persistent hematuria for over 6 months, the biopsy diagnoses were IgA nephropathy in 78 patients, Alport syndrome in 86 patients, TBMD in 50 patients, and no abnormalities in 48 patients. The following approach is suggested when diffuse thin GBM is found in a patient with isolated hematuria: a careful family history and dipstick examination of the parents' urine. An audiogram and eye examination may be indicated, but DNA analysis is not recommended (Box 20-5).

HEMOLYTIC UREMIC SYNDROME (HUS) AND THROMBOTIC THROMBO-CYTOPENIC PURPURA (TTP)

Idiopathic (atypical or non-diarrhea-associated) HUS is a heterogeneous, distinct subgroup of the HUS. The epidemiological, clinical, laboratory, histological, and prognostic features of these patients differ from those with diarrhea-associated HUS. Some are hypocomplementemic with low Factor H concentrations and a pathogenesis that is linked to disorders. Treatment is often difficult because of severe hypertension and progressive renal failure and the possibility of recurrences. Plasmapheresis, although unproven, is still recommended. Post-transplant recurrences are frequent. Using a living-related kidney and calcineurin antagonists increases the chances of a recurrence, whereas pre-transplant nephrectomy may reduce recurrences.

Table 20-3 Mutations in Alport Syndrome		
Alport Syndrome	Gene	Locus
X-linked	Type IV collagen *COL4A5*	Xq22-q23
Autosomal recessive	*COL4A3* or *COL4A4*	2q
Autosomal dominant	*COL4A3* mutation	

Box 20-5 Glomerular Basement Membrane (GBM) Thickness Varies in Children

- 100 to 340 nm at 1 year of age
- 190 to 440 nm >9 years of age
- GBM is thinner in females than males
- Thin basement membranes (TBMs) occur in 5.2–9.2% of the general population
- Local normal ranges should be established

Autosomal Recessive and Autosomal Dominant Inheritance of HUS

The diagnosis of autosomal recessive or autosomal dominant HUS cannot be made without a positive family history, but must be suspected in patients with idiopathic HUS, especially if there is hypocomplementemia and a Factor H deficiency.[18] In the recessive form there are no recognized precipitating events, and no sex or race preferences. Most affected individuals are infants and children. In occasional patients there may be complete resolution, in some there may be several episodes of HUS, and HUS may recur before and/or after renal transplantation. Pregnancy may be a precipitating event in the dominant form in which adults are affected more often than children; there is no sex or race preference. Complete recovery is uncommon. In inherited forms of HUS with Factor H deficiency there is linkage to the Factor H locus on chromosome 1. There is no specific treatment, but fresh-frozen plasma infusions and plasmapheresis are indicated for inherited cases. The prognosis for renal survival is poor. The timing of a renal transplant presents problems, but it is advisable to wait for 6 to 12 months between the occurrence of HUS and the transplant. The patient must be free from all evidence of active disease. Although the use of a living-related donor presents a problem, there are no definite guidelines. There are also no hard data available in regard to the use of cyclosporine A or oral contraceptives. Pregnancy may increase the likelihood of recurrences. Genetic counseling is particularly difficult if the patient is the first affected individual in the family.

Thrombotic Thrombocytopenic Purpura (TTP)

Perturbations in the function of von Willebrand factor (vWF) proteases are the cause of TTP.[19] Patients with acute TTP appear to have an acquired disease with severe deficiency of vWF-cleaving protease caused by IgG antibodies directed against the protease. This deficiency is not detected in TTP patients in remission.

Auto-antibodies to the vWF metalloproteinase occur in patients with ticlopidine- and clopidogrel-associated TTP. Patients with familial forms of TTP have a constitutional lack of the vWF-cleaving protease, ADAMTS13, caused by genetic mutations.

TUBULOINTERSTITIAL DISEASE

Nephronophthisis[3]

Growth retardation, anemia, polyuria and polydipsia, isosthenuria, and potential death from uremia by 4 to 15 years of age characterize familial juvenile nephronophthisis (FJN). The urinalysis is bland, and there is usually no hypertension or proteinuria. There is symmetrical destruction of the kidneys with interstitial cell infiltrates and tubular cell atrophy with cysts arising from the corticomedullary junction. In addition, there are interstitial fibrosis and hyalinized glomeruli. Inheritance is autosomal recessive with a mutated gene, nephrocystin, on chromosome 2q13. There are, however, several additional similar syndromes (Table 20-4). Furthermore, nephronophthisis may be associated with retinal aplasia (Senior–Loken syndrome); cerebellar ataxia, skeletal abnormalities, and cone-shaped epiphyses (Mainzer syndrome); congenital hepatic fibrosis (Boichis syndrome). Nephronophthisis may also be associated with retinal dystrophy and bilateral sensorineural hearing loss.

Biedl–Bardet Syndrome (BBS)

BBS is characterized by mental retardation, retinitis pigmentosa, post-axial polydactyly, obesity, hypogenitalism, and renal disease.[9] All patients have some abnormality in renal structure, function, or both. Most have minor functional abnormalities and radiological appearances of calyceal clubbing or blunting, calyceal cysts or diverticuli. The spectrum of renal lesions ranges from mesangial tissue proliferation to glomerular sclerosis, interstitial scarring, and medullary and cortical cyst formation. Many patients have hypertension, and about 10% progress to end-stage renal disease hemodialysis. Patients with BBS have an increased risk for diabetes

Table 20-4 Classification of Nephronophthisis

Syndrome	Locus
NPHP1 Juvenile nephronophthisis	2q13
NPHP2 Infantile nephronophthisis	9q22-31
NPHP3 Adolescent nephronophthisis	3q21-22
NPHP4 and Senior–Loken syndrome	1p36
Autosomal dominant medullary cystic kidney disease	

mellitus and congenital heart disease. BBS maps to at least six loci: 11q13 (BBS1), 16q21 (BBS2), 3p13-p12 (BBS3), 15q22.3-q23 (BBS4), 2q31 (BBS5), and 20p12 (BBS6).

REFERENCES

1. Barbaux S, Niaudet P, Gubler MC, et al. Donor splice-site mutations in WT1 are responsible for Frasier syndrome. Nature Genet 1997;17:467-470.

2. Cooperstone BG, Friedman A, Kaplan BS. Galloway-Mowat syndrome of abnormal gyral patterns and glomerulopathy. Am J Med Genet 1993;47:250-254.

3. Hildebrandt F, Omram H. New insights: nephronophthisis-medullary cystic kidney disease. Pediatr Nephrol 2001;16: 168-176.

4. Hsu SI, Ramirez SB, Winn MP, et al. Evidence for genetic factors in the development and progression of IgA nephropathy. Kidney Int 2000;57:1818-1835.

5. Kashtan CE. Alport syndrome: an inherited disorder of renal, ocular, and cochlear basement membranes. Medicine 1999;78:338-360.

6. Looij BJ, Jr, Te Slaa RL, Hogewind BL, van de Kamp JJP. Genetic counseling in hereditary osteo-onychodysplasia (HOOD, nail-patella syndrome) with nephropathy. J Med Genet 1988;25:682-686.

7. Monnens L. Thin glomerular basement membrane disease. Kidney Int 2001;60:79.

8. Mothes H, Heidet L, Arrondel C, et al. Alport syndrome associated with diffuse leiomyomatosis: COL4A5-COL4A6 deletion associated with a mild form of Alport nephropathy. Nephrol Dial Transplant 2002;17:70-74.

9. Mykytyn K, Nishimura DY, Searby CC, et al. Evaluation of complex inheritance involving the most common Bardet-Biedl syndrome locus (BBS1). Am J Hum Genet 2003;72: 429-437.

10. Patrakka J, Kestila M, et al. Congenital nephrotic syndrome (NPHS1): features resulting from different mutations in Finnish patients. Kidney Int 2000;58:972-980.

11. Patrakka J, Ruotsalainen V, Reponen P, et al. Recurrence of nephrotic syndrome in kidney grafts of patients with congenital nephrotic syndrome of the Finnish type: role of nephrin. Transplantation 2002;73:394-403.

12. Pelletier J, Bruening W, Kashtan, CE, et al. Germline mutations in the Wilms' tumor suppressor gene are associated with abnormal urogenital development in Denys-Drash syndrome. Cell 1991;67:437-447.

13. Pollak MR. Inherited podocytopathies: FSGS and nephrotic syndrome from a genetic viewpoint. J Am Soc Nephrol 2002;13:3016-3023.

14. Ruf RG, Fuchshuber A, Karle SM. Identification of the first gene locus (SSNS1) for Steroid-Sensitive Nephrotic Syndrome on chromosome 2p. J Am Soc Nephrol 2003;14: 1897-1900.

15. Schumacher V, Scharer K, Wuhl E, et al. Spectrum of early onset nephrotic syndrome associated with WT1 missense mutations. Kidney Int 1998;53:1594-1600.

16. Seri M, Savino M, Bordo D, et al. Epstein syndrome: another renal disorder with mutations in the nonmuscle myosin heavy chain 9 gene. Hum Genet 2002;110: 182-186.

17. Sweeney E, Fryer A, Mountford R et al. Nail patella syndrome: a review of the phenotype aided by developmental biology. J Med Genet 2003;40:153-162.

18. Taylor CM. Hemolytic-uremic syndrome and complement factor H deficiency: clinical aspects. Semin Thromb Hemost 2001;27:185-190.

19. Tsai HM. Advances in the pathogenesis, diagnosis, and treatment of thrombotic thrombocytopenic purpura. J Am Soc Nephrol 2003;14:1072-1081.

CHAPTER 21

Minimal-Change Nephrotic Syndrome

KEVIN E.C. MEYERS M.B., B.Ch. AND

BERNARD S. KAPLAN, M.B., B.Ch.

INTRODUCTION

The nephrotic syndrome is characterized by edema, proteinuria, hypoalbuminemia, and hyperlipidemia. The designation *minimal-change* nephrotic syndrome (MCNS) derives from histopathologic findings of no discernible abnormalities on light microscopy and no immune deposits. By electron microscopy, however, effacement and retraction of podocyte foot processes are seen. Because few patients with presumed MCNS are biopsied, and an objective description of '*minimal*' is difficult, *steroid-sensitive* and *steroid-responsive* nephrotic syndrome more accurately describe the clinical condition. MCNS occurs mainly in children. Patients present with edema after an ill-defined 'upper respiratory tract infection', without gross hematuria, or azotemia. MCNS usually responds to corticosteroid treatment, tends to run a relapsing and remitting course, and rarely progresses to end-stage renal failure. Definitions of remission, relapse, and steroid responses are shown in Box 21-1.

EPIDEMIOLOGY

MCNS occurs mainly between the ages of 2 and 8 years, with a peak at 3 years, and accounts for 60–90% of nephrotic syndrome in children. The incidence is 2 to 7 per 100,000, and the prevalence is 15 per 100,000 children under the age of 16 years.[15] MCNS is uncommon

Box 21-1	Definitions of Response to Treatment for Minimal-Change Nephrotic Syndrome (MCNS)
Remission	Negative or trace urine on dipstick tests for at least 3 days
Relapse	2+ proteinuria for 3 days in a previously negative child
Frequent relapser	Two relapses within 6 months, or three relapses in 1 year
Steroid-responsive	Disappearance of proteinuria within 8 weeks of starting corticosteroids
Steroid-resistant	Failure to induce remission in 8 weeks using conventional doses of corticosteroids
Steroid-dependent	Relapse while trying to wean from corticosteroids or within 2 weeks of discontinuing corticosteroids

Box 21-2 Agents and Conditions Associated with MCNS

Drugs	Gold, penicillamine, ampicillin, mercury, non-steroidal anti-inflammatory drugs, lithium, trimethadione, paramethadione
Allergies	Pollen, milk, pork, house dust, bee stings
Tumors	Hodgkin disease, non-Hodgkin lymphoma, Kimura disease, renal oncocytoma, embryonal cell tumors, bronchogenic carcinoma
Infections	Viral, schistosomiasis, Guillain–Barré syndrome
Skin disorders	Dermatitis herpetiformis, melorheostosis, contact dermatitis
Myasthenia gravis	

Table 21-1 Immunologic Abnormalities in MCNS

Defects in innate immunity	Decreased alternate complement factors B and D
	Decreased opsonization
Defects in specific immunity	*Abnormal humoral immunity*
	Circulating immune complexes
	Decreased immunoglobulin production
	Altered immunoglobulin levels
	Decreased titers of specific antibodies
	Abnormal cell-mediated immunity
	Decreased delayed hypersensitivity reactions
	Decreased proliferative responses to mitogens
	Circulating suppressor lymphokines
	Increased suppressor cell activity

under 12 months, and rare under 6 months of age. Boys are twice as often affected as girls, and the incidence is greater in white and East Asian than in black children. The incidence of MCNS in families is 3.35%. Siblings are affected more often than a parent or child. The presentation and course are similar within families. Many agents and conditions are associated with MCNS; however, there are no proven causes. The most convincing are non-steroidal anti-inflammatory drugs (NSAIDs), lithium, and Hodgkin lymphoma (Box 21-2).

Allergens are implicated in the pathogenesis of MCNS, and there is a higher prevalence of asthma and eczema in patients and their first-degree relatives than in the general population. MCNS may be linked with the major histocompatability complex, but the evidence is weak and many of the proposed associations are inconsistent.

PATHOGENESIS

Immunopathophysiology

The association with atopy and specific antigenic challenges suggests an immunologic basis, but the pathogenesis of MCNS is obscure. T cells are thought to produce a circulating glomerulotoxic lymphokine, but none of the many immunologic abnormalities identified in MCNS actually causes the syndrome (Table 21-1).

Humoral Immunity

Patients are prone to infections, in part because of decreased serum IgG and IgA levels. In contrast, IgM and

IgE levels are elevated. Decreased serum IgG and IgA and increased IgM levels during relapse normalize in remission. B cells from patients with MCNS show impaired immunoglobulin synthesis in response to antigens. There are also lower titers of circulating antibodies to streptococcal and pneumococcal antigens than in equally nephrotic patients with other glomerular lesions. Responses to hepatitis B vaccine are suboptimal. Complement activation and immune complex formation do not have a role in the pathogenesis of MCNS.

Cellular Immunity

In MCNS, the delayed-type hypersensitivity response is decreased.[14] During relapse, the T cells show signs of activation with increased production of interleukin (IL)-1 and IL-2 and IL-13. The latter is an important T-cell cytokine with anti-inflammatory and immunomodulatory functions on B cells and monocytes. IL-13 may stimulate the monocytes' production of a vascular permeability factor that induces proteinuria. T cells may be important in NSAID-associated MCNS in which there is a marked interstitial infiltrate of T cells. Activated T cells in the interstitium may elaborate cytokines that enhance glomerular permeability. Many circulating factors are thought to be present in MCNS (Table 21-2).

Glomerular Pathophysiology

Glomerular capillaries have high-capacity ultrafiltration membranes with low resistance to water flow, in addition to size- and charge-selective filtration barriers that impede the passage of proteins. Transport of polyanions and facilitated filtration of polycations across the glomerular capillary wall are restricted. This suggests that the normal anionic charge barrier is perturbed in MCNS by as much as 50%. Charge selectivity is mainly due to highly sulfated sialoglycoproteins, such as heparan sulfate proteoglycan, in the glomerular basement membrane (GBM)

Table 21-2 Presumed Circulating Factors in MCNS

Factor	Source
Vascular permeability factor (VPF)	Media from stimulated MCNS lymphocytes
Vascular endothelial growth factor (VEGF)	Tumor cells, macrophages
Glomerular permeability factor (GPF)	Media from T-cell hybridomas
Soluble immune response factor (SIRS)	Sera from patients with MCNS
Sulfate turnover factor substance	Media from stimulated MCNS lymphocytes
IL-8	Sera from patients with MCNS
Hemopexin	Sera from patients with MCNS

Box 21-3 Abdominal Pain in MCNS

Pain caused by MCNS	Intestinal wall edema Primary peritonitis
Pain caused by corticosteroids	Gastric irritation Peptic ulcer Acute pancreatitis
Pain not caused by MCNS or its treatment	Acute appendicitis Acute pyelonephritis

and on the surface of endothelial and visceral epithelial cells. The charge barrier may be responsible for the relative impermeability of the GBM to anionic albumin, despite its relatively small molecular size. Alterations in GBM charge may be due to enzymes elaborated by mononuclear cells, or it may be due to circulating highly cationic substances that have not been characterized. Size selectivity is impaired, and foot process effacement may account for the observed decrease in pore density. Changes in foot processes may be related, in part, to a reduction in adhesion proteins anchoring and stabilizing podocytes on the GBM. Changes in nephrin distribution on podocytes in MCNS may be secondary to a component of proteinuria rather than a primary cause of MCNS.

CLINICAL FEATURES

Clinically, the patient looks miserable and complains of fatigue and general malaise. Edema onset is insidious or rapid, and at first is periorbital in the mornings.

The severity and extent of the edema initially fluctuates. During the day, the periorbital swelling decreases and ankle swelling becomes more apparent. There is increasing swelling of the sacral region, genitalia, and abdomen. Severe edema may lead to breakdown of skin and infection. Ascites and/or pleural effusions may cause tachypnea or dyspnea. Ascites also causes a markedly protuberant abdomen and, in some cases, umbilical and inguinal hernias. There may be reduced appetite, colicky abdominal pain, and diarrhea or bulky stools (Box 21-3).

Volume status is assessed by the pulse rate, state of hydration, and orthostatic changes in blood pressure (Box 21-4).

Soft ear cartilages, lusterless hair, and white transverse bands in the nail beds are all consequences of chronic hypoproteinemia. Mild hypertension occurs in 95% of children prior to corticosteroid treatment, and in

19% after remission. Hypertension is occasionally a pressor response to volume depletion, and blood pressure may normalize with volume expansion. However, hypertension is attributed mainly to hypervolemia or loss of antihypertensive substance(s) in the urine. Hypertensive encephalopathy is uncommon and, when it occurs, is the result of corticosteroid treatment. In MCNS, there is oliguria and the urine is foamy and concentrated; gross hematuria is uncommon.

LABORATORY FINDINGS

There are numerous biochemical abnormalities in MCNS. These are the consequences of large urinary losses of albumin and other proteins and of compensatory mechanisms, such as sodium and water retention. The serum albumin concentration is usually less than 2.4 g/dl. The serum albumin concentration, urine protein excretion, and severity of edema are not correlated with each other. There are many lipid derangements, but the hallmark of the syndrome is hypercholesterolemia. Hyperlipidemia occurs during episodes of MCNS, and persists for months after corticosteroids are stopped. The serum sodium concentration is often decreased as a result of free water retention or, less often, because of prolonged sodium restriction, and rarely as a result of acquired adrenal insufficiency. Thrombocytosis can spuriously elevate the measured serum potassium concentration by the in-vitro release of potassium. Serum calcium concentrations are decreased as a consequence of

Box 21-4 Hypovolemia in MCNS[19]

- Hypovolemia can occur in the acute phase of MCNS
- Hypovolemia is usually associated with hemoconcentration and abdominal pain
- Elevated hemoglobin and hyponatremia are the best indicators of hypovolemia
- Consider primary peritonitis and hypovolemia in a child with MCNS and abdominal pain

hypoalbuminemia and urinary losses of 25-hydroxychole-calciferol binding-protein. Serum creatinine concentrations and blood urea nitrogen (BUN) levels are transiently increased in one-third of patients at presentation. The hematocrit is often increased as a result of intravascular volume depletion, and the white cell count and differential are normal. The erythrocyte sedimentation rate is markedly elevated.

Protein excretion is greater than 4 mg/m^2/hour during an episode of MCNS. The standard method for determining the magnitude of proteinuria is to collect urine for 24 hours. However, this is often difficult to do in incontinent children, collection errors are frequent, there is an inherent time delay, and it is difficult to do at home. Urine protein is more easily measured by the dipstick method and by the urine protein:creatinine ratio ($U_{P:C}$) in an early-morning sample. The dipstick test detects albumin, and is less sensitive for low molecular-weight proteins, immunoglobulins, and Bence–Jones protein. Errors arise if the effect of dilution of the urine is ignored, and therefore the test is best done on a concentrated early-morning specimen. In MCNS the dipstick measurement is 4+ (>2000 mg/dl), and the $U_{P:C}$ value is above 1.0.

PATHOGENESIS OF METABOLIC DERANGEMENTS

The serum albumin concentration is the result of a balance between the rate of hepatic synthesis of albumin and the rate of catabolism plus the quantities lost in urine and stool. Edema is the result of an abnormal collection of fluid in interstitial tissues, but the mechanisms underlying the production and maintenance of nephrotic edema are not fully understood.[13] The nephrotic state is dynamic, and different results are obtained because not all studies are conducted at similar stages of the disease. Hypoalbuminemia *per se* may not be the crucial factor because edema does not occur in congenital analbuminemia, or in all cases of nephrotic syndrome. In MCNS, edema occurs when the serum albumin concentration falls to less than 2.0 g/dl, and ascites and pleural effusions develop below a level of 1.5 g/dl. A reduction in intravascular volume results in a decrease in intraglomerular hydraulic pressure, activation of vasoconstrictor mechanisms, and increased efferent arteriolar constriction in an effort to maintain the glomerular filtration rate (GFR). Renal salt and water excretion are impaired in nephrotic syndrome.[16] Volume depletion may cause enhanced proximal tubular sodium retention for restoration of intravascular volume and GFR. In circumstances in which plasma volume is normal or increased, sodium reabsorption may occur in the more distal part of the nephron.

Increased plasma renin activity (PRA) and plasma aldosterone occur more frequently in MCNS than in other forms of nephrotic syndrome. Arginine vasopressin (AVP) levels are increased during edema formation and return to basal levels in remission.

Hyperlipidemia is the result of increased hepatic synthesis of beta-lipoprotein as a result of loss of high-density lipoprotein (HDL) cholesterol and an unidentified substance in the urine, as well as decreased portal vein oncotic pressure. Hypercholesterolemia is almost always a component of MCNS, whereas hypertriglyceridemia occurs with marked reductions in serum albumin concentrations. Cholesterol synthesis is increased, and the serum concentration is inversely related to albumin and oncotic pressure, and correlates with renal albumin clearance. Serum cholesterol levels gradually normalize months after with remission of MCNS. Patients with MCNS are at risk for venous thromboses, but none of the coagulation abnormalities (Box 21-5) correlates directly with a risk for thrombosis.

The serum total calcium level decreases by 0.2 mg/dl for every 1 g/dl decrease in serum albumin concentration. Some patients have low serum ionized calcium concentrations that are out of proportion to the degree

---

Box 21-5 Coagulation Abnormalities

Platelets
  Increased in-vitro platelet aggregability
  Increased platelet adhesion
  Thrombocytosis
Red blood cells
  Reduced erythrocyte deformability
  Increased plasma viscosity
Blood volume
  Volume depletion
Endothelial factors
  Increased von Willebrand factor
  Lysolecithin-enriched LDL impairs nitric oxide production
Hyperfibrinogenemia and increased thrombin formation
  Fibrin deposition
  Increased alpha 2-macroglobulin
  Normal/increased total antithrombolytic activity
  Decreased free protein S
  Functional protein C deficiency
Decreased fibrinolysis
  Decreased plasminogen
  Increased α-2-antiplasmin prevents plasmin-fibrin binding
  Reduced plasminogen-fibrin binding
Urine losses
  Procoagulant and anticoagulant factors
  Antithrombin 3

<table>
<tr><td>

Box 21-6 Causes of Bone Disease in MCNS

- Related to age of onset, duration of illness, frequency of relapses
- Perturbations in the vitamin D-parathyroid hormone axis
- Corticosteroids

</td><td>

Box 21-7 Potential Complications of MCNS

- Infections
- Thrombosis (venous or arterial)
- Protein-losing enteropathy
- Hyponatremia/hypocalcemia/hypokalemia/ hypomagnesemia
- Acute renal failure
- Growth retardation
- Malnutrition
- Hypothyroidism, trace metal deficiency
- Coronary artery disease
- Focal segmental glomerulosclerosis
- Chronic renal failure

</td></tr>
</table>

of hypoalbuminemia, increased parathyroid hormone (PTH) levels, and bone disease. The vitamin-D binding protein (DBP) that transports 25-hydroxycholecalciferol is lost in the urine, and plasma levels of 1,25-dihydroxy-cholecalciferol are normal or decreased (Box 21-6).

In children with MCNS there are urinary losses of thyroid-binding globulin (TBG) and thyroxine (T_4). Although serum TBG and T_4 concentrations are low and thyroid-stimulating hormone (TSH) levels are high, these patients do not have hypothyroidism. Increased urinary loss of ceruloplasmin can cause hypocuprinemia; loss of transferrin can result in anemia; and loss of albumin results in low zinc levels because two-thirds of the circulating zinc is bound to albumin. Zinc deficiency may contribute to growth retardation, immune dysfunction, and delayed wound healing. Additional losses of protein may occur as a result of protein-losing enteropathy and lymphangiectasia in MCNS.

COMPLICATIONS

Patients with MCNS are at increased risk for measles, varicella, and primary peritonitis with encapsulated organisms such as *S. pneumoniae*. The risk of infection is increased by reduced immunity, ascites, and immunosuppressive treatment. Edema and malnutrition may split the skin and predispose patients to cellulitis. Venous and arterial thromboses occur in under 5% of cases, and subclinical pulmonary emboli were detected in 28% of children with MCNS by radionucleotide perfusion studies. Acute renal vein thrombosis can present with flank pain and macroscopic hematuria; hypertension and azotemia may be mild. Treatment is with intravenous heparin followed by coumarin, possibly for many years. Thrombolytic agents lyse clots faster and more completely with less likelihood of re-thrombosis. Chronic renal vein thrombosis is usually asymptomatic. By ultrasonography, the kidney is found to be small, and collateral vessels are seen with renal venography. Renal venography is indicated if there is rapid unexplained deterioration in renal function, acute flank pain, macroscopic hematuria, pleuritic chest pain, or other symptoms suggestive of thromboembolism. Acute renal failure (ARF) is an uncommon complication of MCNS that may occur as a result of severe intravascular volume depletion, bilateral renal vein thrombosis, pyelonephritis, or medications. Acute tubular necrosis is rare in children. ARF usually responds to aggressive therapy with diuretics or corticosteroids. Some patients with ARF may require dialysis, but recovery is usually complete. There are few reports of atherosclerosis and ischemic heart disease in children with MCNS. FSGS may occur subsequently in a small number of patients who previously responded to corticosteroid therapy. Chronic renal failure does not occur in patients with MCNS unless they have developed focal segmental glomerulosclerosis (FSGS) (Box 21-7).

PATHOLOGY

Light Microscopy

Glomeruli appear normal (or nearly so) by light microscopy. The mesangium is considered to be normal if there are two or fewer cells, expanded if there are three cells, and proliferative if there are four or more cells. Mesangial proliferation in the context of MCNS may not be a discrete entity, although these patients are more likely to be corticosteroid-resistant.[9] Even one glomerulus with FSGS portends a more severe prognosis with corticosteroid resistance and progressive azotemia.

Immunofluorescent and Electron Microscopy

Immunofluorescent stains are usually negative for immunoglobulins and complement. Mesangial deposits of IgM with mesangial expansion are seen in a few patients with corticosteroid-dependent nephrotic syndrome.

Electron microscopy shows effacement, retraction and vacuolization of epithelial foot processes. These reversible phenomena occur in association with proteinuria, are not specific for MCNS, and can persist for months after cessation of proteinuria.

MANAGEMENT

General Management

The objectives of treatment are to induce a remission as soon as possible in order to reduce the complications of untreated nephrotic syndrome, to minimize medication side effects, and to provide psychosocial support. We admit the child to hospital when first diagnosed for evaluation, treatment, counseling, and education. Pertinent information is provided and repeated at follow-up visits. Parents and patients are taught how to monitor the condition, and they are provided with an invaluable illustrative booklet. The potential side effects of corticosteroids are explained in detail. Growth in steroid-resistant nephrotic syndrome is mainly affected by the cumulative doses of corticosteroids.

Hypovolemia is corrected with infusions of saline, plasma, or 5% albumin.[19] A sodium-restricted diet of 1–2 g per day reduces edema formation and minimizes the risk of hypertension while on corticosteroids. Protein intake should be in keeping with the recommended daily allowance; a diet which is high in protein is of no benefit. Low-protein diets may reduce albuminuria but can cause malnutrition. Corticosteroids increase the appetite, and calorie intake must be controlled to reduce the likelihood of obesity. Diuretics may be needed in some cases for severe edema, but considerable caution must be exercised, because it is easy to cause hypovolemia and azotemia once a diuresis begins.

Angiotensin-converting enzyme (ACE) inhibitors and angiotensin receptor blockers (ARBs) are prescribed for patients with refractory proteinuria who fail to respond to other therapies.[7] ACE inhibitors and ARBs block the local production and binding of angiotensin II that may contribute to the permeability/selectivity defect. They also affect the size-selective properties of the glomerular capillary wall.

Infections and Immunization

A purified protein derivative (PPD) must be placed before starting treatment with corticosteroids. Varicella infection can cause serious problems in patients receiving corticosteroids or alkylating agents, who must be treated as shown in Box 21-8.

Patients who develop varicella or shingles are treated with acyclovir if they are on high doses of corticosteroids or on an alkylating agent. If exposure to measles occurs, the patient's immune status is checked, quarantine

---

Box 21-8 Treatment of Varicella Exposure During the Previous 96 Hours

- Indications for treatment of a patient on high doses of prednisone >20 mg/m^2 or an alkylating agent:
  - No previous varicella or no serum antibody titers to varicella
- Dose of varicella zoster immune globulin:
  - 125 units/10 kg body weight to a maximum of 625 units

---

measures are instituted, and gamma-globulin is administered. Primary peritonitis is a serious complication that must be treated expeditiously (Box 21-9). Cellulitis is managed in the same way as peritonitis.

There are no criteria for the use of intravenous immunoglobulin. Recommendations include IgG levels under 600 mg/dl in adults, low natural antibody levels, poor response to vaccine, and no protective antibody against the infecting organism. Desensitization, disodium cromoglycate, and an oligoantigenic diet are ineffective forms of therapy.

Glucocorticoids

Corticosteroids (prednisone and prednisolone) remain the treatment of choice for MCNS, despite their side effects and their inability to cure the condition (Figure 21-1). An initial high daily dose of corticosteroids is required to achieve remission.

Typical corticosteroid regimens include:

1. The modified International Study of Kidney Disease in Children (ISKDC) regimen. Prednisone in a dose of 60 mg/m^2 (to a maximum of

---

Box 21-9 Peritonitis in MCNS[8]

- Peritonitis is characterized by abdominal pain (98%), fever (95%), rebound tenderness (85%), and nausea and vomiting (71%)
- Most patients are in relapse or on corticosteroid therapy when peritonitis is diagnosed
- Infiltrates are visible on chest radiographs in many cases
- Antimicrobial therapy should be started in nephrotic children with suspected peritonitis
- Use a combination of penicillin plus an aminoglycoside or a cephalosporin
- This regimen should continue until culture results are available
- Penicillin is sufficient if Gram-positive diplococci are identified in a peritoneal fluid specimen

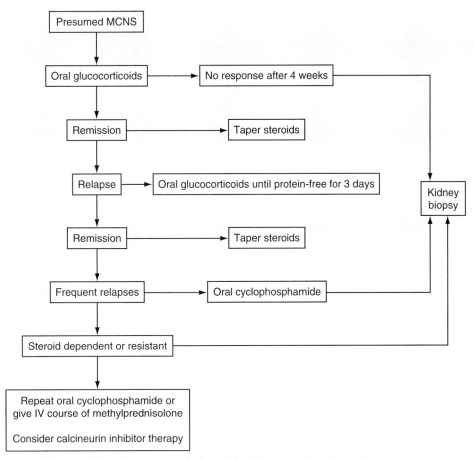

Figure 21-1   Treatment cycle for minimal-change nephrotic syndrome (MCNS).

80 mg/day in children) for 4 weeks followed by 40 mg/m² every second morning for another 4 weeks. The median time from starting treatment to remission is 2 weeks; 95% of patients are in remission by the end of 8 weeks. Urine should be checked for albumin every morning by dipstick testing until the nephrotic syndrome has remitted.

2. Prednisone at a dose of 2 mg/kg ideal body weight, to a maximum of 80 mg/day, or 60 mg/m²/day, until the urine is protein-free for 3 days. Once in remission, the dose is reduced to 40 mg/m² every second morning for 4 weeks.

3. A longer initial course of corticosteroid therapy for 6 weeks. This has not been proven to induce a more prolonged initial remission, and may cause more side effects.

If there is no response by 4 weeks the child is considered to be steroid-resistant. About 80% of patients relapse at least once, 50% have frequent relapses but remain steroid-responsive, and the remainder becomes steroid-dependent.[18] Age, sex, and race as independent variables, do not predict relapses in the first year. However, patients were more likely to be infrequent relapsers if they did not have hematuria and remitted within a week of onset

of therapy.[10] Relapses become less frequent in children as they grow older, and most 'outgrow' the condition after puberty. Corticosteroid-dependence and resistance are more common in patients who relapse within 3 months of the first remission. The first three relapses are managed in the same way as the first episode. Subsequent relapses are treated with more prolonged doses of prednisone every second morning for 6 months at a dose of 0.1 to 0.5 mg/kg, after which the dose is gradually tapered.[6,17]

Alkylating Agents

Alkylating agents can induce prolonged remissions, but are used judiciously because of their potential side effects. The peripheral blood counts must be monitored regularly because of leukopenia. The drug is stopped transiently if the white blood cell count is >4000 per ml.[3] The risk of gonadal toxicity is greatest in postpubertal males. Azoospermia may occur after a cumulative dose of 300 mg/kg for cyclophosphamide and 10 mg/kg for chlorambucil.[4] Doses of cyclophosphamide of 2.5 mg/kg/day for 8-12 weeks usually do not cause alopecia or hemorrhagic cystitis.[1,11] Leukemia is a rare complication. Patients are at risk for developing disseminated varicella while receiving an alkylating agent if they have not previously had varicella or a vaccine. Less frequent complications are nausea, anorexia, and hyperpigmentation. Chlorambucil can cause seizures,[5] and there is no evidence that it is more effective than cyclophosphamide.[2,5]

Longer courses of alkylating agent therapy have a greater likelihood of prolonged remission, and also of side effects. A short course has little benefit because only one-third of children with frequently relapsing nephrotic syndrome remain in remission after 1 year if given cyclophosphamide for less than 6 weeks; two-thirds remain in remission for more than 2 years after 12 weeks of therapy. Remission is not as well maintained with steroid-dependent nephrotic syndrome (SDNS). The current practice is to prescribe 2.5–3 mg/kg for an 8- to 12-week period after remission is induced with corticosteroids. After cyclophosphamide is started, steroid doses are tapered gradually and stopped at 4–6 weeks after the course of cyclophosphamide is completed.

Calcineurin Inhibitors

Calcineurin inhibitors (cyclosporine and tacrolimus) are used to treat steroid-dependent nephrotic syndrome if there are serious side effects of corticosteroids and failure to respond to cyclophosphamide.[12] A kidney biopsy should be performed before starting and after completing a course of a calcineurin inhibitor because it may cause interstitial fibrosis. Contraindications to calcineurin inhibitors treatment are renal insufficiency, severe hypertension, and chronic tubulointerstitial changes. Calcineurin inhibitors are stopped if there is no response by 4 months. The plasma creatinine level, blood pressure, and serum calcineurin level must be monitored regularly. The dose is reduced if the serum creatinine concentration increases by more than 30% above the basal level. The maintenance dose is the lowest effective dose. The calcineurin inhibitors can be tapered and stopped after 1 to 2 years to see if the patient remains in remission. Many patients relapse when the calcineurin inhibitors are tapered or stopped, and they tend to respond less well to a second course of the calcineurin inhibitor.

Controlled studies are required to evaluate the potential value of mycophenolate mofital. Azathioprine, levamisole, vincristine, quinolones, mizoribine, sodium cromoglycate, and immunoglobulin infusions are not effective treatments of MCNS.

OUTCOME

Antibiotics substantially reduce the mortality rate in MCNS, and corticosteroid therapy induces remissions and prevents relapses. Few children die from complications of MCNS or of its treatment. Thrombosis, sepsis, ARF, and cardiovascular disease may result in death. In children who present before the age of 6 years, the incidence of relapses beyond 18 years of age is 5.5%. Untreated proteinuria, in the absence of massive edema, does not always result in an unfavorable outcome.

MAJOR POINTS

- *"Few diseases tax the resources of the practitioner so extensively as the nephrotic syndrome. He must be a combination of infectious disease expert, nutritionist, physiologist, and psychiatrist for the patient and, above all, guide counselor and friend to the parents, who have to live day in and day out, for two or three years with a child who eats poorly and often has periods of irritability or depression, who frequently vomits or has diarrhea, whose appearance may become grotesque at times, and who may become desperately sick with peritonitis and bacteremia at any moment. On the other hand, the satisfaction of seeing a patient restored to normal health after several years of edema is well worth the time and patience required."* Barness
- Onset of nephrotic syndrome may herald an underlying malignancy, may remit with treatment of the tumor, and may relapse with tumor recurrence.
- Edema is frequently misdiagnosed as 'an allergy' and is often treated inappropriately with antihistamines.
- Urine protein must be checked by a dipstick test in any child with periorbital edema.
- The total daily protein excretion can be derived by multiplying the $U_{P:C}$ value by 0.633.
- One-quarter of children with MCNS have microscopic hematuria at the time of diagnosis.
- MCNS induces anxiety in patients and parents because of uncertain etiology, a high likelihood of recurrence, fear of end-stage renal failure, and dislike of corticosteroids.
- Anticipate hypovolemia patients who have any of the following:
  - Peritonitis
  - Marked edema
  - Diarrhea or vomiting
  - Diuretic treatment
- There is no evidence that vaccinations or inoculations precipitate a relapse.
- Decisions to immunize should not be influenced by this issue alone.
- Indications for cyclophosphamide:
  - Frequent relapses while receiving more than 1 mg/kg of prednisone every other day.
  - Serious corticosteroid-induced side effects.

REFERENCES

1. Abeitsgemeinschaft fur Padiatrische Nephrologie. Cyclophosphamide treatment of steroid dependent nephrotic syndrome: comparison of 8-week with 12-week course. Arch Dis Child 1987;62:1102–1106.

2. Abeitsgemeinschaft fur Padiatrische Nephrologie. Effect of cytoxic drugs in frequently relapsing nephrotic syndrome with and without steroid dependence. N Engl J Med 1982; 306:451–454.

3. Abitbol C, Zilleruelo G, Freundlich M, Strauss J. Quantitation of proteinuria with urinary protein/creatinine ratios and random testing with dipsticks in nephrotic children. J Pediatr 1990;116:243–247.

4. Bogdanovic R, Banicevic M, Cvoric A. Testicular function following cyclophosphomide treatment for childhood nephrotic syndrome: long-term follow-up study. Pediatr Nephrol 1990;4:451–454.

5. Elzouki AY, Jaiswal OP. Evaluation of chlorambucil therapy in steroid-dependent and cyclophosphamide-resistant children with nephrosis. Pediatr Nephrol 1990;4:459–462.

6. Elzouki AY, Jaiswal OP. Long-term, small-dose prednisone therapy in frequently relapsing nephrotic syndrome. Clin Pediatr 1988;27:387–392.

7. Garza MB, Guttenberg M, Kaplan BS. Nephrotic syndrome at 5 months: no definitive treatment or complications for 12 years. Pediatr Nephrol 1999;13:604–606.

8. Gorensek MJ, Lebel MH, Nelson JD. Peritonitis in children with nephrotic syndrome. Pediatrics 1988;81:849–856.

9. International Study of Kidney Disease in Children. Nephrotic syndrome in children: prediction of histopathology from clinical and laboratory characteristics at time of diagnosis. Kidney Int 1978;13:159–165.

10. International Study of Kidney Disease in Children. Early identification of frequent relapsers among children with minimal change nephrotic syndrome. J Pediatr 1982;101: 514–518.

11. International Study of Kidney Disease in Children. Prospective controlled trial of cyclophosphamide therapy in children with the nephrotic syndrome. Lancet 1974;2: 413–427.

12. Kitano Y, Norishige Y, Tanaka R, Nakamura M, Ito H. Ciclosporin treatment in children with steroid-dependent nephrotic syndrome. Pediatr Nephrol 1990;4:474–477.

13. Mees EG, Geers AB, Koomans HA. Blood volume and sodium retention in the nephrotic syndrome: a controversial pathophysiological concept. Nephron 1984;6:201–211.

14. Shalhoub RJ. Pathogenesis of lipoid nephrosis: a disorder of T-cell function. Lancet 1974;2:556–559.

15. Schlesinger ER, Sultz HA, Mosher WE, Feldman JG. The nephrotic syndrome: its incidence and implications for the community. Am J Dis Child 1968;116:622–632.

16. Schrier RW. Pathogenesis of sodium and water retention in high-output and low-output cardiac failure, nephrotic syndrome, cirrhosis, and pregnancy. N Engl J Med 1988; 319:1065–1072.

17. Ueda N, Chihara M, Kawaguchi S. Intermittent versus long-term tapering of prednisolone for initial therapy in children with idiopathic nephrotic syndrome. J Pediatr 1988; 112:122–126.

18. Walshaw BL, Hymes LC. Daily single-dose and daily reduced-dose prednisone therapy for children with the nephrotic syndrome. Pediatrics 1989;83:694–699.

19. Wang SJ, Tsau YK, Lu FL, et al. Hypovolemia and hypovolemic shock in children with nephrotic syndrome. Acta Paediatr Taiwan 2000;41:179–183.

Focal Segmental Glomerulosclerosis

BERNARD S. KAPLAN, M.B., B.Ch.

INTRODUCTION

Focal segmental glomerulosclerosis (FSGS) is not a disease, but rather a clinicopathological syndrome. Patients may present with overt features of the nephrotic syndrome, or they may be asymptomatic and the diagnosis is made only after a kidney biopsy in a patient with combinations of isolated proteinuria, hypertension, or chronic renal insufficiency. The histopathologic findings are focal and segmental glomerular sclerosis with foot process effacement. FSGS may be primary (idiopathic) or secondary to numerous and diverse renal conditions as shown in Table 22-1.

There are several morphologic variants of primary and secondary FSGS. FSGS not otherwise specified (NOS) is the predominant lesion in children. There are also perihilar, cellular, tip, and collapsing variants (Table 22-2).

Idiopathic FSGS

Idiopathic FSGS is a primary glomerular disease for which the cause(s) of the chronic, progressive glomerular fibrosis are unknown. Proteinuria, progressive renal insufficiency, and the nephrotic syndrome characterize FSGS. It is the histopathologic lesion in 7–15% of biopsied

Table 22-1	Causes of Focal Segmental Glomerulosclerosis (FSGS)	
Primary FSGS	**Idiopathic**	
Idiopathic nephrotic syndrome	'Minimal change disease', IgM nephropathy, C1q nephropathy, mesangial proliferative glomerulonephritis	
Inherited FSGS	*NPHS2* podocin mutations, *α-actinin 4* mutations, *CD2AP* mutations, *WT1* mutations, mitochondrial DNA mutations	
Glomerular hyperfiltration	Congenital or acquired reduced renal mass, diabetes, sickle cell disease, hypertension, morbid obesity, cyanotic congenital heart disease, glycogen storage disease	
FSGS secondary to inflammation	HIV nephropathy, IgA nephropathy, Henoch–Schönlein nephritis, lupus nephritis, ANCA-positive glomerulonephritis, Shiga toxin-associated hemolytic uremic syndrome, membranous glomerulonephritis	
Medications and drugs	Heroin nephropathy, calcineurin inhibitors, lithium, pamidronate	

ANCA = anti-neutrophil cytoplasmic antibodies.

Table 22-2 The Morphologic Variants of FSGS[9]

Variant	Positive Criteria	Negative Criteria
FSGS (NOS)	• At least one glomerulus with segmental increase in matrix obliterating the capillary lumina • There may be segmental glomerular basement membrane collapse without podocyte hyperplasia	• Exclude perihilar, cellular, tip and collapsing variants
Perihilar variant	• Perihilar sclerosis and hyalinosis involving >50% of segmentally sclerotic glomeruli	• Exclude cellular, tip and collapsing variants
Cellular variant	• At least one glomerulus with segmental endocapillary hypercellularity occluding lumina, with or without foam cells and karyorrhexis	• Exclude tip and collapsing variants
Tip variant	• At least one segmental lesion involving the tip domain (outer 25% of tuft next to origin of proximal tubule) • The tubular pole must be identified in the defining lesion • The lesion must have either an adhesion or confluence of podocytes with parietal or tubular cells at the tubular lumen or neck • The tip lesion may be sclerosing or cellular	• Exclude collapsing variants • Exclude perihilar sclerosis
Collapsing variant	• At least one glomerulus with segmental or global collapse and podocyte hypertrophy/hyperplasia	• None

cases of nephrotic syndrome in children, and in 15–20% of adults. It is frequent in blacks. There is no specific treatment, and FSGS often progresses to end-stage renal disease (ESRD); indeed, it accounts for 20% of children and 5% of adults with ESRD. FSGS can recur after renal transplantation.

EPIDEMIOLOGY

There is a higher incidence of FSGS in children with steroid-dependent or frequently relapsing nephrotic syndrome, and the incidence of FSGS in the pediatric population with nephrotic syndrome is increasing. The odds of a diagnosis of FSGS in a biopsy specimen of a child with nephrotic syndrome are almost three times higher now than before 1990.[2] There is an increased risk and worse outcome of FSGS in blacks compared with non-black children.[22] Black patients with FSGS are older at presentation (mean age 12.7 ± 4.4 years) than non-black patients (mean 5.6 ± 4.6 years) (p <0.001). Increasing age at presentation increases the probability of FSGS in black but not non-black patients (p = 0.04). The 5-year actuarial renal survival of FSGS is worse in black patients (8%) than in non-blacks (31%) (p = 0.01). In Texas, but not in New York, Hispanics have the lowest risk for FSGS and the highest incidence of MCNS. Males are affected slightly more often than females, and blacks more often than whites.[14]

CLINICAL FEATURES

The presenting feature is always proteinuria, often with the features of the nephrotic syndrome (90% of cases).

Many patients, however, have nephrotic range proteinuria without edema or hypoalbuminemia. The proteinuria is not orthostatic, and is usually in excess of 1.5 g per day. Many patients have hematuria (55%) that is usually microscopic, in addition to hypertension (30%) that can be severe. The serum creatinine concentration may be elevated at the time of presentation in 20% of children. Some patients describe a waxing and waning course of periorbital or pedal edema over a period of months. Patients may complain of vague symptoms of malaise and tiredness. There are usually no other symptoms. The clinical signs are edema that ranges from mild periorbital puffiness to massive total body swelling. The edema is dependent, and pitting, and often worsens during the day. Some patients have ascites and labial and scrotal swelling that can be debilitating. There are usually no other clinical signs, except for cardiomegaly or retinal changes in patients with severe and long-standing hypertension. Many patients are obese, but it is unclear whether these constitute a different subset of FSGS or simply the tendency to obesity in the North American population.

LABORATORY INVESTIGATIONS

The initial evaluation includes a careful urinalysis, 24-hour collection for protein excretion, and exclusion of orthostatic proteinuria in non-edematous patients. A complete blood count and measurement of serum electrolyte concentrations, blood urea nitrogen (BUN), and serum creatinine, albumin and cholesterol concentrations should also be included. Anemia that develops before the deterioration of kidney function is a common feature of persistent nephrotic syndrome. Iron stores are depleted (possibly as a result of urinary losses of transferrin), but iron replacement therapy is ineffective. These patients have erythropoietin deficiency with a blunted response to anemia that can be treated with erythropoietin.[10] Serum complement studies, tests for systemic lupus erythematosus and other serological tests can be deferred and tailored to the findings on the kidney biopsy.

PATHOLOGY

Generic FSGS is defined as a discrete segmental consolidation of the glomerular tuft by increased extracellular matrix that results in obliteration of the capillary lumen.[9] The lesions initially affect juxtamedullary glomeruli. Lesions can occur in the vascular pole of the glomerulus or the periphery of the tuft. The latter is more common in children. Podocytes may hypertrophy and increase in number and detach from the glomerular basement membrane (GBM). The mesangium may be hypercellular and expanded. The disease progresses to complete global sclerosis. The GBM is wrinkled; there is accumulation of acellular hyaline material, and adhesions to the Bowman's capsule. Unaffected glomeruli may hypertrophy. There is patchy tubular atrophy, interstitial fibrosis, and even interstitial inflammation.

Focal and segmental deposits of IgM and C3 may be seen by immunofluorescence microscopy in the regions of segmental sclerosis. No deposits are seen by electron microscopy. There are, however, marked changes in the podocytes that include effacement of foot processes and detachment from the GBM.

MORPHOLOGICAL SUBTYPES OR VARIANTS

There are several morphological subtypes of FSGS with possibly different therapeutic approaches and prognoses.[9] The morphologic variants of FSGS are FSGS (NOS, not otherwise specified), perihilar variant, cellular variant, tip variant, and collapsing variant (see Table 22-2).

PATHOGENESIS[15,16,21]

Podocyte injury is implicated in the pathogenesis of primary and secondary types of FSGS. This is especially true for FSGS associated with genetic mutations of the podocin gene. The frequency and speed with which proteinuria recurs in some patients after renal transplant for FSGS support the hypothesis that a circulating factor is responsible for the glomerular injury that leads to FSGS. The presence of a 'permeability factor' is demonstrated in some patients with primary FSGS. A high level has predicted recurrent disease. The mechanism by which the permeability factor injures the podocyte is unknown, but experimental evidence suggests that direct injury to the podocyte can cause both proteinuria and glomerular scarring.

Serial renal biopsies from patients with recurrent FSGS demonstrate a pathogenetic sequence beginning with podocyte pathology that progresses to segmental scars and adhesions. Whereas nephrotic-range proteinuria can appear within minutes of transplantation in recurrent FSGS, glomerular pathology from biopsies performed within 1 month of recurrence sometimes show only foot process effacement. The first lesion seen by light microscopy is segmental collapse of the glomerular capillaries with proliferation and hypertrophy of the surrounding podocytes. Fibrotic scars with adhesions between the involved portions of the glomerulus and Bowman's capsule are not seen until later in the course, and presumably they represent evolution of capillary collapse and podocyte pathology. The injury appears to begin in glomeruli, and specifically in podocytes. This is followed by renal tubular and interstitial injury with tubular dropout, interstitial inflammation, and fibrosis. Proximal tubular protein reabsorption may play an important role in the initiation and progression of the tubulo-interstitial injury. Activation of the renin–angiotensin system with subsequent stimulation of transforming growth factor-β (TGF-β) is also important in the pathogenesis of the fibrosis. Therapy is therefore aimed at reducing protein excretion and blocking angiotensin II production. Glomerular hyperfiltration appears to induce FSGS in cases with congenital or acquired reduced renal mass, diabetes, sickle cell disease, hypertension, morbid obesity, cyanotic congenital heart disease, and glycogen storage disease.

PROGNOSTIC FEATURES

The most important prognostic features at presentation of FSGS are the serum creatinine concentration and the magnitude of proteinuria.[15] Nephrotic-range proteinuria (>3.0–3.5 g/day) is associated with a worse outcome in primary FSGS, with a mean time course to ESRD of 6–8 years. Patients who do not have nephrotic-range proteinuria have a 10-year renal survival of over 80%. Patients with proteinuria in excess of 10 g/day progress rapidly to renal failure in less than 3 years. The patients with 'malignant FSGS' were young, usually hypertensive, had microscopic hematuria, non-selective proteinuria and severe hypercholesterolemia.[4] None responded to treatment with corticosteroids or cytotoxic drugs, and the nephrotic syndrome persisted in some during dialysis and after transplant (Table 22-3).

The prognosis is better in patients who go into remission than those who do not. Fewer than 15% of patients

Table 22-3 Prognostic Features of FSGS[16]

Proteinuria at presentation	Proteinuria >10 g/24 h – ESRD in 5 years
	Non-nephrotic proteinuria – renal survival >80% after 10 years
Serum creatinine at presentation	1.3 mg/dl – poorer renal survival
Histological features that predict a poor prognosis	>20% interstitial fibrosis
	Cellular lesion

who have a complete remission progress to ESRD; up to 50% of nephrotic patients progress to ESRD over 5 years. The best pathologic predictor of poor outcome is the extent of interstitial fibrosis, and not the percentage of segmental or global sclerosis. Spontaneous remission occurs in less than 5% of nephrotic patients with primary FSGS.

Mutations in *NPHS2* that encodes podocin can cause recessive FSGS and FSGS in non-familial cases. These patients are usually resistant to corticosteroids and immunosuppressive agents.[12] The fractional excretion of IgG (FE IgG) may prove to be a useful test to predict whether a patient will enter remission or progress to renal failure, and may be useful as a guide to treatment.[1] The prognosis and response to treatment may also depend on the morphological variant of FSGS (Table 22-4).

DIFFERENTIAL DIAGNOSIS OF PRIMARY FSGS

Minimal Change Disease

The clinical and laboratory features are often indistinguishable. The diagnosis of FSGS is made after a renal biopsy in a patient who is either steroid-resistant or steroid-dependent (see Chapter 21).

Membranous Glomerulonephritis

These patients tend to be older and are usually steroid-resistant (see Chapter 19).

Membranoproliferative Glomerulonephritis

Although these patients often present with the nephrotic syndrome, there are almost always additional nephritic components of hematuria, red blood cell casts, hypertension, azotemia and hypocomplementemia (see Chapter 19).

Mesangial Proliferative Glomerulonephritis[23]

Similarly to FSGS, this describes a histopathologic finding rather than a disease. There is diffuse mesangial cell and matrix expansion with normal glomerular capillary walls and often mesangial deposits of IgM. This finding occurs in 2 to 10% of patients with primary nephrotic syndrome. Clinical presentations include asymptomatic proteinuria, isolated hematuria, proteinuria and hematuria, and nephrotic syndrome. Treatment regimens are similar to minimal change disease and FSGS, but most patients – especially those with severe disease – are non-responsive. Nephrotic patients who respond to treatment are often steroid-dependent or have frequent relapses; those who do not respond are usually found to have FSGS on repeat biopsy and progress to end-stage renal failure (Table 22-5).

GENETIC TYPES OF FSGS[17]

Autosomal recessive steroid-resistant nephrotic syndrome is characterized by onset of proteinuria under the age of 5 years, resistance to corticosteroid treatment, and rapid progression to ESRD. Minimal glomerular changes are seen on early biopsy specimens, and FSGS is

Table 22-4 Response to Treatment Based on Morphological Variant of FSGS

Perihilar variant	• When accompanied by glomerulomegaly, is more common in patients with secondary FSGS caused by glomerular hyperfiltration.	
Cellular variant	• More severe proteinuria • More likely to have nephrotic syndrome • Possibly an earlier stage in FSGS	• May be more likely to respond to treatment with immunosuppressants
Tip variant	• Patients with minimal change nephrotic syndrome who have the tip lesion may progress to FSGS	• 80% responsiveness to corticosteroids [Hogan–Moulton]
Collapsing variant	• HIV must be excluded • More likely to be black • Rapid progression to end-stage renal failure	• Usually does not respond to treatment

Table 22-5   Differential Diagnosis of Primary FSGS

	Differentiating Clinical Features	Differentiating Tests
Minimal change NS	• Younger age at onset • White • No/minimal hematuria, hypertension or azotemia • Steroid-responsive	• Steroid-responsive • If not, renal biopsy
Membranous GN	• Older age at onset • Black • History of hepatitis	• Renal biopsy • Hepatitis serology • Lupus serology
MPGN	• Nephritic presentation	• Renal biopsy • Low serum C3
Mesangial proliferative GN C1q nephropathy	• More likely to have hematuria, hypertension	• Renal biopsy if steroid- resistant
IgM nephropathy	• Corticosteroid-resistant	
Genetic types of FSGS	• May be indistinguishable from idiopathic FSGS • Positive family history	• Renal biopsy if steroid-resistant • DNA studies if available

present later. The causative gene, *NPHS2*, maps to 1q25-q31 and the protein product is called podocin.[3] The identification of mutation allows avoidance of unnecessary immunosuppressive treatment and enables provision of prenatal diagnosis to families at risk. Unfortunately, FSGS may recur after transplantation. The clinical phenotype of patients with NPHS2 mutations but no family history of nephrotic syndrome, is indistinguishable from those with idiopathic FSGS.[6]

Autosomal dominant inheritance of FSGS occurs in families in whom FSGS is linked to at least three loci on chromosomes 1q25-31, 11q22-24, and 9q13. The gene located at 19q13 is *ACTN4*, and encodes α-actinin-4, an actin-binding and cross-linking protein localized to podocytes mainly in the foot processes. Frasier syndrome is characterized by male pseudo-hermaphroditism with complete sex reversal, streak gonads and gonadoblastoma and slowly progressive glomerulopathy. There are intronic mutations in the second splicing site of the *WT1* (Wilms' tumor 1) gene. Autosomal dominant transmission of FSGS occurs in Frasier syndrome (Table 22-6).

TREATMENT

There is no satisfactory treatment of FSGS. Treatment regimens include corticosteroids, pulse alkylating agents,[18] cyclosporine A (CsA), and pulse methylprednisolone. Angiotensin-converting enzyme (ACE) inhibitors and angiotensin II blockers (ARB) are now being added to these regimens, or are being used alone. The following conclusions were reached after a critical evaluation of the levels of evidence for the treatment of FSGS[5]:

1. No prospective studies specifically assess the use of corticosteroids. However, reports of case series support the use of prednisone at an initial dose of 60 mg/day for a minimum of 4 months; patients should not be considered steroid-resistant until a 6-month trial of prednisone has been completed.

2. Patients who are resistant to prednisone therapy or are dependent on corticosteroid therapy may benefit from the use of CsA, but the usefulness of cyclophosphamide, azathioprine, or chlorambucil

Table 22-6   Inherited Types of FSGS

Inheritance of FSGS	Locus	Gene	Gene Product
Autosomal recessive	1q25-31	*SRN1*	CD2-associated protein
Autosomal dominant	1q25-31		
	11q22-24	*ACTN4*	α-actinin-4
	19q13		
Mitochondrial DNA mutations		Mitochondrial tRNA^{Leu} gene (A3243G)	
Frasier syndrome	11p	Dominant negative point mutations of zinc fingers of WT1 protein	

is not clear because few randomized prospective studies have been conducted on which to base any recommendations (Box 22-1).

A renal biopsy should be performed either at the onset of nephrotic syndrome in patients at risk (aged over 8 years, African Americans) or early during the clinical course if there are problems with response to therapy.[2]

Corticosteroids

Patients who receive a course of treatment with corticosteroids are four to ten times more likely to enter remission than untreated patients.[11] No clinical or histological feature at presentation predicts which patients will enter remission, although patients with elevated concentrations of serum creatinine and severe interstitial fibrosis are unlikely to respond to corticosteroids. Therefore, the response to a course of treatment is the best clinical indicator of outcome. Initial treatment for primary FSGS in children consists of prednisone 60–80 mg/day/m^2 in divided doses for 4 weeks, followed by 40 mg/day/m^2 (up to 60 mg/day) in divided doses every second day for 4 weeks, and then either discontinued or tapered over several weeks. The results are disappointing, with a remission rate of less than 30%. Some physicians treat with corticosteroids for up to 6 months in order to achieve a higher rate of remission, but the cushingoid side effects and inhibition of growth can be serious.

Pulse Intravenous Methylprednisolone

This aggressive approach to treatment with very large doses of corticosteroids can induce remissions in a variable percentage of children with FSGS.[13]

Cyclosporine A

Response rates with CsA of 50% to 100% are reported with twice-daily dosing of 5 to 32 mg/kg/day to achieve trough blood levels of 70 to 500 ng/ml. However, this is associated with a high incidence of side effects that include nephrotoxicity, hypertension, gingival hyperplasia, and hirsutism.[7] Therefore, a smaller once-daily dose of 5 mg/kg of cyclosporine A was recommended for the treatment of FSGS. Among 21 children, 11 (52%) had a complete remission, and five (24%) had a partial remission. The total response rate was 76%. The mean time to response was 2.8 ± 0.8 months, and the mean duration of therapy was 20.6 ± 13.7 months. The CsA dosage was tapered or stopped in nine responders; three of these patients maintained remission for 6 to 13 months, and six patients relapsed at 1.5 to 18.7 months (mean 8.7 months). Five of these six patients responded again when the CsA therapy was restarted, or the dosage was increased.[8] Unfortunately, not all patients respond a second time. Secondary resistance to CsA is defined as an initial response to CsA, with relapse on withdrawal of therapy and absent or diminished response on reinstitution of CsA.[19] The presence of FSGS, or of C4 and/or C1q, appears to increase the risk of secondary CsA resistance, and some of these children rapidly progress to ESRD.

Angiotensin-Converting Enzyme Inhibitors

There is limited experience using ACE inhibitors alone in primary FSGS. Their use in FSGS nephrotic patients may reduce proteinuria without inducing a remission or reducing the rate of progression of renal disease (Box 22-2).

> ◤ **MAJOR POINTS** ◢
>
> - Focal segmental glomerulosclerosis (FSGS) is a clinicopathologic syndrome.
> - Primary FSGS is one of the leading causes of ESRD in the United States.
> - Primary FSGS accounts for up to 35% of glomerular lesions in proteinuric children and adults.
> - The prevalence of FSGS in black patients (36–80%) is two- to four-fold that in white patients (14–24%).
> - The incidence of primary FSGS has increased two- to three-fold over the past 20 years.
> - Check for proteinuria by urine dipstick in all patients with periorbital edema before ascribing the puffiness to 'allergies'.
> - FSGS is not part of *a spectrum* of minimal change nephrotic syndrome.
> - Some patients with 'minimal change nephrotic syndrome' *may* develop FSGS.

RECURRENCE POST-TRANSPLANT

FSGS can recur after initial renal transplantation in 30–50% of patients. Patients who have post-transplant recurrence of FSGS have permeability activity defined by measurement of albumin permeability (P[alb]) or glomerular volume variation (GVV).[20] This permeability activity is decreased by plasmapheresis or immunoadsorption, and early use of plasmapheresis in post-transplant recurrence of FSGS may be beneficial.

REFERENCES

1. Bazzi C, Petrini C, Rizza V, et al. Fractional excretion of IgG predicts renal outcome and response to therapy in primary focal segmental glomerulosclerosis: a pilot study. Am J Kidney Dis 2003;41:328–335.
2. Bonilla-Felix M, Parra C, Dajani T, et al. Changing patterns in the histopathology of idiopathic nephrotic syndrome in children. Kidney Int 1999;55:1885–1890.
3. Boute N, Gribouval O, Roselli S, et al. NPHS2, encoding the glomerular protein podocin, is mutated in autosomal recessive steroid-resistant nephrotic syndrome. Nature Genet 2000;24:349–354.
4. Brown CB, Cameron JS, Turner DR, et al. Focal segmental glomerulosclerosis with rapid decline in renal function ('malignant FSGS'). Clin Nephrol 1978;10:51–61.
5. Burgess E. Management of focal segmental glomerulosclerosis: evidence-based recommendations. Kidney Int Suppl 1999;70:S26–S32.
6. Caridi G, Bertelli R, Carrea A, et al. Prevalence, genetics, and clinical features of patients carrying podocin mutations in steroid-resistant nonfamilial focal segmental glomerulosclerosis. J Am Soc Nephrol 2001;12:2742–2746.
7. Cattran DC. Cyclosporine in the treatment of idiopathic focal segmental glomerulosclerosis. Semin Nephrol 2003;23:234–241.
8. Chishti AS, Sorof JM, Brewer ED, Kale AS. Long-term treatment of focal segmental glomerulosclerosis in children with cyclosporine given as a single daily dose. Am J Kidney Dis 2001;38:754–760.
9. D'agati V. Pathologic classification of focal segmental glomerulosclerosis. Semin Nephrol 2003;23:117–134.
10. Feinstein S, Becker-Cohen R, Algur N, et al. Erythropoietin deficiency causes anemia in nephrotic children with normal kidney function. Am J Kidney Dis 2001;37:736–742.
11. Franceschini N, Hogan SL, Falk RJ. Primum non nocere: should adults with idiopathic FSGS receive steroids? Semin Nephrol 2003;23:229–233.
12. Frishberg Y, Rinat C, Megged O, et al. Mutations in NPHS2 encoding podocin are a prevalent cause of steroid-resistant nephrotic syndrome among Israeli-Arab children. J Am Soc Nephrol 2002;13:400–405.
13. Kirpekar R, Yorgin PD, Tune BM. Clinicopathologic correlates predict the outcome in children with steroid-resistant idiopathic nephrotic syndrome treated with pulse methylprednisolone therapy. Am J Kidney Dis 2002;39:1143–1152.
14. Kitiyakara Dagger C, Kopp JB, Eggers Dagger P. Trends in the epidemiology of focal segmental glomerulosclerosis. Semin Nephrol 2003;23:172–182.
15. Korbet SM. Treatment of primary focal segmental glomerulosclerosis. Kidney Int 2002;62:2301–2310.
16. Korbet SM. Angiotensin antagonists and steroids in the treatment of focal segmental glomerulosclerosis. Semin Nephrol 2003;23:219–228.
17. Pollak MR. The genetic basis of FSGS and steroid-resistant nephrosis. Semin Nephrol 2003;23:141–146.
18. Ponticelli C, Passerini P. Other immunosuppressive agents for focal segmental glomerulosclerosis. Semin Nephrol 2003;23:242–248.
19. Sairam VK, Kalia A, Rajaraman S, et al. Secondary resistance to cyclosporin A in children with nephrotic syndrome. Pediatr Nephrol 2002;17:842–846.
20. Savin VJ, McCarthy ET, Sharma M. Permeability factors in focal segmental glomerulosclerosis. Semin Nephrol 2003;23:147–160.
21. Schnaper HW. Idiopathic focal segmental glomerulosclerosis. Semin Nephrol 2003;23:183–193.
22. Sorof JM, Hawkins EP, Brewer ED, et al. Age and ethnicity affect the risk and outcome of focal segmental glomerulosclerosis. Pediatr Nephrol 1998;12:764–768.
23. Wang HY, Li XM. Mesangial proliferative disease. In: Neilson EG, Couser WG (eds), Immunologic Renal Diseases. Lippincott-Raven, New York, 1997, pp. 987–999.

CHAPTER 23

Membranous Nephropathy

LAWRENCE S. MILNER, M.D.

INTRODUCTION

Membranous nephropathy (MN) is an immune complex-mediated injury to the glomerulus that results in proteinuria and nephrotic syndrome. The defining feature of MN is the presence of subepithelial immune deposits adjacent to the glomerular basement membrane (GBM). The pathologic appearance of a thickened GBM gave rise to the term MN.

INCIDENCE

Membranous nephropathy is an uncommon cause of proteinuria and nephrotic syndrome in childhood, and its occurrence is often secondary to an underlying comorbid illness.[3] Geographic variations in the occurrence of MN depend on the regional incidence of coexistent diseases, especially those secondary to infections such as hepatitis B virus, malaria, and syphilis. Children from Africa and Asia, where these infectious diseases are endemic, tend to have a higher incidence of MN; this reflects an increased exposure to these infections. Primary MN is more common in males, and a genetic predisposition is associated with different HLA patterns in various population groups, especially HLA1, B8, and D3 antigens. Furthermore, primary MN has been reported in twins, suggesting a genetic predisposition in susceptible cases.

ETIOLOGY

In *primary* MN there is no known underlying cause, whereas in *secondary* MN there is a coexistent disease (Table 23-1).

PATHOGENESIS

Glomerular accumulation of immune complexes (ICs) is derived from the circulation or by 'in-situ' deposition promoting glomerular injury. In humans with MN the mechanisms of IC accumulation are largely unknown, and the basis for the understanding of subepithelial

179

Table 23-1	Causes of Secondary Membranous Nephropathy (MN)
Infections	
Viral	Hepatitis B, C, HIV
Bacterial	Syphilis
Parasitic	Malaria, schistosomiasis
Auto-immune	SLE, sarcoidosis, thyroiditis
Hematologic	Sickle cell anemia, lymphoma, leukemia
Medications	Penicillamine, gold
Miscellaneous	Solid organ tumors, inflammatory bowel disease

SLE = systemic lupus erythematosus.

immune deposition and proteinuria has been generated from experimental Heyman nephritis, an animal prototype of MN.

In-Situ Immune Complex Deposition

The model of passive Heymann nephritis (PHN) reproduces the accumulation of subepithelial immune deposits by infusing rats with heterologous antibody generated in sheep or rabbits directed against a rat tubular antigen designated as megalin or gp330.[7]

Antibodies to megalin cross-react with similar antigens within the podocytes of rat glomeruli and serve as a 'planted antigen'. Further in-situ accumulation of autologous antibodies produces subepithelial deposits adjacent to the GBM.[18] In human MN, the putative antigen equivalent of megalin is not identified, although a candidate antigen is neutral endopeptidase that occurs in human tubule brush border and on podocytes. Passive transplacental transfer of anti-neutral endopeptidase antibodies caused MN in a neonate.[5]

Complement

Proteinuria in PHN is shown to be complement-dependent, as decomplementation of rats with cobra venom factor abrogates the proteinuria. The attachment of the membrane attack complex (MAC), C_{5b}-9, the terminal component of the complement pathway within the GBM, promotes the development of proteinuria by injuring the membrane.[19]

Cytokines

Cytokine release following IC deposition contributes to glomerular injury in MN. In PHN, insertion of the MAC within membranes activates production of arachidonic acid (a precursor of thromboxane A_2), and increases oxygen free-radicals within glomeruli, thereby aggravating proteinuria.[4,20] Increased production of transforming growth factor β (TGF-β) and tumor necrosis factor (TNF) follows the initial injury, promoting an increase in matrix proteins and subsequent fibrosis.[9,21]

Circulating Immune Complexes

In secondary forms of human MN, glomerular accumulation of ICs may be derived from the circulation. The sites of IC deposition within the glomeruli vary with their size and charge.

PATHOLOGY

The characteristic abnormality seen by light microscopy is thickening of the GBM, with minimal increase in mesangial cellularity. The appearance of a thickened basement membrane with discrete spike formation (using a silver stain) is due to an accumulation of basement membrane-like substances forming around the immune deposits, especially laminin, type 4 collagen, and fibronectin. Electron microscopic findings are typically subepithelial IC deposits. Further incorporation of the immune deposits within the GBM varies with different stages of the disease, and may be helpful in assessing severity and chronicity.[6] Immunofluorescence staining usually detects immunoglobulin G (IgG) – especially IgG 4 – and complement C3 is usually seen in granular and diffuse garland patterns. The deposition of C1Q and extensive deposits of C3 are less common, and if associated with mesangial deposits usually suggest a secondary cause, especially systemic lupus erythematosus (SLE).

The co-deposition of mesangial IgA suggests IgA nephropathy in conjunction with the presence of MN. The presence of interstitial inflammation, interstitial fibrosis, and tubular atrophy signifies a more severe glomerular injury, and usually heralds an inexorable decline in renal function.

CLINICAL FINDINGS

Children with MN often have a secondary cause for their glomerular injury. This requires careful evaluation to detect an underlying comorbid disease (Table 23-2).

History

In neonates with MN, a maternal record is required of prenatal serologic testing for congenital infections, especially syphilis. The immunization status against hepatitis B of infants and children is important. Place of birth, recent travel history, and exposure to medications must be elicited.

Table 23-2	Clinical Differences Between Primary and Secondary MN	
	Primary	Secondary
Nephrotic syndrome	Yes	Yes
Fever	No	Yes (infection/ autoimmune/neoplasia)
Anemia	No	Yes (infection/ autoimmune/neoplasia)
Hepatosplenomegaly	No	Yes (infection/ autoimmune/neoplasia)
Thyromegaly	No	Yes (thyroiditis)
Medication history	No	Yes (gold, penicillamine)

Physical Examination

A physical examination includes an inspection for rash and arthritis. These occur with congenital syphilis, SLE, and sarcoidosis. Lymphadenopathy and/or hepatosplenomegaly suggest an underlying infectious process, hematologic malignancy, or solid tumor. Thyromegaly suggests the presence of an autoimmune thyroiditis.

Renal

Nephrotic syndrome occurs in the majority of children with MN. This is characterized by proteinuria in excess of 40 mg/m^2/hour, edema, and hyperlipidemia. Hypertension occurs in 25% of cases, a few have asymptomatic proteinuria, and many have microscopic hematuria.[13]

Diagnostic Tests

The diagnosis of MN is histopathologic, and is made on a renal biopsy. Serum complement concentrations are usually normal in primary MN, but may be decreased in SLE, hepatitis B MN, and congenital syphilis (Table 23-3).

Table 23-3	Laboratory Evaluation and Differences Between Primary and Secondary MN	
	Primary	Secondary
Treponemal Ab	Negative	Positive (syphilis)
ANA, anti dsDNA Ab	Negative	Positive (SLE)
Serum C3 levels	Normal	Decreased (SLE, syphilis, hepatitis B)
Hepatic enzymes	Normal	Elevated (hepatitis B, C, syphilis, SLE, neoplasia)

ANA = anti-nuclear antibodies; dsDNA = double-stranded DNA.

Secondary Causes of MN

Hepatitis B Viral Infection

Hepatitis B virus (HBV)-induced MN is more common in childhood populations in which the hepatitis B carrier state is endemic, such as in Africa and Asia, where reported incidences range from 0.1 to 15%.[26]

Children with HBV-MN present with proteinuria or nephrotic syndrome that cannot be distinguished from idiopathic nephrotic syndrome. Positive serology for hepatitis s and e antigens, and core antibody, are important findings in HBV-MN. The presence of abnormal liver function tests due to mild hepatitis, as well as depressed complement levels, may help to support a clinical diagnosis of HBV-MN in a child with nephrotic syndrome.[14] The presence of hepatitis B e antigen within the affected glomeruli in children with MN supports the notion that ICs containing e antigen mediate proteinuria in HBV-MN.[11] Studies in primates with HBV-induced glomerular injury showed IgG-bound e antigen in the circulation and within glomeruli.[22] This suggests a possible circulating IC-mediated glomerular injury. However, in humans with HBV-MN a recent study using immunoelectron microscopy showed MAC deposits, co-localized with e antigen within the subepithelial dense deposits, suggesting an in-situ mechanism for IC deposition in HBV-MN.[1] A genetic predisposition to have HBV-MN is suggested by the occurrence of HLA antigens that vary among different population groups.[2] These are thought to control the T-cell immunomodulating response of the host to the offending antigen, in some way predisposing to MN in susceptible individuals. Patients with chronic hepatitis B e antigenemia and positive HBV viral DNA with persistent proteinuria may benefit from alpha interferon therapy to reduce the viral load.[12] The long-term outcome in childhood HBV-MN is good, and there is spontaneous resolution in most affected children. The appearance of hepatitis B e antibodies heralds resolution of the proteinuria.

Syphilis

Neonates and infants with glomerular injury caused by *Treponema pallidum* infection commonly present with nephrotic syndrome and MN. Additional findings are rashes, nasal discharge, hepatosplenomegaly, and periostitis. Some affected infants may be hypertensive.[25,26,28] Abnormal serologic findings are positive VDRL and rapid plasma reagin (RPR) tests, or fluorescent *Treponema* IgM antibodies. Decreased serum complement and elevated serum IgM concentrations are consistent with a response to a congenital infection.

Granular deposits of IgG and complement characterize glomerular ultrastructural findings in congenital syphilis. Treponemal antigens are demonstrated within affected glomeruli in the subepithelial space adjacent to the basement membrane. This predisposes to in-situ IC formation.

Early treatment with penicillin results in the resolution of proteinuria and attenuation of immune-mediated glomerular injury. A recent increase in the incidence of congenital syphilis requires vigilant screening during pregnancy and evaluation of 'at-risk' neonates and infants so that early therapy with penicillin can be given.

Lupus Nephritis

Glomerular injury occurs in up to 75% children with SLE. Clinically, there may be mild glomerulonephritis with microscopic hematuria or acute nephritic or nephrotic syndrome (see Chapter 25).

Drug-Induced MN

MN is most frequently associated with exposure to gold salts, and penicillamine. Captopril, a sulfhydryl-containing angiotensin-converting enzyme (ACE) inhibitor may be a rare cause of MN.[8] Gold treatment may result in tubular deposits and antibodies to renal tubular antigens within glomerular immune complexes.[23] This suggests that primary tubular injury predisposes to immune glomerular deposits in gold-induced proteinuria. Penicillamine-induced injury occurs in up to 20% of patients through penicilloyl moiety hapten-mediated glomerular damage. Discontinuation of the offending drug is required to reverse the proteinuria.

Hematologic/Oncologic Causes of MN

Sickle cell disease may rarely be associated with MN. MN associated with solid tumors is well documented in adults, but is rare in childhood. Proteinuria may precede the diagnosis of an underlying tumor, and its disappearance may coincide with the removal of the tumor. Conversely, reappearance of the tumor may be a sign of tumor recurrence. Neoplasia-induced MN is mediated by tumor-associated antigen that produces circulating or planted antigens. Lymphoma and leukemia are rarely associated with MN.

TREATMENT

Primary MN

Spontaneous resolution of proteinuria in primary MN occurs in up to 20% of affected patients. Hence, controversy exists as to which patients would benefit from immunosuppressive therapy.[17,27] In secondary MN, resolution of the proteinuria usually occurs after removal of the underlying antigenic stimuli precipitating MN.

Specific Therapy

There are no controlled trials in children with MN. Therefore, it is difficult to decide if and when and who

---

Box 23-1   Management of Primary Membranous Nephropathy (Mn)

Non-nephrotic proteinuria
- Observe
- Non-specific therapy: ACE inhibitors

Nephrotic-range proteinuria
- Normal renal function
    i. Pulse steroids IV and oral steroids
- Impaired renal function and/or interstitial inflammation
    i. Corticosteroids and cyclophosphamide
    ii. Cyclosporine if resistant to (i)
    iii. Mycophenolate mofetil if resistant to (i and ii)

---

should be treated. Although the following regimens are used, it is unclear whether or not they are helpful (Box 23-1).

Immunosuppressive Therapy
Glucocorticoids
Intravenous pulsed methylprednisone for three consecutive days followed by daily or an alternate-day oral steroid regimen for up to 6 months may be considered.

Cytotoxic Agents
The addition of cytotoxic agents, such as oral cyclophosphamide daily for 3–6 months in addition to oral steroids has been shown to be effective, with a remission rate of up to 40% in adult studies. Chlorambucil may be substituted for cyclophosphamide, but with possible increased toxicity. Alternate-day oral cytotoxic agents given monthly with alternate-day oral steroids for 6 months also appears to offer a potentially effective therapeutic strategy.

Cyclosporine
Patients resistant to corticosteroid and cytotoxic agents may benefit from cyclosporine A (CsA) therapy. In adults, significant remission (up to 75%) occurs with combined CsA and corticosteroid therapy. However, remission is often not sustained.

Future Immunotherapeutic Strategies
Mycophenolate mofetil (MMF) can be considered as a steroid-sparing agent. The successful use of intravenous gamma-globulin (IVIG) in adults reduces proteinuria in resistant cases.[27]

Secondary MN

Secondary MN associated with an underlying comorbid disease requires directed therapy to eradicate the putative antigenic offender. Hepatitis B-induced MN treated with interferon or other antiviral agents may reduce the viral load and ameliorate the glomerular injury. Infants with congenital syphilis-induced MN respond well to penicillin administered early in the course. Children with MN due to SLE also have a good outcome with immunosuppressive agents, especially if the glomerular injury is a pure membranous lesion without significant mesangial proliferation or sclerosis. In drug-induced MN, elimination of the offending agent results in spontaneous resolution of the condition.

Non-Specific Therapy

Non-specific therapeutic measures may help to reduce proteinuria without necessarily altering IC deposition, but reduces the potential complications of MN.

ACE Inhibitors

The use of ACE inhibitors in MN reduces proteinuria by decreasing efferent arteriolar resistance, thereby reducing intraglomerular hydrostatic pressure, with preservation of podocyte structure.[16] A modest reduction in proteinuria with ACE inhibitors reduces tubular injury by restricting the production of pro-inflammatory substances induced by persistent proteinuria.[10,15,24]

Hypolipemic Agents

Persistent hyperlipidemia occurs in chronic proteinuria, which promotes premature atherosclerosis and glomerulosclerosis, potentially aggravating the glomerular damage. Judicious use of hypolipemic agents may help to control hyperlipemia in MN and prevent these adverse effects.

Antiplatelet Agents

Intravascular thrombosis is an important complication of MN due to a hypercoagulable state. Dipyridamole, a phosphodiesterase inhibitor, is used to prevent intravascular thromboses in MN.

OUTCOME

The outcome of primary MN is generally favorable, as spontaneous remission occurs in up to 40% of cases and there seems to be a reasonably good response to immunotherapy. Chronic renal insufficiency occurs in about 20% of affected patients. Patients with proteinuria of <40 mg/m^2/24 hours and normal renal function have the best outcome. Nephrotic-range proteinuria, especially when associated with impaired renal function, is less responsive to treatment. Glomerulosclerosis, interstitial inflammation, and myofibroblasts indicate a poor outcome with an inexorable decline in renal function. The presence of urinary C5b-9 reflects persistent glomerular

MAJOR POINTS
• Children with membranous nephropathy may have an underlying infectious, autoimmune or neoplastic disease.
• Appropriate serologic testing to exclude causes of MN (syphilis, hepatitis viruses, parasitic infections, SLE) can be carried out after the biopsy confirms the diagnosis of MN.
• Children with non-nephrotic-range proteinuria (<40 mg/m^2/hour) and normal renal function should be observed for spontaneous resolution.
• Children with nephrotic-range proteinuria and or impaired renal function should be considered for immunosuppressive therapy.

activity, while the finding of increased urinary IgG and alpha-1 microglobulin may signify underlying tubulo-interstitial disease. This requires an earlier and more aggressive therapeutic approach.[10]

Relapses occur in up to 30% of patients, and a repeat course of immunosuppressive therapy may result in remission. Long-term follow-up of patients in remission is therefore recommended in order to detect a relapse and to institute early therapy if needed. MN may occur *de novo* in up to 9% of allografts. Recurrence of primary MN is more common than previously appreciated, occurs in up to 29% of allografts, and results in graft failure in up to 50% of cases.

REFERENCES

1. Akano N, Yoshioka K, Aya N, et al. Immunoelectron microscopic localization of membrane attack complex and Hepatitis e antigen in membranous nephropathy. Virchows Arch A Pathol Anat 1989;414:325–330.

2. Bhimma R, Hammond MG, Coovadia HM, et al. HLA class 1 and 2 in Black children with hepatitis B virus-associated membranous nephropathy. Kidney Int 2002;61:1510–1515.

3. Cameron JS. Membranous nephropathy in childhood and its treatment. Pediatr Nephrol 1990;4:193–198.

4. Cattran DC. Idiopathic membranous glomerulonephritis. Kidney Int 2000;59:1983–1994.

5. Debiec H, Guigonis V, Mougenot B, et al. Antenatal membranous glomerulonephritis due to antineutral endopeptidase antibodies. N Engl J Med 2002;345:2053–2060.

6. Ehrenreich T, Churg J. Pathology of membranous nephropathy. Pathol Ann 1986;3:145–186.

7. Farquar MG, Saito A, Kerjaschki D, Orlando RA. The Heymann nephritis antigenic complex: Megalin (gp330) and RAP. J Am Soc Nephrol 1995;6:35–47.

8. Hill GS. Drug-associated glomerulopathies. Toxicol Pathol 1986;14:37–44.

9. Honkanen E, von Willebrand E, Teppo A-M, et al. Adhesion molecules and urinary tumor necrosis factor alpha in idiopathic membranous glomerulonephritis. Kidney Int 1998; 53:909-917.

10. Kon SP, Coupes B, Short CD, et al. Urinary C5b-9 excretion and clinical course in idiopathic human membranous nephropathy. Kidney Int 1995;48:1953-1958.

11. Lai KN, Lai F M-M. Clinical features and the natural course of hepatitis B virus-related glomerulopathy in adults. Kidney Int 1991;40(Suppl. 35):S40-S45.

12. Lin C-Y. Treatment of hepatitis B virus-associated membranous nephropathy with recombinant alpha interferon. Kidney Int 1995;47:225-230.

13. Makker S. Membranous nephropathy. In: Barratt MT, Ellis AD, Harmon WE (eds), *Pediatric Nephrology*, 4th edn. Lippincott Williams & Wilkins, Philadelphia, 719-730, 1999.

14. Milner LS, Dusheiko GM, Jacobs D, et al. Biochemical and serological characteristics of children with membranous nephropathy due to hepatitis B virus infection: correlation with hepatitis B e antigen, hepatitis B DNA and hepatitis D. Nephron 1988;49:184-189.

15. Reichert IJM, Koene RAP, Wetzels JFM. Prognostic factors in idiopathic membranous nephropathy. Am J Kidney Dis 1998;31:1-11.

16. Remuzzi A, Monaci N, Bonassi ME, et al. Angiotensin-converting enzyme inhibition prevents loss of glomerular hydraulic permeability in passive Heymann nephritis. Lab Invest 1999;79:1501-1510.

17. Rose BD, Appel GB. Treatment of membranous nephropathy. Up-to-date in Nephrology and Hypertension. Oct, 2002.

18. Salant DJ, Darby C, Couser WG. Experimental membranous glomerulonephritis in rats: quantitative studies of glomerular immune deposit formation in isolated glomeruli and whole animals. J Clin Invest 1980;66:71-81.

19. Salant DJ, Belok S, Madaio MP, Couser WG. A new role for complement in experimental membranous nephropathy in rats. J Clin Invest 1984;66:1339-1350.

20. Shankland SJ. New insights into the pathogenesis of membranous nephropathy. Kidney Int 2000;57:1204-1205.

21. Shankland SJ, Pippin JJ, Richler RH, et al. Differential expression of transforming growth factor B isoforms and receptors in experimental membranous nephropathy. Kidney Int 1996;50:116-124.

22. Takahashi K, Miyakawa Y, Gotanda T, et al. Shift from free 'small' hepatitis B e antigen to IgG-bound 'large' form in the circulation of human beings and a chimpanzee acutely infected with hepatitis B virus. Gastroenterology 1979; 77:1193-1199.

23. Ueda S, Wakashin M, Wakashin Y, et al. Experimental gold nephropathy in guinea pigs: detection of autoantibodies to renal tubular antigens. Kidney Int 1986;29:539-548.

24. Wang Y, Chen J, Chen L, et al. Induction of monocyte chemoattractant protein-1 in proximal tubule cells by urinary protein. J Am Soc Nephrol 1997;8:1537-1545.

25. Wiggelinkhuizen J, Kaschula ROC, Uys CJ, et al. Congenital syphilis and glomerulonephritis with evidence for immune pathogenesis. Arch Dis Child 1973;48:375-381.

26. Wiggelinkhuizen J, Sinclair Smith C, Tannard LM, Smuts H. Hepatitis B virus associated membranous glomerulonephritis. Arch Dis Child 1983;58:488-496.

27. Yokoyama H, Goshima S, Wada T, et al. The short and long term outcomes of membranous nephropathy treated with intravenous immune globulin. Nephrol Dialysis Transpl 1999;14:2379-2386.

28. Yuceoglu AM, Sagel I, Tresser G, et al. The glomerulopathy of congenital syphilis, a curable immune-deposit disease. JAMA 1974;229:1085-1089.

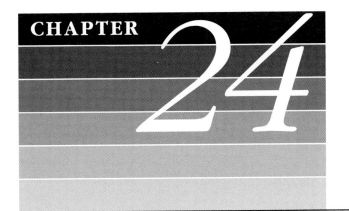

ANCA-Positive Vasculitis/ Pauci-Immune Glomerulonephritis

KEVIN E.C. MEYERS, M.B., B.Ch. AND

JON M. BURNHAM, M.D.

INTRODUCTION

The small vessel vasculitides (SVV) includes a group of diseases characterized by the presence of anti-neutrophil cytoplasmic antibodies (ANCA).[2] ANCA-associated SVV is distinguished from other SVV, including Henoch–Schönlein purpura, cryoglobulinemia and hypersensitivity angiitis by clinical presentation, laboratory studies and pathology.[1,8] The three recognized ANCA-associated vasculitides that may cause renal disease are microvascular polyangiitis (MPA), Wegener granulomatosis (WG) and Churg–Strauss syndrome (CSS) (Table 24-1).[4]

Definitions

SVV differ from medium and large arterial vasculitides by often involving arterioles, venules, and capillaries. Definitions of the SVV are mainly based on histological findings (Box 24-1).

Table 24-1   Presence of Anti-Neutrophil Cytoplasmic Antibodies (ANCA) and Relative Frequency of Kidney and Lung Involvement of the Small Vessel Vasculitides

Small Vessel Vasculitis	Anti-PR3	Anti-MPO	Kidney	Lung
Wegener's granulomatosis	++++	+	++++	++++
Microvascular angiitis	+	+++	++++	++
Churg-Strauss syndrome	+++		+	+++
Henoch-Schönlein purpura	–	–	+++	+
Idiopathic cryoglobulinemia	–	–	++	+
Cutaneous leukoclastic vasculitis	–	–	+	+

Box 24-1   Definitions of the Small Vessel Vasculitides (SVV)

Wegener's granulomatosis
Granulomatous inflammation of respiratory tract and a necrotizing vasculitis that commonly includes the kidney

Microvascular polyangiitis
Necrotizing vasculitis with few or no immune deposits, often involves arterioles, venules and capillaries and is frequently associated with a necrotizing rapidly progressive pauci-immune glomerulonephritis

Churg–Strauss syndrome
Necrotizing eosinophilic vasculitis usually of the lungs with infrequent renal involvement

---

EPIDEMIOLOGY

About 20 per million persons are affected worldwide. There is improved detection and a true increase in the incidence of ANCA-associated vasculitis. The peak incidence is 55 to 70 years, but all ages may be affected and the incidence in childhood is unknown.[13] The immunologic events leading to ANCA production are unknown. *Staphylococcus aureus*, silica exposure, and drugs (e.g., propylthiouracil) may induce vasculitis. Anti-staphylococcal therapy prevents relapses in WG, and carriers are eight-fold more likely to relapse than non-carriers. Patients with abnormal α1-antitrypsin phenotypes have more severe WG and higher mortality rates.

PATHOGENESIS

Anti-Neutrophil Cytoplasmic Antibodies

The pathogenesis of the SVV almost certainly involves ANCA. Patients with SVV are often positive for ANCA. These autoantibodies react with the cytoplasmic constituents of neutrophils and monocytes. ANCA are useful diagnostic markers of SVV, but are usually unhelpful in determining disease activity in response to treatment.

Neutrophils

Glomerular and/or vascular inflammation exposes antigen (i.e., serine proteinase 3; PR3) or myeloperoxidase (MPO) on the surface of cytokine-primed or apoptotic polymorphonuclear neutrophils (PMN). This leads to autoantibody production. ANCA augment endothelial activation, swelling and adherence, promote PMN and monocyte margination, and accentuate platelet deposition.

PMN degranulation, via ANCA ligation, leads to the generation of toxic oxygen metabolites that augments inflammation, and results in necrosis, karyorrhexis, and fibrinous insudation. The inflammatory process then leads to further engagement and activation of primed vascular cells, and the activated participants cause fibrinoid necrosis, and ultimately fibrosis.[6,12]

Endothelia

The endothelium plays a significant role in the pathogenesis of the renal lesions. Endothelial cells provide pro-inflammatory, procoagulant and fibrogenic stimuli through local release of mediators and direct cellular responses. Through an orchestrated and regulated sequence of intracellular processes, these cells actively participate in cellular adhesion, triggering cell–cell interactions, release of inflammatory mediators, and reactive oxygen species. The recruitment of PMN and platelets augments inflammation through direct cellular interactions with release of cytokines and chemokines. This fuels a process that results in vascular occlusion and thrombosis. These intra-capillary PMN are further activated by ANCA and ambient cytokines, such as tumor necrosis factor-α (TNF-α) within lesions (Table 24-2). PMNs produce H_2O_2, which combines with halides to form toxic hypohalous acids. The release of proteases from activated PMN and other cells, together with the hypohalous acids, disrupts the glomerular basement membrane (GBM) and causes lysis of endothelial cells. ANCA-binding to activate PMN within the lesions enhances the inflammatory process by influencing apoptotic events and PMN transit through vessels.

T Cells

T-cell-mediated immunity contributes to the pathogenesis of ANCA-associated vasculitis.[1] Peripheral blood T cells from patients with active or quiescent diseases proliferate in response to PR3 or MPO. T-cell activation persists after disease remission. Two-thirds of patients colonized with *Staph. aureus* carry a strain that

---

Table 24-2   Frequency of Organ Involvement in Wegener's Granulomatosis (WG) and Microvascular Polyangiitis (MPA)

Organ	WG (%)	MPA (%)
Respiratory	90	40
Kidney	80	90
Musculoskeletal	60	60
Gastrointestinal	50	50
CNS	50	30
Skin	40	40

produces T-cell-activating superantigens, and these individuals are more prone to disease flares.

CLINICAL FEATURES

Symptoms and Signs

The presenting symptoms and signs of the SVV are varied because many organ systems may be involved.[7] Over 50% of patients present with a pulmonary-renal syndrome (Table 24-3), and the integumentary, central nervous, ocular, and gastrointestinal systems are variably affected (see Table 24-2). Constitutional symptoms, such as fever, myalgia, weight loss anorexia, and night sweats, occur in over 90% of patients.[11]

Renal

Acute-presentation glomerulonephritis can be fulminant with rapidly progressive renal failure. Most patients with insidious presentation have hematuria, proteinuria, hypertension, and renal insufficiency, although some may present with end-stage renal disease (ESRD). Untreated crescentic glomerulonephritis rapidly progresses to end-stage renal failure.

Respiratory Tract

Upper respiratory tract symptoms include rhinorrhea, sinusitis, epistaxis, otitis media, nasal bridge collapse, and vocal changes with subglottic stenosis. Lung disease presents with cough, hemoptysis, chest pain, and dyspnea. Pulmonary hemorrhage may be life-threatening. Nasal deformity and subglottic stenosis are common in childhood-onset WG. Glomerulonephritis is seen in 77% of patients with WG, and completes the triad of upper and lower airway disease and kidney involvement; however, renal disease is not a pre-requisite for the diagnosis.

Box 24-2 Differential Diagnosis of Renal–Dermal Vasculitic Syndromes

- Anti-neutrophil cytoplasmic antibodies-small vessel vasculitides (ANCA-SVV)
- Systemic lupus erythematosus
- Cryoglobulinemia
- Henoch–Schönlein purpura

Gastrointestinal, Skin, Eyes, Muscles, and Nerves

Disease of the gut results in ischemia and hemorrhage. Ocular involvement includes episcleritis, uveitis, proptosis and optic nerve ischemia. Migratory arthralgias and arthritis occur. Cardiac involvement results in ischemia. Neurological presentation is usually with focal motor or sensory deficits secondary to mononeuritis multiplex. Central nervous system involvement is uncommon. The skin lesion is a leukoclastic vasculitis that produces red macular and papular lesions. There may also be erythematous tender nodules, ulcerations, livedo-reticularis, ecchymoses, and urticaria. Skin-renal involvement occurs in 30% of patients (Box 24-2).

DIAGNOSIS

The diagnosis of ANCA-associated vasculitis is made on the basis of the clinical findings, by biopsy of a relevant involved organ (typically kidney, nasal mucosa, or occasionally lung) and the presence of ANCA. Testing for ANCA using both indirect immunofluorescence and antigen-specific enzyme-linked immunosorbent assay (ELISA) is recommended and provides a high sensitivity (approximately 99%) and good specificity (approximately 70%).[5]

Imaging Studies

In WG, computed tomography scanning or magnetic resonance imaging may reveal interstitial densities consistent with pulmonary vasculitis or hemorrhage. Imaging of the sinus may show sinusitis with nasal septal erosions.

Serological Studies

Appropriate serologic studies include anti-nuclear antibody (Ab) (ANA), dsDNA Ab, anti-GBM Ab, anti-DNase B Ab, ANCA titers, and complement C3 and C4. The ANCA-associated SVV is characterized by normal serum C3 and C4 concentrations. There may be an elevated erythrocyte sedimentation rate (ESR), as well as leukocytosis, thrombocytosis, and anemia.

Table 24-3 Pulmonary–Renal Syndromes in Children

Disease Category	Disorder
Vasculitis	Wegener's granulomatosis
	Microscopic polyangiitis
	Systemic lupus erythematosus
	Henoch–Schönlein purpura
	Post-infectious glomerulonephritis
	Goodpasture syndrome
	Behçet disease
	Rheumatoid arthritis
Infectious	Pneumococcal associated-HUS
Neoplastic	Leukemia
Drugs	Penicillamine

Anti-Neutrophil Cytoplasmic Antibodies

SVV are characterized by the presence of circulating ANCA. The two predominant patterns of ANCA staining seen on indirect immunofluorescence with ethanol-fixed neutrophils are cytoplasmic and peri-nuclear. Approximately 90% of cytoplasmic staining ANCA (C-ANCA) reacts with serine proteinase 3 found within neutrophil azurophilic granules (PR3-ANCA), whereas 90% of the perinuclear staining ANCA (P-ANCA) react with myeloperoxidase found in neutrophil azurophilic granules and in lysosomes (MPO-ANCA) (Box 24-3). Specific and sensitive ELISA testing using purified PR3 and MPO is now available, and this has enhanced sensitivity. Up to 90% of patients with MPA have circulating anti-MPO ANCA by ELISA, whereas 80% of patients with WG have circulating PR3-ANCA.[14]

PATHOLOGY

The characteristic pathologic lesion of the ANCA-associated SVV is fibrinoid necrosis of the capillaries and venules with leukocyte infiltration that includes PMN. Involvement of the arterioles and small arteries is common. The glomerular lesions in MPA typically begin focally and progress through four histologic stages, as seen by light microscopy (Box 24-4). Uninvolved glomerular segments appear normal. Granulomatous lesions may be found on renal or more frequently on pulmonary biopsy of patients with WG. Vascular lesions in other organs are common, with lungs the most frequently affected, although renal involvement may be the only manifestation. The lungs may show multiple necrotizing and non-necrotizing granulomas and vasculitis with irregular endothelial cell proliferation in WG patients. Glomerular crescents are composed of proliferating visceral capsular epithelial cells, of fibrin, basement membrane-like material, and mononuclear cells. Immunofluorescence microscopy of the kidney typically shows little or no deposits, hence the term pauci-immune.[18]

Box 24-3   Clinical Indications for ANCA Testing in Children

- Rapidly progressive glomerulonephritis
- Pulmonary–renal syndrome
- Cutaneous vasculitis with systemic features
- Nodular lung disease
- Upper airway disease, especially where tissue damage is suspected
- Mononeuritis multiplex and peripheral neuropathy
- Retro-orbital mass of unknown etiology

Box 24-4   Histological Stages of Microvascular Polyangiitis (MPA)

- Endothelial activation, swelling, de-adherence, necrosis and platelet deposition
- Focal and segmental inflammation with thrombosis
- Intracapillary infiltration of leukocytes (polymorphonuclear leukocytes/monocytes)
- Extra-capillary accumulation of mononuclear cells in Bowman's space
- Occasional disruption of Bowman's capsule
- Healing through apoptosis, or scarring by sclerosis
- Periglomerular tubulointerstitial inflammation may also be present

---

TREATMENT

Induction and Maintenance Therapy

Initial therapy requires the use of cyclophosphamide and corticosteroids, with additional therapy such as dialysis and or plasmapheresis for patients with life-threatening or organ-threatening disease.[9,10] The risks of maintenance therapy have to be balanced against the risks of disease relapse, which varies from 25 to 50% over a 3- to 5-year period. The combination of prednisone and cyclophosphamide, which is presently considered standard therapy, leads to control of disease in 80–90% of patients. There is little role for the use of prednisone alone as it is associated with a lower remission rate (56% versus 85%), a higher relapse rate, and a higher mortality rate when compared with combined cyclophosphamide and prednisone. Intravenous methylprednisone is prescribed for patients with severe disease who have either rapidly progressive glomerulonephritis (RPGN) or respiratory failure, and this is then followed by oral corticosteroid therapy. Cyclophosphamide is administered either intravenously or orally.[3] The optimal duration of cyclophosphamide therapy varies, and depends on the clinical response. Prolonged treatment is not unusual; however, it is associated with serious side effects. Adults treated with prolonged courses of oral cyclophosphamide have up to a 15% incidence of transitional cell carcinoma of the bladder and an increased incidence of lymphoma; the incidence is lower in children.

In practice, patients who achieve prompt and complete remission within 6 months of initiating therapy can stop treatment, but they require close follow-up. Treatment should be continued for 12 months in those with persistently active disease at 6 months. Azathioprine or methotrexate may be of benefit, either as maintenance therapy to prevent relapse or for patients with normal renal function. Nevertheless, although long-term remission may be achieved, relapses occur in up to 40% of patients. Vasculitic relapses may require repeat courses of prednisone and cyclophosphamide and longer periods of maintenance immunosuppression.

An alternative to azathioprine is methotrexate administered weekly. Methotrexate can be used as induction and maintenance therapy in WG, without threatened vital organ function.[16] Methotrexate is contraindicated with ESRD because of the risks of hepatic and bone marrow toxicity.

Mycophenolate mofetil (MMF) is an alternative to azathioprine. Patients who cannot receive cyclophosphamide and who relapse on azathioprine may respond to MMF. There is however a large variability of plasma concentrations of the drug between individuals, and monitoring of plasma concentrations of MMF should be considered.

The use of cyclosporine as an alternative agent to cyclophosphamide is associated with a higher relapse rate.

Colonization of the upper respiratory tract by *Staph. aureus* may increase the risk of disease relapse, and use of sulfamethoxazole/trimethoprim reduces the risk of respiratory relapse.[15]

Renal Replacement Therapy

Up to 20% of patients with ANCA-associated SVV and glomerulonephritis require dialysis at the time of diagnosis, and half come off dialysis within 8-12 weeks. Dialysis-dependent patients require treatment for at least 8-12 weeks with pulse methylprednisone and oral prednisone. In patients whose renal function improves, the corticosteroid treatment is continued and cyclophosphamide is started. Patients with ESRD in clinical remission with negative or stable ANCA titers are suitable candidates for transplantation. Transplantation should be deferred for patients who have a negative ANCA titer that suddenly increases.[19] Recurrence of disease following transplantation may occur in organs other than the kidney. The relapse rate for WG is appreciably lower in patients receiving azathioprine than in those treated with cyclosporine (20% versus 71%), and a lower recurrence rate occurs when a triple regimen in which azathioprine/MMF or cyclophosphamide is added to cyclosporine/tacrolimus and corticosteroids.

Refractory and Relapsing Disease/Future Therapeutic Options

Standard induction therapy fails to induce remission in approximately 10% of patients. A further difficult patient group comprises those who frequently relapse, necessitating recurrent use of cyclophosphamide. Both of these groups have a high risk of side effects from cyclophosphamide due to the high cumulative dose of

the drug that is accrued. Alternative strategies have involved the use of TNF-α blockade,[17] polyclonal antithymocyte globulin (ATG), monoclonal anti-T-cell antibodies, deoxyspergualin (DSG), immunoablation using high-dose cytotoxic medication followed by stem cell rescue, leflunomide, and blockade of pro-inflammatory cytokines including interleukin-1 and anti-CD20 monoclonal antibody (rituximab) which causes lysis of B cells.

OUTCOME

Treatment has converted this previously rapidly fatal disease into a chronic relapsing disorder that is associated with accumulative morbidity and mortality related to both disease activity and to treatment toxicity. Treatment must be tailored to the acuity and severity of disease, remembering to balance the dangers of disease against those of treatment. Although the average life expectancy without therapy is only 5 months, and 1-year survival is less than 20%, corticosteroids alone doubles life expectancy. The addition of cyclophosphamide results in a 72% decrease in mortality and a 1-year life expectancy of over 80%.

REFERENCES

1. Clayton AR, Savage COS. Evidence for the role of T cells in the pathogenesis of systemic vasculitis. Arthritis Res 2000;2:260-262.
2. Davies DJ, Moran JE, Niall JF, Ryan GB. Segmental necrotising glomerulonephritis with antineutrophil antibody: possible arbovirus etiology. Br Med J 1982;285:606.
3. de Groot K, Adu D, Savage COS. The value of pulse cyclophosphamide in ANCA-associated vasculitis. Meta-analysis and critical review. Nephrol Dial Transplant 2001;16:2018-2027.
4. Falk RJ, Jennette JC. ANCA small vessel vasculitis. J Am Soc Nephrol 1997;8:315-322.
5. Hagen EC, Daha MR, Hermans J, et al. Diagnostic value of standardized assays for anti-neutrophil cytoplasmic antibodies in idiopathic systemic vasculitis. Kidney Int 1998;53:743-753.

6. Harper L, Savage COS. Pathogenesis of ANCA-associated systemic vasculitis. J Pathol 2000;190:349-359.

7. Hattori M, Kurayama H, Koitabashi Y. Antineutrophil cytoplasmic autoantibody-associated glomerulonephritis in children. J Am Soc Nephrol 2001;12:1493-1500.

8. Waldherr R, Wiik A. Nomenclature of systemic vasculitides. Proposal of an international consensus conference. Arthritis Rheum 1994;37:187-192.

9. Nachman PH, Hogan SL, Jennette JC, Falk RJ. Treatment response and relapse in ANCA-associated microscopic polyangiitis and glomerulonephritis. J Am Soc Nephrol 1996;7:33-39.

10. Pusey CD, Rees AJ, Evans DJ, et al. Plasma exchange in focal necrotising glomerulonephritis without anti-GBM antibodies. Kidney Int 1991;40:757-763.

11. Rottem M, Fauci AS, Hallahan CW, et al. Wegener's granulomatosis in children and adolescents: clinical presentation and outcome. J Pediatr 1993;122:26-31.

12. Savage COS, Harper L, Holland M. New findings in pathogenesis of ANCA-associated vasculitis. Curr Opin Rheumatol 2002;14:15-22.

13. Scott DGI. Epidemiology of systemic vasculitis, increasing incidence? Clin Exp Immunol 2000;120(Suppl 1):19-20.

14. Wieslander J, Wiik A. International consensus statement on testing and reporting of antineutrophil cytoplasmic antibodies (ANCA). Am J Clin Pathol 1999;111:507-513.

15. Stegeman C, Cohen Tervaert J, de Jong P, Kallenberg CGM. Trimethoprim-sulfamethoxazole for the prevention of relapses of Wegener's granulomatosis. N Engl J Med 1996; 335:16-20.

16. Stone JH, Tun W, Hellmann DB. Treatment of non-life threatening Wegener's granulomatosis with methotrexate and daily prednisolone as the initial therapy of choice. J Rheumatol 1999;26:1134-1139.

17. Stone JH, Uhlfelder ML, Hellmann DB, et al. Etanercept combined with conventional treatment in Wegener's granulomatosis: a six month open-label trial to evaluate safety. Arthritis Rheum 2001;44:1149-1154.

18. Luqmani RA, Bacon PA, Moots RJ, et al. Birmingham vasculitic activity score (BVAS) in systemic necrotizing vasculitis. Q J Med 1994;87:671-678.

19. Wrenger E, Pirsch JD, Cangro CB, et al. Single-center experience with renal transplantation in patients with Wegener's granulomatosis. Transplant Int 1997;10:152-156.

CHAPTER 25

Systemic Lupus Erythematosus

JON M. BURNHAM, M.D. AND

KEVIN E.C. MEYERS, M.B., B.Ch.

INTRODUCTION

Systemic lupus erythematosus (SLE) is a multisystem autoimmune condition caused by the pathological production of autoantibodies and tissue deposition of immune complexes. Some 15% of SLE patients present in childhood. SLE has a predilection to cause renal disease that is frequently present at diagnosis and is responsible for significant morbidity and mortality. It is essential that all pediatricians should be able to diagnose SLE accurately, and to understand the potential complications and therapeutic options.

EPIDEMIOLOGY

Susceptibility to SLE is the result of a combination of genetic and environmental factors. The incidence is 2–8 per 100,000 and the prevalence is 20–60 per 100,000. Approximately 85% of patients are female. The female:male ratio increases after puberty and before menopause. Males with lupus have increased risks of hypertension, renal insufficiency, glaucoma, thrombosis, and myocardial infarction. In childhood, there is an increased incidence of nephritis, hematological involvement, malar rash, and chorea.[9] Blacks have an increased incidence of nephritis (Box 25-1).

PATHOPHYSIOLOGY

SLE is a complex disorder in which genetic and environmental factors interact to cause immune dysregulation, autoantibody production, immune complex formation, and subsequent inflammation and tissue destruction.[6]

Box 25-1 Factors Associated with an Increased Risk of Developing SLE

Hormonal	Estrogen
Race	Blacks (three-fold greater risk versus whites)
Environmental	Silica dust, hair dyes, solvents, uncooked L-canavanine in alfalfa sprouts
Medications	Procainamide, isoniazid, quinidine, hydralazine, etanercept, infliximab, and minocycline

Different contributions of susceptibility genes and environmental triggers may be responsible for the pleomorphic nature of the illness.

Monozygotic twins and first-degree relatives are at greatly increased risk. Defects in the production of early complement components increase the susceptibility to develop SLE. Certain HLA haplotypes (e.g., DR2, DR3) are associated with SLE, and some extended haplotypes may modify SLE expression (e.g., nephritis). Many non-HLA-associated genes such as Fcγ receptor alleles and cytokine polymorphisms are associated with SLE.

Ultraviolet light can trigger SLE by inducing apoptosis in keratinocytes. During this process, nuclear proteins are transported to the surface of cells and exposed to T cells that may be predisposed to recognize them as autoantigens. Sustained abnormal autoantibody production, complement activation, immune complex formation and clearance are the result of defects of multiple facets of the immune system. B cells are increased in number at all stages of development, are more active in secreting immunoglobulin, and are more responsive to cytokine stimulation. T cells are activated, skewed to a Th2 phenotype, and preferentially support autoantibody production. Suppressor T cells in SLE may enhance the activity of autoreactive B cells, or fail to down-regulate these cells. Fcγ receptor polymorphisms may lead to abnormal clearance of immune complexes by monocytes and macrophages and promote tissue deposition and inflammation.[13]

CLINICAL MANIFESTATIONS

The classification system used to aid diagnosis is shown in Table 25-1.[14] Four of 11 diagnostic criteria must be met to make a definite diagnosis of SLE. The criteria are relatively sensitive and specific in children, but they do not completely account for all the life-threatening,

Table 25-1 American College of Rheumatology Criteria for the Diagnosis of SLE

Malar rash	• Fixed erythema, flat or raised, over the malar eminences, tending to spare the nasolabial folds
Discoid rash	• Erythematous raised patches with adherent keratotic scaling and follicular plugging; atrophic scarring may occur in older lesions
Photosensitivity	• Skin rash as a result of unusual reaction to sunlight, by patient history or physician observation
Oral ulcers	• Oral or nasopharyngeal ulceration, usually painless, observed by physician
Arthritis	• Non-erosive arthritis involving two or more peripheral joints, characterized by tenderness, swelling, or effusion
Serositis	• Pleuritis – convincing history of pleuritic pain or rubbing heard by a physician, or evidence of pleural effusion; or • Pericarditis – documented by ECG or rub, or evidence of pericardial effusion
Renal disorder	• Persistent proteinuria greater than 0.5 g per day, or greater that 3+ if quantitation not performed; or • Cellular casts – may be red cell, hemoglobin, granular, tubular, or mixed
Neurologic disorder	• Seizures or psychosis – in the absence of offending drugs or known metabolic derangements; e.g., uremia, ketoacidosis, or electrolyte imbalance
Hematologic disorder	• Hemolytic anemia – with reticulocytosis; or • Leukopenia – less than 4000 per mm^3 total on two or more occasions; or • Lymphopenia – less than 1500 per mm^3 on two or more occasions; or • Thrombocytopenia – less than 100,000 per mm^3 in the absence of offending drugs
Immunologic disorder	• Positive finding of anti-dsDNA antibodies; or • Positive finding of anti-Smith antibodies; or • Positive finding of antiphospholipid antibodies based on: 　i. abnormal serum level of IgG or IgM anticardiolipin antibodies; or 　ii. positive test result for lupus anticoagulant using a standard method; or 　iii. false-positive serologic test for syphilis know to be positive for at least 6 months and confirmed by *Treponema pallidum* immobilization or fluorescent treponemal antibody absorption test
Antinuclear antibody	• An abnormal titer of antinuclear antibody by immunofluorescence or an equivalent assay at any point in time and in the absence of drugs known to be associated with 'drug-induced lupus' syndrome

Data from Hochberg MC. Updating the American College of Rheumatology revised criteria for the classification of systemic lupus erythematosus [letter]. Arthritis Rheum 1997;40:1725.

painful, debilitating, and disfiguring manifestations of SLE. In addition, a major disease such as nephritis may obscure vague findings, such as poor school performance that may be an important cognitive effect of neuropsychiatric lupus. Subtle, important, disease effects must be pro-actively assessed and treated.

Lupus Nephritis

Lupus nephritis affects 60–80% of pediatric patients, with significant morbidity and mortality.[4] Children may present with the nephritic syndrome, nephrotic syndrome or nephritic-nephrotic syndrome. Variable proteinuria is seen in most patients with lupus nephritis, with greater than 3 g/24 hours in 55% of patients. Microscopic hematuria is found in 79% of patients, and less than 2% have macroscopic hematuria. Hypertension is seen in 40%. Acute renal failure is rare, but the glomerular filtration rate (GFR) is abnormal in about half of the patients. Other renal manifestations of lupus nephritis are tubulo-interstitial nephritis, renal arterial or venous thrombosis, thrombotic microangiopathy as part of thrombotic thrombocytopenic purpura (TTP) and the antiphospho-lipid syndrome (APS). Cystitis may occur as a complication that is independent of cyclophosphamide. Transverse myelitis and inflammatory polyneuropathy may cause a neurogenic bladder.

Clinical Evaluation

Measurement of proteinuria, microscopic analysis for red blood cells, white blood cells and casts, and serum creatinine concentration are followed regularly. Measurement of antibodies directed against double-stranded DNA (anti-dsDNA) and decreased serum levels of complement components C3 and C4 may reflect disease activity. Hypocomplementemia is found in a significantly greater percentage of patients with nephritis (75% versus 49%; $p < 0.01$). These parameters are useful to follow over time, as increasing anti-dsDNA titers and decreasing complement levels may herald a lupus flare, particularly in a patient with established nephritis.

Renal biopsy is indicated for patients with proteinuria greater than 1 g per 24 hours, an active urinary sediment, or an elevated serum creatinine concentration.

Pathology

The World Health Organization (WHO) classification (Table 25-2) stratifies patients for studies in clinical trials, and predicts outcomes. This incorporates findings of light microscopy (LM), immunofluorescence (IF) and electron microscopy (EM), to determine the severity and chronicity of renal damage. The biopsy findings are initially described prior to their allocation to a specific WHO histologic class. LM findings vary from minimal mesangial proliferation to crescentic proliferative necrotizing GN. IF shows

Table 25-2	World Health Organization Classification of Lupus Nephritis
Class I	Normal
Class II	Mesangial glomerulonephritis
Class III	Focal proliferative glomerulonephritis
Class IV	Diffuse proliferative glomerulonephritis
Class V	Diffuse membranous glomerulopathy
Class VI	Glomerular sclerosis

specific patterns of immunoglobulin (IgG, IgM, IgA) and complement (C3, C1q) deposition and differentiates between mesangial and capillary wall immune deposition. When all of these components are present on IF this is called a 'full house' pattern. EM gives ultrastructural information about the presence or absence of immune deposition and their location (i.e., mesangial, subendothelial, subepithelial, or intramembranous).

Normal glomerular architecture is found in 6% of biopsies of lupus nephritis. A focal segmental glomerulo-nephritis (FSGS) and focal proliferative glomerulo-nephritis (FSGN) is present in 23% of children with lupus nephritis. Varying degrees of capillary obliteration, necrosis, proliferation, and scarring may be present. Diffuse proliferative glomerulonephritis (DPGN) is seen in about 43% of biopsy specimens. The glomerulus shows lobular hypercellularity with areas of necrosis, often with crescent formation. Sclerosis indicates chronic scarring. Mesangial hypercellularity is present in FSGS and DPGN. EM reveals mesangial and subendothelial deposition of immune complexes in FSGN and DPGN, with IF positive centrally in the mesangium and peripherally in capillary loops. A membranous glomerulopathy (MGN) may also contain mesangial or more worrisome proliferative lesions in 9% of biopsy specimens. The principal finding in MGN is diffuse, uniform thickening of the GBM, creating a 'wire-loop' appearance on microscopy. EM shows sub-epithelial and intramembranous deposition of immune complexes with BM spikes, the so-called 'spike and dome' pattern. IF reveals a peripheral granular pattern with or without mesangial involvement. Extraglomerular lesions include varying severity of interstitial inflammation and sclerosis, tubular dropout, and vascular changes such as arteritis or thrombotic microangiopathy.

Renal Outcomes

The WHO classification predicts nephritis progression. Up to 75% of children with DPGN develop end-stage renal disease.[17] Clinical markers of adverse renal outcomes include elevated serum creatinine concentration, persistent hypertension, chronic anemia, and nephrotic range proteinuria.[2,8] Data from adult series shows that severe FSGN may have a similar prognosis to DPGN. Renal and patient survival approaches 90% in severe nephritis. Patients with a pure membranous lesion may develop nephrotic syndrome and hypertension, but the long-term outcome is generally good, with few patients progressing to renal failure. Proliferative changes in combination with MPN have a graver prognosis.

Extra-Renal Manifestations

Neuropsychiatric SLE (NP-SLE)

NP-SLE occurs in 30% of children.[4,24] The nomenclature for the classification of 19 neuropsychiatric SLE syndromes is shown in Table 25-3. NP-SLE is associated with anti-neuronal antibodies, antiphospholipid antibodies, and rarely a discrete vasculitis. NP-SLE can be fulminant and life-threatening with seizures, status epilepticus, coma, transverse myelitis and stroke. Or, it may be insidious with psychiatric and cognitive disturbances. Seizures must not be attributed to NP-SLE if a known predisposing factor such as infection or trauma is present. The seizure may be focal or generalized. Cerebrovascular accidents are often the result of the APS. Strokes may be the result of arterial or venous thrombi or emboli from the heart. Acute symptoms such as headache, weakness, altered mental status, and paresis depend on the anatomic location of the thrombus. A small vessel vasculopathy without vasculitis is often found on biopsy or autopsy. Patients with NP-SLE may have frank psychosis with visual, auditory, or tactile hallucinations. Their behavior may be withdrawn, depressed, labile, or disorganized. Depression and anxiety can be part of an adjustment disorder or a maladaptive response to chronic illness. Deteriorating school performance, non-adherence to medical regimens, and altered sleep patterns may be symptoms of organic brain disease.[25] An 'acute confusional state' or delirium may be present at diagnosis, but impairment of memory, concentration, and intellect may be insidious, even in the absence of more overt signs and symptoms of NP-SLE. Tension headaches and migraines are common. A 'lupus headache' is prolonged and intractable. Fatigue, anxiety, and depression are common features in SLE patients with headaches (Box 25-2).

Box 25-2 Useful Tests for Evaluating NP-SLE

- *Lumbar puncture* for infection or bleeds; pleocytosis and/or elevated protein
- *Computed tomography (CT)* for hemorrhage, focal lesions, ventriculomegaly, or atrophy
- *MRI* is more sensitive for detecting white matter lesions and early ischemia[11]
- *MR angiography* for thrombosis of proximal intracranial vasculature. This is not as sensitive as conventional angiography in defining distal abnormalities of small caliber vessels.
- *Electroencephalography (EEG)* may yield normal results
- *Antibodies* include anti-ribosomal P (serum) and anti-neuronal and/or oligoclonal bands (CSF)
- *Neuropsychological testing* is valuable to assess cognitive dysfunction and to develop a plan for specialized attention at school

---

Cardiovascular

Cardiac pathology occurs in 40% of children with SLE.[19] The pericardium, myocardium, conduction system, valves, and coronary arteries are targets. Symptomatic pericarditis occurs in 25% of cases, either in isolation or as part of a generalized serositis. Patients present with precordial pain, radiating to the left shoulder or back that can be associated with fever, cough, or dyspnea. There may be tachycardia, distant heart sounds, and a friction rub. Electrocardiography reveals low voltages, mild ST-segment elevation, and T-wave inversion. Chest X-radiography shows an enlarged cardiac silhouette, and an echocardiogram is diagnostic. The pericardial fluid is exudative. Cardiac tamponade occurs in less than 1% of patients. The pathogenesis of the cardiomyopathy is multifactorial: it may be an autoimmune phenomenon, or it may be secondary to atherosclerosis, hypertension, or antimalarial therapy. Presenting symptoms include dyspnea, orthopnea, cough, palpitations, and exercise intolerance. A physical examination reveals tachycardia, an S_3

Table 25-3 Defined Neuropsychiatric Syndromes in SLE

Central Nervous System		Peripheral Nervous System
Aseptic meningitis	Acute confusion	Guillain–Barré syndrome
Cerebrovascular disease	Anxiety disorder	Autonomic disorder
Demyelinating syndrome	Cognitive dysfunction	Mononeuropathy
Headache	Mood disorder	Myasthenia gravis
Chorea	Psychosis	Cranial neuropathy
Myelopathy	Seizures	Plexopathy
		Polyneuropathy

gallop, and rales. Chest X-radiography shows cardiac enlargement, with varying degrees of pulmonary edema. Echocardiography shows diminished ventricular systolic function. Heart block (1st, 2nd, and 3rd degree), atrial fibrillation, and atrial or premature ventricular contractions may be the result of an autoimmune phenomenon. In the neonatal lupus syndrome, transplacental transfer of maternal autoantibodies (anti-SS-A, SS-B) may cause congenital complete heart block. Valvular disease is a common finding, but may be asymptomatic and unrelated to overall lupus activity. In adults, valvular abnormalities were found in 61% and 53% of lupus patients on an initial and follow-up transesophageal echocardiography, respectively. The mitral and aortic valves are most commonly affected. Libmann–Sachs endocarditis is a non-infectious inflammatory condition in SLE that can simulate bacterial disease. Dyslipidemia, premature atherosclerosis, and myocardial infarction are complications of juvenile SLE.[10] The dyslipidemia may be secondary to the underlying disease, corticosteroid use, or both. An increased carotid intima-media wall thickness can occur in young lupus patients with nephrotic-range proteinuria.

Respiratory

The pleura, lung parenchyma, pulmonary vasculature, and respiratory muscles may become involved in the disease process.[7] Pleuritis is the most common pulmonary manifestation. It may be clinically silent, but often causes fever, cough, dyspnea, and chest pain on deep inspiration. Physical findings include a pleural friction rub and diminished breath sounds. Chest radiography may reveal a pleural effusion. This is typically exudative (Box 25-3).

Lupus pneumonitis is potentially fulminant. It presents with fever, cough, dyspnea, chest pain, and unilateral or bilateral infiltrates. This must be distinguished from infection often as a diagnosis of exclusion. Pathologic features are non-specific, but immunofluorescence may reveal immune deposition. Alveolar hemorrhage can be catastrophic and is often associated with nephritis. Hemoptysis occurs in 50% and often progresses to respiratory failure. Pulmonary hypertension may be the result of chronic thromboembolic disease or parenchymal lung disease, and is associated with antiphospholipid antibodies and Raynaud's phenomenon.

Shrinking lung syndrome is characterized by progressive dyspnea and exercise intolerance, with elevated hemidiaphragms on chest radiography. The etiology may be respiratory muscle weakness secondary to myopathy or neuropathy. Asymptomatic alterations in pulmonary function testing have been noted commonly with restriction and diminished diffusion capacity.[7]

Hematologic

Lupus commonly affects the hematologic system, resulting in aberrant production or accelerated destruction of leukocytes, platelets, or erythrocytes. The cytopenias may be specifically autoimmune, or the result of more complex phenomena such as TTP or a hemophagocytic syndrome. Thrombocytopenic patients with APS are at risk of thrombosis, despite markedly low platelet counts. In a study of childhood-onset TTP, 26% fulfilled the American College of Rheumatology (ACR) criteria for the diagnosis of SLE, and 23% were found to have incipient SLE (Box 25-4).[3]

Musculoskeletal

Limb and joint pain is seen in the majority of children with SLE, and is often the presenting complaint. Symptoms of inflammatory joint pain include morning stiffness and gelling (pain with rest, for example after a long class or automobile trip). In contrast, mechanical joint pain usually improves after a period of rest. The patient may have arthralgias – that is, joint pain without objective signs of

---

Box 25-3	Causes of Pleural Effusions in Patients with Lupus

- Pleuritis
- Pulmonary embolism
- Pulmonary hemorrhage
- Infection
- Pneumonitis
- Congestive heart failure
- Hypoalbuminemia

Box 25-4	Hematologic Abnormalities in SLE
Leukopenia	(<4000 per mm^3) and lymphopenia (<1500 per mm^3) in about 50% of cases
Neutropenia	In 15% secondary to anti-neutrophil antibodies, anti-G-CSF antibodies, myelofibrosis, marrow aplasia, or increased apoptosis
Thrombocytopenia	In 10% at presentation and 25% overall
Anemia	• Anemia of chronic disease in one-third of patients • Iron deficiency in one-third of patients • Autoimmune hemolytic anemia in one-sixth of patients • Chronic renal failure • Anti-erythropoietin antibodies in one-fifth of patients

inflammation, such as swelling, effusion, deformity, or limitation of range of motion. Arthritis, in which objective signs are present, may involve any number of joints, may be symmetric, additive, or migratory. Characteristically, erosions do not develop, nor does chronic loss of function. Ligamentous laxity in the joints of the hand is characteristic of lupus.

Inflammatory myositis is rare in lupus but may be indicative of an overlap syndrome, such as mixed connective tissue disease (MCTD). Proximal muscles are more commonly affected, as in dermatomyositis. Creatine kinase, aldolase, aspartate aminotransferase, and lactate dehydrogenase may be elevated. Infectious causes (influenza B) and medications (HMG-CoA reductase inhibitors) can also cause myositis.

Osteopenia and osteoporosis are common, and result from underlying disease activity, diminished weight-bearing activity, malnutrition, amenorrhea, corticosteroid use, and cytokine effects on bone. Avascular necrosis (AVN) is a serious complication in 15% of patients.[20,21] The pain is usually a deep ache that may awaken the patient, with or without movement. AVN occurs in one or both femoral heads and also in the knees, shoulders, elbows, and ankles. SLE AVN is associated with corticosteroid use, arthritis, and cytotoxic therapy. The hip must be imaged to assess for early, asymptomatic involvement in patients diagnosed with AVN in a joint other than the hip. MRI is the most sensitive modality.

Gastrointestinal

Abdominal pain is a difficult complaint to assess in lupus as its underlying cause may be benign or catastrophic.[26] The symptoms and signs of acute abdominal processes may be masked in patients on corticosteroids. The abdominal complications of SLE are listed in Table 25-4.

Pancreatitis is a life-threatening complication of lupus, antiphospholipid antibodies, glucocorticoids, or azathioprine. It typically presents with epigastric pain that radiates to the back with fever and emesis and progression to hypovolemic shock.

Mesenteric vasculitis, with or without bowel infarction, and mesenteric thrombosis are difficult to differentiate. Presenting symptoms and signs are fever, vomiting, diarrhea with or without blood, abdominal pain, distention, quiet bowel sounds and rebound tenderness. X-radiography and computed tomography scanning may reveal bowel wall edema, or air–fluid levels. In extreme cases of suspected bowel infarction, visceral angiography is helpful to define the location of an arterial thrombus. Liver enzyme abnormalities occur in one-third of patients, but this rarely progresses to liver failure.

Dermatologic

Mucocutaneous involvement in lupus is common (75%), and a variety of eruptions are seen (Box 25-5). Four of 11 ACR criteria for the diagnosis of lupus involve the skin and mucosal surfaces of the mouth and nose (e.g., malar and discoid rashes, photosensitivity, and oral or nasal ulceration).[16] Some patients with cutaneous lesions do not fulfill ACR criteria for the diagnosis of SLE and are labeled 'Cutaneous Lupus Erythematosus.'

SEROLOGIC EVALUATION

Positive tests for: (1) antinuclear antibodies (ANA); and (2) an 'immunologic disorder' (anti-dsDNA, anti-Smith antibodies (anti-Sm), anti-cardiolipin antibody (anti-CL), lupus anticoagulants, and a false-positive rapid plasma reagin (RPR) test comprise two of the 11 ACR criteria for the diagnosis of SLE. There are, however, many other autoantibodies with pathologic significance in lupus.[12]

Table 25-4 Gastrointestinal and Hepatic Manifestations of SLE	
Pharyngitis	Mesenteric vasculitis
Dysphagia	Bowel infarction/perforation
Esophagitis	Pancreatitis
Peptic ulcer	Hepatomegaly
Peritonitis	Jaundice
Protein-losing enteropathy	Hepatitis
Ulcerative/lupus colitis	Budd–Chiari syndrome

Box 25-5 Dermatologic Manifestations of SLE

- Malar rash or 'butterfly rash' is erythematous, raised, and spares the nasolabial folds
- Discoid lupus appears on sun-exposed areas, is discrete, often annular with scale, and can leave scars
- Subacute cutaneous lupus erythematosus is papulosquamous; it can be confused with psoriasis
- Photosensitivity
- Oral/nasal ulceration is usually painless
- Cutaneous vasculitis/purpura
- Livedo reticularis is a lacy rash that is often seen with APS
- Periungual erythema
- Alopecia can be marked and may be secondary to cyclophosphamide
- Raynaud's phenomenon is a painful condition that may cause digital ulceration. Finger(s) become white, blue, and/or red
- Rare manifestations are bullae, panniculitis, urticaria, Sweet syndrome

Table 25-5 Antinuclear Antibodies (ANA) Patterns

All of these patterns occur in SLE

Peripheral ('rim')	Autoimmune hepatitis (less common)
Homogenous	Autoimmune hepatitis
Speckled	Mixed connective tissue disease, scleroderma, Sjögren syndrome
Nucleolar	Scleroderma, dermatomyositis
Centromere	CREST (calcinosis, Raynaud's phenomenon, esophageal dysmotility, sclerodactyly, telangiectasis)

Antinuclear Antibodies

Antibodies to nuclear antigens are the *sine qua non* of lupus. The patient's serum is exposed to a standardized cell line (HEp-2, human epithelial cell tumor), and immunofluorescence microscopy is performed. When an ANA is positive, the result is expressed as a titer. In the general population, the ANA will be positive at a titer of 1:40 in about 25–30% of cases and 1:160 in 5%.

ANA testing has a sensitivity approaching 95%, but the positive predictive value is low in unselected persons.

No pattern is specific for lupus or related conditions with the exception of the peripheral, or 'rim' pattern in patients with anti-dsDNA antibodies (Table 25-5).

Antibodies to dsDNA

Anti-dsDNA antibodies are specific for lupus, although some patients with autoimmune hepatitis are positive.[22] These antibodies are associated with the development of lupus nephritis, and rising anti-dsDNA titers in conjunction with falling serum complement levels may predict an impending lupus flare. Periodic monitoring of anti-dsDNA concentrations is routine in the care of lupus patients. These autoantibodies are pathogenic and have been eluted from renal lesions.

Antibodies to Extractable Nuclear Antigens (ENAs)

A variety of ENAs may yield clinically relevant information. Anti-Smith (anti-Sm) is found in 20–30% of lupus patients, and is associated with MGN. Antibodies to a specific ribonucleoprotein (anti-RNP) may correlate with lung, muscle, esophageal, and joint involvement in lupus, and are positive in high titers in mixed connective tissue disease. Anti-SS-A (Ro) and anti-SS-B (La) are positive in 40% and 15% of lupus patients, respectively. They are also positive in Sjögren syndrome, subacute cutaneous lupus erythematosus, and congenital complete heart block in neonatal lupus. Anti-Scl-70 is directed

against topoisomerase I, and may be present in high titers in individuals with scleroderma. Anti-Jo1, which is found to bind histidine tRNA synthetase, has been linked to lung disease, particularly in dermatomyositis. Anti-histone antibodies are seen with drug-induced lupus.

Complement

Individuals with deficiencies of early complement components have an increased risk of developing lupus, but decreases in serum complement levels are most often a sign of active disease. Total serum hemolytic complement activity (CH50) is useful in the identification of complement deficiencies. CH50, C3, and C4 are decreased in active SLE.

MANAGEMENT OF LUPUS

The optimal care of children with lupus starts with counseling patients and their families about the disease, with special attention to health maintenance measures, emotional support, recognition of disease complications, and education concerning medication side effects and adherence. Given the relatively small number of children with lupus, there are no randomized placebo-controlled trials of pharmacologic therapies. Treatment strategies are often extrapolated from studies in adults, or are based on anecdotal reports. A list of common drugs and dosages is given in Table 25-6.

Table 25-6 Medications and Dosages in the Treatment of Lupus

Hydroxychloroquine	5.0–6.5 mg/kg/day up to 400 mg/day
Aspirin (prophylaxis)	3–5 mg/kg/day up to 81 mg/day
Prednisone/Prednisolone	1–2 mg/kg/day as starting dose. Increased doses increases efficacy and side effects
Methylprednisolone	30 mg/kg/day IV for up to 3 days (pulse dosing)
Methotrexate	Up to 1 mg/kg/week, subcutaneous route preferred
Azathioprine	1 mg/kg/day as starting dose, up to 3 mg/kg/day maintenance dose
Mycophenolate mofetil	1200 mg/m²/day (b.i.d.) up to 2 g/day. The starting dose depends on the WBC count
Cyclophosphamide Must ensure adequate hydration to prevent hemorrhagic cystitis	IV: 750 mg/m²/month increasing to 1 g/m² if WBC count is >2500 per mm³ at nadir Oral: 1–3 mg/kg/day (q.d.) depending on WBC count as above

Health Maintenance

The lives of both the family and the child are up-ended with the diagnosis of a chronic illness. Matters of healthy living which were previously taken for granted, such as diet, exercise, and sun protection become more important. The pediatrician should play a role in assuring that proper adaptations are made for school (e.g., two sets of books, no timed tests, extra time between classes, early tutoring if school days are missed, appropriate physical education classes), so that chances of success are maximized. Children on corticosteroids may have difficulty with their peers if they gain weight and develop cushingoid features. Early onset of atherosclerotic disease requires monitoring of fasting serum cholesterol, LDL, HDL, and triglycerides. Regular aerobic exercise, weight loss, cessation of smoking, and a diet low in fat should be encouraged. A nutritional evaluation and institution of a National Cholesterol Education Program (NCEP) Step I diet is recommended for hyperlipidemia. There are no formal recommendations for cholesterol-lowering medications in childhood lupus. Patients on long-term glucocorticoid therapy appear to be at particular risk for bone problems. Adequate weight-bearing exercise, calcium (minimum 1200 mg/day), and vitamin D intake (plain or activated, particularly if on chronic glucocorticoids) is encouraged, and a DXA scan should be performed periodically. There are no data available on the long-term effects of bisphosphonates in adolescents for the treatment and prevention of osteoporosis. Contraception should be discussed with fertile female lupus patients. Oral contraceptives containing estrogen may be unsafe for patients at risk for thrombosis, and low estrogen or progesterone-only methods should be used. Patients on warfarin, methotrexate, or cyclophosphamide must be counseled about teratogenic side effects. Alternative therapies must be initiated if a patient intends to become pregnant. Pregnancy is inadvisable in active disease. Sun avoidance and protection are important. Patients are encouraged to wear hats, long pants, and long sleeves. Routine application of sunscreen with UVA and UVB protection is imperative, and the sun protection factor (SPF) should be 15 or greater. Children need to be reminded to reapply the sunscreen after swimming, or activities that cause sweating.

The administration of killed or component vaccines has not been shown to precipitate lupus flares. Yearly influenza vaccination is recommended. If the patient is immunocompromised, pneumococcal vaccination with the pneumococcal conjugate and polysaccharide vaccine is recommended (as per AAP guidelines). Live vaccines, such as the Varicella vaccine, MMR (measles, mumps and rubella), and oral poliovirus vaccine (OPV) may be dangerous in immunocompromised hosts, and may cause true infections.

Pneumocystis carinii (PCP) infections occur in lupus. Prophylaxis should be considered for glucocorticoid-treated patients, particularly those who are lymphopenic and are receiving other immunosuppressive medications, such as cyclophosphamide. Since sulfonamides may cause lupus flares, dapsone or monthly inhaled pentamidine are alternative options for PCP prophylaxis.

Conservative Therapies

Mild manifestations of lupus, such as skin or musculoskeletal disease, often respond to conservative pharmacologic therapies. Topical corticosteroid preparations may be used for cutaneous lesions. Low potency, nonfluorinated steroid creams should be used on the face to avoid atrophy and telangiectasias. Medium-potency fluorinated formulations can be used on the limbs and trunk. Intralesional steroid injections may be useful for refractory discoid lesions.

Non-steroidal anti-inflammatory drugs (NSAIDS; e.g., ibuprofen, naproxen) may be used for the treatment of musculoskeletal pain, serositis, and headaches. Side effects are common, however, and include gastritis, ulcers, stomatitis, hepatitis, and renal insufficiency. Therefore, NSAIDS must be used with caution in patients with lupus nephritis. Antimalarial drugs, primarily hydroxychloroquine, are used for the treatment of dermatologic manifestations, constitutional symptoms, arthralgias/arthritis, and may be protective against thrombosis. Proven to have a sun-blocking, steroid-sparing effect, antimalarials appear to reduce the incidence of lupus flares. Side effects include nausea, abdominal cramps, diarrhea, and pigment changes of the hair or skin. Formal ophthalmologic screening including visual field testing is recommended every 6 months to 1 year to screen for alterations in visual acuity, corneal pigment deposition, and retinopathy. Hydroxychloroquine can precipitate hemolysis in individuals with glucose 6-phosphate dehydrogenase (G6PD) deficiency. Careful management of hypertension in patients with nephritis is of the utmost importance, as sustained hypertension is a predictor of poor renal outcome. Angiotensin-converting enzyme (ACE) and angiotensin receptor inhibitors are the mainstay of therapy, particularly because of their beneficial effects in proteinuric patients.

Immunosuppressive Medications

Immunosuppressive medications are used to obtain rapid control of a lupus flare, and to maintain remission, particularly in patients with more severe manifestations. None of the medicines is curative, and all have benefits and risks.

Systemic Corticosteroids

These are potent immunosuppressives that have a rapid onset of action. The prolonged use of corticosteroids can

Table 25-7   Side Effects of Glucocorticoid Therapy for Lupus

Weight gain	Myopathy	Cataracts
Cushingoid features	Osteopenia	Glaucoma
Acne	Avascular necrosis	Mood alteration
Hirsutism	Glucose intolerance	Psychosis
Striae	Hypertension	Adrenal suppression
Pancreatitis	Atherosclerosis	Infection
Gastritis/peptic ulcer		

cause many side effects (Table 25-7). For a lupus flare, the initial oral dose is usually 1-2 mg/kg/day. The tapering schedule depends on the indication and the patient, but usually occurs over 3 months. Methylprednisolone may be used as a 'pulse' in a high dose of 30 mg/kg up to 1 g, intravenously for 3 days for severe disease manifestations, such as lupus nephritis or NP-SLE. Additional immunosuppressive agents are used to maximize disease control and maximize the likelihood that a patient will tolerate a careful reduction in the daily steroid dose. Thus, these medications have beneficial effects that are independent of steroids, but they are also steroid-sparing agents.

Methotrexate
Methotrexate is an inhibitor of the enzyme dihydrofolate reductase, and has anti-inflammatory and immunosuppressive properties. Common indications are arthritis, serositis, and refractory cutaneous disease in SLE. There is also a corticosteroid-sparing effect in thrombocytopenic patients. Side effects are relatively uncommon and include oral ulcers, fatigue, headache, abdominal discomfort, alopecia, myelosuppression, hepatitis, and rarely pneumonitis. Oral supplementation of folic acid can minimize hepatotoxicity and mucositis.

Azathioprine and Mycophenolate Mofetil
Azathioprine and mycophenolate mofetil (MMF) are used to treat some non-renal manifestations, but they are not as efficacious as cyclophosphamide for inducing a remission of severe lupus nephritis.[5] They are useful corticosteroid-sparing agents, and may help maintain renal remission. Side effects include myelotoxicity, hepatitis, nausea, vomiting, diarrhea, hypersensitivity reactions, and possibly lymphoproliferative malignancies.

Cyclophosphamide
Cyclophosphamide is used to treat severe complications of lupus, and is the most effective therapy for proliferative glomerulonephritis. In long-term studies, cyclophosphamide is more effective (90%) than steroids alone (20%) or with azathioprine (60%) in the prevention of renal failure.[23] Cyclophosphamide when given monthly as an IV pulse for 6 months for proliferative

nephritis, followed by an infusion every 3 months for 3 years, results in a decrease in renal biopsy activity, and allows for a systematic reduction in corticosteroid dose.[17] Cyclophosphamide may have beneficial effects on mortality.[1] This agent is increasingly used in NP-SLE, although there are no carefully constructed trials. Side effects include nausea, vomiting, hemorrhagic cystitis, alopecia, amenorrhea, infertility, and late onset of bladder cancer and hematologic malignancies. MESNA and careful hydration can prevent hemorrhagic cystitis.

Overview of Therapy for Lupus Nephritis
Mesiangial inflammation does not require any specific treatment. Patients with proliferative glomerular lesions (FSGN, DPGN) are treated with glucocorticoids and cyclophosphamide. There is an increased risk of a renal flare off therapy in patients with a partial response to long-term therapy, who usually have low C4 levels and who are usually black.[15] The risk of an early transition after 6 months of cytotoxic therapy with azathioprine or MMF, when compared to long-term therapy, has not been clearly established with controlled studies, but may be substantial. Therapeutic options for pure membranous nephritis include steroids and either azathioprine, MMF, or cyclophosphamide (Figure 25-1).

Dialysis and Transplantation
Acute renal failure (ARF) may require temporary dialysis, and ESRD requires permanent renal replacement therapy. Lupus is usually inactive on chronic dialysis, and prednisone therapy is usually sufficient for mild flares. Thrombosis of vascular access is a problem, but patients are candidates for either hemodialyis (HD) or peritoneal dialysis (PD).

Pediatric recipients of renal allografts usually do well. The cross-matching of sera may be difficult because of prior transfusions or autoantibodies, and allograft thrombosis is more common especially when antiphospholipid antibodies are present. Patients with APS should be anti-coagulated after transplant. Lupus recurrence in the allograft is <1%, and is almost never associated with graft loss. Triple immunosuppression is suitable, and cyclosporine monotherapy should be avoided as it not a good suppressant of autoimmunity. Overall, outcome is similar to patients with other causes of ESRD.

ANTIPHOSPHOLIPID SYNDROME (APS)
Children with lupus appear to be at particular risk for thrombosis because of a propensity to develop APS.[18] Primary APS is seen in patients without underlying autoimmune conditions, whereas secondary APS occurs in patients with rheumatologic conditions. Autoantibodies

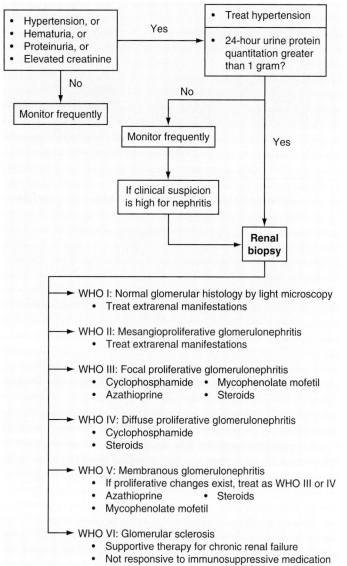

Figure 25-1   Overview of therapy for lupus nephritis.

may induce a prothrombotic state, with the risk of arterial and venous thromboses and morbidity in pregnancy. The diagnosis of APS is made in an individual who has a thrombosis, or specific morbidity in pregnancy, and has specific laboratory abnormalities (Table 25-8).

Pathophysiology

The autoantibodies responsible for APS are 'lupus anticoagulants,' or are directed against cardiolipin (anti-CL, a mitochondrial phospholipid) and β2-glycoprotein-1 (anti-β2-GP1, a phospholipid-binding protein). Lupus anticoagulant antibodies create a peculiar in-vitro prolongation of the activated partial thromboplastin time (aPTT). Prolongation of the clotting time does not correct with the addition of normal plasma, but normalizes with the addition of excess phospholipid. Non-pathogenic anti-CL antibodies may be seen in a variety of infectious diseases,

but in lupus they are clearly pathogenic and titers correlate with risk. Anti-β2-GP1 antibodies are also indicative of an increased risk of thrombosis. Laboratory studies useful in the diagnosis of APS are shown in Table 25-9. Endothelial cell activation, interference with the coagulation cascade, and oxidant-mediated endothelial injury are important in the pathogenesis of APS.

Clinical Manifestations

Less serious manifestations are Raynaud's phenomenon and livedo reticularis. Serious complications are deep venous thrombosis, pulmonary embolus, Budd–Chiari syndrome, and major arterial thromboses. Renal involvement also occurs as a thrombotic microangiopathy. APS in lupus is linked to neuropsychiatric disease, in particular transverse myelitis, myocardial infarction, retinal vasculitis, Libmann–Sacks endocarditis,

Table 25-8	Antiphospholipid Syndrome Diagnostic Criteria*

Clinical Event	Laboratory Abnormality
Vascular thrombosis • Arterial–venous: small-vessel	Anticardiolipin antibodies • IgM or IgG • Moderate to high levels on two or more occasions at least 6 weeks apart
Pregnancy morbidity • One or more unexplained death of a morphologically normal fetus after 10 weeks' gestation; or • One or more premature births of normal neonate before 34 weeks' gestation; or • Three or more unexplained consecutive spontaneous abortions before 10 weeks' gestation	Lupus anticoagulant antibodies • Detected on two or more occasions at least 6 weeks apart

*The diagnosis of APS requires one clinical event and one laboratory criterion. These are not necessarily related in time.

pancreatitis, thrombocytopenia, TTP, and other vascular events. Catastrophic APS refers to thromboses of predominantly small vessels, in at least three organ systems, over days to weeks.

Therapy

Lupus patients who have not experienced a thrombotic event, but have a lupus anticoagulant, or antibodies to ACL, anti-β2-GP1, or a false-positive RPR, are managed with prophylactic low-dose aspirin anti-platelet therapy. Anti-platelet therapy is contraindicated if the platelet count is below 60,000 per mm^3. The elimination of risk factors for thrombosis, such as estrogen-containing contraceptives, is important. For those who have a thrombosis, unfractionated or low molecular-weight heparin is used for anticoagulation, followed by maintenance with warfarin. The current recommendation is life-long

Table 25-9	Laboratory Assays Useful in the Diagnosis of Antiphospholipid Syndrome

Antibodies	Functional Measures of Lupus Anticoagulant
Anticardiolipin antibody (IgG, IgM) Anti-β2-glycoprotein-1 (IgG, IgM) Rapid Plasma Reagin (RPR)	aPTT Dilute Russell's Viper Venom Time (DRVVT)

aPTT = activated partial thromboplastin time.

MAJOR POINTS

- The optimal care of a patient with SLE requires a multidisciplinary endeavor that involves primary care pediatricians; pediatric rheumatologists, nephrologists, dermatologists, cardiologists, pulmonologists, and neurologists; nurses, nutritionists, physical therapists, psychologists, and social workers.
- Lupus hepatitis should not to be confused with type-1 autoimmune hepatitis, or 'lupoid hepatitis'. Such patients may be positive for ANA and sometimes anti-dsDNA. These individuals also have autoantibodies to smooth muscle and mitochondrial antigens, and rarely meet ACR criteria for the diagnosis of SLE.
- A positive ANA must be viewed with great skepticism in the absence of other signs or symptoms of SLE or of other autoimmune conditions, such as juvenile rheumatoid arthritis.
- A diagnosis of SLE may be difficult – because presenting complaints such as fatigue, weight loss, fever, rash, and arthritis are non-specific, and because lupus can affect any organ system.

anticoagulation, given the high risk of recurrent thrombosis if anticoagulation is discontinued. Plasmapheresis in conjunction with immunosuppression is used in catastrophic APS.

REFERENCES

1. Bansal VK, Beto JA. Treatment of lupus nephritis: a meta-analysis of clinical trials. Am J Kidney Dis 1997;29: 193-199.

2. Baqi N, Moazami S, Singh A, et al. Lupus nephritis in children: a longitudinal study of prognostic factors and therapy. J Am Soc Nephrol 1996;7:924-929.

3. Brunner HI, Freedman M, Silverman ED. Close relationship between systemic lupus erythematosus and thrombotic thrombocytopenic purpura in childhood. Arthritis Rheum 1999;42:2346-2355.

4. Cameron JS. Lupus nephritis in childhood and adolescence. Pediatr Nephrol 1994;8:230-249.

5. Chan TM, Li FK, Tang CS, et al. Efficacy of mycophenolate mofetil in patients with diffuse proliferative lupus nephritis. Hong Kong-Guangzhou Nephrology Study Group. N Engl J Med 2000;343:1156-1162.

6. Cooper GS, Dooley MA, Treadwell EL, et al. Hormonal, environmental, and infectious risk factors for developing systemic lupus erythematosus. Arthritis Rheum 1998;41: 1714-1724.

7. Delgado EA, Malleson PN, Pirie GE, et al. The pulmonary manifestation of childhood onset systemic lupus erythematosus. Semin Arthritis Rheum 1990;19:285-293.

8. Emre S, Bilge I, Sirin A, et al. Lupus nephritis in children: prognostic significance of clinicopathological findings. Nephron 2001;87:118-126.

9. Font J, Cervera R, Espinosa G, et al. Systemic lupus erythematosus (SLE) in childhood: analysis of clinical and immunological findings in 34 patients and comparison with SLE characteristics in adults. Ann Rheum Dis 1998;57:456-459.

10. Galaschi F, Ravelli A, Martignoni A, et al. Nephrotic-range proteinuria, the major risk factor for early atherosclerosis in juvenile onset systemic lupus erythematosus. Arthritis Rheum 2000;43:1405-1409.

11. Gonzalez-Crespo MR, Blanco FJ, Ramos A, et al. Magnetic resonance imaging of the brain in systemic lupus erythematosus. Br J Rheumatol 1995;34:1055-1060.

12. Hahn BH. Antibodies to DNA. N Engl J Med 1998;338:1359-1368.

13. Hahn BH. Pathogenesis of systemic lupus erythematosus. In: Ruddy S, Harris ED, Sledge CB (eds), *Kelley's Textbook of Rheumatology*, 6th edn. WB Saunders Company, Philadelphia, 2001.

14. Hochberg MC. Updating the American College of Rheumatology revised criteria for the classification of systemic lupus erythematosus [letter]. Arthritis Rheum 1997;40:1725.

15. Illei GG, Takada K, Parkin D, et al. Renal flares are common in patients with severe proliferative lupus nephritis treated with pulse immunosuppressive therapy: long-term follow up of a cohort of 145 patients participating in randomized controlled studies. Arthritis Rheum 2002;46:995-1002.

16. Iqbal S, Sher MR, Good RA, et al. Diversity in presenting manifestations of systemic lupus erythematosus in children. J Pediatr 1999;135:500-505.

17. Lehman TJ, Onel K. Intermittent intravenous cyclophosphamide arrests progression of the renal chronicity index in childhood systemic lupus erythematosus. J Pediatr 2000;136:243-247.

18. Levine JS, Branch DW, Rauch J. The antiphospholipid syndrome. N Engl J Med 2002;346:752-763.

19. Moder KG, Miller TD, Tazelaar HD. Cardiac involvement in systemic lupus erythematosus. Mayo Clin Proc 1999;74:275-284.

20. Petri M. Musculoskeletal complications of systemic lupus erythematosus in the Hopkins Lupus Cohort: an update. Arthritis Care Res 1995;8:137-145.

21. Petri M. Hopkins Lupus Cohort: 1999 Update. Rheum Dis Clin North Am 2000;26:199-213.

22. Solomon DH, Kavanaugh AJ, Schur PH, et al. Evidence-based guidelines for the use of immunologic tests: antinuclear antibody testing. Arthritis Rheum 2002;47:434-444.

23. Steinberg AD, Steinberg SC. Long-term preservation of renal function in patients with lupus nephritis receiving treatment that includes cyclophosphamide versus those treated with prednisone only. Arthritis Rheum 1991;34:945-950.

24. Steinlin MI, Blaser SI, Gilday DL, et al. Neurologic manifestations of pediatric systemic lupus erythematosus. Pediatr Neurol 1995;13:191-197.

25. Turkel SB, Miller JH, Reiff A. Case series: neuropsychiatric symptoms with pediatric systemic lupus erythematosus. J Am Acad Child Adolesc Psychiatr 2001;40:482-485.

26. Wallace DJ. Gastrointestinal and hepatic manifestations. In: Wallace DJ, Hahn BH (eds), *Dubois' Lupus Erythematosus*, 5th edn. Williams & Wilkins, Baltimore, 1997.

CHAPTER 26

Hemolytic Uremic Syndrome: Stx HUS

HOWARD TRACHTMAN, M.D. AND

BERNARD S. KAPLAN, M.B., B.Ch.

INTRODUCTION

The landmark event in the history of hemolytic uremic syndrome (HUS) was the isolation of a toxin that was cytopathic to Vero cells from the stool of patients with diarrhea-associated (D+) HUS.[1] This toxin was linked to antecedent infection with *Escherichia coli* O157:H7.[8]

Definitions

HUS is a disease phenotype characterized by acute renal injury, thrombocytopenia, and anemia with fragmentation of erythrocytes. The kidney dysfunction may be manifest as hematuria and/or proteinuria and/or azotemia. Most cases of HUS occur after a prodromal diarrheal illness, and therefore are called 'D+HUS'. The term 'Stx HUS' is more precise than D+HUS because it informs on the mechanism of disease. Atypical, hereditary, and secondary forms of HUS are discussed in Chapter 27.

EPIDEMIOLOGY

The incidence of Stx HUS in the United States is 1 to 3 per 100,000 population per year.[2] Stx HUS occurs at any age, but peaks between 6 months and 4 years. It occurs mainly in summer, sporadically, and in clusters. A number of outbreaks have been reported in the popular media because of linkage to unusual foods or beverages (cider, deer jerky) or to distinctive settings (water parks, petting zoos) (Table 26-1). In most cases of Stx HUS a source of the disease is not identified.

PATHOPHYSIOLOGY

Microbiology

The proximate cause of Stx HUS is infection with Shiga toxin-producing organisms.[13]

Escherichia coli (STEC)

The most common of these strains, *E. coli* O157:H7, is characterized by an inability to ferment sorbitol on sorbitol-MacConkey agar plates.[13] More than 90% of all cases of Stx HUS are caused by *E. coli* O157:H7. Several other Shiga toxin-producing bacteria such as Non-O157 strains of *E. coli* (O126, O111), *S. dysenteriae*, and *Aeromonas* species are implicated as causes of HUS.

Table 26-1	Sources of STEC Infection Leading to Hemolytic Uremic Syndrome (HUS)
Foods	Ground meat, sausages, deer venison, jerky, turkey, poultry, vegetables (bean sprouts, radishes, alfalfa sprouts)
Beverages	Water, apple cider, cow's and goat's milk
Activities	Paddling and swimming pool water
Person-to-person spread	
Direct animal contact	Petting zoos
Urinary tract infections caused by STEC	

Tests used to diagnosis STEC infection are summarized in Box 26-1.

Cattle are the major reservoir of STEC, and fecal shedding is the primary route of environmental contamination. Between 1 and 5% of cattle herds are colonized with STEC, though this varies among countries and seasons. Sheep, deer, turkey, dogs, and birds are also carriers of STEC. The absence of disease in animal hosts is attributed to the lack of a toxin-binding receptor on the gastrointestinal epithelial cell membrane; as a result, Stx cannot enter the bloodstream.

Any food, beverage, or water source that comes into contact with fecal material from a STEC-excreting animal, or direct contact with the animal, can be the vehicle for introduction of disease into humans (see Table 26-1). Stx HUS is a rare complication of urinary tract infections, and routine screening of urine cultures for STEC is not warranted.

STEC are readily killed by heating to 140–160°C for 5–10 minutes, exposure to low doses of ionizing radiation, or treatment with standard bactericidal detergents. However, STEC can survive exposure to low temperature, acidic pH, or extremes in osmolality, and are also difficult to eradicate from stored foods.

Box 26-1 Tests Used to Make the Diagnosis of Stx HUS

- Stool culture for *E. coli* O157:H7 (Sorbitol-MacConkey plate)
- Direct assay for free Stx in stool
- Polymerase chain reaction for Stx genes in stool
- Serum levels of antibodies to *E. coli* O157 antigen
- Salivary levels of antibodies to *E. coli* O157 antigen

Shiga Toxin (Stx)

STEC cause HUS by elaborating Stx.[1] Stx is a member of the α1-β5 family of toxins that are composed of five binding non-toxic B-subunits and a single cytotoxic A-subunit moiety. Two varieties of Stx cause human disease: Stx 1 is nearly identical to classic Shiga toxin and Stx2, the amino acid sequence of which is 60% homologous to classic Stx. Clinical isolates of STEC associated with Stx HUS are more likely to produce only Stx 2 or a combination of Stx 1 and Stx 2. Immunization studies in experimental animals indicate that there may be cross-reactivity among anti-Stx antibodies. This finding may explain why recurrent disease is rare after an episode of Stx HUS.

Stx initially crosses the gastrointestinal epithelium following a transcellular pathway, and enters the bloodstream. Stx binds to polymorphonuclear leukocytes by a membrane-associated Stx receptor with an affinity constant that is 1000-fold lower than the binding molecule on the endothelium.[14] This permits the leukocyte to transport Stx from the gastrointestinal tract and to unload Stx in the peripheral circulation. The leukocyte-associated Stx levels are elevated for up to 6 days after the onset of Stx HUS.

Stx binds to a globotriaosylceramide receptor, Gb_3, on the endothelial cell surface. The toxin is taken up by the endothelial cell via pinocytosis in clathrin-coated pits, and then transported in a retrograde fashion to the Golgi apparatus where the active enzymatic portion of Stx is released. The A-subunit cleaves a specific adenine residue from the 28S ribosomal subunit and thereby inhibits protein synthesis. This causes endothelial cell death, with resultant tissue ischemia and organ failure. There is local activation of coagulation and fibrinolytic cascades that may augment tissue damage. The process can occur throughout the vasculature and cause systemic disease. Abnormalities in the von Willebrand factor-cleaving protease are not implicated in the pathogenesis of Stx HUS.[15]

Cytokines

Toxin-induced injury is also mediated by the release of inflammatory cytokines. Stx promotes secretion of tumor necrosis factor-α (TNF-α) by endothelial and renal tubular epithelial cells. Stx also stimulates the production of the chemokines, interleukin (IL)-8 by polymorphonuclear leukocytes and monocyte chemoattractant protein-1 by monocytes. These cytokines help to up-regulate expression of the Gb_3 receptor.[9]

PATHOLOGY

The renal histopathology is characterized by a glomerular thrombotic microangiopathy (TMA) and congested, rather than ischemic, glomeruli. The changes are capillary wall thickening, endothelial cell swelling, and narrowing, or thrombosis of the capillary lumens. There is often thrombosis of preglomerular arterioles that is more common at the hila of glomeruli but is sometimes also seen proximally, including in the interlobular arteries. Cortical infarcts with extensive thrombosis are less commonly seen.

At autopsy, patients with HUS have fibrin/red cell-rich thrombi that are largely confined to kidneys. This is in contrast to patients with thrombotic thrombocytopenic purpura (TTP) in whom platelet-rich thrombi are present, in decreasing severity, in the heart, pancreas, kidney, adrenal gland, and brain.

The ultrastructural changes are swollen endothelial cells with formation of a subendothelial space containing fibrin, cellular deposits, lipids, and platelet fragments.[5,6,11]

CLINICAL PRESENTATION

There are several poorly defined risk factors for progression from enteritis to HUS (Boxes 26-2 and 26-3). Antibiotic treatment of bloody diarrhea may be a risk factor for development of Stx HUS, but this is controversial.[12,17] In-vitro data suggest that exposure of STEC to trimethoprim-sulfamethoxazole or quinolone may provoke plasmid DNA injury and stimulate Stx release.

Disease Presentation

Stx HUS usually presents abruptly with pallor, malaise, and a decrease in urine output within 48 hours of the diagnosis. The most serious problem is the onset of acute renal failure (ARF) that manifests with hypertension, and signs and symptoms of extracellular fluid volume overload. Sudden onset of pallor begins a few days after cessation or improvement of gastrointestinal symptoms. This is often followed by increasing edema and, occasionally, by mild jaundice, petechiae, or seizures. Hypertension, with or without congestive heart

---

Box 26-2   Timeline of the Disease[3,7,16]

- The interval between the ingestion of an inoculum of STEC and onset of gastrointestinal symptoms is usually 24–72 hours
- Enteritis begins as watery diarrhea and progresses to frankly bloody stools in >90% of cases. After a 2- to 6-day latency period, 5–15% of patients with STEC enteritis develop Stx HUS

Box 26-3   Risk Factors for Progression from STEC Infection to Stx HUS

- Young age – under 1 year
- Fever during the prodromal enteritis
- Use of antimotility drugs to treat diarrhea
- Leukocytosis
- Treatment of enteritis with antibiotics or antimotility agents

---

failure and pulmonary venous congestion, may result in part from excessive fluid administration before recognition of oliguria.

Gastrointestinal

Gastrointestinal symptoms are abdominal pain, vomiting, and diarrhea, usually with bloody and/or mucoid stools. Stx HUS can occur in the absence of diarrhea and may be associated with a urinary tract infection. Colonic symptoms mimic ulcerative colitis, appendicitis, intussusception, rectal prolapse, gastroenteritis, or acute bacterial enterocolitis. Acute colitis is usually transient, but may be complicated by toxic megacolon or bowel wall necrosis. Hepatomegaly is common. Colonic gangrene is difficult to diagnose and has a poor prognosis. An abdominal plain film radiograph shows gas accumulation in the colon and bowel wall thickening. Barium enema or sigmoidoscopy is rarely indicated. Hypoalbuminemia is caused mainly by a protein-losing enteropathy. Pancreatic dysfunction causes marked elevation of serum amylase and lipase levels, and islet cell necrosis results in hyperglycemia with low insulin levels.

Renal

Oligoanuria occurs in half the cases, and some have non-oliguric renal failure. Microscopic hematuria is more frequent than macroscopic hematuria. Blood pressure is usually normal at the onset, but often increases after a blood transfusion. Fluid overload causes edema, hypertension, and heart failure. Urinalysis shows red blood cells and various casts. Biochemical changes of renal dysfunction are increased serum levels of creatinine, potassium, phosphorus, hydrogen ion, uric acid, and blood urea nitrogen (BUN). The serum potassium concentration may be low initially as a result of gastroenteritis. Hyperkalemia may develop with reduced glomerular filtration rate, hemolysis, and transcellular shifts caused by acidosis. Serum concentrations of sodium, calcium, bicarbonate, and albumin are low, especially in severely ill patients. Serum levels of cholesterol, triglycerides, and phospholipids may be elevated. A renal biopsy is rarely indicated in Stx HUS.

Hematologic

Hemolytic anemia varies from slight decreases in hemoglobin concentration to levels of 3 g/dl. There is no correlation between the severity of hemolysis and of renal failure. Repeated episodes of hemolysis may occur during the first few weeks. The erythrocytes are fragmented as a result of a microangiopathic injury and/or peroxidative damage. Serum levels of lactic dehydrogenase and unconjugated bilirubin are increased, along with the reticulocyte count. Haptoglobin levels are decreased and the Coombs' tests are usually negative. A leukocytosis occurs during the first week. Thrombocytopenia lasts for up to 2 weeks, and is not related to the course of the renal disease.

Neurologic

Neurologic symptoms are irritability, somnolence, behavioral changes, restlessness, seizures, ataxia, dizziness, tremors, and twitching. Stx-induced injury, hyponatremia, hypocalcemia, markedly increased BUN and accelerated hypertension may cause central nervous system injury. Magnetic resonance imaging is sensitive for early detection of structural lesions. Brain edema and microthrombi are found in some cases at autopsy.

Cardiopulmonary

Cardiovascular abnormalities usually result from volume overload, but some patients have myocarditis, or cardiogenic shock caused by microthrombi, cardiomyopathy, or aneurysms. A few patients have features of adult respiratory distress syndrome.

Outcome

Almost 20% of patients with Stx HUS have at least one serious complication. The mortality rate during an acute episode is 3-5%. Risk factors for more severe Stx HUS and an adverse outcome are female gender, persistent fever, leukocytosis, prolonged gastrointestinal disease, severe colitis with rectal prolapse, and neurological complications.[4,10] Complete recovery occurs in 64% of patients, chronic renal insufficiency with hypertension in 4%, late sequelae in 12%, and end-stage renal disease in 9%. Recurrent episodes of Stx HUS are uncommon. It is unusual for Stx HUS to recur after renal transplantation (Table 26-2).

Table 26-2 Extra-Renal Complications of HUS

Central nervous system	Coma, thrombotic or hemorrhagic stroke, cortical blindness, seizures
Pancreas	Pancreatic insufficiency, diabetes mellitus
Intestine	Perforation, necrosis, intussusception, stricture
Gallbladder	Hydrops

TREATMENT[3,7,16]

Management of ARF

The biochemical abnormalities require meticulous medical management, including restricted intake of fluids, salt, and potassium, aggressive control of even mildly elevated blood pressure levels, and administration of loop diuretics to maintain urine output. ARF develops in 40-50% of children with Stx HUS. This is of sufficient severity to warrant temporary renal replacement therapy. The indications for initiating dialysis are based on concurrent medical complications or anuria rather than on BUN level and serum creatinine concentration.

Peritoneal dialysis is the preferred modality. However, if there is bowel gangrene or severe metabolic disturbances, hemodialysis or hemofiltration are indicated.

General Medical Management

Sufficient calories and protein are provided to reverse the high catabolic state. If severe vomiting interferes with feeding, then intravenous administration of ondansetron, 0.15 mg/kg/dose every 4 hours can be given. If gastrointestinal disease interferes with enteral feeding, intravenous hyperalimentation is required. Antimotility agents should not be prescribed because they delay clearance of the Stx from the gastrointestinal tract. Enteric precautions should be implemented in children with Stx HUS to prevent person-to-person transmission of the disease. Surgery may be required to repair bowel wall gangrene or perforation or other gastrointestinal complications. Surveillance should be maintained for pancreatitis and insulin-requiring diabetes mellitus. Transfusions of packed red blood cells should be administered only if the hemoglobin is below 6-7 g/dl, or if there is evidence of compromised cardiovascular status. Platelets should be infused only if there is active hemorrhage or an invasive procedure is required. The dosage of antibiotics, anticonvulsant agents, or other medications should be adjusted to the level of kidney function.

Box 26-4 Ineffective Treatments of Stx HUS

- Anticoagulants – heparin
- Fibrinolytics – streptokinase
- Passive immunization to neutralize Stx – intravenous IgG
- Infusion of fresh-frozen plasma
- Anti-inflammatory agents – corticosteroids
- Anti-platelet drugs – aspirin and dipyridamole
- High-dose furosemide infusions to maintain urine flow
- Plasma exchange or plasmapheresis
- Antioxidants
- Oral toxin-binding agents – SYNSORB Pk®

Specific Medical Therapy

There is no specific therapy for Stx HUS, and treatment consists of careful supportive care until the disease resolves. None of the treatments listed in Box 26-4 is effective in the treatment of Stx HUS. Despite the absence of a specific treatment that is proven to be effective, physicians continue to prescribe unproven treatments for children with this disease. Among the first 82 children enrolled in the multicenter trial of SYNSORB Pk®, 20 were given unproven treatments: two received intravenous IgG, two were treated with corticosteroids, and 13 with anti-platelet drugs, while plasmapheresis was used in three cases.

Table 26-3 Strategies for Preventing Stx HUS

Primary care measures	• Hand washing when preparing food • Cleaning of all cooking surfaces • Cooking meat at high enough temperatures, such as 140–160°C for a sufficient time (e.g., 10–15 minutes) to cook beef thoroughly • Isolation of patients with bloody diarrhea or STEC infection • Timely reporting of cases of STEC enteritis and Stx HUS
Public health measures	• Implementation of bacterial detection techniques in all foods • Switch from grain to hay feed before animal slaughter • Inoculation of animals with probiotic organisms • Irradiation of foods • Immunization against Shiga toxin antigens

PREVENTIVE STRATEGIES

Because of the accelerated course of the illness in most children with Stx HUS, it may be difficult to implement effective treatment early enough to ameliorate the disease. Therefore, it is necessary to design strategies to prevent this disease (Table 26-3).

MAJOR POINTS

- Stx HUS is the most common cause of acute renal failure in previously healthy children.
- It is transmitted via any food or beverage that is contaminated by Shiga toxin-producing strains of *E. coli.*
- In the absence of a proven specific therapy, treatment is intensive supportive care.
- Stx HUS can be prevented by careful food preparation, hand washing, cleaning of food preparation surfaces, and thoroughly cooking meat at sufficient temperatures to kill the Stx-producing *E. coli.*
- STEC infection and Stx HUS are *reportable* diseases in all 50 states in the United States.
- Affected cases must be reported to the health department.
- Contacts who develop diarrhea must be evaluated.
- STEC are virulent because the inoculum of bacteria that can cause disease is very low, often less than microorganisms.
- The current consensus is that antibiotics should be prescribed with caution for children with STEC hemorrhagic colitis, unless there is invasive bacterial disease.
- Stx HUS is a systemic disease with widespread but variable extra-renal organ involvement.
- There are no indications for a coagulation work-up in Stx HUS.
- Repeated episodes of hemolysis may occur during the first few weeks.
- The severity of anemia does not correlate with severity of renal disease.
- A leukocytosis occurs during the first week.
- Thrombocytopenia lasts for up to 2 weeks.
- Thrombocytopenia does not correlate with the course of the renal disease.
- A renal biopsy is rarely indicated in Stx HUS.
- In the absence of serious extra-renal events, anuria for 24 hours, or oliguria (<0.5 ml/kg/h) for 48–72 hours, dialysis can be deferred despite markedly elevated BUN and serum creatinine concentrations.[3]
- The impulse to use plasmapheresis should be resisted; it is not effective in Stx HUS.
- Plasmapheresis is labor-intensive and costly.

DIFFERENTIAL DIAGNOSIS

Stx HUS must be differentiated from idiopathic or atypical types of HUS, *S. pneumoniae*-associated HUS, hereditary HUS, and thrombotic thrombocytopenic purpura (see Chapter 27).

REFERENCES

1. Andreoli SP, Trachtman H, Acheson DWK, et al. Hemolytic uremic syndrome: epidemiology, pathophysiology, and therapy. Pediatr Nephrol 2002;17:293-298.

2. Bender JB, Hedberg CW, Besser JM, et al. Surveillance for *Escherichia coli* O157:H7 infections in Minnesota by molecular subtyping. N Engl J Med 1997;337:388-394.

3. Bhimma R, Coovadia HM, Adhikari M, et al. Re-evaluating criteria for peritoneal dialysis in 'classical' (D+) hemolytic uremic syndrome. Clin Nephrol 2001;55:133-142.

4. Cimolai N, Morrison BJ, Carter JE. Risk factors for the central nervous system manifestations of gastroenteritis-associated hemolytic-uremic syndrome. Pediatrics 1992;90:616-621.

5. Hosler GA, Cusumano AM, Hutchins GM. Thrombotic thrombocytopenic purpura and hemolytic uremic syndrome are distinct pathologic entities. A review of 56 autopsy cases. Arch Pathol Lab Med 2003;127:834-839.

6. Inward CD, Howie AJ, Fitzpatrick MM, et al. Renal histopathology in fatal cases of diarrhoea-associated haemolytic uraemic syndrome. British Association for Paediatric Nephrology. Pediatr Nephrol 1997;11:556-559.

7. Kaplan BA, Meyers KE, Schulman SL. The pathogenesis and treatment of hemolytic uremic syndrome. J Am Soc Nephrol 1998;9:1126-1133.

8. Karmali MA, Petric M, Lim C, et al. The association between idiopathic hemolytic uremic syndrome and infection by Verotoxin-producing *Escherichia coli*. J Infect Dis 1985;151:775-782.

9. Litalien C, Proulx F, Mariscalco MM, et al. Circulating inflammatory cytokines in hemolytic uremic syndrome. Pediatr Nephrol 1999;13:840-845.

10. Lopez EL, Devoto S, Fayad A, et al. Association between the severity of gastrointestinal prodrome and long-term prognosis in classic hemolytic-uremic syndrome. J Pediatr 1992;120:210-215.

11. Richardson SE, Karmali MA, Becker LE, et al. The histopathology of the hemolytic uremic syndrome associated with verocytotoxin-producing *Escherichia coli* infections. Hum Pathol 1988;19:1102-1108.

12. Safdar N, Said A, Gangnon RE, et al. Risk of hemolytic uremic syndrome after antibiotic therapy treatment of *Escherichia coli* O157:H7 enteritis: a meta-analysis. JAMA 2002;288:996-1001.

13. Tarr PI, Neill MA. *Escherichia coli* O157:H7. Gastrol Clin North Am 2001;30:735-751.

14. Te Loo D, Van Hinsburgh V, Van den Huvel L, et al. Detection of verocytotoxin bound to circulating polymorphonuclear leukocytes of patients with hemolytic uremic syndrome. J Am Soc Nephrol 2001;12:800-806.

15. Tsai HM, Chandler WL, Sarode R, et al. Von Willebrand factor and Von Willebrand factor-cleaving metalloprotease in *Escherichia coli* O157:H7-associated hemolytic uremic syndrome. Pediatr Res 2000;49:653-659.

16. Trachtman H, Christen C. Hemolytic uremic syndrome: current understanding of the pathogenesis and therapeutic trials and interventions. Curr Opin Pediatr 1999;11:162-168.

17. Wong CS, Jelacic S, Habeeb RL, et al. The risk of hemolytic-uremic syndrome after antibiotic treatment of *Escherichia coli* O157:H7 infections. N Engl J Med 2000;342:1930-1936.

SUGGESTED READING

Kaper JB, O'Brien A (eds), Escherichia coli *O157:H7 and other Shiga-Toxin-Producing* E. coli *strains*. American Society of Microbiology Press, Washington, DC 364-373, 1998.

Kaplan BS, Trompeter RS, Moake J. *Hemolytic Uremic Syndrome and Thrombotic Thrombocytopenic Purpura*. Marcel Dekker, Inc., New York, 1992.

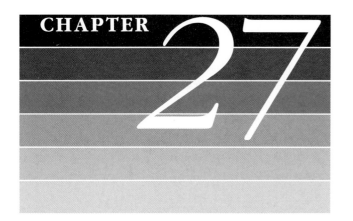

CHAPTER 27

Classification of the Hemolytic Uremic Syndromes and Thrombotic Thrombocytopenic Purpura

BERNARD S. KAPLAN, M.B., B.Ch.

Introduction
Hemolytic Uremic Syndrome (HUS)
    Infectious Causes of HUS
        Shiga Toxin-Associated HUS (Stx HUS)
        Streptococcus pneumoniae-Associated HUS
        Capnocytophaga canimorsus
        Human Immunodeficiency Virus (HIV)-Associated HUS
    Idiopathic or Atypical HUS
    Hereditary HUS
    Associations (Secondary HUS)
    Medication- and Treatment-Associated HUS
Thrombotic Thrombocytopenic Purpura (TTP)

INTRODUCTION

Stx HUS is discussed in detail in Chapter 26. The purposes of the present chapter are to describe the classification of HUS and TTP, and to describe some of the conditions that are similar to Stx HUS. The hemolytic uremic syndromes (HUS) are a group of conditions with similar clinical, biochemical and histopathologic abnormalities with many different causes and pathogenetic mechanisms. Thrombotic thrombocytopenic purpura (TTP) forms another group of conditions with clinical, biochemical and histopathologic abnormalities that are similar to those that are found in HUS. An etiologic classification of HUS is shown in Box 27-1.

HEMOLYTIC UREMIC SYNDROME (HUS)

Infectious Causes of HUS

HUS usually follows an infection with shiga toxin-producing bacteria, but can also be caused by neuraminidase-producing bacteria and viruses (Box 27-2). Possible but unproven infectious causes include *Salmonella typhi*, *Clostridium difficile*, β-hemolytic *Streptococcus*, and viruses other than HIV.

Shiga Toxin-Associated HUS (Stx HUS)

The term 'Stx HUS' is more precise than 'D+,' 'typical-,' or 'post-diarrheal HUS'.[6] Stx HUS follows infection with shiga toxin-producing bacteria that include *Escherichia coli* (STEC) and *Shigella dysenteriae* type 1.[1]

Stx HUS is discussed in detail in Chapter 26, but two points need to be stressed: first, HUS is not TTP (Box 27-3); and second, the clinician must have a high index of suspicion for the onset of HUS (Box 27-4).

Streptococcus pneumoniae-Associated HUS

HUS may complicate *S. pneumoniae* infections.[3] Although the clinical outcome was poor in early reports, the outcomes have improved in recent years.[10] In addition, there are patients with milder involvement. The HUS occurs in patients with otitis media, pneumonia with or without empyema, and meningitis. Young children are mainly affected, renal disease is often severe, and survivors may have chronic renal insufficiency as well as the complications of the pneumococcal infection such as neurological deficits and chronic lung disease. The death rate, which was once 50%, has decreased in some series but not in others.[10] Improved outcome is probably because fresh-frozen plasma is no longer used and washed red cells are infused, thereby reducing the risks of transfusing anti-Thomsen–Friedenreich (TF) antibodies exposed on the surfaces of erythrocytes and platelets by neuraminidase produced by the organism. In a series of 11 patients with *S. pneumoniae*-associated HUS,[9] three died from meningitis and one from

---

Box 27-1   Etiologic Classification of Hemolytic Uremic Syndrome (HUS)

- Infection causes of HUS
- Idiopathic (atypical) HUS
- Hereditary HUS (familial HUS)
- Associations (secondary HUS)
- Medication- or treatment-associated HUS

Box 27-3   HUS is not TTP

Any patient who develops acute onset of hemolytic anemia with fragmented erythrocytes, thrombocytopenia, and renal injury, during or after bloody diarrhea, whether a child or an adult, whether or not there is a fever, and with and without CNS involvement – has HUS and *not* TTP.

---

neurological sequelae after a partial recovery of renal function. The mean duration of dialysis was 32 days in patients with acute renal failure (ARF) who survived the acute infectious period. Cortical necrosis was documented in five of six kidney specimens. Among the seven surviving patients, five developed end-stage renal failure after 4 to 17 years.[10]

Capnocytophaga canimorsus

This is an uncommon cause of HUS that follows dog bites.[9] The offending organism is a fastidious Gram-negative rod that produces neuraminidase, so that HUS possibly is caused by exposure of the TF antigen.

Human Immunodeficiency Virus (HIV)-Associated HUS

Few cases of HIV-associated HUS have been reported in children,[16] in contrast to the large numbers of reports in adult patients. In a representative large series of 92 adults aged between 21 to 51 years and with HIV infection, 32 (35%) developed HUS.[11] Males outnumbered females in a ratio of 31 to 1. The interval between HIV diagnosis and onset of HUS ranged from 9 months to 5 years. The renal lesions were usually mixed glomerular/arteriolar lesions. Treatment remains unsatisfactory in that seven patients died within 2 months, although outcomes may be improving with the use of dialysis and fresh-frozen plasma and/or plasmapheresis.

Idiopathic or Atypical HUS

Idiopathic (atypical, non-diarrhea-associated D-HUS is a heterogeneous subgroup of HUS that differs from diarrhea-associated HUS on epidemiologic, clinical, laboratory, histological, and prognostic grounds.[5]

Increasingly sophisticated studies are showing that many patients with atypical HUS have a genetic form of the syndrome.[13] Atypical cases of HUS share a number of characteristics with inherited HUS. These include the possibilities of recurrent episodes before and/or after transplantation, and deficiencies of complement. In addition, the renal histopathologic findings show predominantly arteriolar involvement, and the prognosis is often poor with severe hypertension and progression to end-stage renal failure.

Hereditary HUS

The diagnosis of hereditary HUS cannot be made in the absence of a positive family history. Hereditary HUS must be suspected in patients with idiopathic or atypical HUS, especially if there is hypocomplementemia and/or a Factor H deficiency.[13] HUS can be inherited as either an autosomal recessive or as an autosomal dominant trait. In the recessive form there are no recognized precipitating events, but episodes may follow non-specific viral infections. There are no sex or race preferences. Affected individuals are usually infants and children. The outcome may vary greatly and include complete resolution, several episodes of HUS either before renal transplantation

---

Box 27-2   Infectious Causes of HUS

Shiga toxin-producing bacteria
- *E. coli* 0157:H7 and other serotypes
- *Shigella dysenteriae* type 1
- *Aeromonas*
- *Citrobacter freundii*

Neuraminidase-producing bacteria
- *Streptococcus pneumoniae*
- *Capnocytophaga canimorsus*

Viruses
- Human immunodeficiency virus

Box 27-4   Stx HUS Must be Suspected in Any Patient:

- with diarrhea, and whose urine volume does not increase when rehydrated
- with pallor or edema during or after bloody diarrhea
- with seizures during or after bloody diarrhea
- with anemia and fragmented erythrocytes, thrombocytopenia, and renal injury

and/or after transplantation.[7,8] Some patients have hypocomplementemia with low Factor H concentrations, and the pathogenesis may be linked to disorders of complement. Two groups of mutations have been detected in hereditary and atypical cases: (i) mutations in the C-terminal region involved in binding of factor H to solid-phase C3b and to negatively charged cellular structures; and (ii) mutations that introduce premature stop codons that interrupt translation of Factor H.[12]

There is no satisfactory treatment. Moreover, treatment is extremely difficult because of severe hypertension and a course that is often indolent. Plasmapheresis is recommended, although its value has not been proven and the frequency and duration of treatment are not known. Characteristically, families with inherited HUS tend to show extreme anxiety (Box 27-5).

Post-transplant recurrences are frequent. Using a living-related kidney and calcineurin antagonists increases the chances of a recurrence, whereas pre-transplant nephrectomies may reduce this possibility.

Adults are affected more often when HUS is inherited in an autosomal dominant mode. There is no sex or race preference. A number of patients have manifested the condition in association with pregnancy, but this may differ even within a family. Complete recovery is uncommon.[17] The pathogenesis of both the autosomal recessive and dominant forms of HUS may be related, in some families, to Factor H deficiency with linkage to the Factor H locus on chromosome 1q (Box 27-6).

There is no specific treatment, but fresh-frozen plasma infusions and plasmapheresis are indicated for autosomal dominantly inherited cases. The prognosis for renal survival is dismal, and for patient survival is poor. It is advisable to wait for 6 to 12 months between the occurrence of HUS and a renal transplant. The patient must be free from all evidence of active disease. There appears to be an increased risk of post-transplant recurrences with donors from relatives, use of cyclosporine A, and pregnancy.[4] There are no established guidelines, and genetic counseling is even more difficult if the patient is the first affected individual in the family.

Associations (Secondary HUS)

HUS is associated with – or complicates the course of – many unrelated conditions. A partial list includes pregnancy, solid organ transplant, bone marrow transplant, malignancy, leukemia, systemic lupus erythematosus, systemic sclerosis, Sjögren's syndrome, membranoproliferative glomerulonephritis, pancreatitis, and Denys–Drash syndrome. That HUS has occurred in each of these circumstances is beyond doubt. However, the relationship between HUS and some of these conditions is extremely complicated. For example, HUS during or after pregnancy has not been proven to be caused by pregnancy *per se*, but has occurred in women who have had a mutation in the Factor H locus or in others with an *E. coli* O157:H7 infection. Patients with a malignancy complicated by HUS have been treated with antineoplastic drugs that are themselves implicated as causes of HUS. Chronic myeloid leukemia and HUS are reported in patients treated with interferon-α. HUS following bone marrow transplantation may be related in part to the dose of total body irradiation. HUS following kidney transplantation may be the result of a recurrence of an inherited type of HUS, or the use of a calcineurin anti-rejection drug.

Medication- and Treatment-Associated HUS

Many agents and treatments are associated with HUS. These include cyclosporine A, FK-506, OKT3, mitomycin-C, oral contraceptives, quinine, irradiation, interferon-α, and crack cocaine.

THROMBOTIC THROMBOCYTOPENIC PURPURA (TTP)

Stx HUS differs fundamentally from TTP in regard to etiology, pathogenesis, and outcome.[14] The term 'HUS/TTP' confuses the approach to the diagnosis, treatment (Box 27-7), and outcome of these different conditions.

Box 27-7   Treatment of TTP

Acute TTP with IgG inhibitors against metalloproteinase	Plasmapheresis
TTP caused by ticlopidine or clopidogrel	Plasmapheresis
TTP caused by ADAMTS13 deficiency	Fresh-frozen plasma infusions

There are abnormalities in the function of von Willebrand factor (VWf) proteases in TTP, but not in HUS. Patients with acute TTP have a severe deficiency of VWf-cleaving protease caused by inhibitory activity against the protease. This deficiency is not detected in patients with TTP who are in remission. The inhibitors are IgG antibodies that can be removed by plasmapheresis.

Patients with familial forms of TTP have a constitutional defect in VWf-cleaving protease activity, and do not have an inhibitor of the enzyme. These findings are in contrast to those in HUS in which some patients with inherited HUS had normal or slightly decreased levels of activity of VWf-cleaving protease during the acute episode. ADAMTS13 is a member of the ADAMTS family of zinc metalloproteinase genes. Proteolysis of VWf and/or other ADAMTS13 substrates is required for normal vascular homeostasis. The molecular mechanism responsible for this type of TTP is a number of mutations in the ADAMTS13 gene on chromosome 9q34.[8]

Therefore, non-familial TTP appears to result from an inhibitor of VWf-cleaving protease, whereas the familial form is caused by a constitutional deficiency of the protease with a mutation of a metalloproteinase gene.

TTP may be caused by the antiplatelet agents ticlopidine and clopidogrel.[2,15] Autoantibodies to the VWf metalloproteinase were demonstrated in patients who developed ticlopidine-associated TTP; this led to the same type of VWf abnormalities observed in patients with idiopathic acute TTP. The findings suggest that failure to process large and unusually large VWf multimers *in vivo* caused binding of VWf to platelets, systemic platelet thrombosis, and TTP.

MAJOR POINTS

- TTP and HUS although similar, are different disorders with different causes, treatments and prognoses.[6,14]
- Stx HUS is a post-infectious, multi-system syndrome, defined by acute onset of hemolytic anemia with fragmented erythrocytes, thrombocytopenia, and renal injury.
- Although many patients are often very ill, the prognosis is usually good.
- *S. pneumoniae*-associated HUS and the inherited types of HUS are sometimes included in the subgroup of atypical HUS, but should be considered separately.
- Fresh-frozen plasma is indicated for the treatment of TTP caused by an inherited deficiency of ADAMTS13.

REFERENCES

1. Azim T, Rashid A, Qadri F, et al. Antibodies to Shiga toxin in the serum of children with Shigella-associated haemolytic uraemic syndrome. J Med Microbiol 1999; 48:11-16.

2. Bennett CL, Connors JM, Carwile JM, et al. Thrombotic thrombocytopenic purpura associated with clopidogrel. N Engl J Med 2000;342:1773-1777.

3. Brandt J, Wong C, Mihm S, et al. Invasive pneumococcal disease and hemolytic uremic syndrome. Pediatrics 2002; 110:371-376.

4. Ducloux D, Rebibou JM, Semhoun-Ducloux S, et al. Recurrence of hemolytic-uremic syndrome in renal transplant recipients: a meta-analysis. Transplantation 1998;65: 1405-1407.

5. Fitzpatrick MM, Walters MD, Trompeter RS, et al. Atypical (non-diarrhea-associated) hemolytic-uremic syndrome in childhood. J Pediatr 1993;122:532-537.

6. Kaplan BS, Meyers KW, Schulman SL. The pathogenesis and treatment of hemolytic uremic syndrome. J Am Soc Nephrol 1998;9:1126-1133.

7. Kaplan BS, Papadimitriou M, Brezin JH, et al. Renal transplantation in adults with autosomal recessive inheritance of hemolytic uremic syndrome. Am J Kidney Dis 1997;30: 760-765.

8. Levy GG, Nichols WC, Lian EC, et al. Mutations in a member of the ADAMTS gene family cause thrombotic thrombocytopenic purpura. Nature 2001;413:488-494.

9. Mulder AH, Gerlag PG, Verhoef LH, et al. Hemolytic uremic syndrome after *Capnocytophaga canimorsus* (DF-2) septicemia. Clin Nephrol 2001;55:167-170.

10. Nathanson S, Deschenes G. Prognosis of *Streptococcus pneumoniae*-induced hemolytic uremic syndrome. Pediatr Nephrol 2001;16:362-365.

11. Peraldi MN, Maslo C, Akposso K, et al. Acute renal failure in the course of HIV infection: a single-institution retrospective study of ninety-two patients and sixty renal biopsies. Nephrol Dial Transplant 1999;14:1578.

12. Richards A, Buddles MR, Donne RL, et al. Factor H mutations in hemolytic uremic syndrome cluster in exons 18-20, a domain important for host cell recognition. Am J Hum Genet 2001;68:485-490.

13. Rougier N, Kazatchkine MD, Rougier JP, et al. Human complement factor H deficiency associated with hemolytic uremic syndrome. J Am Soc Nephrol 1998;9: 2318-2326.

14. Tsai HM. Advances in the pathogenesis, diagnosis, and treatment of thrombotic thrombocytopenic purpura. J Am Soc Nephrol 2003;14:1072–1081.

15. Tsai HM, Rice L, Sarode R, Chow TW, Moake JL. Antibody inhibitors to von Willebrand factor metalloproteinase and increased binding of von Willebrand factor to platelets in ticlopidine-associated thrombotic thrombocytopenic purpura. Ann Intern Med 2000;132:794–799.

16. Turner ME, Kher K, Rakusan T, et al. A typical hemolytic uremic syndrome in human immunodeficiency virus-1-infected children. Pediatr Nephrol 1997;11:161–163.

17. Kaplan BS, Leonard M. Autosomal dominant hemolytic uremic syndrome: variable phenotypes and transplantation. Pediatr Nephrol 2000;14:464–468.

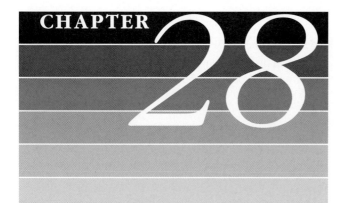

CHAPTER 28

Polycystic Kidney Diseases

KATHERINE MacRAE DELL, M.D.

INTRODUCTION

The polycystic kidney diseases are a heterogeneous group of inherited disorders characterized by cystic changes in the kidneys (Table 28-1).[6] The two major inherited types are autosomal recessive polycystic kidney disease (ARPKD) and autosomal dominant polycystic kidney disease (ADPKD). Other forms include glomerulocystic kidney disease (GCKD) and cystic dysplasia, either primary or associated with congenital syndromes.

AUTOSOMAL RECESSIVE POLYCYSTIC KIDNEY DISEASE (ARPKD)

ARPKD is a genetic disorder characterized by polycystic kidneys and the liver lesion of congenital hepatic fibrosis. It has also been called 'infantile' polycystic kidney disease or Potter's type I polycystic kidney disease,[5] but these terms are no longer used. The majority of children with ARPKD present as newborns or infants, although a subset of children is diagnosed during childhood.

Genetics and Pathogenesis

ARPKD occurs with an estimated incidence of between 1 in 10,000 and 1 in 40,000 live births.[5,20] The true incidence may be greater however, because severely affected neonates may die before receiving a definitive diagnosis. ARPKD is inherited in an autosomal recessive fashion. Parents of children with ARPKD are 'obligate' heterozygote (carriers) and are unaffected. Families with one affected child have a 25% chance of having another affected child, and unaffected siblings of ARPKD patients have a 67% chance of being carriers. ARPKD affects males and females equally, and affects all ethnic and racial groups (Box 28-1).[5]

Research in several animal models has demonstrated abnormalities in expression of the epidermal growth factor receptor (EGFR) and one or more of its ligands, which may contribute to cyst formation and expansion.[6] In addition, the proteins encoded by two murine ARPKD genes, Oak Ridge polycystic kidney disease (orpk; TgN737) and congenital polycystic kidney disease (cpk), were localized to the primary cilia present on the surface of renal tubule cells. Polycystin 1 and 2, the abnormal proteins in ADPKD, are also localized to the primary cilia. It has been hypothesized that cyst formation in ARPKD may be related to altered cilia structure and/or function, including potential chemosensor or mechanosensor functions.[13] Whether this emerging 'cilia hypothesis' proves to be the key to the understanding of ARPKD (or ADPKD) pathogenesis remains to be determined.

Table 28-1 Differential Diagnosis of Cystic Kidneys in Children

Polycystic kidneys	• Autosomal recessive polycystic kidney disease • Autosomal dominant polycystic kidney disease • Glomerulocystic kidney disease

Diffuse cystic dysplasia	• Non-syndromic
	  • Inherited
	  • Sporadic
	• Syndromic

Acquired cystic kidney disease[*]	
Simple cyst[*]	

[*]Rare in children.

Box 28-2 Clinical Features of ARPKD

- Flank masses
- Hypertension
- Pyuria
- Hyponatremia
- Renal insufficiency
- Respiratory insufficiency
- Hepatosplenomegaly[*]
- Esophageal varices[*]
- Hypersplenism[*]

[*]Less common in neonates/infants

Pathology

There are lesions in the kidney and liver only. The kidneys are uniformly enlarged, but usually do not demonstrate discrete macroscopic cysts. Histologically, the cystic kidney disease is confined to the collecting tubules. Fusiform cystic dilatations ('microcysts' <2 mm) are oriented in a radial fashion from the cortex to the medulla.[11] There is no evidence of renal dysplasia.[11,14] 'Macrocysts' (usually >2 cm), are more characteristic of ADPKD, but may become evident in ARPKD as the disease progresses. The hepatic pathology consists of a characteristic 'ductal plate' lesion consisting of periportal fibrosis and bile duct proliferation. A severe form of the biliary lesion, in which the bile ducts are markedly dilated, is called 'Caroli's disease.'[20]

Clinical Features

Patients typically present in the newborn period or infancy with large, palpable flank masses.[3,14,20] Many patients are now diagnosed *in utero* by prenatal -

Box 28-1 Genetics of Autosomal Recessive Polycystic Kidney Disease (ARPKD)[16,19]

- Mutation on chromosome 6p21
- Mutated gene is PKHD1 (polycystic kidney and hepatic disease)
- Protein product is fibrocystin/polyductin
- Fibrocystin/polyductin may function as a receptor
- There is no predominant mutation in affected kindreds
- Mechanisms whereby the gene defect results in kidney and liver disease is undefined

ultrasonography. There may be a history of oligohydramnios. Renal manifestations include varying degrees of renal impairment and oliguria, hypertension and electrolyte disturbances, especially hyponatremia (Box 28-2).[3,14,20]

Newborns may have significant oliguria even in the presence of apparently normal or mildly impaired renal function. The diminished urine output may improve with improvements in respiratory status. Although most neonates with ARPKD have evidence of renal insufficiency, few require dialysis in the newborn period. Hypertension is usually present, and may be severe, requiring treatment with several antihypertensive medications at a very early age to attain adequate control. Impaired urinary concentrating ability is very common. Pyuria may represent a urinary tract infection, or the urine may be sterile.

Respiratory distress is a common finding in newborns with ARPKD, and is a major cause of mortality in the newborn period. This may be due to several factors. Pulmonary hypoplasia occurs as the result of oligohydramnios. There may be additional features of the oligohydramnios sequence, including the Potter facies, limb contractures and hip dislocation. Furthermore, the massively enlarged kidneys may cause significant impairment in diaphragmatic excursion resulting in respiratory embarrassment. Infants with ARPKD may develop pneumothoraces, respiratory distress syndrome, and pneumonia.

Clinical evidence of hepatic disease (e.g., hepatomegaly) may not be present in about 50% of newborns with ARPKD, despite the fact that the ductal plate lesion is invariably present on microscopic examination. With progressive disease, the hepatic abnormalities become more clinically evident. A small subset of patients with ARPKD will present as older infants and children with primarily evidence of hepatic involvement including hepatosplenomegaly and esophageal varices and variceal bleeding. In fact, polycystic kidneys may be an incidental finding during imaging studies for hepatomegaly.

Imaging Studies

Ultrasound examination shows very enlarged and echogenic kidneys, with loss of normal corticomedullary differentiation (Figure 28-1). Discrete cysts are generally not seen; however, with progressive disease, 'macrocysts' may be evident. The hepatic ultrasound may be normal in the newborn and young child. Radiographic abnormalities of the liver, when present, include hepatomegaly, splenomegaly, increased echogenicity, and poor visualization of peripheral portal veins. A small subset of patients will have radiographic evidence of dilated hepatic bile ducts (Caroli's disease). Macroscopic liver cysts – a more common finding in ADPKD – occur rarely in ARPKD. There may be choledochal cysts.

Diagnosis

The diagnosis of ARPKD is generally made on the basis of clinical findings, especially bilateral flank masses, respiratory distress and hypertension in an infant (Box 28-3).

Although liver and kidney biopsies are diagnostic, these procedures are not used routinely in establishing the diagnosis of ARPKD, except in rare instances. Several inherited and acquired conditions (Box 28-4) may present in the neonate with features similar to those of ARPKD, including flank masses and enlarged, diffusely echogenic kidneys on ultrasound.[11]

Increasing numbers of ARPKD patients are detected *in utero*. Findings on prenatal ultrasound suggestive of ARPKD include kidney enlargement, oligohydramnios,

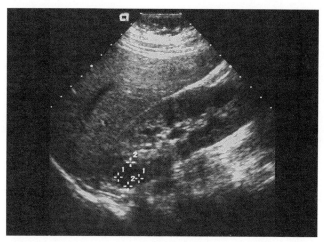

Figure 28-2 Autosomal dominant polycystic kidney disease. Renal ultrasound (left kidney) of a 13-year-old with ADPKD demonstrates the presence of multiple discrete cysts, the largest measuring 1.2 × 1.2 cm. The kidney is enlarged (kidney size = 11.7 cm, normal for age = 8.3–11.3 cm). The contralateral kidney is also enlarged, and shows multiple cysts of varying sizes.

and the absence of urine in the bladder. These findings may be present in the second trimester, and may be detected by screening ultrasound at 18–20 weeks' gestation. However, not all patients will have clinical evidence of disease at that time, and the typical features of ARPKD may not be present until after 30 weeks. With improvements in fetal ultrasonography, however, it is likely that the rates of detection in the first or second trimester will improve.[6]

Prenatal genetic diagnosis of ARPKD is available in families with an affected child, using linkage analysis. In informative families, the detection rate with this method is over 95%. Currently, direct mutation analysis is not available for clinical use, but may be in the future.[5]

Treatment, Complications, and Prognosis

There are no disease-specific therapies for ARPKD at present. Treatment is generally focused on managing the

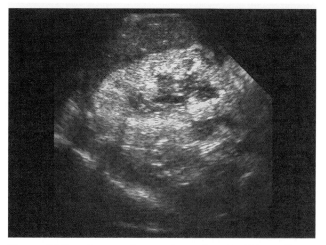

Figure 28-1 Autosomal recessive polycystic kidney disease (ARPKD). Renal ultrasound (right kidney) of a neonate with ARPKD demonstrates the typical radiographic features including renal enlargement, markedly increased echogenicity, and loss of corticomedullary differentiation (kidney size = 6.5 cm, normal for age = 3.9–5.1 cm). The contralateral kidney shows similar abnormalities.

Box 28-3 Criteria for Diagnosis of ARPKD[20]

- Typical radiographic features of ARPKD
- Presence of one or more additional findings including:
  - absence of renal cysts in both parents;
  - a previously affected sibling;
  - parental consanguinity; and
  - clinical, laboratory or pathologic features of hepatic fibrosis

Box 28-4 Differential Diagnosis of Enlarged Echogenic Kidneys in the Neonate

- ARPKD
- ADPKD
- GCKD
- Diffuse cystic dysplasia
- Congenital nephrotic syndrome
- Transient nephromegaly of the newborn
- Contrast nephropathy
- Renal vein thrombosis

respiratory distress, hypertension, electrolyte abnormalities, and the sequelae of acute or chronic renal insufficiency. With the advent of modern neonatal intensive care units and the improvements in ventilator support, survival of neonates with ARPKD has improved. Nevertheless, respiratory failure remains a leading cause of mortality for severely affected infants. At present, it is difficult to predict at birth which newborns with ARPKD requiring mechanical ventilation have degrees of pulmonary hypoplasia that are not compatible with life. Confounding issues include pulmonary edema, volume overload, surfactant deficiency in premature neonates, and respiratory impairment from massive kidney enlargement. Some authors advocate performing unilateral nephrectomy or bilateral nephrectomy with dialysis support to allow optimal ventilation and the assessment of long-term pulmonary prognosis.

The hypertension may be severe, and require several medications for adequate control. Although elevated plasma renin levels are not consistently demonstrated in these patients,[14] the hypertension is usually responsive to angiotensin-converting enzyme (ACE) inhibitors, which are considered first-line therapy. Additional therapy with calcium channel blockers or diuretics is often required. Hyponatremia may require modifications in sodium and water intake.[14] The urine-concentrating defect may result in recurrent episodes of volume depletion that must be monitored closely during episodes of intercurrent illnesses. The concentrating defect also causes primary enuresis that may be refractory to treatment. Patients with metabolic acidosis should receive bicarbonate supplementation. Urinary abnormalities are also common. Patients may have pyuria with or without evidence of urinary tract infection (UTI). Those with UTI should undergo standard evaluation including renal ultrasound and voiding cystourethrogram. Hematuria and/or proteinuria may occur, but these are not prominent features of ARPKD.

Feeding difficulties and poor growth are often present.[14,20] These may be due to increased metabolic

demands and poor feeding associated with renal insufficiency. In addition, massively enlarged kidneys may cause impingement on the stomach, resulting in early satiety and the development or exacerbation of gastroesophageal reflux. Nasogastric or gastrostomy tube feedings may be necessary in order to deliver sufficient calories.

Renal replacement therapy, in the form of dialysis or transplantation, is indicated when patients progress to end-stage renal disease (ESRD). Peritoneal dialysis is the preferred modality, particularly in young children. The presence of hepatosplenomegaly or a past history of prior abdominal surgery (such as nephrectomy) generally does not preclude the use of peritoneal dialysis.

With the advances in renal replacement therapy and improved patient survival, the hepatic manifestations and complications are becoming more prominent, and may dominate the clinical picture in an older child or adolescent.[6] Portal hypertension is common, and patients should be monitored regularly by a pediatric gastroenterologist. Potential complications include bleeding esophageal varices, portal thrombosis, and hypersplenism resulting in chronic thrombocytopenia, anemia, and leukopenia. Patients with varices generally undergo periodic endoscopy and may require banding or other therapy. Bacterial cholangitis is a potentially life-threatening complication.

In patients with severe portal hypertension, portosystemic shunting may be indicated. However, recent studies have reported the occurrence of hepatic encephalopathy in patients with portosystemic shunts who subsequently progressed to ESRD. The precise mechanism for the encephalopathy is unknown, but is thought to be due to impaired renal clearance of toxins shunted away from the liver. With the increasing use of living-relation liver donation, liver transplant has been advocated as an alternative to shunting in patients with severe portal hypertension.

Two recent experimental studies in mice raise the possibility that novel therapies directed at the function of the EGFR or one of its ligands may help to slow kidney and/or liver disease progression in ARPKD.[7,18] Additional studies are needed to determine if these novel therapies are safe and effective in the treatment of children with ARPKD and other polycystic kidney diseases.

The prognosis for patients with ARPKD has improved significantly, although the disease continues to have significant morbidity and mortality. Although published data suggest that neonatal survival is approximately 70%, it is likely with the newer neonatal intensive care therapy that this number is higher.[17,20] Longitudinal studies suggest that 50–80% of patients with ARPKD are alive at 15 years.[14,17] Although most patients with ARPKD have some degree of renal impairment, some may not require dialysis or renal transplantation until late childhood or adolescence. A subset of patients will also require liver transplantation and, as noted previously, with improved renal survival the hepatic disease becomes more prominent. Of those patients who undergo renal transplantation for ARPKD, it has been reported that up to 36% of them will die in the first 5 years after transplant, the majority from complications directly attributable to their liver disease.[15]

AUTOSOMAL DOMINANT POLYCYSTIC KIDNEY DISEASE (ADPKD)

ADPKD is a systemic disease characterized by polycystic kidneys and variable abnormalities of abdominal organs, the heart, and the vasculature.[10] The term 'adult' polycystic disease is no longer used because ADPKD can present in individuals from birth to adulthood.

Genetics

The incidence of ADPKD is approximately 1 in 1000, making it the most common genetic kidney disease and one of the most common genetic diseases overall.[12,13] It is inherited in an autosomal dominant fashion with considerable variability in disease expression, even within the same family. Children with an affected parent have a 50% chance of developing the disease. Males and females are affected, although the disease phenotype may be more severe in the former. ADPKD occurs in all races. It is an uncommon cause of ESRD in pediatrics, but accounts for 5-10% of ESRD in adults.

Two major disease-causing genes have been identified and characterized. *PKD1* mutations account for the majority of ADPKD (85%), whereas a smaller percentage of patients (15%) have *PKD2* mutations. Linkage to *PKD1* and *PKD2* has not been confirmed in a very small subset of families. Therefore, a third PKD locus, *PKD3*, is postulated. About 10% of patients do not have a positive family history of ADPKD and are presumed to have a new mutations.[12]

The gene that is mutated for PKD1 is localized to chromosome 16p13.3. It encodes a large protein, polycystin 1; this is a membrane-bound protein that mediates cell–cell and/or cell–matrix interactions. Polycystin 1 may serve as a receptor for an as-yet unidentified ligand.

Polycystin 1 is expressed in kidney, other abdominal organs, and the vasculature, and has a role in the development of the kidneys, heart, vasculature, and pancreas.[13]

The gene that is mutated for PKD2 is localized to chromosome 4q13-q23 and encodes the smaller protein, polycystin 2 that is a voltage-gated ion channel.[13]

Pathogenesis and Pathology

The mechanism whereby mutations in either of these two genes result in progressive cyst formation or vasculature abnormalities remains unknown. Polycystin 1 and 2 interact with each other and may be components of a larger multi-protein complex. Polycystin 1 may have a role in regulating the cation channel function of polycystin 2. The variability in expression has been postulated to be due to a second-hit mechanism. This hypothesis arose out of the observation that, although renal tubular cells harbor the same mutation, only a small subset develops cysts. Detailed genetic analysis demonstrated that some of the cyst-lining epithelial cells had evidence for loss of heterozygosity – that is, they had mutations in *PKD* genes on each allele. Why some cells might be susceptible to such a second hit remains unknown.[13]

Renal cysts in ADPKD may occur throughout the nephron. The cysts progressively enlarge, and eventually become disconnected from the tubular lumen. Cyst expansion requires both proliferation of the tubular epithelial cells as well as active secretion of chloride into the cyst lumen. Therefore, it has been hypothesized that *CFTR*, the mutated gene in cystic fibrosis (CF) has a role in modifying disease expression. Several kindreds with both CF and PKD have been reported. However, the presence of one or two copies of the mutant CF gene has not been shown consistently to affect disease progression.

Clinical Features

In children, ADPKD may be asymptomatic or may present with hypertension, urinary tract infection, or gross hematuria.[9] The extra-renal manifestations of ADPKD are uncommon in children. Patients who become symptomatic during childhood typically do so during adolescence. A small subset may present in the newborn period with clinical features indistinguishable from those of ARPKD (Table 28-2).[11]

Hypertension is a common presenting feature, and appears to be due to activation of the renin–angiotensin–aldosterone axis, possibly due to impaired local renal blood flow from expanding cysts. Gross hematuria may occur, particularly after a seemingly minor flank trauma. Alternately, it may be a symptom of a kidney stone or urinary tract infection, both of which can occur at increased frequency in patients with ADPKD. Most children with ADPKD have normal renal function, although renal insufficiency may be seen rarely. There may be a urine-concentrating defect and flank pain from kidney enlargement or cyst hemorrhage.

Extra-renal manifestations of ADPKD include cyst formation in the liver, pancreas, and reproductive organs.[10]

Table 28-2   Clinical Features of ADPKD

Renal	Extra-renal
Hypertension	Hepatic, pancreatic, ovarian and seminal vesicle cysts**
Urinary tract infection/pyuria	Mitral valve prolapse
Gross or microscopic hematuria	Cerebral aneurysms**
Flank masses*	Gastrointestinal diverticuli**
Urolithiasis**	
Renal insufficiency**	

*Rare in older children, more common in neonates.
**Rare in children.

Gastrointestinal diverticuli may also be present. These complications are rare in children. However, up to 15% of children may have an increased rate of mitral valve prolapse.[9] Furthermore, increased left ventricular mass has been demonstrated in children with ADPKD, even before the development of hypertension. Endocardial fibroelastosis is rarely reported in children.

Also rare in children are vascular abnormalities. Aneurysms occur anywhere along the aorta, and potentially are life-threatening conditions. Cerebral aneurysms are a dreaded complication of ADPKD, and familial clustering of ruptured aneurysms occurs.[1]

Diagnosis

Specific diagnostic criteria for ADPKD in children have not been established. Prenatal diagnosis may be suspected in fetuses with enlarged kidneys. In pediatric patients known to be at-risk for ADPKD (those with a parent with ADPKD and a resultant 50% risk of disease), the finding of one cyst or bilateral echogenic cysts (in the newborn) is diagnostic.[9,12] Since simple cysts are rare in children (unlike adults, in whom one or two cysts might be considered a normal finding), the finding of a single cyst in a child not known to be at risk should raise the suspicion of PKD and merit further investigation. It is not uncommon for children to be diagnosed with ADPKD when one or more cysts of the kidney are detected as an incidental finding during radiographic evaluation for an unrelated problem.

Both parents of a child with ADPKD should undergo screening ultrasonography. Because ADPKD is a slowly progressive disease and adults may not become symptomatic until the third or fourth decade of life, the finding of a normal ultrasound in parents who are aged less than 30 years does not preclude the diagnosis of ADPKD. Moreover, the grandparents should also be considered for screening by ultrasound.[6] Conversely, because adults in their 20s and 30s may not be symptomatic, parents of children with ADPKD may be unaware that they are affected. In fact, a small subset of adults with ADPKD is diagnosed as part of the evaluation of cystic kidneys in their child.

A genetic diagnosis is possible in both PKD1 and PKD2 families by linkage analysis. In large informative families, the accuracy of diagnosis is >90%, but only about 50% of families have sufficient numbers of affected and unaffected members able or willing to be tested.[12] Considerable advances have been made in techniques of direct mutation analysis. However, because of the complexity of the *PKD1* gene, the accuracy of these techniques remains to be determined. An up-to-date listing of laboratories performing genetic testing is available at http://www.geneclinics.org.

The issue of screening presymptomatic children who have a parent with ADPKD remains controversial. In most instances of adult-onset diseases without specific therapies, the general consensus is that presymptomatic children should not be screened.[12] The ethical dilemma is that of allowing an adult to act in the best interests of a child without knowing what the child might really want to have done. In the case of ADPKD, because of its relatively slow progression, the finding of a normal renal ultrasound may be falsely reassuring. Alternately, the finding of cysts in an otherwise asymptomatic child may have significant psychosocial and financial implications. Diagnosing ADPKD in a presymptomatic individual may not always be in that person's best interests. A more prudent approach would be to check the urine, blood pressure, and serum creatinine concentration and proceed with imaging studies only if any of these are abnormal. Such at-risk children, however, should undergo regular monitoring of blood pressure and urinalysis. Because of the complexities of these issues, practitioners should refer these individuals to a pediatric nephrologist before undertaking any diagnostic studies of presymptomatic children.

Treatment and Prognosis

There are no disease-specific therapies for ADPKD. Although a number of dietary and pharmacologic therapies, such as a soy protein diet and lipid-lowering agents, have been studied in ADPKD, none has consistently been shown to significantly impact disease progression in humans.[4] Infants with ADPKD are managed in much the same way as those with ARPKD, including control of hypertension, close attendance to electrolyte and renal function, and monitoring of growth and development.[6] In the older child, treatment focuses on the management of renal-related complications, since extra-renal manifestations (except for mitral valve prolapse) are generally rare in children. As with any other kidney disease, control of hypertension is essential. ACE inhibitors (or angiotensin II receptor blockers) are generally first-line therapy. However, it has not been clearly established whether these agents carry any additional benefit over other anti-hypertensive agents in their impact on disease progression. UTI is common in ADPKD, and because the cysts may be discontinuous with the tubular lumen, treatment requires the use of antibiotics that penetrate the cyst lumen. Cyst infection may be particularly problematic for the same reason, and localized cyst infection may be present despite the finding of a negative urine culture. Conversely, pyuria may be seen in the absence of infection, further complicating the clinical picture. In addition, agents traditionally used to treat UTIs – including cephalosporins and aminoglycosides – are generally ineffective in penetrating cysts. Antibiotics such as ciprofloxacin and sulfonamides are more effective, and should be used for the treatment of suspected UTI in ADPKD patients, particularly those who have persistent pain or fever. Rarely, persistently infected cysts require laparoscopic drainage.

Flank pain, due to cyst expansion, can be significant and debilitating. Short-term narcotic administration may be necessary, but chronic use should be avoided because of the risk of dependence or addiction. Referral to a pain management team may be helpful. Patients with one or more very large cyst may be candidates for laparoscopic cyst decortication. Routine radiographic screening for cerebral aneurysms is generally not recommended. Although magnetic resonance angiography (MRA) will detect the majority of aneurysms, the finding of a negative study does not preclude their subsequent development. MRA is generally reserved for symptomatic patients (such as those with recurrent headache) or those with a family history of cerebral aneurysm.

Approximately 50% of patients with ADPKD will progress to ESRD.[10,12] Patients with PKD1 typically progress to ESRD about 15 years prior to those with PKD2 (mean age 53 years versus 69 years). However, it should be stressed that individual disease courses may vary significantly. In addition, genotype–phenotype correlations have not been established, so identifying the patient's specific mutation may not be helpful in determining his or her prognosis. Children with certain clinical findings, such as multiple cysts with hypertension, may be at increased risk for more rapid disease progression.[8] Despite the high likelihood of progression to ESRD in adulthood, the majority of pediatric patients with ADPKD maintain normal renal function during the course of childhood.

GLOMERULOCYSTIC KIDNEY DISEASE

Glomerulocystic kidney disease (GCKD) is a relatively rare heterogeneous group of inherited and non-inherited cystic kidney diseases characterized by cysts restricted to the glomeruli.[2] It may occur as a subset of ADPKD. Alternately, it may occur as an isolated renal disease, either as a sporadic or a non-syndromal heritable disorder. GCKD may also occur as a major component of various malformation syndromes.

With the exception of GCKD occurring as a component of ADPKD, the genetics of the disorder are not fully defined. Familial GCKD with isolated renal disease is inherited in an autosomal dominant fashion in some instances. A clinically distinct subset of GCKD is the hypoplastic variant, a rare autosomal dominant disorder reported in only a few kindreds. A disease-causing gene for this variant is the hepatocyte nuclear factor-1beta, which encodes a protein of the same name that functions as a transcription factor. However, the mechanism by which this abnormal protein results in cyst formation remains to be determined. GCKD is a major component of a number of congenital syndromes including Trisomy 13, short rib-polydactyly, brachymesomelia-renal syndrome and orofaciodigital syndrome, type I. It is a minor component of several other syndromes such as Zellweger syndrome.[6]

The pathogenesis of GCKD remains undefined. In most forms of GCKD, the kidneys are enlarged. Cystic involvement in GCKD may involve both kidneys equally, or be asymmetric. Microscopic examination demonstrates dilated Bowman's spaces with primitive-appearing glomeruli. The remaining portions of the nephron are generally uninvolved until late in the disease course, when tubular atrophy and interstitial fibrosis may be evident. Both sporadic forms of GCKD and the GCKD form of ADPKD are associated with hepatic abnormalities in a minority of patients. In the hypoplastic GCKD variant, the kidneys are small. Histologically, there is evidence of glomerular cysts with abnormal collecting systems and abnormal (or absent) papillae.

Patients with primary GCKD usually present with hypertension and variable degrees of renal insufficiency.

Those with GCKD associated with congenital syndromes will present with features of their respective syndromes. GCKD typically presents in infancy with enlarged flank masses and may be indistinguishable clinically from patients with ARPKD or early-onset ADPKD. A smaller percentage of patients with GCKD present as adults with features more typical of ADPKD, such as hypertension, flank pain, and hematuria. An autosomal dominant pattern of inheritance may be seen in this latter group. Since several of the case series describing these kindreds were published prior to the availability of genetic testing for ADPKD, it is difficult to determine if this group actually represents the GCKD form of ADPKD.

Ultrasound studies show that patients with sporadic or inherited GCKD have enlarged echogenic kidneys with evidence of small cortical cysts. Patients with the hypoplastic variant generally have small kidneys on imaging studies.

The heterogeneity of GCKD and the variability in clinical course makes it difficult to determine the prognosis. However, although the hypoplastic variant may show evidence of renal insufficiency early in life, the subsequent progression of renal disease is slow.

CYSTIC DISEASES ASSOCIATED WITH CONGENITAL SYNDROMES

Polycystic kidneys may occur as a major or minor component of many inherited and sporadic congenital syndromes. In the majority of cases, the kidneys demonstrate histologic evidence of cystic dysplasia, rather than true PKD. Specific details of cystic dysplasia are addressed in Chapter 29. Examples include Meckel, Jeune, and Ivemark syndromes. The Online Mendelian Inheritance in Man (OMIM) database (http://www3.ncbi. nlm.hih.gov/OMIM) provides an updated list and description of inherited disorders associated with polycystic cystic kidneys and/or diffuses cystic dysplasia.

Patients with cystic kidneys associated with congenital syndromes may present as infants with signs and symptoms that may be initially confused with ARPKD, including bilateral enlarged flank masses, hypertension, renal insufficiency, and variable degrees of the oligohydramnios sequence. The hallmark of syndromic cystic diseases, however, is the presence of extra-renal features of the underlying syndrome, thus highlighting the importance of a careful physical examination in all patients with suspected polycystic kidneys. Other congenital renal lesions, such as obstructive uropathy, can often be associated with cystic changes and enlarged kidneys, but these are easily distinguishable by ultrasonography.

Two specific inherited syndromes associated with polycystic kidneys bear mention, in part, because the associated abnormalities may not be fully evident when the kidney disease is first detected. Tuberous sclerosis (TS) is associated with both ADPKD and GCKD. In the case of the former, several families have been identified in which TS and severe childhood-onset ADPKD occur in the same patient. Genetic analysis of these families has demonstrated linkage to the chromosome 16 region that contains the genes for both TS and ADPKD (PKD1). Additional investigations showed that these patients have large deletions that span both genes, resulting in a contiguous gene syndrome. Von Hippel–Lindau disease

---

MAJOR POINTS

- Referral to a pediatric nephrologist is recommended for all children with suspected PKD.
- Both ARPKD and ADPKD can present in the fetus, newborn, older child or adolescent, although ARPKD occurs more commonly than ADPKD in neonates and young infants.
- The mutated genes for both ARPKD (*PKHD1*) and ADPKD (*PKD1, PKD2*) have now been identified, although the pathogenesis of both disease types has not been fully defined.
- Several inherited and non-inherited disorders may present as bilateral enlarged echogenic kidneys in the neonate.
- Polycystic kidneys (diffuse cystic dysplasia) are a component of a variety of congenital syndromes. Detailed family histories and physical examinations are key to identifying this group of patients.
- Disease in ARPKD is confined to the kidneys and liver, whereas ADPKD is a systemic disease with potential involvement of multiple organs.
- ARPKD patients with ductal plate fibrosis may not present with the typical features of cholangitis such as abnormal liver enzymes and fever. Instead, they may have unexplained recurrent episodes of fever with Gram-negative bacteremia.
- Renal ultrasonography of the parents may help to distinguish ADPKD from ARPKD in a child with polycystic kidneys. The finding of a negative ultrasound in a parent aged under 30 years, however, does not exclude the diagnosis of ADPKD.
- Routine ultrasonography of an asymptomatic child who has a parent with ADPKD is generally not recommended. Referral to a pediatric nephrologist is recommended for all asymptomatic patients at risk for ADPKD for whom radiographic imaging or genetic testing is being considered.
- The diagnosis of ADPKD in a presymptomatic individual may impose psychological and financial burdens.

is an autosomal dominant disorder characterized by renal cell carcinoma, pheochromocytoma and eye, spine and brain hemangioblastomas. Cysts in the kidneys and pancreas may also be seen, and can occasionally be confused with ADPKD. A detailed family history is essential to identify these patients.

Morbidity and mortality of children with ARPKD and early-onset ADPKD has improved over the past few decades with modern obstetrical and neonatal intensive care, careful attention to growth and development, improved control of hypertension, and advances in renal replacement therapy. However, both diseases continue to be important causes of ESRD in the pediatric (and adult) populations. The challenge remains to identify therapies that will slow or prevent progression of disease. Although currently not available, it is hoped that with the advances made in the understanding of genetics and pathogenesis of these diseases, newer, disease-specific therapies may become available in the future.

REFERENCES

1. Belz MM, Hughes RL, Kaehny WD, et al. Familial clustering of ruptured intracranial aneurysms in autosomal dominant polycystic kidney disease. Am J Kidney Dis 2001; 38:770-776.

2. Bernstein J. Glomerulocystic kidney disease – nosological considerations. Pediatr Nephrol 1993;7:464-470.

3. Cole BR, Conley SB, Stapleton FB. Polycystic kidney disease in the first year of life. J Pediatr 1987;111:693-699.

4. Davis ID, MacRae Dell K, Sweeney WE, Avner ED. Can progression of autosomal dominant or autosomal recessive polycystic kidney disease be prevented? Semin Nephrol 2001;21:430-440.

5. Dell KM, Avner ED. Autosomal recessive polycystic kidney disease. GeneClinics: Clinical Genetic Information Resource [database online]. Copyright, University of Washington, Seattle. Available at http://www.geneclinics.org, 2001.

6. Dell KM, Avner ED. Polycystic kidney disease. In: Avner ED, Harmon W, Niadet P (eds), *Pediatric Nephrology*, 5th edn. Lippincott, Williams & Wilkins, Philadelphia, 2003.

7. Dell KM, Nemo R, Sweeney WE, Jr., et al. A novel inhibitor of tumor necrosis factor-alpha converting enzyme ameliorates polycystic kidney disease. Kidney Int 2001;60: 1240-1248.

8. Fick-Brosnahan GM, Tran ZV, Johnson AM, et al. Progression of autosomal dominant polycystic kidney disease in children. Kidney Int 2001;59:1654-1662.

9. Fick GM, Duley IT, Johnson AM, et al. The spectrum of autosomal dominant polycystic kidney disease in children. J Am Soc Nephrol 1994;4:1654-1660.

10. Gabow P. Autosomal dominant polycystic kidney disease. N Engl J Med 1993;329:332-342.

11. Guay-Woodford LM, Galliani CA, Musulman-Mroczek E, et al. Diffuse renal cystic disease in children: morphologic and genetic correlations. Pediatr Nephrol 1998;12: 173-182.

12. Harris PC, Torres VE. Autosomal dominant polycystic kidney disease. GeneClinics: Clinical Genetic Information Resource [database online]. Copyright, University of Washington, Seattle. Available at http://www.geneclinics. org, 2002.

13. Igarashi P, Somlo S. Genetics and pathogenesis of polycystic kidney disease. J Am Soc Nephrol 2002;13:2384-2398.

14. Kaplan BS, Fay J, Shah V, et al. Autosomal recessive polycystic kidney disease. Pediatr Nephrol 1989;3:43-49.

15. Khan K, Schwarzenberg SJ, Sharp HL, et al. Morbidity from congenital hepatic fibrosis after renal transplantation for autosomal recessive polycystic kidney disease. Am J Tranplant 2002;2:360-365.

16. Onuchic LF, Furu L, Nagasawa Y, et al. PKHD1, the polycystic kidney and hepatic disease 1 gene, encodes a novel large protein containing multiple immunoglobulin-like plexin-transcription-factor domains and parallel beta-helix 1 repeats. Am J Hum Genet 2002;70:1305-1317.

17. Roy S, Dillon MJ, Trompeter RS, Barratt TM. Autosomal recessive polycystic kidney disease: long-term outcome of neonatal survivors. Pediatr Nephrol 1997;11:302-306.

18. Sweeney WE, Chen Y, Nakanishi K, et al. Treatment of polycystic kidney disease with a novel tyrosine kinase inhibitor. Kidney Int 2000;57:33-40.

19. Ward CJ, Hogan MC, Rossetti S, et al. The gene mutated in autosomal recessive polycystic kidney disease encodes a large, receptor-like protein. Nature Genet 2002;30: 259-269.

20. Zerres K, Rudnik-Schoneborn S, Deget F, et al. Autosomal recessive polycystic kidney disease in 115 children: clinical presentation, course and influence of gender. Arbeitsgemeinschaft fur Padiatrische, Nephrologie. Acta Paediatr 1996;85:437-445.

Developmental Abnormalities of the Kidneys

BERNARD S. KAPLAN, M.B., B.Ch.

INTRODUCTION

Prenatal ultrasonography, improved ventilator and nutritional support, and progress in dialysis techniques for newborns and renal transplantation for young children have changed the natural history of many developmental abnormalities of the kidneys. A team approach is needed to evaluate carefully the information obtained from many sources in order to manage optimally a newborn with a genetic or developmental disorder of the kidneys. Errors occur when there are insufficient data, inadequate communication, and poor understanding of the natural history of these disorders. Many newborns that previously might have died can now be dialyzed (albeit with difficulty) and transplanted when they reach about 10 kg body weight. A precise diagnosis should be made before starting dialysis, because some problems impose enormous ethical, emotional, and financial burdens on families. The diagnosis depends on the evaluation of the prenatal history, results of fetal ultrasonography, family history, clinical examination, imaging studies of the infants and parents when indicated, laboratory studies (including DNA tests if available), and interpretation of pathology (Box 29-1). Ear abnormalities and single umbilical arteries are often cited as reasons to exclude a renal anomaly, but these associations are quite uncommon. Autosomal recessive polycystic kidney disease (ARPKD) and autosomal dominant polycystic kidney disease (ADPKD, PKD) are described in detail elsewhere (see Chapter 28), and will only be alluded to in this chapter.

223

Box 29-1   Guiding Principles in Abnormalities of the Kidneys

- Few genetic renal disorders are confined to the kidneys
- Many syndromes have renal involvement
- Urogenital ultrasonography should be performed in all newborns with multiple defects
- Ultrasonography features can change over time
- Variable expression of congenital renal defects may occur within a family, and among kindreds

---

Box 29-2   Features of Multicystic Kidney

- Usually unilateral
- No continuity between glomeruli and calyces
- The kidney does not function
- The contralateral kidney may be normal, absent, hydronephrotic, ectopic, or dysplastic
- There may be vesicoureteric reflux

CLASSIFICATION

There are many classifications of cystic and dysplastic kidneys. Some classify according to gross features such as abnormalities of position (ectopic kidney, horseshoe kidney), size (hypoplastic kidneys), abnormal development (dysplasia), or presence of cysts (multicystic, polycystic). Within each category the abnormalities may be sporadic or inherited.

Abnormalities of Position

Ectopic kidney, horseshoe kidney, and crossed fused ectopia are abnormalities in position of the kidney(s). Unless associated with dysplasia, vesicoureteric reflux (VUR), or obstruction, there are few long-term effects. These kidneys are at risk for the same problems as those in normal positions, although a pelvic horseshoe kidney may cause problems in pregnant women. Horseshoe kidney occurs with increased frequency in Turner syndrome and other syndromes. A voiding cystourethrogram should be performed to exclude vesicoureteric reflux, and a radionuclide scan carried out if there is evidence on ultrasonography of obstruction.

Multicystic Kidney

A multicystic kidney is the result of abnormal metanephric differentiation. This is the second most common cause of a flank mass in the newborn. The prevalence rate is 1 in 4300. A true multicystic kidney is usually a sporadic, non-syndromal, congenital anomaly. The diagnosis is made *in utero* by prenatal ultrasonography or by detection of an abdominal mass, or by the evaluation of a urinary tract infection (UTI). Multicystic kidney is rarely the cause of symptoms in the newborn. Multicystic kidney must be differentiated from obstructive cystic renal dysplasia associated with hydronephrosis and other causes of obstructive uropathy by performing a

radionuclide scan. The multicystic kidney does not function. The contralateral kidney is usually normal, but in up to 50% of the cases the other kidney may be absent, hydronephrotic, ectopic, have VUR, and occasionally it may be dysplastic. Most patients are followed by yearly ultrasonography. Spontaneous involution often occurs without complications of infection, bleeding, or malignancy (Box 29-2).[2,3,24]

Renal Adysplasia and Dysplasia

Adysplasia encompasses a spectrum of renal anomalies that include renal agenesis, hypoplasia, and dysplasia.[3,16] This may occur sporadically, in a patient, as an inherited defect without other major abnormalities, or as part of a syndrome. Adysplasia and dysplasia can be the result of a single autosomal recessive or dominant gene disorder, multifactorial inheritance, chromosomal disorders, or in-utero infections or toxins.[11] One kidney may be absent ('A' for agenesis), and the contralateral kidney may be normal or dysplastic. Both may be dysplastic but have sufficient function to sustain life for variable periods of time. The clinical picture depends on the severity of the renal anomaly, whether it is unilateral or bilateral, and the presence of associated anomalies. Prenatal diagnosis by ultrasonography is possible, especially if there is oligohydramnios or associated anomalies such as limb deformations (Box 29-3).

Unilateral Renal Agenesis

Unilateral renal agenesis is usually an isolated, non-syndromal, sporadic abnormality that is detected during

---

Box 29-3   Features of Renal Cystic Dysplasia

- May be unilateral or bilateral
- Kidneys may or may not be cystic
- Disorganized architecture
- Often contains ectopic tissues (cartilage, muscle)
- Reduced renal function

prenatal ultrasonography. Unilateral renal agenesis is a more important finding if the solitary kidney is abnormal, or is part of a syndrome, or is an expression of hereditary renal dysplasia. The incidence is 1 in 500–800 live births. If the solitary kidney is normal, there is little risk of chronic renal failure. The newborn must be examined carefully for additional anomalies – cleft palate, preauricular pits, cardiac and vertebral defects, and müllerian duct aplasia. A voiding cystourethrogram (VCUG) should be performed to exclude VUR. No evaluations are needed after 1 year of age if renal function is normal and renal ultrasonography shows normal kidney growth, no cysts, and compensatory hypertrophy.

Bilateral Renal Agenesis

Bilateral renal agenesis occurs as an isolated, non-syndromal, sporadic abnormality detected during prenatal ultrasonography. It can also be a component of a syndrome such as the branchio-otorenal dysplasia (BOR) syndrome, or a feature of hereditary renal adysplasia. There can be variable expression within a family, and both autosomal recessive and dominant inheritance occur. The incidence is about 1 in 3000 births. Bilateral renal agenesis is an important cause of the oligohydramnios sequence (Potter syndrome), in which decreased amniotic fluid causes uterine compression of the fetus. This produces the Potter facies with wide-set eyes, a prominent skin fold that extends from medial canthus to cheek, a parrot-beak nose, pliable low-set ears, and receding chin (Boxes 29-4 and 29-5). There are lower-limb deformations and a narrow, small chest with pulmonary hypoplasia. The newborn infant is anuric, and dies from azotemia and pulmonary insufficiency.

Isolated Dysplasia and Adysplasia

The incidence of non-syndromal bilateral renal dysplasia is about 15 per 100,000 newborns.[13] Modes of transmission are autosomal dominant inheritance and multifactorial inheritance. There may be incomplete penetrance and variable expression so that a parent and siblings may be unaffected, have unilateral dysplasia, or

---

Box 29-5	Causes of the Oligohydramnios Sequence
Obstructive uropathy	Posterior urethral valves
	Prune belly syndrome
Renal anomalies	Bilateral renal agenesis
	Bilateral renal cystic dysplasia
	Renal tubular dysgenesis
	Autosomal recessive polycystic kidneys
	Autosomal dominant polycystic kidneys
Chronic leakage of amniotic fluid	

unilateral agenesis. Sporadic adysplasia may be caused by a new mutation or inheritance of the gene(s) from a non-manifesting parent. First-degree relatives should be screened by ultrasonography if genetic counseling is requested. The empiric risk of bilateral renal adysplasia for future siblings is 3.5%.[6] The recurrence risk increases if two siblings are affected.

Dysplasia and Adysplasia in Regional Defects

Renal adysplasia occurs in prune belly syndrome (PBS) and posterior urethral valves (PUV), possibly as a result of obstructive uropathy. The renal pathology ranges from minor anomalies to severe dysplasia with or without cysts.

Prune Belly Syndrome (PBS)

The features of PBS are deficient abdominal wall muscles, unilateral or bilateral undescended testes, and urinary tract abnormalities. Females are rarely affected, but may have uterine or vaginal anomalies. PBS is also associated with lower-intestinal tract malrotation and atresias, lower-limb deformations, and cardiovascular defects.

Posterior Urethral Valves (PUV)

PUV are characterized by urethral valves, either a flap valve or a diaphragm in the prostatic urethra, and features of obstructive uropathy.

A dilated prostatic urethra, megacystis, and mega-ureters can occur in both conditions. The most frequent clinical presentation in the newborn of both conditions consists of features of the oligohydramnios sequence. The survival of newborns with PBS or PUV depends on the severity of pulmonary hypoplasia and the severity of renal dysplasia. PBS or PUV are usually isolated occurrences, although PUV may occur in families and in malformation syndromes.

Box 29-4	Features of the Oligohydramnios Sequence (Potter Syndrome)

- Deformation of the limbs
- Pulmonary hypoplasia
- Flat face, beaked nose and low-set ears
- Ears appear big because they are simple

Dysplasia and Adysplasia with Multiple Congenital Anomalies

Branchio-Otorenal Dysplasia (BOR Syndrome)[15]

The incidence of this condition is 1 in 40,000 of the population, and it occurs in 2% of profoundly deaf children. Renal abnormalities include bilateral renal agenesis, bilateral hypoplasia or dysplasia, unilateral renal agenesis with contralateral hypoplasia or dysplasia, ureteropelvic obstruction, and VUR. The kidneys may be normal. Renal function ranges from normal to severe reduction in glomerular filtration rate. Extra-renal manifestations are preauricular pits, malformations in the external, middle, and inner ear; and hearing loss. There may be cervical fistulas or cysts. Inheritance is autosomal dominant, with high penetrance and variable expression. One mutant gene, *EYA1*, is on chromosome 8q13.3. The prognosis depends on the severity of the renal disorder.

Mayer–Rokitansky–Kuster–Hauser Syndrome

This syndrome appears to be sporadic in most cases, but may be associated with a mutation in the gene encoding the hepatocyte nuclear factor (HNF)-1beta. The features are renal adysplasia with Müllerian anomalies of vaginal atresia and bicornuate or septated uterus.[22] Fallopian tubes, ovaries, and broad and round ligaments are normal. There is a normal female karyotype, and normal secondary sexual development.

Acrorenal Syndromes

Ectodermal Dysplasia-Ectrodactyly-Cleft Lip and/or Palate (EEC 1) Syndrome

In this condition there are combinations of urogenital defects, ectrodactyly affects, ectodermal dysplasia, clefting, lachrymal ducts anomalies, and conductive hearing loss. Inheritance is autosomal dominant, with variable penetrance and expression.

VACTERL/VATER Association

This is defined by combinations of <u>v</u>ertebral anomalies, <u>a</u>nal atresia, <u>c</u>ongenital cardiac disease, <u>t</u>racheo-<u>e</u>sophageal fistula, <u>r</u>enal abnormalities, and radial-<u>l</u>imb dysplasia. VACTERL is usually sporadic. Patients with features of VACTERL must be tested for Fanconi anemia.

Fanconi Anemia (Pancytopenia) Syndrome (FA)

Congenital malformations occur in 60% of cases. Affected patients may have renal malformations, short stature, café-au-lait spots, radial-ray abnormalities, gastrointestinal, microcephaly, skeletal abnormalities; in males there are also genital anomalies, hypogonadism, and infertility. There is chromosomal instability and mutagen hypersensitivity in cells. Inheritance is autosomal recessive, with variable expression and mutations in one of at least seven different genes.[14]

Thrombocytopenia Absent Radius Syndrome (TAR)

Renal anomalies may occur in this syndrome.

Townes–Brocks Radial-Ear-Anal-Renal Syndrome (TBS)

The clinical features of this syndrome include broad, bifid, or triphalangeal thumb; flat thenar eminences; small, 'lop,' or 'satyr' external ear, preauricular pits or tags; sensorineural hearing loss; and imperforate or stenotic or anteriorly placed anus. Renal and urological anomalies encompass renal hypoplasia, renal dysplasia, unilateral renal agenesis, horseshoe kidney, PUV, uretero-vesical reflux, and meatal stenosis.[19] Inheritance is dominant, with a defect in the gene encoding SALL1 on chromosome16q12.1.

POLYCYSTIC KIDNEYS

The term *polycystic kidney* is applied to both autosomal recessive and autosomal dominant polycystic kidneys. There are at least two cysts in one kidney and one in the other, or three cysts in one kidney. There is no renal dysplasia, and there is continuity of the lumen of the nephron from the uriniferous space to the urinary bladder. Patients with tuberous sclerosis, orofacial-digital syndrome, and Hadju–Cheney syndrome may have various kinds of cystic kidneys including polycystic kidneys. Autosomal recessive and autosomal dominant polycystic kidney disease (ARPKD and ADPKD) are discussed in Chapter 28. Tuberous sclerosis is also discussed in Chapter 28, but its details are reiterated in this chapter to reinforce the importance of thinking about this important condition in patients with various types of cystic kidney diseases.

Tuberous Sclerosis (TS)

TS is characterized by hamartomata in numerous organs. Rarely, polycystic or unilateral cystic disease is found in a newborn in which a diagnosis of TS is made later (Table 29-1). In TS, the renal cysts are identical to simple cysts or to dominant polycystic disease in their appearances in ultrasonographic, intravenous urography, and computed tomography scans. Nonsymptomatic renal lesions, cysts and/or angiomyolipomas, occur in about 60% of individuals with TS.[9] Skin lesions occur in 96%, and additional problems are epilepsy, learning difficulties, and behavioral problems. 'Ash leaf' hypopigmented nevi may be the only skin

Table 29-1 Syndromes with Polycystic Kidney Disease that Resemble Autosomal Recessive Polycystic Kidney Disease (ADPKD)

Condition	MIM#	Locus	Mutated Product	Inheritance
Polycystic kidney disease PKD1	179,300	16p13.3-p13.12	Polycystin	AD
Polycystic kidney disease PKD2	179,300	4q13-q23	Polycystin	AD
Tuberous sclerosis TSC2	191,100	16p13.3	Tuberin	AD
Tuberous sclerosis TSC1	191,100	9q34	Hamartin	AD
Von Hippel-Lindau disease vHL		Xp22		AD
Oral-facial digital syndrome OFD1	311,200			XL
Hadju-Cheney syndrome				XL

MIM# = Mendelian Inheritance in Man number; AD = autosomal dominant; XL = X-linked.

manifestation of TS in infants, and babies with polycystic kidneys must be examined for these nevi under ultraviolet light. Shagreen patches and adenoma sebaceum develop before the age of 14 years; nail fibromata appear after 5 years. Ventricular rhabdomyomas and seizures may occur in infancy. Patients usually survive to adolescence and adulthood, but those with early-onset polycystic kidneys may develop end-stage renal failure. Inheritance is autosomal dominant, with variable expression within a family, non-penetrance of the gene, or germinal mosaicism. A parent with the gene may appear unaffected, so the parents must also be examined clinically and by imaging studies for stigmata of TS. TS is linked in half the cases to a gene *TSC1* ('hamartin') on chromosome 9q34. In other patients TS is linked to a marker gene, *TSC2* ('tuberin'), near the locus for PKD 1 on chromosome 16p13.3.[23]

CYSTIC KIDNEYS WITH AUTOSOMAL RECESSIVE INHERITANCE

Meckel Syndrome

In Meckel syndrome (MKS 1, MKS 2), polycystic kidneys are an obligatory feature; a consistent feature is hepatic fibrosis with variable reactive ductule proliferation, dilation, and portal fibrosis (Box 29-6).[7] Other features include a sloping forehead, posterior encephalocele, microphthalmia, postaxial polydactyly, and ambiguous genitalia. Some 50% of MKS patients have oligohydramnios, with perinatal death. The incidence of MKS is 1 in 9000. Inheritance is autosomal recessive, with variable expression within and among families.[12] Gene loci are on chromosomes 17q22-q23 (MKS 1) and 11q13 (MKS 2).[18] Prenatal diagnosis is possible by ultrasonography and by the detection of increased alpha-fetoprotein levels in amniotic fluid.

Jeune Asphyxiating Thoracic Dystrophy Syndrome

The inheritance of asphyxiating thoracic dystrophy syndrome is autosomal recessive with variable expression (Box 29-7). There are respiratory distress, dysostoses, renal cystic disease, and congenital hepatic fibrosis. Dysostoses include short ribs, small and long thoracic cage, small pelvis, trident acetabular margins, short and thick second and third phalanges, cone-shaped epiphyses, handle-bar clavicle, and mesomelic shortening of the limbs.[10] Three different morphologic lesions of the kidneys have been described: (1) dilated proximal and distal tubules and Bowman capsule with interstitial fibrosis; (2) cystic dysplasia and disorganized renal

Box 29-6 Conditions with Abnormal Kidneys and Congenital Hepatic Fibrosis (CHF)

- CHF and polycystic kidneys
- Autosomal recessive polycystic kidneys
- Autosomal dominant polycystic kidneys
- CHF and hereditary tubulointerstitial nephritis
- Juvenile nephronophthisis
- Biedl–Bardet syndrome
- Jeune syndrome (asphyxiating thoracic chondrodystrophy)
- CHF and hereditary renal dysplasia
- Meckel syndrome
- Chondrodysplasia syndromes
- Renal-hepatic-pancreatic cystic dysplasia (Ivemark syndrome)
- Zellweger syndrome
- COACH syndrome (hypoplasia of Cerebellar vermis, Oligophrenia, congenital Ataxia, Coloboma, and Hepatic fibrosis)

architecture; and (3) chronic tubulointerstitial disease resembling juvenile nephronophthisis. Survivors have metaphysical dysplasia with short-limb dwarfism, and may progress to end-stage renal failure. Prenatal diagnosis by ultrasonography is possible by 18 weeks' gestation.

Renal-Hepatic-Pancreatic Dysplasia (Ivemark Syndrome)

The inheritance of Ivemark syndrome is autosomal recessive. Patients may have the oligohydramnios sequence, and the kidneys may be dysplastic with peripheral cortical cysts, primitive collecting ducts, glomerular cysts, and metaplastic cartilage.[5] There is fibrosis of the liver and pancreas. Most patients die from respiratory insufficiency during the newborn period.

HYPOPLASTIC KIDNEYS

Hypoplastic kidneys are small, have fewer calyces, and may be dysplastic (Table 29-2). Simple hypoplasia, oligomeganephronia, and renal dysplasia are the types of small kidneys that are seen in the newborn. Oligomeganephronic kidneys are small, and have a decreased number of enlarged glomeruli, but this is probably not a specific clinicopathologic entity. In simple hypoplasia, the renal architecture is normal, but there are decreased numbers of reniculi and small nephrons.

Table 29-2 Differential Diagnosis of Small Kidneys

Congenital	Acquired
Inherited	Chronic pyelonephritis
Syndromal	Chronic glomerulonephritis
Dysplastic	Renovascular accident
Cystic-dysplastic	
Reflux with cystic dysplasia	
Hypoplastic	
Glomerulocystic	
Oligomeganephronia	
Nephronophthisis	

GLOMERULOCYSTIC KIDNEYS

In the purest form of glomerulocystic kidney, there are dilated Bowman spaces, with few or no cysts in the tubule.[4] The rest of the renal architecture is normal. The kidneys may be large or small. The liver is normal. Glomerular cysts are also seen in obstructive uropathy, in autosomal dominant polycystic kidneys, in association with malformations of other organs, in dysplastic kidneys, and in infants whose mothers received phenacetin or indomethacin during pregnancy. Glomerular cysts are often subcapsular and may contain more than one glomeruloid structure. Glomerulocystic kidneys may occur sporadically. An autosomal dominant inheritance is found in some kindred, in association with mutations in the gene encoding hepatocyte nuclear factor (HNF)-1beta and early-onset diabetes.

DYSGENETIC KIDNEYS

Congenital Hypernephronic Nephromegaly with Tubular Dysgenesis

This is a rare autosomal recessive condition with late-onset oligohydramnios after 24 weeks of gestation; there are large non-functioning kidneys,[1] and the calvaria is abnormal (Box 29-8). By using ultrasonography, the kidneys are seen to be enlarged symmetrically, and the corticomedullary junction is poorly defined. There is an apparent increase in the number of glomeruli, and there are immature tubules without proximal convolutions. Prenatal diagnosis is not possible before 20 weeks' gestation. In all cases, the patients have died during the neonatal period.

IN-UTERO EXPOSURE TO TERATOGENS

Urogenital anomalies are found occasionally in infants exposed *in utero* to teratogens, although no convincing proof of a cause-and-effect relationship has been provided for associations in many of the single case reports (Box 29-9).

Box 29-9 Urogenital Anomalies Possibly Caused by In-Utero Exposure to Teratogens

- ACE inhibitor embryopathy[17]
- Valproic acid and other anticonvulsant agents
- Cocaine (and polydrug) use
- Indomethacin may cause renal dysgenesis
- Lead exposure and VACTERL association
- Phenacetin and salicylate may cause glomerulocystic disease
- Warfarin and unilateral renal agenesis

OVERGROWTH SYNDROMES

Beckwith–Wiedemann syndrome, Simpson–Golabi–Behmel syndrome and Perlman syndrome are overgrowth syndromes, with overlapping features and kidneys that may be abnormal at birth.

Beckwith–Wiedemann Syndrome

Features of this condition include nephromegaly, Wilms' tumor, medullary renal cysts, caliceal diverticula, hydronephrosis, and nephrolithiasis.[8] The syndrome is caused by a mutation of a gene encoding a human cyclin-dependent kinase inhibitor, p57 (*KIP2*) on chromosome 11p15.5. Patients should be screened using renal ultrasound for Wilms' tumor at 3-monthly intervals for the first 7 years of life.

Perlman Syndrome with Renal Hamartomas, Nephroblastomatosis, and Fetal Gigantism

Features of this syndrome include polyhydramnios, macrosomia, and bilateral nephromegaly with nephroblastomatosis, visceromegaly, cryptorchidism, diaphragmatic hernia, interrupted aortic arch, hypospadias, and polysplenia and renal findings of dysplasia, microcysts, and nephrogenic rests.[20] Inheritance is autosomal recessive.

Simpson–Golabi–Behmel Syndrome, Type 1; SGBS1

Features include pre- and postnatal overgrowth, 'coarse' face, hypertelorism, broad nasal root, cleft palate, full lips with a midline groove of the lower lip, grooved tongue with tongue tie, prominent mandible, congenital heart defects, arrhythmias, supernumerary nipples, splenomegaly, large dysplastic kidneys, cryptorchidism, hypospadias, skeletal abnormalities and

postaxial hexadactyly. Inheritance is X-linked. Some cases are caused by a mutation in the gene for glypican-3, which maps to Xq26. A second SGB syndrome locus (SGBS2 is located on Xp22).[6]

INBORN ERRORS OF METABOLISM

Glutaric Aciduria Type II (Multiple Acyl-CoA-Dehydrogenase Deficiencies)

In glutaric aciduria Type II, the deficiencies in mitochondrial enzymes (electron transfer flavoprotein or electron transfer ubiquinone oxoreductase) are inherited as autosomal recessive traits. This is a rare condition. Clinical features are prematurity, hypotonia, hepatomegaly, nephromegaly, craniofacial anomalies, rocker bottom feet, anterior abdominal wall defects, and external genital anomalies. An odor of sweaty feet may be present. Within 24 hours, there is severe hypoglycemia but no ketosis, a metabolic acidosis with an increased anion gap, and mild hyperammonemia. Organic acids are elevated in the urine, cerebrospinal fluid, and blood. Renal cystic dysplasia occurs in many cases.[25] Prenatal diagnosis may be possible by assaying the enzyme in amniocytes or elevated glutaric acid in amniotic fluid. Prenatal ultrasonography may show enlarged cystic kidneys. Treatment is unsuccessful, and death occurs in days to months.

Zellweger Cerebrohepatorenal Syndrome

The clinical features of Zellweger cerebrohepatorenal syndrome, an autosomal recessive condition, are similar to those of glutaric aciduria Type II. In addition, there may be nystagmus, cataracts (sometimes oil droplets), pigmentary retinopathy, optic disc pallor, and stippled epiphyses of patella and acetabulum. There is no abnormal odor. The kidneys are enlarged. All peroxisomal functions are abnormal. Cortical renal cysts, brain heterotopias, abnormal gyri, absent corpus callosum, and micronodular cirrhosis are seen at post-mortem examination. Prenatal diagnosis is possible by enzyme assays in amniocytes or in chorionic villus cells. Most affected infants die by the age of 6 months, but those with a milder form survive into their teens with deafness, retardation, and seizures.

Carbohydrate-Deficient Glycoprotein Syndrome

Multiple renal microcysts are found in the carbohydrate-deficient glycoprotein syndrome.[21] There is multisystem involvement with olivopontocerebellar atrophy, retinitis pigmentosa, testicular atrophy, hypothyroidism, and immune deficiency. Several glycoproteins are deficient in their carbohydrate moieties. Inheritance is autosomal recessive, and the prognosis is variable.

> **MAJOR POINTS**
>
> - Definition of polycystic renal disease.
> - Many cysts in both kidneys.
> - There is no dysplasia.
> - There is continuity between glomeruli and calyces.
> - The kidneys may be very large.

REFERENCES

1. Allanson JE, Hunter AGW, Mettler GS, Jiminez C. Renal tubular dysgenesis: a not uncommon autosomal recessive syndrome. A review. Am J Med Genet 1992;43:811–814.

2. Atiyeh B, Husmann D, Baun M. Contralateral renal abnormalities in multicystic-dysplastic kidney disease. J Pediatr 1992;121:65–67.

3. Bernstein J. The multicystic kidney and hereditary renal adysplasia. Am J Kidney Dis 1991;17:495–496.

4. Bernstein J. Glomerulocystic kidney disease – nosological considerations. Pediatr Nephrol 1993;7:464–470.

5. Bernstein J, Chandra M, Cresswell J, et al. Renal-hepatic-pancreatic dysplasia: a syndrome reconsidered. Am J Med Genet 1987;26:391–403.

6. Brzustowicz LM, Farrell S, Khan MB, et al. Mapping of a new SGBS locus to chromosome Xp22 in a family with a severe form of Simpson–Golabi–Behmel syndrome. Am J Hum Genet 1999;65:779–783.

7. Cobben JM, Breuning MH, Schoots C, et al. Congenital hepatic fibrosis in autosomal dominant polycystic kidney disease. Kidney Int 1990;38:880–885.

8. Choyke PL, Siegel MJ, Oz O, et al. Nonmalignant renal disease in pediatric patients with Beckwith–Wiedemann syndrome. Am J Roentgenol 1998;171:733–737.

9. Cook JA, Oliver K, Mueller RF, et al. A cross-sectional study of renal involvement in tuberous sclerosis. J Med Genet 1996;33:480–484.

10. Donaldson MDC, Warner AA, Trompeter RS, et al. Familial juvenile nephronophthisis, Jeune's syndrome and associated disorders. Arch Dis Child 1985;60:426–434.

11. Egli F, Stalder G. Malformations of kidney and urinary tract in common chromosomal aberrations: I. Clinical studies. Humangenetik 1973;18:1–15.

12. Fraser FC, Lytwyn A. Spectrum of anomalies in the Meckel syndrome, or: "Maybe there is a malformation syndrome with at least one constant anomaly." Am J Med Genet 1981;9:63–73.

13. Holmes LB. Prevalence, phenotypic heterogeneity and familial aspects of bilateral renal agenesis/dysgenesis. In: Liss AR (ed), *Genetics of Kidney Disorders*. Alan R. Liss, New York, 1989, pp. 1–11.

14. Joenje H, Patel KJ. The emerging genetic and molecular basis of Fanconi anaemia. Nature Rev Genet 2001;2:446–457.

15. Kumar S, Deffenbacher K, Marres HA, et al. Genomewide search and genetic localization of a second gene associated with autosomal dominant branchio-oto-renal syndrome: clinical and genetic implications. Am J Hum Genet 2000;66:1715–1720.

16. Moerman P, Fryns J-P, Sastrowijoto SH, et al. Hereditary renal adysplasia: new observations and hypotheses. Pediatr Pathol 1994;14:405–410.

17. Pryde PG, Sedman AB, Nugent CE, et al. Angiotensin-converting enzyme inhibitor fetopathy. J Am Soc Nephrol 1993;3:1575–1582.

18. Roume J, Genin E, Cormier-Daire V, et al. A gene for Meckel syndrome maps to chromosome 11q13. Am J Hum Genet 1998;63:1095–1101.

19. Salerno A, Kohlhase J, Kaplan BS. Townes–Brocks syndrome and renal dysplasia: a novel mutation in the SALL1 gene. Pediatr Nephrol 2000;14:25–28.

20. Schilke K, Schaefer F, Waldherr R, et al. A case of Perlman syndrome: fetal gigantism, renal dysplasia, and severe neurological deficits. Am J Med Genet 2000;91:29–33.

21. Strom EH, Stromine P, Westvik J, et al. Renal cysts in the carbohydrate-deficient glycoprotein syndrome. Pediatr Nephrol 1993;7:253–255.

22. Tarry WF, Duckett JW, Stephens FD. The Mayer–Rokitansky syndrome: pathogenesis, classification and management. J Urol 1986;136:648–652.

23. van Slegtenhorst M, Nellist M, Nagelkerken B, et al. Interaction between hamartin and tuberin, the TSC1 and TSC2 gene products. Hum Mol Genet 1998;7:1053–1057.

24. Wacksman J, Phipps L. Report of the multicystic kidney registry: preliminary findings. J Urol 1993;150:1870–1872.

25. Wilson GN, de Chadarevian J-P, Kaplan P, et al. Glutaric aciduria type II: review of the phenotype and report of an unusual glomerulopathy. Am J Med Genet 1989;32:395–401.

SUGGESTED READING

Bingham C, Ellard S, Cole TR, et al. Solitary functioning kidney and diverse genital tract malformations associated with hepatocyte nuclear factor-1beta mutations. Kidney Int 2002;61:1243–1251.

Coppin B, Moore I, Hatchwell E. Extending the overlap of three congenital overgrowth syndromes. Clin Genet 1997;51:375–378.

Kaplan BS, Kaplan P, Ruchelli E. Hereditary and congenital malformations of the kidneys. Perinat Clin North Am 1992;19:197.

Pohl M, Bhatnagar V, Mendoza SA, et al. Toward an etiological classification of developmental disorders of the kidney and upper urinary tract. Kidney Int 2002;61:10–19.

Woolf AS, Feather SA, Bingham C. Recent insights into kidney diseases associated with glomerular cysts. Pediatr Nephrol 2002;17:229–235.

Disorders of Renal Tubular Function

BERNARD S. KAPLAN, M.B., B.Ch.

INTRODUCTION

Prenatal

Some renal tubular disorders may be suspected and confirmed *in utero*. A prenatal diagnosis, however, requires chorionic villus sampling or amniocentesis. Therefore, this can only be performed after the diagnosis of the condition in an older sibling.

Neonatal

A diagnosis of a renal tubular disorder cannot be made without an appreciation of normal renal maturation. Premature newborns (and even full-term newborns) can waste sodium and chloride and have variable combinations of aminoaciduria, glucosuria, phosphaturia, impaired potassium excretion, reduced reabsorptive capacity for sodium bicarbonate, and an inability to concentrate the urine maximally. In healthy newborns, these are transient aberrations that are usually isolated and do not cause problems. An exception is the low bicarbonate threshold in preterm infants that may cause a mild metabolic acidosis during the first few months of life. Very low-birth-weight newborns may have non-oliguric hyperkalemia, in part secondary to decreased Na^+K^+-ATPase activity, which increases with maturation. Therefore, except in specific circumstances, it is not necessary to embark on a full-scale evaluation (Box 30-1).

Postnatally, the possibility of a tubular disorder may arise when abnormal blood gas and electrolyte results are obtained. The initial manifestations of a renal tubular disorder may not include all the findings associated with the disorder. Three constellations of fluid and electrolyte

Box 30-1   Metabolic Causes of Jaundice in the Newborn

- Hereditary fructose intolerance (HFI)
- Galactosemia
- Tyrosinemia type 1

imbalances should alert a neonatologist to the possibility of a disorder of renal tubular function. The combination of *metabolic acidosis*, *hyperkalemia*, and *hyponatremia* is seen in renal dysplasias, obstructive uropathy (especially if complicated by a urinary tract infection), pseudohypoaldosteronism and congenital adrenal hyperplasia, can present with these abnormalities. Metabolic acidosis, *hypokalemia*, and *hypophosphatemia* are the characteristic findings seen in patients with the renal tubular Fanconi syndrome. *Metabolic alkalosis*, hypokalemia, and hyponatremia occur in the Bartter syndromes.

Important clinical clues for the presence of a renal tubular disorder are poor feeding, unexplained vomiting, dehydration, failure to thrive, drowsiness, irritability, tetany, seizures, and unexplained icterus. Isolated proximal renal tubular acidosis (RTA) is uncommon, and the need for large quantities of bicarbonate to correct a hyperchloremic metabolic acidosis is a clue to the diagnosis. Fructose intolerance and galactosemia must be considered in a jaundiced newborn that has Fanconi syndrome. Hypophosphatemia and renal phosphate wasting are manifestations of X-linked hypophosphatemic rickets, but it is uncommon for this to be diagnosed in a newborn. Hyperchloremic metabolic acidosis with a decrease in the unmeasured anion gap and in the absence of diarrhea raises the possibility of distal RTA. Distal RTA rarely presents in the neonatal period, however. Pseudohypoaldosteronism, Bartter syndromes, and renal adysplasias must be considered in newborns with severe hyponatremia and renal salt wasting. Infants with Bartter syndrome are hypokalemic, whereas those with renal adysplasia, pseudohypoaldosteronism, and the renal tubular hyperkalemia syndromes are hyperkalemic. Hematuria, renal calculi, and nephrocalcinosis with hypercalciuria can occur in newborns with and without prolonged use of furosemide. Primary hyperoxaluria type 1 may present in the newborn period with acute renal failure and nephrocalcinosis.[11]

Infants and Children

Important clues to the presence of a renal tubular disorder in infants and children, in addition to any of the above, are rickets, polydipsia, and polyuria. There are also symptoms and signs that are specific for different syndromes.

Examples are photophobia and retinopathy in cystinosis, Kaiser–Fleisher rings in Wilson disease, hepatocellular carcinoma in tyrosinosis type I.

RENAL FANCONI SYNDROME OF PROXIMAL TUBULAR DYSFUNCTION

Renal Fanconi syndrome is characterized by generalized proximal renal tubular dysfunction with impaired net reabsorption of amino acids, bicarbonate, glucose, phosphate, urate, sodium, potassium, magnesium, calcium, and low-molecular-weight proteins. Renal excretion of these solutes and water is increased, and the serum concentrations of some are variably reduced. Hypophosphatemia results in vitamin D-resistant rickets, and bicarbonaturia causes a hyperchloremic metabolic acidosis. The clinical manifestations of renal Fanconi syndrome may include polyuria, dehydration, metabolic acidosis, and glycosuria. These features are often asynchronous. Growth retardation and rickets mostly occur later in infancy. (Table 30-1.)

Cystinosis

Affected individuals appear normal at birth, and develop manifestations of the renal Fanconi syndrome between 6 and 12 months of age. The diagnosis should be considered if there are features of the renal Fanconi syndrome in a patient with combinations of failure to thrive, photophobia, and rickets (Box 30-2). Inheritance is autosomal recessive. There is defective lysosomal transport of cystine. The cystinosis gene, *CTNS*, maps to

Table 30-1   Causes of Proximal Renal Tubular Dysfunction

Idiopathic Fanconi Syndrome	
Inherited causes	• Cystinosis, hereditary fructose intolerance
	• Galactosemia, tyrosinemia (type I)
	• Oculocerebrorenal syndrome (Lowe syndrome), Fanconi–Bickel syndrome
	• Mitochondrial cytopathies[5]
Toxins	• Cadmium, lead, mercury, platinum, uranium
Medications	• Aminoglycosides, cisplatin, ifosfamide, 6-mercaptopurine, outdated tetracycline
Immunologic injury of the proximal tubules	• Interstitial nephritis • Renal transplantation • Malignancies
Immunological (mainly in adults)	• Multiple myeloma, amyloidosis, light-chain nephropathy, benign monoclonal gammopathy

- Renal Fanconi syndrome
- Rickets
- Growth failure
- Hypothyroidism
- Photophobia
- Distal myopathy, cardiomyopathy
- Impairments in spatial processing
- End-stage renal failure usually by 10 years if not treated with cysteamine

chromosome 17p13, and encodes an integral membrane protein, cystinosin.[32] Cystinosis can be diagnosed *in utero* by cystine measurements in chorionic villi by 9 weeks of age.[30] Early and adequate treatment with oral cysteamine retards progression to end-stage renal failure, and administration of 0.55% cysteamine eyedrops from 1 year of age dissolves the corneal cystine crystals.[12] Although cystinosis does not recur after renal transplantation, patients may have many other extra-renal complications (Box 30-3).[12]

Hereditary Fructose Intolerance

Hereditary fructose intolerance (HFI) presents in newborns fed sucrose or fructose in formula, antibiotics, fruit juices, or honey. The symptoms are poor feeding, vomiting, and failure to thrive.[2] The diagnosis can be made by molecular analysis of the aldolase-B gene in blood.[6] Inheritance is autosomal recessive.

Galactosemia

Classic galactosemia deficiency can manifest in neonates with vomiting, diarrhea, hyperbilirubinemia with jaundice, hepatomegaly, ascites, and *E. coli* sepsis a few days after starting milk ingestion. Cataracts are

| Box 30-3 | **Post-Transplant Extra-Renal Complications of Cystinosis** |

- Progressive, distal myopathy, muscle wasting
- Primary hypogonadism in males
- Swallowing difficulty
- Retinal blindness
- Diabetes mellitus
- Pulmonary dysfunction
- Pancreatic exocrine dysfunction
- Brain calcifications
- CNS deterioration

| Box 30-4 | **Clinical Features of Tyrosinemia Type 1** |

Failure to thrive	Hepatomegaly
Fever	Acute liver failure
Fanconi syndrome	Hepatic carcinoma
Renal rickets	Ascites
Vomiting	Coagulopathy
Diarrhea	Chronic liver failure
Jaundice	

occasionally detectable by slit-lamp examination in neonates. This autosomal recessive disease is caused by deficient activity of galactose-1-phosphate uridyl transferase (GALT) as a result of mutations at the *GALT* gene on chromosome 17q.[33] Two other autosomal recessively inherited disorders of galactose metabolism (transferase and epimerase deficiency) occur more rarely. Newborn screening programs include tests for detection of galactosemia. The diagnosis is suggested by demonstrating increased concentrations of galactose in blood and urine and confirmed by showing deficient red blood cell galactose 1-phosphate uridyltransferase (or galactokinase).

Tyrosinemia Type 1

Tyrosinemia type 1 is caused by deficiency in the gene for fumarylacetoacetate hydrolase on chromosome 15q23-q25. Tyrosinemia type 1 is an important cause of neonatal jaundice, renal Fanconi syndrome and hepatocellular carcinoma (Box 30-4).[34] It is also one of the causes of unexplained hypertension and of bilateral nephromegaly. Patients can be treated successfully with 2-(2-nitro-4-trifluoromethylbenzoyl)-1,3 cyclohexane dione (NTBC), together with dietary restriction of phenylalanine and tyrosine. This may prevent liver failure, but not hepatocellular carcinoma.[10]

Renal Glycosuria

Renal glycosuria is autosomal recessive with mild glycosuria in heterozygotes. There is a low renal threshold for glucose, with urine losses of glucose despite normal blood glucose concentrations. Intermittent or constant renal glycosuria can be detected in newborns that have the rare and possibly autosomal recessive condition of glucose and galactose malabsorption.

CYSTINURIA

In cystinuria, there is increased renal excretion of cystine, ornithine, arginine, and lysine, and the intestinal absorption of these four compounds is decreased. Renal calculi form because of increased excretion of cystine that is poorly soluble at normal urine pH. Cystine stones are often resistant to lithotripsy. There are three distinct phenotypes based on the urinary excretion of cystine in obligate heterozygotes: Type I (silent carriers); Type II (marked elevation); and Type III (mild elevation). All three types of cystinuria are clinically the same – autosomal recessive, and allelic. Cystinuria type I is caused by a mutation in the *SLC3A1* amino acid transporter gene on chromosome 2p16.3. Cystinuria II is incompletely recessive, with a mutation on 19q13.1. Cystine stones often can be dissolved and new stones often prevented by maintaining a high fluid intake. Regular treatment with penicillamine is effective, and side effects are not severe enough to prevent its use. However, an early diagnosis is important, and cystinuria should be considered in all persons, of any age, who form urinary stones.

RENAL TUBULAR ACIDOSIS (RTA)

Primary RTA is characterized by chronic hyperchloremic metabolic acidosis associated with an inability to acidify the urine. It may be a primary disorder, or secondary to acquired renal injury. Primary RTA is not associated with the renal Fanconi syndrome. Primary RTA is separated into three main types:[24] proximal RTA (pRTA) (Type 2); distal RTA or 'classic' RTA (Type 1); and hyperkalemic RTA (Type 4).

Primary Proximal Renal Tubular Acidosis

Proximal renal tubular acidosis (pRTA) is an integral feature of the renal Fanconi syndrome, and primary pRTA is extremely uncommon. pRTA is the result of an inability to reabsorb filtered bicarbonate in the proximal tubule with bicarbonate wasting and hyperchloremic metabolic acidosis and normal distal tubular acidification. Therefore, when the filtered bicarbonate is reclaimed up to the maximal renal tubular reabsorptive capacity for a patient with pRTA, the urine pH is appropriate for the severity of the metabolic acidosis, with values below 5.3. When pRTA occurs as an isolated defect, it is usually transient.

Distal Renal Tubular Acidosis

Clinical manifestations of the distal renal tubular acidosis (dRTA) are anorexia, failure to thrive, hypotonia, a persistently low serum bicarbonate, elevated serum chloride, inappropriately high urine pH, and, in some cases, nephrocalcinosis. Additional findings are decreased urinary excretion of titratable acid, NH_4^+ (ammonium), and citrate. Some patients have congenital high-frequency nerve deafness. Untreated patients develop rickets.[7] dRTA is often considered in the differential diagnosis of a neonate with a non-anion gap acidosis, but there are few reports of dTRA in neonates.[7,24] The possibility of distal RTA can be inferred from calculating the rate of excretion of NH_4^+. This can be determined indirectly by calculating the urinary net charge or urine anion gap:[14] $Na^+ + K^+ + NH_4^+ = Cl^- + 80$. The kidney is not the cause of the acidosis if the Cl^- (chloride) is greater than the sum of the Na^+ (sodium) + K^+ (potassium). If the $Na^+ + K^+$ is greater than Cl^- (chloride), then the urinary NH_4^+ may be less than 80 mmol per day, in keeping with dRTA.[8] The diagnosis of dRTA is often made erroneously in patients with a hyperchloremic metabolic acidosis who have an 'inappropriate' urine pH over 6, and who have diarrhea.[17] Regardless of whether a transient or permanent form of distal RTA is suspected, adequate amounts of alkali, either as bicarbonate or citrate, in doses of 2–3 mEq/kg/day are required to maintain a normal serum bicarbonate concentration.[16] This can be withdrawn after several months to challenge the diagnosis, or the infant can be allowed to outgrow the dose. Challenging with an ammonium chloride loading test is not necessary because the diagnosis can be inferred from indirect tests such as the urine anion gap.

There are at least two autosomal recessively inherited forms of dRTA. In dRTA *without* nerve deafness, the mutated gene is located on chromosome 7q33-34; the gene product is the 116-kDa B-subunit of the apical pump (*ATP6B1*). dRTA *with* nerve deafness[20] is caused by mutations in *ATP6B1*, located on chromosome 2p13, and encoding the B-subunit of the apical proton pump mediating distal nephron acid secretion.

BARTTER SYNDROME

Bartter syndrome is a congenital chronic tubular disorder characterized by hypokalemic metabolic alkalosis, polyuria, salt wasting, hyperkaluria, and hyperaldosteronism. There is resistance to the pressor effect of angiotensin, juxtaglomerular apparatus hyperplasia and increased renal renin production. Some patients have hypercalciuria and nephrocalcinosis. There are at least three clinical subtypes of the Bartter syndromes with marked phenotypic variations within each subtype. Each subtype, however, has hypokalemic metabolic alkalosis and Antenatzl Hyperczlciuric Varizat (HP/BS) renal salt wasting (Box 30-5).

Antenatal Hypercalciuric Variant (H Ps/aBS)

The antenatal hypercalciuric variant is a life-threatening neonatal disorder. There are combinations of polyhydramnios, premature delivery, hypokalemia, hypercalciuria, metabolic alkalosis, fever, vomiting, diarrhea and failure to thrive, hyposthenuria, and nephrocalcinosis. Inheritance is autosomal recessive, with mutations in the gene for the furosemide-sensitive NaK-2Cl-cotransporter NKCC2 (*SLC12A1*) or the inwardly rectifying potassium channel, subfamily J, member 1, ROMK (*KCNJ1*) on chromosome 11q24.[18] Because classic Bartter syndrome can also be caused by a mutation in either of these genes, the antenatal and classic forms may be different manifestations of severity of the same disorder. In addition, there are neonates who have homozygous gene mutations linked to chromosome 1p31, which do not respond to indomethacin treatment, and have a more severe variant with marked delays in growth and motor development, chronic renal failure, and congenital deafness.[19] There is no cure for Bartter syndrome. Treatment with inhibitors of prostaglandin synthesis improves polyuria, corrects biochemical abnormalities, and permits satisfactory growth and development. Nephrocalcinosis may not improve.[26]

Classic Bartter Syndrome (cBS)

The clinical phenotype varies from episodes of neonatal severe volume depletion with hypotension and hypokalemia in mildly symptomatic patients diagnosed in adolescence. Serum magnesium levels are normal (Box 30-6).

Gitelman Variant of Bartter Syndrome (GS)

The Gitelman variant usually does not present in neonates.[3] Hypocalciuria and hypomagnesemia are

specific clinical features of Gitelman syndrome. The Gitelman variant is caused by mutations in the gene for the thiazide-sensitive NaCl-cotransporter NCCT (*SLC12A3*) of the distal tubule located on chromosome 16q13.

RENAL TUBULAR HYPERKALEMIA

Causes of renal tubular hyperkalemia (RTH) are shown in Box 30-7. RTH is defined by an inappropriately low urine potassium concentration in the face of hyperkalemia, renal salt wasting, and metabolic acidosis.[27] The serum creatinine concentration is often increased because of volume depletion as in pseudohypoaldosteronism or congenital adrenal hyperplasia, reduced nephron mass as in renal adysplasia, and obstruction with posterior urethral valves.

Pseudohypoaldosteronism

There are two syndromes of aldosterone resistance: pseudohypoaldosteronism type I and pseudohypoaldosteronism type II.[15] Furthermore, there are two clinically and genetically distinct types of type I pseudohypoaldosteronism: renal pseudohypoaldosteronism and multiple organ pseudohypoaldosteronism.[31] Pseudohypoaldosteronism may be inherited as an autosomal dominant and as an autosomal recessive trait. In the dominant form of pseudohypoaldosteronism type I there are mutations in the gene *MLR*, encoding the mineralocorticoid receptor. In the recessive form of pseudohypoaldosteronism type I there are mutations in the genes *SNCC1A*, *SNCC1B*, and *SCNN1G*, which encode subunits of the epithelial Na+ channel.[28]

Renal Pseudohypoaldosteronism Type I

Renal pseudohypoaldosteronism type I usually presents in early infancy, and is characterized by diminished renal tubular responsiveness to aldosterone with hyponatremia, hyperkalemia, markedly elevated plasma aldosterone, and hyper-reninemia. The clinical expression ranges from severely affected patients who die in infancy to asymptomatic individuals. Symptomatic patients are treated with sodium supplementation, which usually is no longer necessary by the age of 2 years.

Multiple Organ Pseudohypoaldosteronism Type I

Multiple organ pseudohypoaldosteronism type I is characterized by impaired responsiveness to aldosterone in salivary and sweat glands, renal tubules, and colonic mucosal cells. The course is protracted, with life-threatening episodes of salt wasting.

Pseudohypoaldosteronism Type II (Gordon Hyperkalemia-Hypertension Syndrome)

The features are hyperkalemia, despite a normal glomerular filtration rate, hypertension, variable mild hyperchloremia, metabolic acidosis, and suppressed plasma renin activity.[29] The metabolic abnormalities are corrected by treatment with thiazide diuretics. There are no reports of neonatal presentation.

CONGENITAL NEPHROGENIC DIABETES INSIPIDUS (NDI)

NDI is caused by either congenital or acquired insults to the kidneys (Box 30-8). In X-linked NDI, there is insensitivity of the distal nephron to the antidiuretic effect of vasopressin. This results in an inability to concentrate urine, and the consequent excretion of large quantities of hypotonic urine.[4,35] Affected neonates may be irritable, feed poorly, fail to gain weight, and have unexplained dehydration and fevers. Serum concentrations of sodium, chloride, creatinine, and blood urea nitrogen (BUN) are elevated, and serum levels of vasopressin are normal or increased. There is a blunted response of plasma factor VIII, von Willebrand factor, and plasminogen activator after administration of 1-desamino-8-D-arginine vasopressin (DDAVP). Treatment with hydrochlorothiazide (3 mg/kg/day) and amiloride

---

<table>
<tr><td>**Box 30-8**</td><td>**Causes of Nephrogenic Diabetes Insipidus (NDI)**</td></tr>
</table>

- *Electrolyte abnormalities*: hypokalemia, hypocalcemia
- *Medications*: aminoglycosides, amphotericin B, lithium
- *Renal defects*: tubular interstitial inflammation, obstruction, dysplasia
- *Congenital NDI*: X-linked, autosomal recessive

(0.3 mg/kg/day) may be preferable to hydrochlorothiazide and indomethacin because indomethacin can cause gastric bleeding.[25] Treatment can prevent dehydration, electrolyte imbalances, cerebral calcification and seizures, and result in normal growth, but patients continue to have polydipsia and polyuria.

About 90% of patients with inherited NDI have the X-linked form caused by mutations in the arginine vasopressin receptor 2 gene (*AVPR2*) that codes for the V2 receptor located in chromosomal region Xq28.[4,25] Males are much more severely affected than females. In fewer than 10% of the families, the inheritance of NDI is either autosomal recessive or autosomal dominant.[22] Mutations occur in the aquaporin-2 gene (*AQP2*) on chromosome 12q13 that codes for the vasopressin-sensitive water channel.[13] The reliability of prenatal diagnosis of the X-linked form of NDI is about 96%.

HYPOMAGNESEMIA

Hypomagnesemia is most often detected in patients on intensive care units. Hypomagnesemia causes neuromuscular irritability, cardiac arrhythmias, and increased sensitivity to digoxin. Refractory hypokalemia and hypocalcemia can be caused by concomitant hypomagnesemia, and can be corrected with magnesium therapy. There are several rare inherited and many acquired causes of renal magnesium wasting, as well as gastrointestinal causes (Table 30-2).[1,9]

Secondary Hypocalcemia

Hypomagnesemia with secondary hypocalcemia is characterized by early onset, the inheritance is autosomal recessive, and the mutation is linked to chromosome 9q12-22.2.[36] Affected individuals have severe hypomagnesemia and hypocalcemia soon after birth. This causes seizures and tetany, and requires life-long magnesium supplementation. The disorder is caused by a defect in the intestinal absorption of magnesium.

Isolated Renal Magnesium Wasting

Hypomagnesemia with isolated renal magnesium wasting is autosomal recessive, with linkage to chromosome 11q23.[23] Some of these individuals have tetany and convulsions, but others may be asymptomatic.

Hypercalciuria and Nephrocalcinosis

Hypomagnesemia with hypercalciuria and nephrocalcinosis is autosomal recessive.[21] The mutation of the

Table 30-2   Causes of Hypomagnesemia

Causes	Inherited	Acquired
Renal	• Hypomagnesemia with isolated renal magnesium wasting • Hypomagnesemia with hypercalciuria and nephrocalcinosis • Variable hypomagnesemia with hypoparathyroidism • Gitelman syndrome	• Post-obstructive diuresis • Post-acute tubular necrosis • Renal transplantation • Interstitial nephropathy
Medications		• Aminoglycosides, cisplatin, diuretics, amphotericin b, cyclosporine, pentamidine, foscarnet
Gastrointestinal	• Hypomagnesemia with secondary hypocalcemia	• Protein-calorie malnutrition • Mg-free intravenous fluids • Mg-free total parenteral nutrition • Chronic watery diarrhea • Steatorrhea • Short bowel syndrome • Bowel fistula • Continuous nasogastric suctioning
Non-renal		• Diabetes mellitus • Lymphoma

claudin 16 gene, which codes for a tight junctional protein (Paracellin-1) that regulates paracellular Mg^{2+} transport in the loop of Henle, is linked to chromosome 3q27.

Variable Hypomagnesemia with Hypoparathyroidism

Variable hypomagnesemia with hypoparathyroidism can present with transient neonatal seizures.[37] The inheritance is autosomal dominant. Inactivating mutations of the extracellular Ca^{2+}/Mg^{2+}-sensing receptor (*Casr*) gene are linked to chromosome 3q13.3-21.

MAJOR POINTS

- A low serum bicarbonate concentration in an infant or child is often the result of technical errors. These include:
  - using a tight tourniquet;
  - obtaining blood by squeezing a finger stick; and
  - not assaying the sample expeditiously.
- An infant or child who has failure to thrive, the combination of a low serum bicarbonate concentration, high serum chloride concentration, and an inappropriate urine pH, is more likely to have diarrhea than dRTA.
- Fructose-containing foods must be withdrawn from the diet as soon as HFI is suspected.
- In galactosemia, milk and milk-containing products must be withdrawn from the diet.
- Similar features to Bartter syndrome occur with loop diuretic treatment and congenital chloride diarrhea.

Gitelman Syndrome

Gitelman syndrome is a recessive form of hypomagnesemia caused by mutations in the distal tubular NaCl cotransporter gene, *SLC12A3*, at chromosome 16q13.

REFERENCES

1. al-Ghamdi SM, Cameron EC, Sutton RA. Magnesium deficiency: pathophysiologic and clinical overview. Am J Kidney Dis 1994;24:737-752.

2. Ali M, Rellos P, Cox TM. Hereditary fructose intolerance. J Med Genet 1998;35:353-365.

3. Bettinelli A, Ciarmatori S, Cesareo L, et al. Phenotypic variability in Bartter syndrome type I. Pediatr Nephrol 2000;14:940-945.

4. Bichet DG, Oksche A, Rosenthal W. Congenital nephrogenic diabetes insipidus. J Am Soc Nephrol 1997;8:1951-1958.

5. Biervliet JPAM, Bruinvis L, Ketting D, et al. Hereditary mitochondrial myopathy with lactic aciemia, a De Toni-Fanconi-Debre syndrome, and a defective respiratory chain in voluntary striated muscle. Pediatr Res 1977;11:1088-1093.

6. Brooks CC, Tolan DR. Association of the widespread A 149 P hereditary fructose intolerance mutation with newly identified sequence polymorphisms in the aldolase gene. Am J Med Genet 1993;52:835-840.

7. Caldas A, Broyer M, Dechaux M, et al. Primary distal tubular acidosis in childhood: clinical study and long-term follow-up of 28 patients. J Pediatr 1992;121:233-241.

8. Carlisle EJF, Donnelly SM, Halperin ML. Renal tubular acidosis (RTA): recognize the ammonium defect and pHorget the urine pH. Pediatr Nephrol 1991;5:242.

9. Cole DE, Quamme GA. Inherited disorders of renal magnesium handling. J Am Soc Nephrol 2000;11:1937-1947.

10. Croffie JM, Gupta SK, Chong SK, Fitzgerald JF. Tyrosinemia type 1 should be suspected in infants with severe coagulopathy even in the absence of other signs of liver failure. Pediatrics 1999;103:675-678.

11. Ellis SR, Hulton SA, McKiernan PJ, et al. Combined liver-kidney transplantation for primary hyperoxaluria type 1 in young children. Nephrol Dial Transplant 2001;16:348-354.

12. Gahl WA, Thoene JG, Schneider JA. Cystinosis. N Engl J Med 2002;347:111-121.

13. Goji K, Kuwahara M, Gu Y, et al. Novel mutations in aquaporin-2 gene in female siblings with nephrogenic diabetes insipidus: evidence of disrupted water channel function. J Clin Endocrinol Metab 1998;83:3205-3209.

14. Goldstein MB, Bear R, Richardson RM, et al. The urine anion gap: a clinically useful index of ammonium excretion. Am J Med Sci 1986;282:198-202.

15. Hanukoglu A. Type I pseudohypoaldosteronism includes two clinically and genetically distinct entities with either renal or multiple organ defects. J Clin Endocrinol Metab 1991;73:936-944.

16. Igarashi T, Sekine Y, Kawato H, et al. Transient neonatal distal renal tubular acidosis with secondary hyperparathyroidism. Pediatr Nephrol 1992;6:267-269.

17. Izraeli S, Rachmel A, Frishberg Y, et al. Transient renal acidification defect during acute infantile diarrhea: the role of urinary sodium. J Pediatr 1990;117:711-716.

18. Jeck N, Derst C, Wischmeyer E, et al. Functional heterogeneity of ROMK mutations linked to hyperprostaglandin E syndrome. Kidney Int 2001;59:1803-1811.

19. Jeck N, Reinalter SC, Henne T, et al. Hypokalemic salt-losing tubulopathy with chronic renal failure and sensorineural deafness. Pediatrics 2001;108:E5.

20. Karet FE. Inherited distal renal tubular acidosis. Am Soc Nephrol 2002;13:2178-2184.

21. Kari JA, Farouq M, Alshaya HO. Familial hypomagnesemia with hypercalciuria and nephrocalcinosis. Pediatr Nephrol 2003;18:506-510.

22. Knoers NV, Deen PM. Molecular and cellular defects in nephrogenic diabetes insipidus. Pediatr Nephrol 2001;16:1146-1152.

23. Meij IC, Saar K, van den Heuvel LP, et al. Hereditary isolated renal magnesium loss maps to chromosome 11q23. Am J Hum Genet 1999;64:180-188.

24. McSherry E, Morris RC, Jr. Attainment of normal stature with alkali therapy in infants and children with classic renal tubular acidosis. J Clin Invest 1978;61:509-527.

25. Morello JP, Bichet DG. Nephrogenic diabetes insipidus. Annu Rev Physiol 2001;63:607-630.

26. Mourani CC, Sanjad SA, Akatcherian CY. Bartter syndrome in a neonate: early treatment with indomethacin. Pediatr Nephrol 200;14:143-145.

27. Rodriguez-Soriano J. Potassium homeostasis and its disturbances in children. Pediatr Nephrol 1995;9:364-374.

28. Rodriguez-Soriano J. New insights into the pathogenesis of renal tubular acidosis – from functional to molecular studies. Pediatr Nephrol 2000;14:1121-1136.

29. Schambelan M, Sebastian A, Rector FC, Jr. Mineralocorticoid-resistant renal hyperkalemia without salt wasting (type II pseudohypoaldosteronism): role of increased renal chloride reabsorption. Kidney Int 1981;19:716-727.

30. Smith ML, Pellett OL, Cass MM, et al. Prenatal diagnosis of cystinosis utilizing chorionic villus sampling. Prenat Diagn 1987;7:23-26.

31. Strautnieks SS, Thompson RJ, Gardiner RM, Chung E. A novel splice-site mutation in the gamma subunit of the epithelial sodium channel gene in three pseudohypoaldosteronism type 1 families. Nature Genet 1996;13:248-250.

32. Town M, Jean G, Cherqui S, et al. A novel gene encoding an integral membrane protein is mutated in nephropathic cystinosis. Nature Genet 1998;18:319-324.

33. Tyfield L, Reichardt J, Fridovich-Keil J, et al. Classical galactosemia and mutations at the galactose-1-phosphate uridyl transferase (GALT) gene. Hum Mutat 1999;13:417-430.

34. Vanden Eijnden S, Blum D, Clercx A, et al. Cutaneous porphyria in a neonate with tyrosinaemia type 1. Eur J Pediatr 2000;159:503-506.

35. van Lieburg AF, Knoers NV, Monnens LA. Clinical presentation and follow-up of 30 patients with congenital nephrogenic diabetes insipidus. J Am Soc Nephrol 1999;10:1958-1964.

36. Walder RY, Landau D, Meyer P, et al. Mutation of TRPM6 causes familial hypomagnesemia with secondary hypocalcemia. Nature Genet 2002;31:171-174.

37. Winter WE, Silverstein JH, Maclaren NK, et al. Autosomal dominant hypoparathyroidism with variable, age-dependent severity. J Pediatr 1983;103:387-390.

PART III

CHAPTER 31

Acute Renal Failure

JOSEPH T. FLYNN, M.D., M.S.

INTRODUCTION

Acute renal failure (ARF) is defined as the sudden suppression of normal kidney function so that the renal regulation of internal homeostasis is compromised.[20] ARF has a rapid onset, and is potentially reversible. This contrasts with chronic renal failure, which has a gradual onset, progresses over time, and is irreversible.

EPIDEMIOLOGY AND ETIOLOGY

The incidence of ARF in children is unknown. ARF constituted 7% of all referrals to a pediatric nephrology service over a 20-year period.[21] In the general pediatric population, ARF is uncommon. The incidence of ARF in neonates[1] and children in intensive care units is higher than in regular units (Box 31-1).

ARF is categorized by the degree of impairment of urine output, and by the underlying cause or mechanism. Categorization by the amount of urine output (Table 31-1) is important because this may impact on the clinical course: patients with non-oliguric ARF have lower complication rates and better survival than those with oliguric ARF. ARF can also be classified as pre-renal ARF, post-renal ARF, and intrinsic ARF. In pre-renal ARF, renal function is initially normal, but compromised renal perfusion leads to renal failure. Pre-renal ARF is reversible in its early stages, but can progress to intrinsic ARF because of compromise of renal perfusion and therefore must be treated promptly (Table 31-2). In post-renal ARF, the kidney function is initially normal but obstruction to urine flow causes ARF. This type of ARF is important to identify quickly because it typically reverses with relief of obstruction. However, post-renal ARF can also progress to intrinsic ARF if not corrected promptly (Table 31-3).

Intrinsic ARF occurs when the kidneys themselves are primarily affected by a process that causes loss of renal function. These processes include glomerular, tubular, interstitial and vascular disorders (Table 31-4). Acute tubular necrosis (ATN) is the final common pathway for ischemic, anoxic, toxic, or obstructive injury to the renal tubules. ATN is characterized by a rapid decline in glomerular filtration rate (GFR) and signs of tubular cell injury, including oliguria, anuria, polyuria, and electrolyte disorders. Important nephrotoxins are listed in Table 31-5.

PATHOGENESIS OF ARF

ARF results from insults to the kidney that primarily affect either renal blood flow or tubular function. Decreased renal blood flow results from renal vasoconstriction; the resultant renal ischemia leads to

---

Box 31-1   Patients at Increased Risk of Acute Renal Failure (ARF)

- Post-surgical patients
- Patients with sepsis
- Patients with underlying chronic renal disease
- Patients with cardiac disease
- Newborns requiring intensive care

---

decreased GFR. Possible mechanisms responsible for the vasoconstriction include adrenergic stimulation, failure of renal prostaglandin production, and increased angiotensin II formation. Tubular cell death is the other major mechanism responsible for producing ARF. Although the term 'acute tubular necrosis' is used clinically to describe the results of tubular cell injury, apoptosis (programmed cell death) is the major mechanism responsible for tubular cell death. The first wave of apoptosis occurs within a day of the acute insult; this leads to a loss of epithelial cells and exacerbation of renal dysfunction. The second wave of apoptosis occurs after 5–7 days, when regeneration and recovery have begun. This limits excessive proliferation and facilitates remodeling of the tubules. ARF appears to be initiated by vascular mechanisms, and seems to be maintained by tubular cell apoptosis once ARF is established.[14]

Reduction in GFR is a consequence of tubular obstruction by intraluminal debris (dead tubular cells or casts) and back-leak of glomerular filtrate into the peritubular capillaries. Proximal tubular dilatation, intraluminal casts, debris and tubular back-leak of glomerular filtrate have been demonstrated in clinical and experimental settings. These processes are interrelated in the complex pathogenesis of ARF (Figure 31-1).

CLINICAL ASPECTS OF ARF

The clinical course of ARF is divided into three phases (Box 31-2). In the initiation phase, ischemia, inflammation and/or toxic substances damage renal cells and the

---

Table 31-1   Categorization of ARF by Amount of Urine Output

Category	Child	Adult
Anuric	<0.2 ml/kg/h	<100 ml/day
Oliguric	<1.0 ml/kg/h	<400 ml/day
Non-oliguric	>1.0 ml/kg/h	>400 ml/day
High-output	>2.0 ml/kg/h	>400 ml/m^2/day

Table 31-2   Pre-Renal Causes of ARF in Children

Category	Cause
Volume depletion	• Severe diarrhea
	• Protracted vomiting
	• Osmotic diuresis
	• Diuretics
	• Extensive burns
	• Hemorrhage
Decreased effective blood volume	• Septic shock
	• Anaphylaxis
	• Nephrotic syndrome
Cardiac failure	• Anatomic malformation
	• Arrhythmia
	• Cardiomyopathy
	• Tamponade
	• Post-cardiac surgery

---

patient begins to display symptoms of ARF, such as a decrease in urine output. This phase is important to identify because intervention may prevent progression to established, intrinsic ARF.

Renal injury continues during the maintenance phase, producing additional damage. Oliguria and azotemia are invariably present, and ARF is considered established once this phase is entered. Renal function slowly returns to normal in the recovery phase of ARF. The onset of the recovery phase is often heralded by the development of a brisk diuresis.

Complications of ARF

Metabolic complications of ARF include hyperkalemia, metabolic acidosis, hyperphosphatemia, hypocalcemia, and uremia. With the exception of hyperkalemia,

---

Table 31-3   Post-Renal Causes of Acute Renal Failure in Children

Site	Cause
Kidney	• Ureteropelvic junction obstruction
	• Trauma
	• Nephrolithiasis (bilateral)
	• Neoplasm
Ureters	• Intra-abdominal neoplasms
	• Bilateral primary megaureter
	• Trauma
	• Retroperitoneal fibrosis
Bladder/urethra	• Posterior urethral valves
	• Nephrolithiasis
	• Foreign body
	• Neoplasm

Table 31-4	Intrinsic Causes of ARF in Children
Indication	**Symptom**
Glomerular	Post-infectious glomerulonephritis
	Lupus nephritis
	Henoch–Schönlein purpura
	IgA nephropathy
	Crescentic glomerulonephritis
	SBE-associated nephritis
Vascular/hemodynamic	Hemolytic-uremic syndrome
	Renal venous thrombosis
	Vasculitis
	Malignant hypertension
	Non-steroidal anti-inflammatory drugs (NSAIDs)
	ACE inhibitors
Tubular (ATN)	Uncorrected pre-renal or post-renal ARF
	Asphyxia/hypoxemia
	Obstruction by crystals – uric acid
	Medications
	Toxins
	Tumor-lysis syndrome
Interstitial nephritis	Allergic interstitial nephritis
	Malignant infiltration
	Pyelonephritis
	Sarcoidosis

SBE = subacute bacterial endocarditis; ATN = acute tubular necrosis.

most of these complications are not life-threatening. Systemic complications include fluid overload, hypertension, anemia, altered mental status, increased susceptibility to infection, bleeding, and gastrointestinal problems. Impaired immune function and indwelling lines and catheters have important roles in causing infection; this is the most common extra-renal complication, and is responsible for most deaths in ARF. Anemia can be caused by suppression of erythropoiesis, hemolysis, blood loss from hemorrhage or phlebotomy, and hemodilution. There is usually a leukocytosis, even in the absence of infection. A bleeding diathesis can develop from uremic platelet dysfunction, Factor VIII dysfunction, and thrombocytopenia.

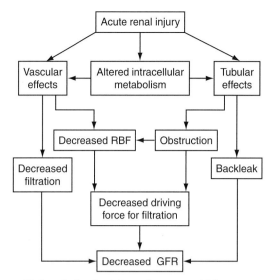

Figure 31-1   Pathophysiology of acute renal failure. RBF = renal blood flow.

Gastrointestinal manifestations range from uremic symptoms such as anorexia, nausea, and vomiting, to severe erosive gastrointestinal ulcers that may be secondary to stress. These ulcers may lead to significant gastrointestinal bleeding, and occur so frequently that the routine use of H_2-receptor blockers or other preventative measures are warranted.

Short- and Long-Term Outcome of ARF

The short-term mortality from ARF remains close to 50% of those patients who require dialysis, even in the most technologically advanced pediatric centers.[3,6] Patients typically die from the underlying cause of the ARF, or from failure of an organ other than the kidneys (Box 31-3).[8]

Few data are available on the long-term outcome of ARF in children. The study by Georgaki-Angelaki et al. is compromised by low patient numbers and the inclusion of children with many different causes of ARF.[12]

Table 31-5	ARF Caused by Toxins or Medications	
Toxins	Heavy metals	Lead, gold, platinum, mercury
	Chelating agents	EDTA
	Organic solvents	Carbon tetrachloride, ethylene glycol
	Crystals	Oxalic acid, uric acid
	Pigments	Hemoglobin, myoglobin
Antibiotics	Interstitial nephritis	Methicillin, ampicillin, amoxicillin, cephalosporins, fluoroquinolones
	Direct tubular damage	Aminoglycosides, amphotericin B
	Tubular obstruction by crystals	Acyclovir, cephalexin
	Unknown mechanism	Vancomycin
Other agents		Radiocontrast agents, ACE inhibitors, chemotherapeutic agents, NSAIDs, cyclosporine, tacrolimus

---

Box 31-2   Phases of ARF

- Initiation phase
- Maintenance phase
- Recovery phase

DIAGNOSTIC APPROACH TO ARF

The clinical approach to ARF begins with a careful history and physical examination. The patient's recent medical history should be reviewed, with particular attention to the use of medications, the presence of infection, and trauma. The past medical history should be reviewed to determine whether there are underlying or predisposing conditions. A careful assessment of the fluid intake and urine output must be made to assist in management. Appropriate orders should be given for the strict monitoring of fluid intake and output.

The physical exam should begin with review of the patient's vital signs, particularly weight, blood pressure, and heart rate. Body weight should be obtained at least daily, and even twice daily in infants or in patients with polyuric acute renal failure. The general apperance of the patient should be assessed for pallor or edema. Careful pulmonary and cardiac examinations should be performed to determine the degree of fluid overload (if present), and how well the patient is being perfused. The abdominal examination may help in diagnosis as well, particularly if a mass or hepatosplenomegaly is present.

Laboratory studies should include serum concentrations of electrolytes, blood urea nitrogen (BUN), creatinine, calcium, phosphorus, albumin, and uric acid. Hemoglobin, hematocrit, and platelet counts are determined. Liver enzyme tests are indicated if there is a history of anoxia or hepatic disease. Serologic studies should be obtained if indicated by signs of acute glomerulonephritis. Urine studies are always indicated. These should include urinalysis, sodium, creatinine,

---

Box 31-3   Predictors of Poor Prognosis in Children with ARF

- Presence and duration of anuria
- Persistent hypotension and/or hypovolemia
- Multi-organ system failure
- Coma
- Severe trauma
- Need for mechanical ventilation

Table 31-6   Differential Diagnosis of ARF According to Urinary Indices

	Pre-Renal ARF	Intrinsic ARF
Urine sodium (mmol/l)	<10	>10
Specific gravity	>1.018	<1.010
Urine:serum creatinine ratio	>40	<40
FENa$^+$		
Children (%)	<1	>2
Neonates (%)	<3	>3
Urine osmolality (mOsm/kg)	>500	<350
Sediment	Usually normal	Active with many casts

FENa$^+$ = fractional excretion of sodium; Na$^+$ = sodium.

and osmolality. The fractional excretion of sodium (FENa$^+$) can then be calculated:

$$FENa^+ = \frac{Urine/Serum\ Sodium \times 100}{Urine/Serum\ Creatinine}$$

The results of the FENa$^+$ and other laboratory studies can be used to help differentiate between pre-renal and intrinsic types of ARF (Table 31-6).

The two most helpful imaging studies are chest radiography and renal ultrasound, which should be obtained in all patients with ARF. Chest radiography helps to assess whether there is significant fluid overload. Renal ultrasound is most useful diagnostically, especially if urinary obstruction or renal venous thrombosis are being considered as possible causes of the ARF. A full abdominal ultrasound or computed tomography of the chest or abdomen should be obtained as indicated by the history and physical examination.

INTERVENTION TO PREVENT OR AMELIORATE THE PROGRESSION OF EARLY ARF

It is occasionally possible to intervene early in the course of ARF to prevent progression to established renal failure, and thereby avoid renal replacement therapy. In other patients at high risk of developing ARF, it may be possible to avert the development of ARF if the predisposing factors are correctly identified and acted upon. These potential interventions can be divided into those proven to be effective, those proven ineffective, and those that remain experimental.

Effective or Possibly Effective Interventions

Early pre-renal ARF is the most obvious clinical situation in which ARF may be prevented. The goal is to restore renal perfusion in order to prevent progression to intrinsic ARF. The first step is fluid resuscitation with one or more boluses, preferably of normal saline. In addition, maintenance fluid requirements and replacement of on-going losses should be provided during fluid resuscitation. However, if ARF is established, fluid must be restricted to prevent fluid overload.

The administration of furosemide may help to maintain urine output in the early stages of ARF. Effects of furosemide or other diuretics may include increased intratubular pressure, thereby preventing tubular obstruction; increased intraluminal osmolality, thereby decreasing back-leak of glomerular filtrate; and increased renal blood flow, thereby reducing ischemic injury.[5,20]

In some patients, diuretics convert ARF from oliguric to non-oliguric, which reduces the complications of ARF. Diuretics should only be given during the initial phase of ARF; using them during the maintenance phase will have no benefit, and may be harmful (furosemide is ototoxic). Patients with ARF do not respond normally to diuretics, and require higher doses to produce a response. If furosemide is used for example, a loading dose of 2–4 mg/kg should be given, followed immediately by a continuous infusion of 0.25–1.0 mg/kg/hour.[5] This should be discontinued if there is no improvement in urine output within 1–2 hours.

Inotropic agents such as dobutamine may be given to improve cardiac output, or norepinephrine may be given to induce peripheral vasoconstriction, thereby increasing the effective blood volume of the central circulation. These agents may help to avert ARF by improving renal perfusion.

ARF may also be prevented by relieving acute urinary obstruction. The site of obstruction should be established by ultrasound, and an appropriate drainage catheter should be placed. A pediatric urologist and/or interventional radiologist must be consulted promptly. Post-obstructive diuresis should be successfully managed with milliliter-for-milliliter urine replacement and frequent electrolyte monitoring.

In patients with chronic renal insufficiency it is important either to avoid, or to monitor levels of, potential nephrotoxins when such agents are clinically indicated. The administration of normal saline prior to amphotericin B reduces its nephrotoxicity, and should be carried out in all patients. Acetylcysteine administration prior to radiocontrast agents may prevent contrast nephropathy.[18,19]

Ineffective Interventions

Dopamine may occasionally be useful when clearly there is diminished renal perfusion, such as in an infant or small child who receives a kidney from an adult donor. The doses should not be greater than 5 μg/kg/minute, because higher doses cause renal vasoconstriction.

However, randomized studies have failed to demonstrate a benefit of dopamine in other forms of ARF.[4]

Atrial natriuretic peptide (ANP) is another agent that was thought to have a potential role in the management of ARF. However, in a multicenter, randomized, double-blind trial of ANP in critically ill patients with ATN, ANP failed to improve the overall rate of dialysis-free survival, although patients who already had oliguria at the time of randomization did appear to derive some benefit from ANP.[2] This positive finding was offset by a worsening of outcome in non-oliguric patients, who apparently experienced a hypotensive response to ANP that may have exacerbated their renal dysfunction.

Experimental Interventions

Fenoldopam, a dopamine receptor agonist, appears to be a promising potential therapy for ARF, but its effects require further study.

MANAGEMENT OF ESTABLISHED ARF

Conservative Measures

Management of ARF begins with the conservative measures outlined in Table 31-7. First and foremost among these is fluid restriction, which in oliguric patients is vitally important to prevent the fluid overload that can lead to pulmonary edema or hypertension. Fluid restriction is less critical in non-oliguric patients. To maintain an even fluid balance, the amount of fluid administered to the patient should be equal to their fluid losses. Insensible water losses should be calculated and given as 5% or 10% dextrose in water at a constant rate. Urine output should be replaced with equivalent volumes of 0.5 normal saline (if urine electrolyte results are available, a custom urine replacement solution can be given with the same sodium concentration as the patient's urine).

If there are other sources of fluid loss such as bleeding or oozing from surgical wounds, those losses should also be replaced with packed red blood cells or 5% albumin respectively, to prevent hypovolemia. Insensible water losses are reduced if the patient is being mechanically ventilated because of administration of humidified air.

If the patient is hypervolemic, net fluid loss can be accomplished by replacing a fraction of the insensible water losses, and/or a fraction of the urine output.

Metabolic Acidosis
Treatment of metabolic acidosis is important to restore a normal pH for normal metabolism and to help prevent hyperkalemia by shifting excess potassium intracellularly. Sodium citrate solution or sodium bicarbonate tablets are given to correct the serum bicarbonate

Table 31-7 Conservative Management of Acute Renal Failure

Problem	Approach	Comments
Fluid overload	Fluid restriction: D5W at insensible rate (35 ml/100 kcal) Half-normal saline to replace urine output ml-for-ml	Monitor other sources of fluid loss and replace as appropriate
Uremia	Dietary protein restriction to RDA for age	Provide adequate non-protein calories to promote anabolism
Metabolic acidosis	Alkali supplementation: intravenous bicarbonate or oral sodium citrate	Watch for development of hypernatremia if giving bicarbonate repeatedly
Hyperkalemia	Acute emergencies: Calcium gluconate 0.5–1.0 ml/kg/dose Continuous albuterol by inhalation Less urgent situations: Insulin + glucose infusion $NaHCO_3$/alkali administration Sodium polystyrene resin, 1 g/kg/dose	Stabilizes cardiac cell membranes Shifts potassium into cells Requires careful glucose monitoring Redistribution of potassium May be given orally or rectally
Hyperphosphatemia	Phosphate binders Dietary protein/phosphorous restriction	Avoid aluminum-containing agents
Nutritional support	Modest dietary protein restriction Provision of adequate (100–120% of RDA) non-protein calories	Use high-calorie, low protein enteral formulas Benefits of TPN unclear

D5W = 5% dextrose in water; RDA = recommended daily allowance; TPN = total parenteral nutrition.

concentration, but if oral medications cannot be taken, then intravenous sodium bicarbonate should be administered. Dialysis may be needed if the administration of alkali fails to correct the acidosis.

Hyperkalemia

Hyperkalemia is the most serious metabolic complication of ARF. Treatment options can be divided into those that redistribute potassium within the body, and those that remove it from the body. Calcium administration is crucial for stabilizing the cardiac action potential but does not treat the hyperkalemia.

Redistributive measures are albuterol, bicarbonate, and insulin plus glucose infusions. Albuterol, by stimulating beta-2 receptors on cell membranes, causes potassium to be transported from the serum back into the cells. Inhaled albuterol acts within 10–30 minutes, its effects last for 2–4 hours, and it can be quickly administered in an intensive care unit. Indeed, this should be the first measure instituted when hyperkalemia is detected.

Sodium bicarbonate is an effective treatment for hyperkalemia, takes effect within 30 minutes, and lasts for 1–2 hours. A drawback to bicarbonate is that its use may result in fluid overload or hypernatremia.

The administration of insulin plus glucose infusions also requires large quantities of fluid. Insulin shifts potassium intracellularly by stimulating beta-receptors on cell membranes. Glucose must be administered with insulin to prevent hypoglycemia. Insulin lowers the serum

potassium within 30 minutes, and the effect lasts for up to 2–4 hours. The serum potassium may rise rapidly shortly after the infusion is stopped.

Potassium can also be removed via the gastrointestinal tract, the kidneys, or by dialysis. Sodium polystyrene resin (Kayexalate®) removes potassium by exchanging it with sodium; a dose of 1 g/kg usually lowers the serum potassium by 1.0 mEq/l within about 2 hours. Serum potassium is reduced more rapidly when Kayexalate® is given orally than rectally, although both routes are effective. Doses can be repeated at 4- to 6-hour intervals, but hypernatremia is a potential adverse effect that is more likely to occur with repeated doses. If the patient is not anuric, loop diuretics may be given to encourage the excretion of potassium.

Dialysis is the definitive method of potassium removal, but usually is not the first choice in an urgent situation because of the time required to achieve access and to set up the necessary equipment.

Hypocalcemia

Possible causes of hypocalcemia in ARF include hyperphosphatemia, vitamin D deficiency, parathyroid hormone (PTH) resistance, and hypoalbuminemia. Serum ionized calcium is a better reflection of physiologically active calcium than total serum calcium. Hypocalcemia usually is mild, and responds to the correction of hyperphosphatemia and administration of calcium in the diet. Severe hypocalcemia can cause tetany, and should be treated with intravenous calcium gluconate or calcium chloride.

Hyponatremia

Hyponatremia is usually iatrogenic and is managed by fluid restriction because it is caused by the excessive administration of free water. Occasionally, correction of the serum sodium is necessary with a carefully calculated infusion of 3% sodium chloride. This should only be done if there are symptoms of hyponatremia such as altered mental status or seizures.

Hyperphosphatemia

Hyperphosphatemia is caused by decreased renal phosphate excretion. Dietary phosphate intake should be restricted, and oral phosphate binders should be given to increase intestinal phosphate excretion. Aluminum-containing binders should be avoided because absorbed aluminum can lead to significant adverse effects in bone and the brain. Calcium carbonate is the easiest phosphate binder to administer to children because it is available commercially in both liquid and chewable tablet forms. Sevelamer is less potent than other phosphate binders, and is only available as a tablet that cannot be chewed or crushed.

Uremia

Uremia is the most difficult metabolic complication of ARF to control with conservative measures. The usefulness of dietary restriction for increased BUN is limited by the need to provide adequate protein to meet the child's anabolic needs. Protein intake should not be limited to less than 1.0 g/kg/day in children, although the limit of 0.8 g/kg/day used in adults can be considered for older teenagers. However, it is typical for patients with ongoing ARF to become progressively more uremic despite these measures. The magnitude in rise in BUN is one of the indications for initiating dialysis.

A relatively high caloric intake of 80–100 cal/kg/day must be provided to promote anabolism. Although no clinical study has demonstrated a beneficial impact of total parenteral nutrition (TPN) on survival in patients with ARF, TPN with a high concentration of dextrose is the most effective way to adequately nourish the critically ill child with ARF. Enteral feedings should be used if the child can tolerate this, and a nasogastric feeding tube may be needed. High-calorie formulas designed for patients with renal insufficiency such as Suplena® or Renalcal® can provide adequate calories in the lowest possible volume of fluid.

Management of Hypertension

Most instances of hypertension in ARF are caused by fluid overload. The prevention of fluid overload will prevent hypertension in some patients, but if hypertension develops despite fluid restriction, then antihypertensive medications will be needed (Table 31-8). Diuretics may help in non-oliguric patients and in those with acute glomerulonephritis. Vasodilators, preferably by intravenous administration, are the best choice in most patients. If the hypertension is severe, or if there are signs of malignant hypertension, a continuous infusion of an intravenous antihypertensive agent should be started. Nicardipine is usually the best choice because it is an arterial vasodilator and can be precisely titrated to the desired effect. Labetalol is also effective, but may be contraindicated if the patient has asthma or congestive heart failure. Sodium nitroprusside should be considered a last resort in ARF because cyanide accumulation develops more rapidly with reduced renal function. It causes venous as well as arterial vasodilatation that may result in decreased preload, thereby compromising renal perfusion. A potential drawback of continuous infusions in patients with ARF is that they may contribute to the development of fluid overload if they are diluted in a large volume of carrier fluid. This can be avoided by administering an undiluted antihypertensive agent with a syringe pump (which is commonly done with labetalol), or by using a higher concentration of the medication than usually recommended.

If a continuous antihypertensive therapy is not clinically indicated, then intermittently administered agents may be used. Acceptable intravenous agents include hydralazine and labetalol. Diazoxide is no longer recommended as a first-line agent because of unpredictable effects in terms of the magnitude and duration of blood pressure reduction. Oral agents may be used if the patient is not critically ill; these include clonidine, isradipine, hydralazine, and minoxidil. Angiotensin-converting enzyme inhibitors should be avoided in ARF because they reduce the glomerular filtration pressure and increase the chances of hyperkalemia. Doses for all of these medications are shown in Table 31-8.

Renal Replacement Therapy

When conservative measures fail to control the manifestations of ARF, renal replacement therapy becomes necessary.[9-11,15-17,20] Indications for renal replacement therapy are summarized in Box 31-4.

Anecdotal experience suggests that children may tolerate higher levels of BUN than adults before developing uremic symptoms. However, there is also evidence to suggest that early initiation of dialysis, before severe symptoms develop, may improve patient outcome. In many patients it is impossible to provide adequate nutritional support while they are oliguric because of the need for fluid restriction; although provision of nutrition alone is a controversial indication

Table 31-8   Drugs for the Management of Hypertension in Acute Renal Failure

Drug	Class	Dose	Route	Comments
Clonidine	Central alpha agonist	0.05–0.1 mg/dose	Oral	Side effects include dry mouth and sedation
Esmolol	Beta blocker	Infusion: 100–500 mcg/kg/min	IV infusion	Very short-acting
Fenoldopam	Dopamine receptor agonist	0.2–0.8 mcg/kg/min	IV infusion	May also improve renal blood flow
Hydralazine	Vasodilator (arteriolar)	IV: 0.2–0.6 mg/kg/dose PO: 0.25–1.0 mg/kg/dose	IV bolus or PO	Should be given every 4 hours when given IV
Isradipine	Calcium channel blocker	0.05–0.15 mg/kg/dose	Oral	Oral suspension can be compounded
Labetalol	Alpha and beta blocker	IV: 0.20–1.0 mg/kg/dose Infusion: 0.25–3.0 mg/kg/hr	IV bolus or infusion	Asthma, heart failure relative contraindications
Monoxidil	Vasodilator (arteriolar)	0.1–0.2 mg/kg/dose	Oral	Most potent vasodilator; may not take effect for 1–2 hours
Nicardipine	Calcium channel blocker	Infusion: 1–4 mcg/kg/min	IV infusion	May cause reflex tachycardia
Sodium nitroprusside	Vasodilator (arteriolar and venous)	Infusion: 0.3–10 mcg/kg/min	IV infusion	Thiocyanate toxicity with prolonged use

Abbreviations used in table: IV, intravenous; PO, oral; mcg, micrograms: mg, milligrams.

Box 31-4   Indications for Dialysis in ARF

- Fluid overload with pulmonary edema and/or respiratory failure or compromise
- Encephalopathy, pericarditis, or bleeding
- Metabolic disturbances: hyperkalemia, acidosis, hyperphosphatemia
- Intoxications: lithium, methyl alcohol, salicylate, others
- Inborn errors of metabolism: urea cycle defects
- Nutritional support (controversial)

---

for dialysis, there are patients in whom this may be justifiable.

One of the most important factors to consider is the patient's hemodynamic status (Table 31-9). Patients who are hypotensive or hemodynamically unstable cannot tolerate rapid correction of fluid overload, and therefore traditional intermittent hemodialysis (HD) is not indicated.

Peritoneal dialysis (PD) is the most common renal replacement modality used in infants and children with ARF[10] (see Chapter 36). HD offers several potential advantages over PD in ARF, most notably the ability to rapidly correct fluid overload, hyperkalemia, and metabolic acidosis[11] (see Chapter 35). Access-related problems are the most vexing aspect of pediatric HD in ARF and chronic renal failure. Continuous hemofiltration (HF) is rapidly becoming a commonly employed modality for the management of ARF in pediatrics[7,11,13,15] (see Chapter 35). A theoretical advantage of HF is

---

Table 31-9   Dialysis Modality in Pediatric Acute Renal Failure

Primary Goal of Dialysis	Hemodynamic Status	Modality
Fluid removal	Normotensive	Intermittent HD (with isolated UF)
	Hypotensive	Continuous HF or PD
Urea clearance	Normotensive	Intermittent HD or PD
	Hypotensive	Continuous HF or PD
Treatment of hyperkalemia	Normo- or hypotensive	Intermittent HD
Correction of metabolic acidosis*	Normotensive	Any
	Hypotensive	Continuous HF or PD
Treatment of hyperphosphatemia	Normo- or hypotensive	Any; continuous HF possibly superior

HD = hemodialysis; HF = hemofiltration; PD = peritoneal dialysis; UF = ultrafiltration.
*Bicarbonate dialysate preferred in patients with hepatic failure and/or lactic acidosis.

MAJOR POINTS

- The most common form of ARF in children is pre-renal ARF, usually resulting from dehydration, sepsis or blood loss.
- Other important forms of ARF that occur commonly in children include hemolytic–uremic syndrome, acute glomerulonephritis, and obstruction of the GU tract.
- Major complications of ARF include fluid overload, hyperkalemia, metabolic acidosis, hyperphosphatemia, uremia, anemia and infection.
- The short-term outcome of ARF in children is similar to that in adults and depends on the underlying cause of ARF and whether dialysis is necessary.
- Intervention early in the course of ARF may prevent the development of oliguria and may reduce the morbidity and mortality of ARF.
- Accurate monitoring of fluid balance is of primary importance in managing ARF and should include frequent weights, precise accounting of all sources of fluid intake, including IV medications, and all types of fluid loss, especially non-urinary fluid losses.
- For patients with pre-renal ARF, fluid resuscitation should be attempted first, as this may prevent the development of acute tubular necrosis (ATN).
- Diuretics may be helpful in converting oliguric ARF to non-oliguric ARF, but if there is no response to initial attempts at diuretic therapy, they should not be continued.
- Multiple studies have failed to demonstrate a benefit for routine administration of 'renal-dose' dopamine in ARF; however, the dopamine receptor agonist fenoldopam shows promise as a potential means of increasing renal blood flow in ARF.
- The decision to initiate dialysis depends on the overall clinical status of the patient, not on an absolute level of BUN or creatinine.
- Usual indications for initiation of dialysis in children with ARF include fluid overload, metabolic complications unresponsive to conservative measures, and symptomatic uremia
- Peritoneal dialysis, hemodialysis and continuous veno-venous hemofiltration can all be used to manage children with ARF when dialysis becomes necessary; the choice of which modality to use depends on clinical and technical factors.

the continuous removal of cytokines and other inflammatory mediators involved in the pathogenesis and maintenance of ARF.

REFERENCES

1. Airede A, Bello M, Weerasinghe HD. Acute renal failure in the newborn: incidence and outcome. J Paediatr Child Health 1997;33:246–249.
2. Allgren RL, Marbury TC, Rahman SN, et al. Anaritide in acute renal failure. N Engl J Med 1997;336:828–834.
3. Arora P, Kher V, Rai PK, et al. Prognosis of acute renal failure in children: a multivariate analysis. Pediatr Nephrol 1997;11:153–155.
4. Australian and New Zealand Intensive Care Society Clinical Trials Group. Low-dose dopamine in patients with early renal dysfunction: a placebo-controlled randomized trial. Lancet 2000;356:2139–2143.
5. Brater DC. Diuretic therapy. N Engl J Med 1998;339:387–395.
6. Bunchman TE, McBryde KD, Mottes TE, et al. Pediatric acute renal failure: outcome by modality and disease. Pediatr Nephrol 2001;16:1067–1071.
7. Bunchman TE, Maxvold NJ, Barnett J, et al. Pediatric hemofiltration: Normocarb dialysate with citrate anticoagulation. Pediatr Nephrol 2002;17:150–154.
8. Ehrich JHH. Acute renal failure in infants and children. Int J Artif Organs 1996;19:121–123.
9. Flynn JT. Causes, management approaches and outcome of acute renal failure in children. Curr Opin Pediatr 1998;10:184–189.
10. Flynn JT, Kershaw DB, Smoyer WE, et al. Peritoneal dialysis for management of pediatric acute renal failure. Perit Dial Int 2001;21:390–394.
11. Flynn JT. Choice of dialysis modality in pediatric acute renal failure. Pediatr Nephrol 2002;17:61–69.
12. Georgaki-Angelaki HN, Steed DB, Chantler C, et al. Renal function following acute renal failure in childhood: a long-term follow-up study. Kidney Int 1989;35:84–89.
13. Goldstein SL, Currier H, Graf JM, et al. Outcome in children receiving continuous venovenous hemofiltration. Pediatrics 2001;107:1309–1312.
14. Lameire N, Vanholder R. Pathophysiologic features and prevention of human and experimental acute tubular necrosis. J Am Soc Nephrol 2001;12:S20–S32.
15. Maxvold NJ, Smoyer WE, Gardner JJ, et al. Management of acute renal failure in the pediatric patient: hemofiltration vs. hemodialysis. Am J Kid Dis 1997;30(Suppl. 4):S84–S88.
16. Parekh RS, Bunchman TE. Dialysis support in the pediatric intensive care unit. Adv Ren Replace Ther 1996;3:326–336.
17. Schiffl H, Lang SM, Fischer R. Daily hemodialysis and the outcome of acute renal failure. N Engl J Med 2002;346:305–310.
18. Solomon R. Contrast-medium-induced acute renal failure. Kidney Int 1998;53:230–242.
19. Tepel M, van der Giet M, Schwarzfeld C, et al. Prevention of radiographic-contrast-agent-induced reductions in renal function by acetylcysteine. N Engl J Med 2000;343:180–184.
20. Thadhani R, Pascual M, Bonventre JV. Acute renal failure. N Engl J Med 1996;334:1448–1460.
21. Williams DM, Sreedhar SS, Mickell JJ, et al. Acute kidney failure: a pediatric experience over 20 years. Arch Pediatr Adolesc Med 2002;156:893–900.

Chronic Renal Failure

BERNARD S. KAPLAN, M.B., B.Ch. AND

KEVIN E.C. MEYERS, M.B., B.Ch.

INTRODUCTION

Chronic renal failure (CRF) refers to the progressive and usually inexorable loss of renal function as a result of injury to the kidneys. All patients with CRF have *chronic renal disease* (CRD), but not all of those with CRD are in CRF (Boxes 32-1 and 32-2).

Box 32-1 Definitions of Chronic Kidney Disease

- GFR ≤ 60 ml/min/1.73 m^2 for ≥ 3 months; or
- pathological abnormalities; or
- abnormal findings in urine or blood; or
- abnormal imaging studies

Box 32-2 Definition of Kidney Failure

GFR <15 ml/min/1.73 m^2 with signs and symptoms of uremia or the need for dialysis/transplant for treatment of complications of decreased GFR that increase risks of mortality and morbidity.

End-stage renal disease (ESRD) is difficult to define; the condition generally refers to a level of reduction in renal function that requires the initiation of dialysis or transplantation (Box 32-3).

DEFINITION OF CHRONIC RENAL FAILURE

Early diagnosis of CRD is important because it may be possible to retard the course of progression of kidney

---

Box 32-3 End-Stage Renal Disease (ESRD)

- ESRD is an administrative term in the United States, and is based on the conditions stipulated for payment of healthcare by the Medicare ESRD Program
- ESRD does not specifically refer to a level of GFR, but to the time at which the occurrence of signs and symptoms of kidney failure necessitate initiation of replacement therapy
- ESRD includes patients treated by dialysis or transplant, regardless of their GFR level

---

Table 32-1 Stages of Chronic Renal Disease

Stage	Description	GFR (ml/min/1.73 m^2)
1	Kidney damage with normal or increased GFR	≥90
2	Kidney damage with mildly decreased GFR	60–89
3	Moderate decrease in GFR	30–59
4	Severe decrease in GFR	15–29
5	Kidney failure	≤15 (or on dialysis)

GFR = glomerular filtration rate.

disease, to treat co-morbid problems earlier, and to improve the outcomes and quality of life of all patients with kidney disease, long before dialysis or renal transplant is necessary (The Kidney Disease Outcomes Quality Initiative, or K/DOQI).[10] The presence of CRD must be established on the basis of kidney damage and level of kidney function as reflected by the glomerular filtration rate (GFR), regardless of any etiological or pathological diagnosis (Table 32-1). However, this should not preclude attempts to make a precise diagnosis for specific treatment, prognosis, and genetic counseling. In addition, the patient must be assessed for co-morbid conditions and complications of decreased kidney function. CRD and hypertension increase the risks of loss of kidney function and cardiovascular disease. Therefore, individuals with hypertension should be evaluated for CRD because hypertension is a cause and consequence of CRD. It is possible to have a GFR 60 to 89 ml/min/1.73 m^2 without kidney damage. This is referred to as 'decreased GFR,' and may result from age (infants), vegetarian diets, unilateral nephrectomy, extracellular fluid volume depletion, or heart failure (Table 32-2).

Table 32-2 Normal Glomerular Filtration Rate (GFR) Values in Pediatrics

Age	GFR (ml/min/1.73 m^2)*
One week	40.6±14.8
2 to 8 weeks	65.8±24.8
>8 weeks	95.7±21.7
2 to 12 years	133.0±27.0
13 to 21 years (males)	140.0±30.0
13 to 21 years (females)	126.0±22.0

*Values are mean ± SD.

EVALUATION OF CHRONIC RENAL DISEASE

Chronic kidney disease is evaluated by the excretion of protein (and/or albumin) and by the estimation of GFR. Proteinuria is an early and sensitive marker of kidney damage. Albumin is the most abundant urine protein in most types of chronic kidney disease, and low molecular-weight globulins are the most abundant urine proteins in some types of chronic kidney disease. *Proteinuria* includes albuminuria, increased urinary excretion of specific proteins, and increased excretion of total urine protein. *Albuminuria* refers to increased urinary albumin excretion. *Microalbuminuria* refers to excretion of small but abnormal amounts of albumin. Less than 1% of children have persistent proteinuria, and the prevalence of increased urine albumin excretion on initial screening varies from 1% to 10%. Glomerular integrity can be assessed by dividing albumin clearance by creatinine clearance in spot urine samples; this provides a better marker of glomerular permeability to albumin than the 24-hour albumin excretion rate.[2]

GFR is the best measure of overall kidney function. In children, this is usually estimated by the convenient (but unreliable) Schwartz formula[11] that tends to underestimate the true GFR. Normal GFRs vary according to age, gender, and body size (see Table 32-2). Adult values for mean GFR are reached by two years of age. The prevalence of decreased GFR in children is not known. Several imaging studies are used judiciously to assist in diagnosing CRD in neonates and children (Box 32-4).

Chronic Renal Disease in Neonates and Infants

Neonates with prenatal renal abnormalities whose serum creatinine concentrations rise rapidly after birth do not have 'acute renal failure' but CRD, because the failure started *in utero*.[5] CRD in the neonate usually results from inherited disorders or congenital abnormalities. Neonatal acute renal failure from perinatal asphyxia

Box 32-4 Imaging Studies that may be Requested in CRF

- X-radiography of the hands and hips
- DXA scan
- Renal and bladder ultrasound
- Voiding cystourethrogram (VCUG)
- Computed tomography scan; magnetic resonance imaging
- Radionuclide studies

or bilateral renal venous thromboses may progress to CRF. The natural history and treatment of some renal disorders are altered by prenatal diagnosis and treatment. In addition, genetic renal disorders are rarely isolated abnormalities and are often components of many syndromes. Conversely, neonates with multiple congenital defects often have renal involvement. Renal function often improves in the first year of life even in neonates with marked reductions in GFR.

Causes of CRD in neonates, infants and children are shown in Table 32-3. These conditions have been reviewed in greater detail in other chapters. It is important to note that not all renal abnormalities classified as CRD result in CRF. Examples include unilateral multicystic kidney and unilateral renal adysplasia.

Table 32-3	Causes of Chronic Renal Disease in Children
Congenital abnormalities	Multicystic kidney
	Renal adysplasia/dysplasia
Obstructive uropathies	Urethral atresia
	Posterior urethral valves
	Uretero-pelvic junction obstruction
Cystic kidney diseases	Autosomal recessive polycystic kidney disease
	Autosomal dominant polycystic kidney disease
	Glomerulocystic kidney diseases
Dysgenetic kidneys	Autosomal recessive renal tubular dysgenesis
Congenital nephrotic syndrome	Autosomal recessive (Finnish type)
	Diffuse mesangial sclerosis
	Denys–Drash syndrome
	Galloway–Mowat syndrome
Neonatal acute renal injury	Asphyxia
	Renal venous thromboses
Glomerulonephritis	Lupus nephritis
	IgA nephropathy
	Henoch-Schönlein nephritis
	Crescentic glomerulonephritis
	Alport syndromes
Nephrotic syndrome	Focal segmental glomerulosclerosis
	Membranoproliferative glomerulonephritis
	Membranous glomerulopathy
Hemolytic uremic syndromes	Stx HUS
	Factor H HUS
Tubulointerstitial diseases	Medications
	Infections
	Cystinosis, hyperoxaluria
	Nephronophthisis
	Pyelonephritis
Renal transplantation	Chronic rejection
	Immunosuppressive agents
	Recurrence

SYMPTOMS AND SIGNS OF CRF IN CHILDREN

There are few symptoms or signs of CRF in children. Rather, there may be *indicators* of chronic renal disease. Antenatal pointers to CRD include oligohydramnios, polyhydramnios, and abnormal antenatal ultrasound findings. The presence of a syndrome should prompt a physical examination to evaluate the kidneys and urinary tract, for example in the BOR syndrome, Townes–Brocks syndrome or Biedl–Bardet syndrome. Defined conditions that are associated with CRD include cystinosis and cystinuria. Incidental findings such as single umbilical artery, hypospadias and low-set ears are rarely important signs of CRD. An incidental episode, such as dehydration, may result in the measurement of the serum creatinine concentration, and this may be the first indication of CRF.

It is important to obtain a careful family history (see Chapter 3). Failure to thrive is an important sign of CRD in infants and young children. Most of the symptoms are vague and non-specific. Fatigue, headaches, anorexia, nausea, and vomiting occur late in the course of CRF. Pruritis and peripheral neuropathy are uncommon. Polydipsia, polyuria, and nocturia occur in tubulointerstitial conditions, renal adysplasias, and posterior urethral valves. Older children and adolescents may present with delayed puberty, forgetfulness and falling grades at school. Some children present with pallor and others with rickets. Edema and/or hypertension are often the first signs of CRD. Congestive heart failure, pericarditis, and peripheral neuropathy are uncommon in children with CRF (Table 32-4).

METABOLIC ABNORMALITIES IN CRF

Hyponatremia

Hyponatremia can occur as a result of excess free water ingestion in a patient with a reduced GFR, or reduced salt intake in a salt-losing nephropathy. A salt-losing syndrome with tubular resistance to aldosterone can occur in infants aged under 3 months with congenital urinary tract malformations and acute pyelonephritis.[9] Sodium chloride should not automatically be restricted in CRD unless there is hypertension, edema, or volume expansion.

Hyperkalemia

Hyperkalemia is the result of reduced GFR, metabolic acidosis, activation of the renin-angiotensin-aldosterone system, reduced flow rate of distal tubular fluid, and medications such as angiotensin-converting enzyme inhibitors. Hyperkalemia plays a pivotal role in potassium

Table 32-4	Complications of CRF
Cardiopulmonary	Hypertension
	Pulmonary edema
	Congestive heart failure
	Uremic pericarditis
Gastrointestinal	Anorexia
	Decreased growth
	Nausea, vomiting
	Weight loss
	Gastroesophageal reflux disease (GERD)
	Bleeding
	Esophagitis, gastritis, duodenal ulcers, colitis
Neuromuscular	Myopathy
	Peripheral neuropathy
	Encephalopathy
Psychological	School failure
	Forgetfulness
Dermatologic	Sallow color
	Pruritus
	Dermatitis
Hematological	Bleeding
	Platelet dysfunction
	Anemia
Immunological	Delayed wound healing
	Infections
Sexual	Menstrual abnormalities
	Impotence

homeostasis in renal insufficiency by stimulating potassium excretion. In patients with CRF, a new steady state develops in which extracellular [K$^+$] rises to the level needed to stimulate K$^+$ excretion so that it again matches intake. When this new steady state is achieved, the plasma [K$^+$] remains stable unless dietary intake increases, GFR falls, or drugs disrupt the new balance.[3] Patients with CRD and hypokalemia must not be given boluses of potassium, because the serum potassium concentration may increase too quickly.

Metabolic Acidosis

Metabolic acidosis may be the result of proximal tubular wasting of bicarbonate and, more commonly, decreased distal excretion of hydrogen ion as a result of reduced nephron mass. Metabolic acidosis has role in initiating a muscle-wasting syndrome in CRF with a loss of lean body mass and a negative nitrogen balance.[1] Metabolic acidosis alters vitamin D and parathyroid hormone (PTH) levels, and is another cause of bone disease in CRF.[7]

Hyperuricemia

Hyperuricemia is rarely a problem in patients with CRF. In familial juvenile gouty nephropathy (FJGN),

hyperuricemia is out of proportion to the reduction in GFR. Early treatment with allopurinol may retard progression to end-stage renal failure in these patients.[8]

Hypocalcemia

Hypocalcemia is caused by perturbations in the calcium-parathyroid-calcitriol axis. Serum calcium levels are affected by the level of kidney function, and low concentrations in serum calcium become evident when the GFR is <30 ml/min/1.73 m^2. Some infants with CRF initially may have elevated serum calcium concentrations. Patients with nephrotic syndrome are hypocalcemic because less albumin is available for calcium binding.

Hyperphosphatemia

Hyperphosphatemia is the result of reduced GFR, with decreased excretion of phosphate. This results in secondary hyperparathyroidism, and this in turn contributes to renal osteodystrophy. The threshold level of GFR, at which serum phosphorus levels start to increase, ranges from 20 to 50 ml/min/1.73 m^2. Higher calcium-phosphorus products and increased prevalence of an elevated calcium-phosphorus product occur with lower GFRs (Box 32-5). Calcium-phosphorus precipitation in the kidneys secondary to elevated phosphorus levels may hasten the loss of kidney function. Calciphylaxis or extraosseous calcification of soft tissue and vascular tissue is uncommon in children.

RENAL OSTEODYSTROPHY

Bone disease and disorders of calcium and phosphorus metabolism develop during the course of CRD. Radiological and histological changes of bone disease are demonstrated in 40% of patients with severely decreased kidney function, and almost 100% of those in kidney failure. However, abnormalities leading to bone disease begin to occur at earlier stages of CRD. Elevated levels of PTH and phosphorus, reduced levels of calcium, and reduced urinary phosphate excretion occur when the GFR is <70 ml/min/1.73 m^2.

Box 32-5	Complications of Abnormal Calcium-Phosphorus Metabolism

- Renal osteodystrophy
- Calciphylaxis
- Coronary artery calcification

Classification: High- and Low-Bone Turnover

Renal osteodystrophy can be classified as: high bone turnover and high PTH levels (osteitis fibrosa), and mixed lesion; or low bone turnover and low or normal PTH levels.

Low-bone turnover disease is further divided into two subgroups, both of which are characterized by a decrease in bone turnover or remodeling, with a reduced number of osteoclasts and osteoblasts, and decreased osteoblastic activity.

Osteomalacia

This may be the result of vitamin D deficiency, excess aluminum, or metabolic acidosis. In osteomalacia there is an accumulation of unmineralized bone matrix, or increased osteoid volume.

Adynamic Bone Disease

In this condition bone volume and mineralization are reduced. This may be caused by excess aluminum ingestion or oversuppression of PTH production with calcitriol (dihydroxyvitamin D_3).[12]

Secondary Hyperparathyroidism

Bone disease caused by secondary hyperparathyroidism is the consequence of abnormal mineral metabolism:

- Decreased renal function reduces phosphorus excretion and increases phosphorus retention
- Elevated serum phosphorus concentrations directly suppress calcitriol production
- Reduced renal mass decreases calcitriol production
- Decreased calcitriol production with consequent reduced calcium absorption from the gastrointestinal tract contributes to hypocalcemia. An abnormal calcium-phosphorus balance leads to an elevated calcium-phosphorus product, and this also contributes to hypocalcemia[4]
- Hypocalcemia, reduced calcitriol synthesis, and elevated serum phosphorus concentrations stimulate the production of PTH and the proliferation of parathyroid cells,[6] resulting in secondary hyperparathyroidism
- High PTH levels stimulate osteoblasts, and this results in a high bone turnover
- High bone turnover leads to irregularly woven abnormal osteoid, fibrosis, and cyst formation, which result in decreased cortical bone and bone strength and an increased risk of fracture (Box 32-6).

Box 32-6 Complications of Secondary Hyperparathyroidism

- Renal osteodystrophy bone pain, fractures, growth retardation
- Cardiac calcification of cardiac muscle and coronary arteries, myocardial dysfunction
- Neuromuscular impaired neurological and skeletal muscle unction
- Hematopoietic anemia

ANEMIA

This usually develops during the course of CRD, and may be associated with adverse outcomes. The hemoglobin level must be measured in patients with a GFR <60 ml/min/1.73 m^2, and the anemia must be evaluated and treated (Figure 32-1). If there is a low hemoglobin level, then the iron stores (serum ferritin, transferrin saturation levels) must be measured. Erythropoietin levels are less useful because they are often not appropriately elevated, despite low hemoglobin levels. There is no quantitative definition of anemia in CRD, because 'acceptable' hemoglobin levels are not defined for patients with CRD. It is important to define anemia relative to physiological norms rather than payment rules.[14]

Anemia may result from reduced renal erythropoietin synthesis and/or inhibitors of erythropoiesis. However, anemia in CRD may also result from blood loss, decreased hemoglobin synthesis, or hemolysis (Box 32-7). The severity of anemia in CRD disease is related to the duration and extent of kidney failure. The prevalence of anemia increases when the GFR is below about 60 ml/min/1.73 m^2. Low hemoglobin levels are associated with higher rates of hospitalizations, cardiovascular disease, cognitive impairment, and increased mortality rates. Measures of iron stores, ferritin, and transferrin saturation, are not consistently associated with the level of GFR. Ferritin levels in patients with reduced GFR may represent total body iron status, or they may be markers of inflammation and are not useful in measuring iron stores, or in predicting the relation of hemoglobin to kidney function. Transferrin saturation, in combination with serum iron and ferritin levels, is helpful in diagnosing functional iron deficiency.

GROWTH FAILURE

This is a major obstacle to the full rehabilitation of children with CRF. Factors that contribute to impaired linear growth are protein and calorie malnutrition, metabolic

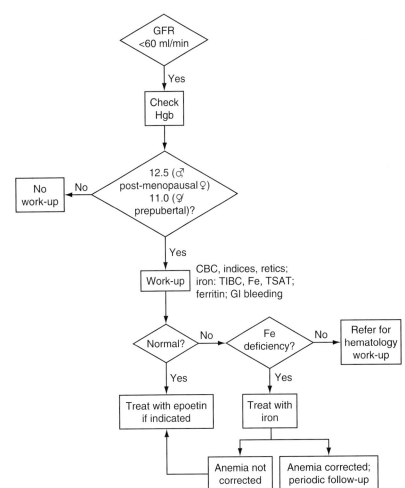

Figure 32-1 Evaluation of anemia in patients with chronic kidney disease. TIBC = total iron-binding capacity; TSAT = transferrin saturation.
Modified from National Kidney Foundation: Guidelines for anemia of chronic kidney disease. In: NKF-K/DOQI Clinical Practice Guidelines. NKF K/DOQI Guidelines, 2000. http://www.kidney.org/professionals/doqi/guidelines/doqiupan_i.html#1.

acidosis, growth hormone resistance, anemia, and renal osteodystrophy. Although therapeutic interventions such as recombinant human growth hormone (rhGH),[13] recombinant human erythropoietin, and calcitriol have made substantial contributions, the optimal therapeutic strategy remains to be defined. Growth failure can persist in many children with CRF and in those treated with maintenance dialysis. In addition, the increasing prevalence of adynamic bone disease and its effect on growth has raised concern about the continued generalized use of calcitriol in children with CRF. Parathyroid hormone-related protein (PTHrP) and the ratio of PTH to PTHrP receptor have critical roles in the regulation of endochondral bone formation. PTH/PTHrP receptor mRNA expression is down-regulated in the kidneys and growth plate cartilage of animals with renal failure. Differences in the severity of secondary hyperparathyroidism influence growth plate morphology and the expression of selected markers of chondrocyte proliferation and differentiation. These findings suggest potential molecular mechanisms whereby cartilage and bone

development may be disrupted in children with CRF and thereby contribute to diminished linear growth.

There is also reduced production of insulin-like growth factor-1 (IGF-1) in response to endogenous or exogenous growth hormone and reduced expression of

---

Box 32-7   Causes of Anemia in Chronic Kidney Disease

- Low erythropoietin levels
- Functional or absolute iron deficiency
- Blood loss – occult or overt
- Uremic inhibitors – parathyroid hormone, spermine
- Aluminum toxicity
- Medications
- Reduced half-life of circulating red blood cells
- Folate or vitamin B_{12} deficiencies
- Concurrent underlying hematological problems
- Copper toxicity

MAJOR POINTS

- Adverse outcomes of chronic kidney disease may often be prevented or delayed through early detection and treatment.
- Earlier stages of chronic kidney disease may be detected through routine laboratory measurements.
- PTH levels are elevated in patients with decreased GFR, and likely are the earliest marker of abnormal bone mineral metabolism.
- The intact PTH (iPTH) test is the most reliable measure of PTH levels.
- Hyperkalemia is a medical emergency, and must be treated appropriately.
- In mild hyperkalemia: restrict potassium; bind dietary potassium; correct metabolic acidosis; and increase urinary K^+ excretion with furosemide.
- In moderate/severe hyperkalemia: infuse glucose and insulin; initiate acute dialysis if unresponsive to medical treatment.
- Patients with CRD whose hemoglobin levels are lower than physiological norms are anemic.

growth hormone mRNA. The expression of IGF-binding proteins further reduces growth hormone availability and action. Metabolic acidosis reduces the pulsatile secretion of growth hormone in children with CRF. Treatment with rhGH overcomes the tissue resistance.

REFERENCES

1. Bailey JL, Mitch WE. Metabolic acidosis as a uremic toxin. Semin Nephrol 1996;16:160-166.

2. Barratt TM, McLaine PN, Soothill JF. Albumin excretion as a measure of glomerular dysfunction in children. Arch Dis Child 1970;45:496-501.

3. Gennari FJ, Segal AS. Hyperkalemia: an adaptive response in chronic renal insufficiency. Kidney Int 2002;62:1-9.

4. Hsu CH. Are we mismanaging calcium and phosphate metabolism in renal failure? Am J Kidney Dis 1997;29:641-649.

5. Kaplan BS, Kaplan P. Chronic renal disease in the neonate. In: Spitzer A (ed), Intensive Care of the Fetus and Neonate. Mosby, St. Louis, 1996, pp. 1070-1078.

6. Kates DM, Sherrard DJ, Andress DL. Evidence that serum phosphate is independently associated with serum PTH in patients with chronic renal failure. Am J Kid Dis 1997;30:809-813.

7. Kraut JA. Disturbances of acid-base balance and bone disease in end-stage renal disease. Semin Dial 2000;13:261-266.

8. McBride MB, Rigden S, Haycock GB, et al. Presymptomatic detection of familial juvenile hyperuricaemic nephropathy in children. Pediatr Nephrol 1998;12:357-364.

9. Melzi ML, Guez S, Sersale G, et al. Acute pyelonephritis as a cause of hyponatremia/hyperkalemia in young infants with urinary tract malformations. Pediatr Infect Dis J 1995; 14:56-59.

10. Patel SS, Kimmel PL, Singh A. New clinical practice guidelines for chronic kidney disease: a framework for K/DOQI. Semin Nephrol 2002;22:449-458.

11. Schwartz GJ, Haycock GB, Edelmann CM, Jr, Spitzer A. A simple estimate of glomerular filtration rate in children derived from body length and plasma creatinine. Pediatrics 1976;58:259-263.

12. Sherrard DJ, Hercz G, Pei Y, et al. The spectrum of bone disease in end-stage renal failure – An evolving disorder. Kidney Int 1993;43:436-442.

13. Warady BA. Growth retardation in children with chronic renal insufficiency. J Am Soc Nephrol 1998;9(12 Suppl.): S85-S89.

14. Yorgin PD, Belson A, Al-Uzri AY, Alexander SR. The clinical efficacy of higher hematocrit levels in children with chronic renal insufficiency and those undergoing dialysis. Semin Nephrol 2001;21:451-462.

SUGGESTED READING

http://www.kidney.org/professionals/doqi/guidelines/doqi_uptoc.html.

CHAPTER 33

Management of Chronic Renal Failure

BERNARD S. KAPLAN, M.B., B.Ch. AND

KEVIN E.C. MEYERS, M.B., B.Ch.

INTRODUCTION

'Progression of renal disease' refers to an irreversible decline in glomerular filtration rate (GFR) as a result of structural damage to the renal vasculature, tubules, or interstitium. Renal disease usually progresses slowly, with a loss of GFR of about 3 ml/min each year. Therefore, even small improvements in the slowing of renal disease progression may provide large benefits.[6] Before accepting the diagnosis of chronic renal failure (CRF) or end-stage renal failure (ESRF), patients and their parents have mixed emotions of anger, disbelief, or a sense of futility. Knowing that something may be done to slow the progression of the renal failure may offer some hope. Achieving blood pressure and dietary goals slowed progression of renal disease (as indicated by GFR) by an average of about 1 ml/min per year (MDRD study in adults). For each 1 gram of reduction in proteinuria after 4 months of the interventions, subsequent GFR decline was slowed by about 1 ml/min per year (MDRD study in adults). Avoidance of excessive fluid intake (MDRD study) slowed the progression of renal disease by as much as 1–1.5 ml/min per year. Additional measures may add further to renoprotection, and there are no reasons to suggest that the therapies are mutually antagonistic. Although the multiple-risk-factor intervention strategy may be beneficial, it is not clear how much benefit can be achieved. To do that requires a prospective trial in which patients are randomized to usual care or to the multiple-risk-factor intervention. However, because it is unlikely that such a study will be undertaken in the near future, nephrologists must make prudent decisions regarding their patients, and may have to use evidence that is not conclusive.

ROLE OF THE PHYSICIAN OF RECORD

A team approach is essential for the optimal care of a patient with chronic renal disease (CRD), chronic renal failure (CRF), and especially end-stage renal disease (ESRD) (Box 33-1).

Successful, optimum care requires both the input of many individuals and also an attending physician of record who coordinates care and provides the family with information.

The nature of the condition must be explained in simple language that is not condescending. Patience is important, because the terms are new and the family is bombarded by the realization that their child is going to be chronically ill. Fathers initially often intellectualize the problem. The parents' hopes are being dashed, and the physician is the dasher of hopes – the bearer of bad news. Therefore, the physician must not be angry with the parents if they become hostile. There should be as few people as possible in a room when bad news is imparted. The physician should be optimistic but realistic, and leave room for hope, but should not try to be unrealistically optimistic. There is no need to cover everything at the first encounter. The problem should be managed in a rational way, by making the baby as comfortable as possible and by treating everything that can be treated by conventional means, until the parents have made a decision regarding dialysis and transplantation. The physician should gently explain that the child will feel pain, and that he or she may suffer from the treatment, that there are no guarantees of success, and that there will be major disruptions to the family's life. The family should be encouraged to obtain a second opinion. The physician must not pass moral judgments. Access to other parents whose children have, or have had, similar problems should be offered, but this must comply with HIPAA guidelines. The physician should not be afraid of long periods of silence. The physician must never take away all hope from a family. Present and

potential symptoms and signs must be explained. These are initially nausea, vomiting, poor appetite, metabolic acidosis, hyponatremia, and hyperkalemia. Later complications may include hypertension, anemia, growth retardation, developmental delay, osteodystrophy, and acute urinary tract infections with or without septicemia.

NUTRITION

The approach to nutritional management is summarized in Box 33-2, and is discussed more fully in Chapter 10.

Fluid intake should not be restricted, unless there is edema or congestive heart failure. Many patients have an impaired ability to concentrate urine and hence suffer from polydipsia and polyuria. This can cause nocturnal enuresis and even daytime accidents. Fluids should be restricted if the patient is edematous, or if there is a dilutional hyponatremia.

There is no need to restrict sodium intake unless the patient is edematous or hypertensive. Potassium intake should only be restricted if there is an elevated serum potassium concentration. Carefully review each of the

---

Box 33-1 The Renal Failure Team

Nephrologists	Nurses	Nutritionists
Pediatricians	Clinical nurse	Social workers
Specialty services	specialists	Psychologists
Urologists	Dialysis nurses	Play therapists
Transplant surgeons	Transplant	Fellows
Radiologists	coordinators	Interns
Pathologists	Secretaries	Residents
	Phlebotomists	
	Laboratory	
	technicians	

Box 33-2 Guidelines of Nutritional Management[13]

- The best way to prevent early growth failure in children with CRD is by using specified nutrition, appropriate buffer, activated vitamin D, and calcium-containing phosphate binders as needed
- Supplemental sodium and water in children with polyuria and intravascular volume depletion may prevent growth failure
- Cow's milk is detrimental in this group of individuals because of high solute and protein load, often causing intravascular volume depletion, hyperphosphatemia, and acidosis
- In children with <50% of normal GFR, PTH levels must be measured
- Activated vitamin D therapy should be started if PTH is elevated to more than two to three times normal
- Thereafter, careful monitoring of calcium, phosphorus, and PTH is crucial to prevent renal osteodystrophy, low turnover bone disease, and hypercalcemia with hypercalciuria and nephrocalcinosis
- Children with tubular defects with severe polyuria also may benefit from low-solute, high-volume feedings
- All physicians caring for children with renal disease should have pediatric nephrology consultation available
- Prevention of growth failure is much more cost-effective than pharmacologic therapy

medications that are being taken because some drugs such as angiotensin-converting enzyme (ACE) inhibitors and spironolactone may cause hyperkalemia in a patient with reduced GFR. The correction of a metabolic acidosis will help to reduce the serum potassium concentration. Metabolic acidosis can usually be managed by giving sodium bicarbonate in a dose of 2–3 mEq/kg each day, split into three or four doses. It is never necessary to restrict calcium intake, as additional calcium not only helps to increase the serum calcium concentration but also helps to bind phosphorus. It is important to prescribe preparations that do not contain any magnesium or aluminum. Serum magnesium levels tend to be increased in CRD and CRF, except in very rare conditions.

Maintaining normal serum phosphorus concentrations is one of the major challenges in the management of CRF. This is done initially by dietary restriction of phosphorus, but is rarely successful and consequently phosphate binders are used. In this respect, calcium carbonate is cheap and efficient, but is often poorly tolerated by patients because of the taste. In addition, this can cause hypercalcemia in some patients. Sevelamer hydrochloride (Renagel®) is a calcium-free, aluminum-free phosphate binder that shows promise for long-term phosphorus control in patients with ESRD.[10] Unlike calcium-based phosphate binders, sevelamer hydrochloride may not reduce single-dose iron absorption.[7]

RENAL OSTEODYSTROPHY

Renal osteodystrophy must be prevented, and treated if present, by restricting phosphate, providing adequate calcium, using calcitriol carefully, and correcting metabolic acidosis.[11] This can be an extremely difficult balancing act:

- Although phosphate must be restricted, this can lead to severe phosphate depletion and rickets in infants with CRF
- Many calcium-containing phosphate binders also contain aluminum, which aggravates renal osteodystrophy
- Hypercalcemia may occur as a result of the use of calcium-containing phosphate binders, especially if calcitriol is also administered
- Sevelamer hydrochloride comes in large capsules that may be difficult to swallow
- Calcitriol may cause adynamic bone disease if parathyroid hormone (PTH) is zealously suppressed

ANEMIA

Hemoglobin levels must be measured regularly at 6- to 12-monthly intervals in all individuals with CRD.

The hemoglobin level usually declines over time with deterioration of kidney function. Anemia must be evaluated in all patients with a GFR <60 ml/min/1.73 m^2. The anemia must be assessed in relation to the patient's symptoms and findings, and the impact of anemia on co-morbid conditions and other complications of decreased kidney function such as tiredness, memory loss, and heart failure. Treatment appropriate to the etiology of the anemia may include iron supplementation, iron plus erythropoietin, and folic acid and vitamin B$_{12}$ if needed. Anemia is treated with erythropoietin and iron supplements when the hemoglobin level is below 10 g/dl. The initial dose of erythropoietin is 100 units per/kg per week, and the dose of elemental iron is 2–3 mg/kg per day. Failure to respond to erythropoietin may be the result of infection, chronic inflammation, hyperparathyroidism, insufficient doses of erythropoietin, aluminum toxicity, and iron deficiency. The long-term administration of erythropoietin is not associated with accelerated deterioration of renal function,[11] but may be complicated by hypertension.[2]

GROWTH

Before initiating growth hormone treatment for growth retardation, assiduous treatment of co-existing renal osteodystrophy and provision of optimal nutritional intake should be accomplished.[13] This may be difficult to achieve because of decreased appetite, nausea and vomiting. Growth loss in infants with CRF occurs during the first 6 months of life when nutrient intakes are poorly controlled, and therefore requirements may need to exceed recommended daily averages. Feeding by nasogastric or gastrostomy tubes may be needed. There are no established guidelines for optimum dietary protein requirements in neonates, infants and children with CRF. Inadequately treated bone disease has a negative impact on linear growth. Calcitriol and calcium-containing phosphate binder therapy must be monitored carefully by measurements of serum calcium and PTH levels. Vomiting is a frequent problem that can be treated with antiperistaltic agents, and some infants may require a fundal plication.

In children with CRF caused by polyuric, salt-wasting diseases, growth may be impeded if sodium and water losses are not corrected with low-caloric-density, high-volume, sodium-supplemented feedings.[9]

The results of 10 randomized controlled trials involving 481 children with CRF[14] showed that treatment with rhGH (28 IU/m^2/wk) resulted in a significant increase in height standard deviation score at 1 year (four trials, weighted mean difference [WMD] = 0.77, 95% CI = 0.51 to 1.04), and a significant increase in height velocity at 6 months (two trials, WMD = 5.7 cm/year, 95% CI 4.4 to 7.0) and 1 year (two trials, WMD = 4.1 cm/year,

95% CI 2.6 to 5.6). The authors of this meta-analysis concluded that, on average, 1 year of treatment with 28 IU/m^2 per week rhGH in children with CRF results in an increase of 4 cm per year in height velocity above that of untreated control subjects, and that there is no demonstrable benefit for longer courses or higher doses of treatment.[14] rhGH treatment also results in a significant improvement of adult height in children with CRF. The eventual height benefit of extended rhGH treatment is 1.0 to 1.5 standard deviations on average. Prepubertal rhGH treatment has a beneficial effect on final height; the efficacy of rhGH during puberty is less evident.[4] There are additional benefits of rhGH therapy. One dose of 28 IU/m^2 per week restores previously disproportional body structure and shape in children with CRF.[16] There are few adverse effects of this treatment.[3]

RENOPROTECTION

CRF invariably leads to ESRF and replacement therapy with dialysis and renal transplant.[6] Hebert et al. carefully describe the concept of renoprotection in their seminal review in 2001.[6] They hypothesize that the benefit of multiple-risk-factor interventions to retard progression of renal disease is the summation of multiple small beneficial effects. This approach is aimed mainly at preventing renal disease progression in adults, but it can be modified – with important caveats – for children. Some of these caveats are listed in Box 33-3.

ACE inhibitors may slow the progression of renal disease, but they rarely stop progression when used alone. Therefore, a multiple-risk-factor intervention strategy was developed based on inhibiting the progression mechanisms that are common to most forms of progressive renal disease. Each intervention is prioritized and assigned a level of recommendation. This is based on its proven value or use that is plausibly effective and prudent. This approach may provide hope for patients who feel that nothing can be done to prevent an inexorable progression

---

Box 33-3 Special Considerations in the Application of the Principles of Renoprotection in Pediatrics

- Infants and children need adequate protein and calories for growth
- Infants with renal dysplasia may need extra salt because of salt wasting
- Teenage girls must be warned that ACE inhibitors can cause an embryopathy
- Children with UTIs may need to drink large quantities of fluid

---

to ESRF. The proposed renoprotective strategies are based on clinical and experimental studies on the mechanisms of renal disease progression. The interactions of these mechanisms are complex. For example, blood pressure control might slow progression of renal disease, not only by reducing blood pressure, but also by decreasing proteinuria. Because of the uncertainty of how simultaneously deployed renoprotective mechanisms interact, both the proven and plausible mechanisms and interventions are listed and their possible modes of action are discussed.

Renoprotective strategies are not recommended for conditions in which there is little or no increased risk for progressive renal disease. The most important of these in pediatrics is steroid-responsive minimal change disease in the absence of persistent proteinuria or corticosteroid resistance. They are not recommended for conditions that cause acute renal failure with the expectation of nearly complete recovery of kidney function. These include acute post-infectious glomerulonephritis, acute obstructive uropathy, and acute tubular necrosis from toxins or ischemia. Shiga toxin-associated hemolytic uremic syndrome may be an exception, especially if the serum creatinine concentration does not return to normal or if proteinuria persists.[8]

LEVELS OF INTERVENTION

For mechanisms of renal disease progression and treatment, four levels of intervention with 18 interventions are identified. There are four interventions in each of levels 1 and 2. Most patients can achieve most of the L1 and L2 interventions. There are 10 interventions in level 3, and many of these can be achieved.

Treat Hypertension (Level 1)

Hypertension induces arteriolar nephrosclerosis, but the glomeruli are spared unless the hypertension is severe. When hypertension is superimposed on intrinsic renal disease, the resulting arteriolar nephrosclerosis adds to renal disease progression. In proteinuric renal disease, hypertension creates a vicious cycle, promoting the progression of renal disease.

Treatment

It is important to restrict salt intake and to encourage weight loss in obese individuals. If possible, dihydropyridine calcium channel blockers (D-CCBs) should not be used in chronic renal failure because they are not antiproteinuric and may worsen proteinuria. The D-CCBs are more effective antihypertensives than their non-dihydropyridine counterparts (ND-CCBs), but they may blunt the renal protection provided by

ACE inhibitor therapy. Minoxidil may cause hair growth and also worsen proteinuria. If the goals of blood pressure control are not achieved with quadruple therapy, the issues of compliance and secondary hypertension must be addressed.

The following sequence is the approximate level of recommendation:
1. ACE inhibitor, diuretic, β-blocker, and D-CCB.
2. ACE inhibitor, diuretic, β-blocker, and minoxidil.
3. ACE inhibitor, diuretic, β-blocker, and α-1-receptor blocker. The addition of D-CCB or minoxidil will increase the effectiveness of this combination.

Reduce Proteinuria (Level 1)

Hormonal replacement with erythropoietin, calcitriol, and growth hormone have had a great impact on the outcome of ESRD. The careful management of patients with CRD and CRF may not only retard the progression of CRD, but also have major impacts on the success of dialysis and transplantation on selective contains toxic or inflammatory systems that promote the progression of renal disease. Glomerular injury inflicted on podocytes worsens the proteinuria. Tubular injury is the result of C5b-9 deposition, inflammatory cell infiltration, and free-radical formation (induced by Fe^{3+}). Tubular epithelial hyperplasia results from growth factors and mitogens induced by proteinuria through complement and by filtered insulin-like growth factor-1 (IGF-1). Proximal tubular epithelial cell hyperplasia encroaches on the tubular lumen in proteinuric renal disease. In addition, these compounds induce tubulo-interstitial fibrosis by proteinuria-induced TGF-β and endothelin-1 (ET-1).

Treatment with ACE inhibitors may reduce proteinuria and therefore inhibit the progression of renal disease.

Role of Angiotensin II

Angiotensin II promotes renal disease progression by inducing glomerular hypertension, glomerular hypertrophy, and glomerular sclerosis.

Treatment

The renoprotective effects of ACE inhibitors in diabetic and non-diabetic nephropathies are independent of their antihypertensive effects. There are broad health benefits from prolonged ACE inhibitor therapy, and no identifiable health risks. In non-diabetic nephropathy, ACE inhibition is renoprotective independent of blood pressure control, but this is only in patients with nephrotic-range proteinuria. However, ACE inhibition is also renoprotective independently of blood pressure control in nephropathies with <3 g of protein per day. Enalapril, captopril, benazepril, and ramipril are all renoprotective in humans. The amount of ACE inhibitor therapy needed to achieve renoprotection is modest (daily treatment with 3.0 mg ramipril, 5 mg enalapril and 10 mg benazepril, or 25 mg captopril three times each day).

The goal of ACE inhibition is to reduce proteinuria goal below 1 g per 24 hours. Improved blood pressure control and decreased proteinuria are evidence that ACE-inhibitor therapy is providing renoprotection. ACE inhibitor therapy can be renoprotective, even with serum creatinine concentrations as high as 2.5 mg/dl. However, ACE inhibitors may cause hyperkalemia. If the 24-hour urine for potassium exceeds 50 mEq, a reduction in potassium intake should prevent serious hyperkalemia. However, if hyperkalemia occurs when a 24-hour urine for potassium was <40 mEq, it is unlikely that hyperkalemia can be avoided by dietary measures alone. If diuretic therapy or sodium bicarbonate therapy does not reduce hyperkalemia, ACE inhibition should be stopped and angiotensin receptor blocker (ARB) therapy should be used because the latter is less likely to cause hyperkalemia. The serum creatinine concentration usually increases slightly with initiation of ACE-inhibitor therapy. The latter approach and a low-protein diet have additive effects on reducing proteinuria and slowing the decline in GFR.

Principles of ARB Therapy

ARBs are similar to ACE inhibitors in their antiproteinuric and antihypertensive effects, but they are less likely to cause cough, angioedema, or hyperkalemia. ARBs suppress fibrogenic and inflammatory mechanisms similar to ACE inhibitors. It is unknown whether ARBs are renoprotective in humans, but they are recommended for patients who suffer side effects with ACE inhibitors. ACE-inhibitor therapy alone, or ARB therapy alone, have theoretical therapeutic loopholes, and combining them has theoretical advantages. Chymase is not inhibited by ACE-inhibitor therapy, and therefore angiotensin II can still be generated on this treatment. This loophole does not apply to ARB therapy because these agents directly block the angiotensin II type 1 (AT1) receptor. ARBs do not inhibit the degradation of bradykinin, which may have an important antihypertensive effect. In contrast to ACE inhibitors, ARBs do not significantly suppress aldosterone production. Because aldosterone induces tissue fibrosis, ACE inhibitors that suppress aldosterone would be advantageous.

Control Hyperglycemia (Level 1)

Hyperglycemia causes glomerular hyperfiltration, hypertrophy, and hypertension. This is rarely a problem in non-diabetic CRF patients. The hemoglobin A1C goal for type 1 diabetics should be within two percentage points of the upper limits of normal for the particular hemoglobin A1C assay.

Reduce Protein Intake (Level 1)

Increased protein intake acutely increases GFR and increases protein excretion in proteinuric individuals. The mechanisms include increased renin and eicosanoid production and the effects of individual amino acids, including that of L-arginine, on nitric oxide production.

Treatment

Protein restriction slows progression of renal disease (as GFR) by about 0.5 ml/min per year. When patients are instructed in a dietary protein intake of 0.6 g/kg ideal body weight per day, the average dietary protein intake achieved is 0.7–0.8 g/kg ideal body weight per day. This, and lower levels of dietary protein intake, are associated with slowed renal disease progression. Although there are no known risks to a low-protein diet in adults, one must proceed with caution in children. Children require at least their required daily allowance of protein calories.[15] Patients with heavy proteinuria require an increase of 1 g per day for each gram of proteinuria in excess of 3 g per 24 hours.

Correct Anemia (Level 2)

Anemia contributes to cardiovascular morbidity and mortality, and so may accelerate the progression of renal disease.

Treatment

Correction of anemia by erythropoietin therapy may slow the progression of renal disease. High-dose vitamin C therapy to augment iron absorption and to reduce oxidant stress is not recommended because it might lead to deposition of calcium oxalate in tissues and in turn to increased aluminum absorption. Vitamin E mitigates oxygen stress and hence may be beneficial.

Reduce Salt Intake

Increased salt intake can override the antiproteinuric effect of ACE-inhibitor and calcium channel blocker therapy.

Treatment

Salt should only be restricted in children with advanced CRF, or if hypertension is present.

Reduce Fluid Intake

Increased fluid intake is associated with a more rapid decline in GFR, especially in autosomal dominant polycystic kidney disease (ADPKD) patients.[5] The high urine volumes are also associated with maintained or increased blood pressures and greater use of diuretics.

High urine volumes could not be explained by more aggressive renal disease causing a renal concentrating and salt-wasting defect and polyuria. If chronically high urine volume promotes progression of renal disease, the effect may be due to adverse effects of increased intratubular pressure caused by high urine volume.

Treatment

Fluid intake must be individualized in children. There is a general misconception held by lay people and many professionals that large quantities of fluid are required in order to *flush out the kidneys*. Chronic high fluid intakes should not be recommended for patients with CRF, especially those with polycystic kidney disease (PKD).[5]

Control Hyperlipidemia (Level 1 for General and Level 2 for Renal Benefit)

Hyperlipidemia is associated with progressive glomerular injury. Hypercholesterolemia induces an atherosclerotic process in the renal microvasculature analogous to that in larger vessels. Hypercholesterolemia and glomerular hypertension may act synergistically to initiate structural injury.[1] However, there are no definitive controlled clinical trials in patients that demonstrate a benefit from lipid control on the progression of renal disease.

Treatment

Controlling blood lipids may slow the progression of diabetic and non-diabetic renal disease. Low levels of high-density lipoprotein cholesterol is an independent risk factor for progression of renal disease. HMG-CoA reductase inhibitors have anti-inflammatory effects by blocking NF-κB activation, a transcription factor for inflammatory pathways, including the chemokine MCP-1 that is expressed in inflammatory and non-inflammatory renal diseases.

Avoid Cigarette Smoking

Cigarette smoking induces vasoconstrictor, thrombotic, and direct toxic effects on the vascular endothelium. Smoking is an independent risk factor for progression of inflammatory renal disease (IgA nephritis), non-inflammatory renal disease (PKD), and diabetic nephropathy.

Treatment
The best treatment is to avoid or quit smoking.

Control Hyperhomocysteinemia (Level 2 for General and Level 3 for Renal Benefit)

Hyperhomocysteinemia is a risk factor for atherothrombosis and microalbuminuria in diabetic nephropathy, possibly because of oxidant stress-induced endothelial injury.

Treatment

It is difficult to normalize plasma homocysteine in patients with advanced renal insufficiency.

Control Increased Endogenous Insulin (Increased C-Peptide) (Level 3)

In experimental models of insulin resistance, high plasma insulin levels (and/or triglycerides) induce glomerular sclerosis. This might explain the association of microalbuminuria with insulin resistance in non-obese subjects, and the increased incidence of focal and segmental glomerulosclerosis in obese individuals and blacks.

Treatment

Weight reduction in obese patients and exercise may decrease insulin resistance in patients with elevated C-peptide levels.

Avoid NSAIDs (Level 2)

NSAIDs may cause acute and usually reversible renal failure[12] and interstitial nephritis. It is not clear whether chronic daily use of NSAIDs causes progressive nephrotoxicity.

Treatment

In patients with CRD or CRF and chronic pain, either acetaminophen, propoxyphene, or tramadol are recommended.

Control Hyperphosphatemia (Level 1 for General and Level 3 for Renal Benefit)

Hyperphosphatemia may promote progression of renal disease by deposition of calcium-phosphorus in the kidneys and/or by secondary hyperparathyroidism.

Treatment

The serum phosphorus concentration should be kept within the normal range by dietary phosphorus restriction and phosphate binders.

Avoid Potassium Depletion (Level 1 for General and Level 3 for Renal Benefit)

Progressive renal interstitial fibrosis may be associated with sustained potassium depletion possibly by induction of growth factors and TGF-β.

Treatment

In patients with chronic severe hypokalemia there is progressive renal failure caused by tubular interstitial disease. Chronic hypokalemia may also promote cyst growth in normal kidneys and in PKD.

REFERENCES

1. Anderson S, King AJ, Brenner BM. Hyperlipidemia and glomerular sclerosis: an alternative viewpoint. Am J Med 1989;87:34N-38N.
2. Brandt JR, Avner ED, Hickman RO, Watkins SL. Safety and efficacy of erythropoietin in children with chronic renal failure. Pediatr Nephrol 1999;13:143-147.
3. Fine RN, Ho M, Tejani A, Blethen S. Adverse events with rhGH treatment of patients with chronic renal insufficiency and end-stage renal disease. J Pediatr 2003;142:539-545.
4. Haffner D, Schaefer F. Does recombinant growth hormone improve adult height in children with chronic renal failure? Semin Nephrol 2001;21:490-497.
5. Hebert LA, Greene T, Levey A, et al. High urine volume and low urine osmolality are risk factors for faster progression of renal disease. Am J Kidney Dis 2003;41:962-971.
6. Hebert LA, Wilmer WA, Falkenhain MF, et al. Renoprotection: one or many therapies? Kidney Int 2001;59:1211-1226.
7. Malluche HH, Mawad H. Management of hyperphosphataemia of chronic kidney disease: lessons from the past and future directions. Nephrol Dial Transplant 2002;17:1170-1175.
8. Mujais S, Henderson L. The uremic syndrome: therapeutic-evaluative discordance. Kidney Int 2003;63(Suppl. 84): 2-5.
9. Parekh RS, Flynn JT, Smoyer WE, et al. Improved growth in young children with severe chronic renal insufficiency who use specified nutritional therapy. J Am Soc Nephrol 2001;12:2418-2426.
10. Pruchnicki MC, Coyle JD, Hoshaw-Woodard S, Bay WH. Effect of phosphate binders on supplemental iron absorption in healthy subjects. J Clin Pharmacol 2002; 42:1171-1176.
11. Sanchez CP. Prevention and treatment of renal osteodystrophy in children with chronic renal insufficiency and end-stage renal disease. Semin Nephrol 2001;21: 441-450.

12. Schaller S, Kaplan BS. Acute nonoliguric renal failure in children associated with nonsteroidal antiinflammatory agents. Pediatr Emerg Care 1998;14:416-418.

13. Sedman A, Friedman A, Boineau F, Strife CF, Fine R. Nutritional management of the child with mild to moderate chronic renal failure. J Pediatr 1996;129:S13-S18.

14. Vimalachandra D, Craig JC, Cowell CT, Knight JF. Growth hormone treatment in children with chronic renal failure: a meta-analysis of randomized controlled trials. J Pediatr 2001;139:560-567.

15. Wingen AM, Fabian-Bach C, Schaefer F, Mehls O. Randomised multicentre study of a low-protein diet on the progression of chronic renal failure in children. European Study Group of Nutritional Treatment of Chronic Renal Failure in Childhood. Lancet 1997;19;349: 1117-1123.

16. Zivicnjak M, Franke D, Ehrich JH, Filler G. Does growth hormone therapy harmonize distorted morphology and body composition in chronic renal failure? Pediatr Nephrol 2000;15:229-235.

PART *IV*

CHAPTER 34

Peritoneal Dialysis and Hemodialysis

KEVIN E.C. MEYERS, M.B., B.Ch.

INTRODUCTION

During the past 15 years, an increasing number of infants and young children with end-stage renal disease (ESRD) have been started on dialysis. The incidence of children entering ESRD is 11 to 15 per million of the population per year, and patients aged under 20 years account for 1.3% of ESRD cases on dialysis in the USA. In 1976, shortly after the development of chronic ambulatory peritoneal dialysis (CAPD), peritoneal dialysis (PD) was recognized as having special value for children.[1] This type of PD offers the child and family greater freedom, despite the possible complications of bacterial peritonitis from catheter and tunnel contamination. Numerous studies have been performed to define the concept of adequacy of dialysis and removal of toxins and water. Since 1980, PD has been widely used in children,[1] and the technique remains an invaluable alternative therapy to hemodialysis (HD), especially in smaller children because of the small size of blood vessels required for vascular access. In larger children, PD permits consistent school attendance and travel for family vacations. In contrast to adults, PD is now the predominant method of dialysis in children.

INDICATIONS FOR DIALYSIS

The choice of dialysis depends on the child's age, the renal disease, socioeconomic factors, and the physician and family preference.[3] Some 50% of children on chronic dialysis have congenital or hereditary renal disorders (Table 34-1),[2] in contrast to adults in whom 80% have an acquired renal disease.

Table 34-1 Primary Diagnoses in Pediatric Dialysis Patients (Rounded off to the Nearest Percentage)

Diagnosis	Proportion (%)
Renal adysplasia/hypoplastic/dysplasia	16
Focal segmental glomerulosclerosis	15
Obstructive uropathy	14
Vasculitis	8
Hemolytic uremic syndrome	4.5
Chronic glomerulonephritis	4
Reflux nephropathy	3.5
Polycystic kidney disease	3
Membranoproliferative glomerulonephritis types I and II	3
Prune belly syndrome	2.5
Medullary cystic disease	2.5
Congenital nephrotic syndrome	2
Interstitial nephritis	2
Familial nephritis	1.5
Idiopathic crescentic glomerulonephritis	1.5
Cystinosis	1.5
Denys–Drash syndrome	1.0
Sickle cell nephropathy	0.5
Oxalosis	0.5
Other	15.5

Acute Dialysis

The indications for initiating dialysis in children (Table 34-2) with acute renal failure are similar to those in adults.[5]

Acute PD is usually preferred for infants and young children because of ease of access, simplicity of equipment, rapidity with which severe hyperkalemia is corrected, and efficacy in the face of hemodynamic instability. Hemodialysis is favored when the peritoneal membrane cannot be used because of abdominal surgery. Continuous hemofiltration (CVVHD) or hemodiafiltration (CVVHDF) can be effective in a critically ill infant or child with hemodynamic instability.[5] Most poisons are best removed with hemodialysis. Hemodialysis or CVVHD are used to treat hyperammonemia and inborn errors of metabolism.

Chronic Dialysis

Chronic dialysis is started when the creatinine clearance is below 10 ml/min/1.73 m^2, and earlier in infants who have reduced growth velocity, poor head growth or delayed milestones.[6] Peritoneal dialysis (Automated Peritoneal Dialysis [APD] or Continuous Ambulatory Peritoneal Dialysis [CAPD]) is the technique of choice for treating chronic renal failure in children. APD is favored for all age groups (Box 34-1).[4]

CAPD is useful for children and adolescents. Although CAPD does not depend on an electrical source, it requires repeat access to the dialysis catheter with the risk of breaking the sterile barrier. It also needs additional school nursing support. An assurance of adherence must be obtained in adolescents who choose home PD. During adolescence, the requirement for a permanent intra-abdominal catheter may adversely affect body image, and must be accounted for when choosing this form of dialysis. However, in reality this also pertains equally to hemodialysis access.

Box 34-1	Benefits of Automated Peritoneal Dialysis (APD)
APD can be performed at night	School attendance is optimized
There is a one 'on–off' procedure	Scrutiny by peers is avoided
The risk of peritonitis is minimized	Precise dwell volumes are ensured
Working parents prefer APD	Oral nutrition is improved

HEMODIALYSIS

There is a curvilinear relationship between blood urea clearance and blood flow in children on hemodialysis. The clearance curves for a particular dialyzer must be known in order to estimate urea clearance at a given blood flow rate. The clearance may plateau at relatively low blood flow rates with a small dialyzer. With high-efficiency dialyzers, the urea clearance can approach 90% at blood flow rates below 150 ml/min (Figure 34-1).

The Gambro C3® and Fresenius 2008® series machines are useful for dialyzing children weighing less than 20 kg. Older children can be dialyzed with many other machines. Dialysis can be performed with single needles, for which adapters are available. However, these add to the extracorporeal blood volume and increase recirculation. Hollow-fiber dialyzers can be used for infants or children, while flat-plate dialyzers are no longer available. The priming volume (dialyzer plus tubing) must be less than 10% of the blood volume. Low-volume tubing is available for pediatric dialysis, and this reduces the priming volume, but it also restricts the blood flow rates. In order to avoid excessive fluid removal, 'volumetric' ultrafiltration is prescribed and is monitored by pre- and post-dialysis bed-scale weights accurate to 5.0 g. Vascular access may be either temporary or permanent (Table 34-3). Single- and double-lumen catheters are available for temporary dialysis, and these can be inserted via the internal jugular or femoral vessels; the subclavian route is avoided whenever possible because of a high rate of thrombosis. Venous cuffed cannulae provide permanent access for infants and children aged less than 6 years. Arteriovenous fistulae (AVF) are the preferred method of vascular access in children and adolescents. When AVF placement fails, polytetrafluoroethylene grafts (Gortex®) or central cuffed venous cannulae can be used.

Infants and children are prone to develop complications of the disequilibrium syndrome, hypotension,

Table 34-2	Indications for Dialysis
Absolute Indications	**Relative Indications**
Hyperkalemia with ECG abnormalities	BUN >120 mg/dl
Congestive cardiac failure caused by fluid overload	Organic acidemia
Severe hypertension caused by fluid overload	
Severe uremic pericarditis	
Uremic encephalopathy	

BUN = blood urea nitrogen.

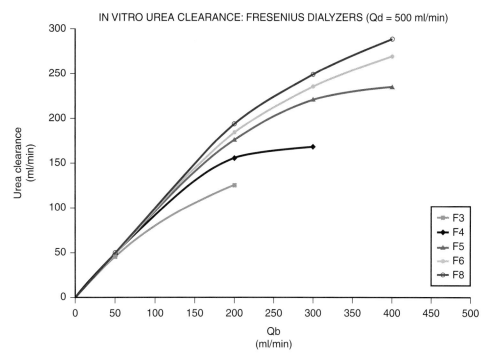

Figure 34-1 Urea clearance curves for various dialyzers. Urea clearance decreases in the smaller dialyzers with blood flow rates (Qb) above 50-100 ml/min. Qd = dialysis rate.

and hypothermia. Chronic hemodialysis treatments are given three times each week. The dialyzer and blood flow rate should result in a urea clearance of at least 3.5 ml/min/kg. The required amount of dialysis per session should be at least KT/V = 1.3 (Box 34-2). Higher-efficiency dialyzers can be used to improve solute clearance.[9] Pre- and post-dialysis serum urea nitrogen values are monitored to verify dialysis efficacy. Urea nitrogen

removal should achieve a urea reduction ratio (URR) of 70-85% (URR = {1 − [U_{post}/U_{pre}]} × 100). Heparinization is used to prevent clotting, the initial loading dose of heparin being 10-20 U/kg. The activated clotting time (ACT) or whole blood clotting time is maintained at 125-150%, by giving either additional boluses of 5-10 U/kg of heparin or a constant infusion of heparin (Box 34-3).

Table 34-3 Suggested Vascular Access Catheter Sizes

Patient Body Weight (kg)	Catheter	Modality	Insertion Site
1-3	*18-14 G single lumen, 3-8 cm length	CAVHD	*Femoral artery/vein
			*Umbilical artery/vein (newborns)
			*Femoral vein
			*Internal/external jugular vein
	*18-14 G single lumen, 3-8 cm length	CVVHD	*Subclavian vein
	*6.5-7.0 Fr, dual lumen		
>3-12	*16-14 G single lumen, 3-8 cm length	CAVHD	*Femoral artery/vein
	*16-14 G single lumen, 3-8 cm length	CVVHD	*Femoral vein
			*Internal/external jugular vein
	*6.5-8.0 Fr dual lumen		*Subclavian vein
>12-35	*5 Fr single lumen	CAVHD	*Femoral artery/vein
			*Femoral vein
	*5 Fr single lumen		*Internal/external jugular vein
	*8.0-9.0 Fr dual lumen	CVVHD	*Subclavian vein
>35	*5-8 Fr single lumen	CAVHD	*Femoral artery/vein
			*Femoral vein
	*5-8 Fr single lumen	CVVHD	*Internal/external jugular vein
	*9.0-11.5 Fr dual lumen		*Subclavian vein

*Vascular access for hemofiltration in children: selection depends on the physician's assessment of safety for a particular patient.
CAVHD = continuous arteriovenous hemodialysis; CVVHD = continuous venovenous hemodialysis.

Box 34-2 Calculation of *KT/V*: the Required Amount of Hemodialysis per Session for Three Sessions per Week:

If the required amount of dialysis is expressed as KT/V

Where K is urea clearance in liters/hour (assuming no residual renal function $K_R = 0$)

T is the session length in hours

V is the urea space

If $K = 3.5$ ml/min/kg = 0.21 l/h/kg, and V is set to the volume of the total body water (0.6 × kg), then

$1.3 = K \times T/V = (0.21 \times kg) \times T/(0.6 \times kg) = T \times 0.21/0.6$

$T = 1.3/0.35 = 3.7$ hours per session

CONTINUOUS HEMOFILTRATION/DIALYSIS

Continuous hemofiltration/dialysis and its applications are discussed in detail in Chapter 35. Continuous therapy is indicated for hemodynamically unstable, critically ill patients. Complications are infrequent, but they include inadequate access, bleeding around the access site, patient removal of the line, line sepsis, hemofilter membrane rupture, hypotension, hyponatremia, hypocalcemia, hyperkalemia, hemolysis, and seizures.

Box 34-3 Usual Settings for Hemodialysis

Dialyzer and tubing	Less than 10% of the patient's blood volume
Blood flow rate	Calculated to provide a urea clearance of 1.5–2.0 ml/kg/min for the first few sessions, and to provide a urea clearance of 3.0 ml/kg/min thereafter
Session length	2–3 hours for the first few sessions, 3–4 hours thereafter
Prophylactic mannitol	0.5–1.0 g/kg (mannitol is seldom required with a graded increase in dialysis)
Dialysis sodium	At or above the serum sodium concentration (sodium modeling)
Dialysis potassium	According to serum potassium concentration
Dialysis solution flow rate	500 ml/min to 800 ml/min
Ultrafiltration	Individualized

PERITONEAL DIALYSIS

The surface area of the peritoneal membrane as a percentage of the body weight is higher in infants and children than in adults, and approximates the body surface area. This large surface area allows for rapid and efficient equilibration of solutes. Shorter dwell times result in increased urea clearance and better fluid removal. The same solutions are used for children and adolescents. Larger bag volumes are used for APD. Tubing with smaller volumes is required for cyclers to minimize recirculation volumes when the volumes exchanged are less than 800 ml per cycle.

Acute Peritoneal Dialysis

Temporary catheters are now used infrequently. They are placed over a guidewire after first filling the abdomen with dialysate. A single- or double-cuffed Tenckhoff catheter for chronic use is inserted if more than 3 days of dialysis are anticipated. Three sizes of Tenckhoff Catheter® are available: neonatal (<3 kg), pediatric (3–10 kg), and adult (>10 kg). There are no data that support the contention that newer catheter designs are superior to the Tenckhoff catheter.[7] Catheters for chronic dialysis are inserted under general anesthesia. The peritoneum around the catheter must be sealed with a purse-string suture with the cuff immediately proximal to the peritoneum. The exit site must face inferolaterally in order to minimize the risk of exit-site infection (Figure 34-2). When double-cuffed catheters are used, the second cuff must be at least 2 cm from the exit site in order to prevent cuff extrusion. A partial omentectomy is recommended in all children to prevent catheter obstruction (Box 34-4).

Continuous Ambulatory Peritoneal Dialysis (CAPD)

Young children require five to six exchanges per day to control the biochemical abnormalities of uremia, and to achieve adequate fluid removal.

Box 34-4 Usual Settings for Acute Peritoneal Dialysis

Exchange volumes	20 to 50 ml/kg
Cycle times	30 to 60 minutes
Inflow/dwell times	25 to 50 minutes
Drain times	5 to 15 minutes
Dialysis dextrose	Concentration is chosen according to the amount of ultrafiltration that is required (1.5%, 2.5%, and 4.25% solutions)

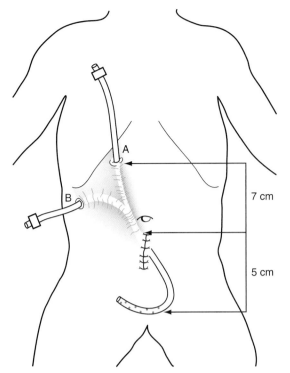

Figure 34-2 Correct Tenckhoff catheter positioning. A single cuff is positioned at the middle arrow. The exit site may need to be at point *A* in the infant, but this increases the risk of exit site infection. The exit site should point inferolaterally in the older child point *B*, and can be tunneled even lower than is shown. When a double-cuffed catheter is used the second cuff should be positioned at least 2 cm proximal to the exit site to avoid extrusion and reduce risk of infection.

Automated Peritoneal Dialysis (APD)

Five or more 2-hour nocturnal exchanges are used for adolescents. Infants require more frequent shorter cycles. A one-half-volume dwell or no dwell during the day helps to prevent a sensation of fullness, facilitates food intake, and reduces the occurrence of leaking and hernias. The advantages and disadvantages of long-term PD are shown in Table 34-4.

Dialysis requirements vary among and within individuals based on differences of solute mass and transfer rates in patients receiving long-term PD. The standardized peritoneal equilibrium test (PET) for adults was developed to allow for the characterization and comparison of basic information on solute transport rates of the peritoneal membrane (Box 34-5). Based on the kinetics of solute equilibration between dialysate and plasma (the D/P ratio), reference curves have been developed upon which individualized dialysis can be prescribed in adults. The pediatric PET procedure has been standardized in a small number of patients. More accurate characterization of the peritoneal membrane in pediatric patients and rational clinical application of the PET require publication of pediatric reference curves determined from larger numbers of children. Complications associated with PD are similar for children and adults (Box 34-6).

RECOMBINANT HUMAN ERYTHROPOIETIN (rhEPO)

CRF in children is associated with the development of a normochromic, normocytic, hypoproliferative anemia. The pathogenesis of the anemia is multifactorial. Anemia is more pronounced in children on HD than on PD, and this often resulted in dependency on blood transfusion. Uremia complicated by severe anemia is responsible for reduced physical work capacity, disturbed well-being, mental changes and dialysis discomfort. The use of rhEPO prevents anemia and avoids blood transfusions. Potential causes contributing to anemia should be investigated before starting rhEPO therapy (Table 34-5). Initial doses of rhEPO are 125 to 275 U/kg per week; maintenance doses are smaller (Box 34-7). Intravenous administration is preferred while on HD, although subcutaneous administration allows up to a 50% reduction in dose. Children on PD are given subcutaneous rhEPO once or twice a week. A non-responder is a

Table 34-4 Advantages and Disadvantages of Long-Term Peritoneal Dialysis in Children	
Advantages	**Disadvantages**
Vascular access is not required	Peritonitis (one episode per 10–19 patient–months of dialysis)
Less antihypertensive medication	
Independence	Exit-site and tunnel infections
Daily routine normalized	Burnout of parents or caregivers
Relatively safe and simple procedure	Development of hernias
Continuous fluid and biochemical homeostasis	Decreased appetite from glucose absorption and a feeling of abdominal fullness
Fewer dietary and fluid restrictions	
Applicable to infants	Body image disturbances from the external catheter and protruding abdomen
Better growth	

Box 34-5   Adequacy of Peritoneal Dialysis[4,8]

Adequacy of dialysis is assessed using actual ultrafiltration, *KT/V* of ≥2.1 and the peritoneal equilibrium test (PET).

Box 34-6   Complications of Peritoneal Dialysis

Infections of exit site, tunnel, peritonitis	Metabolic (hyponatremia/ hypernatremia,
Hernias	hypokalemia/hyperkalemia,
Hypervolemia	hyperglycemia,
Leak	hyperlipidemia
Lower back pain	Anorexia
Burnout	Hypotension
	Increased mortality in infants dialyzed more than once each year

Box 34-7   rhEPO Dosing

Response dose (starting dose)	125–275 U/kg per week
Correction dose	~80% response dose
Sustaining dose	~30–60% response dose

Monitor the hemoglobin and reticulocyte count every 2 weeks to adjust rhEPO doses.

Table 34-5   Evaluation of Anemia

Cause	Investigation
Hemolysis	Lactate dehydrogenase (LDH)
Blood loss	Stools for occult blood, calculation of blood draw volumes
Hyperparathyroidism	Intact parathyroid hormone levels (PTH ratio)
Iron deficiency	Serum ferritin, serum iron, TIBC, % saturation
Folate/B$_{12}$ deficiency	Serum folate, B$_{12}$
Aluminum toxicity	Serum aluminum
Infection	Cultures, C-reactive protein

TIBC = total iron-binding capacity.

Table 34-6   Side Effects of Recombinant Human Erythropoietin (rhEPO) Administration

Side effect	Pre-dialysis (%)	CAPD (%)	HD (%)
Hypertension	10	30	33
Hyperkalemia >6.0 mEq/l	4	36	24
Hyperphosphatemia >6.5 mEq/l	4	52	18
Thrombocytosis >500,000 per μl	0	20	25

CAPD = chronic ambulatory peritoneal dialysis; HD = hemodialysis.

child requiring blood transfusions despite 3 months of rhEPO with a dose of more than 750 U/kg per week. Iron supplementation (2 mg/kg/day) is required for most children receiving rhEPO. Arterial hypertension is the most frequent adverse reaction of rhEPO therapy (Table 34-6). rhEPO results in better physical and psychosocial adaptation of children on dialysis, and this in turn enhances the patient's quality of life.

RECOMBINANT HUMAN GROWTH HORMONE (rhGH)

Many factors contribute to growth failure in CRF (Box 34-8), but the underlying mechanisms are incompletely understood. rhGH enhances growth in children with renal insufficiency who are on dialysis.

Box 34-8   Factors Contributing to Growth Failure in Children with Chronic Renal Failure

Age at onset of primary renal failure	Tubular losses of potassium, sodium, water
Cause of primary renal disease	Anemia
Genetic potential	Infection, inflammation
Degree of renal impairment	Psychosocial problems
Inadequate calorie and protein intake	Growth hormone inhibition, hypothyroidism
Renal osteodystrophy	Corticosteroids
Metabolic acidosis	

RENAL OSTEODYSTROPHY

Renal osteodystrophy affects skeletal growth and maturation. Disorders of vitamin D metabolism, especially calcitriol, play a key role in the development of secondary hyperparathyroidism. Serum concentrations of calcium, phosphate, parathyroid hormone, and alkaline phosphatase must be monitored. Adjustments of calcium and vitamin D intake are required to keep the serum calcium concentration in the upper normal reference range. Hyperphosphatemia must be controlled by dietary phosphate restriction and oral phosphate binders. Phosphate restriction in children is difficult to achieve because protein is needed for growth. Calcium acetate (PhosLo®), calcium carbonate (Tums®), and sevelamer (Renagel®) are used as phosphate binders. Calcium acetate does not have to be chewed with meals.

NUTRITION

The recommended energy intake is age-dependent and should meet recommended daily requirements (RDA). Additional calories cause obesity rather than growth. The RDA for infants is 100 kcal/kg per day. The RDA for older children varies from 40 to 70 kcal/kg per day. Infants usually require gavage (nasogastric) feeding to attain sufficient calorie intake. The optimal protein intake for children is not known, but should be 2.0-2.5 g/kg per day for infants, and 1.0-1.5 g/kg per day for children. Protein loss during PD with long dwells should be accounted for and replaced in the diet. The volume of urine (residual renal function) and dialysis modality influence fluid, sodium, and potassium restrictions. Restrictions are less severe when PD is used. The protein intake is individualized to provide for normalization of serum albumin concentration in patients who are not nephrotic.

Box 34-9 Dialysis and Transplantation

- Normal growth and development cannot be achieved with even the best dialysis
- Renal transplantation is better than dialysis for optimal quality of life, rehabilitation, and improved survival for children with ESRD[10]

MAJOR POINTS

- The type of dialysis *does not* affect the outcome of renal transplantation.
- Aluminum-containing compounds must not be used for chronic control of hyperphosphatemia
- Calcium citrate must be avoided because it markedly increases aluminum absorption.

DIALYSIS AND TRANSPLANTATION

A normal physiological state cannot be achieved by peritoneal or hemodialysis (Box 34-9).

REFERENCES

1. Alexander SR. Peritoneal dialysis in children. In: Nolph KD (ed), *Peritoneal Dialysis*, 3rd edn. Kluwer, Dordrecht, 1989.

2. Avner ED, Chavers B, Sullivan EK, Tejani A. Renal transplantation and chronic dialysis in children and adolescents; the 1993 annual report of the North American Pediatric Renal Transplant Cooperative Study. Pediatr Nephrol 1995;9:61-73.

3. Fine RN. A symposium on: Advances in pediatric dialysis. Semin Dialysis 1994;7.

4. Flynn JT, Warady BA. Peritoneal dialysis in children: challenges for the new millennium. Adv Ren Replace Ther 2000;7:347-354.

5. Flynn JT. Choice of dialysis modality for management of pediatric acute renal failure. Pediatr Nephrol 2002; 17:61-69.

6. Goldstein SL. Hemodialysis in the pediatric patient: state of the art. Adv Ren Replace Ther 2001;8:173-179.

7. Harvey EA. Peritoneal access in children. Perit Dial Int 2001;21(Suppl. 3):S218-S222.

8. Morgenstern BZ, Mahoney DW, Warady BA. Estimating total body water in children on the basis of height and weight: a reevaluation of the formulas of Mellits and Cheek. J Am Soc Nephrol 2002;13:1884-1888.

9. Sharma AK. Reassessing hemodialysis adequacy in children: the case for more. Pediatr Nephrol 2001;16:383-390.

10. Sherman NJ. Pediatric dialysis. In: Nissenson AR, Fine RN (eds), *Dialysis Therapy*, 2nd edn. Mosby-Yearbook, St Louis, 1993, pp. 345-385.

CHAPTER 35

Dialysis: Hemodiafiltration

MINI MICHAEL, M.B.B.S, F.R.A.C.P. AND

STUART L. GOLDSTEIN, M.D.

Introduction

History

Definitions

    Continuous Renal Replacement Therapy (CRRT)

        Molecular Transport Mechanisms

        Diffusion

        Convection

        Ultrafiltration

        Adsorption

        Sieving Coefficient

        Slow Continuous Ultrafiltration (SCUF)

    Continuous Arteriovenous Hemofiltration (CAVH)

    Continuous Arteriovenous Hemodialysis (CAVHD)

    Continuous Venovenous Hemofiltration (CVVH)

    Continuous Venovenous Hemodialysis (CVVHD)

    Continuous Venovenous Hemodiafiltration (CVVHDF)

CRRT Equipment

    Machines

    Vascular Access

    Blood Pump and Extracorporeal Circuit

    Prescription

    Solutions

    Anticoagulation

Nutrition and CRRT

Indications for CRRT

Non-Renal Indications of CRRT

    Inborn Errors of Metabolism

    Lactic acidosis

    Intoxications

    Tumor Lysis Syndrome

Drug Management During CRRT

Complications

    Filter Clotting

    Membrane Reactions

    Temperature Control

    Nutrient and Electrolyte Losses

Outcome

INTRODUCTION

Continuous renal replacement therapy (CRRT) encompasses a variety of extracorporeal techniques for supporting critically ill children with acute renal failure (ARF), oliguria, and fluid overload. Prior to the introduction of CRRT techniques, critically ill children with ARF and fluid overload were treated with hemodialysis (HD) or peritoneal dialysis (PD). Critically ill children with hemodynamic instability may not tolerate rapid fluid removal by conventional HD treatment, which occurs over 3–4 hours. Peritoneal dialysis treatment often yields less solute clearance; moreover, patients with respiratory failure may not tolerate fluid in the peritoneum.[6] The introduction of CRRT has been a revolutionary step in the management of critically ill children with ARF, as the CRRT treatments occur continuously, allowing for fluid removal in children with hemodynamic instability.

HISTORY

CRRT development dates back to the mid-1960s, when Henderson described a renal replacement therapy technique called diafiltration, which relied solely on ultrafiltration (UF), using membranes that were more permeable to water and small solutes compared to standard hemodialysis membranes. The technique came to be known later as hemofiltration. Henderson showed that, by pumping blood at high flow rates through an extracorporeal circuit containing a highly permeable filter, large volumes of plasma ultrafiltrate could be generated. During the late 1970s, Kramer first used continuous hemofiltration as a treatment for ARF, and showed that the heart could provide sufficient flow to produce UF by placing the hemofilter between the

274

arterial and venous catheters. This technique was then termed continuous arteriovenous hemofiltration (CAVH).

In 1980, Paganini introduced slow continuous ultra-filtration (SCUF) for patients with ARF and fluid over-load. In 1983, Geronemus and Schneider introduced continuous arteriovenous hemodialysis (CAVHD), in which dialysate fluid is passed through the filtrate compartment continuously to enhance the solute removal. In 1985, Lieberman used the SCUF technique to treat an anuric neonate with ARF and fluid overload, which was the first reported case of the use of contin-uous hemofiltration technology to treat a pediatric patient. In the following year, Ronco provided the first description of the use of continuous arteriovenous hemofiltration (CAVH) in neonates. The transition from CAVH to continuous venovenous hemofiltration (CVVH) using pumped hemofiltration systems in children was made during the early 1990s.

DEFINITIONS

Continuous Renal Replacement Therapy (CRRT)

CRRT is defined as any extracorporeal blood purifica-tion therapy intended to substitute for impaired renal function over an extended period of time, and prescribed for 24 hours per day.[1] In general, CRRT may be divided into the seven basic modalities, and defini-tions of each are detailed below.[1] The molecular trans-port mechanism employed with each modality is described first.

Molecular Transport Mechanisms

There are a number of key scientific principles used to accomplish the goals of CRRT. Understanding the principles of diffusion, ultrafiltration, convection and adsorption leads to the prescription of appropriate ther-apy or combination of therapies for a particular clinical setting.

Diffusion

Diffusion refers to the movement of solutes from an area of higher concentration to an area of lower concentration, across a semipermeable membrane. Current CRRT filters are constructed of a hollow fiber design, with blood being pumped inside the fiber. During conventional hemodialysis or CRRT dialytic ther-apies, the addition of a countercurrent balanced elec-trolyte solution to the extraluminal space of the dialyzer creates the concentration gradient, leading to diffusion of small solutes from the blood across the fiber membrane.

Convection

Convection refers to the movement of solutes across a semipermeable membrane where solute is transported together with solvent, otherwise called 'solvent drag,' by means of filtration in response to a transmembrane pres-sure gradient.

With hemofiltration (HF), the removal of solutes occurs via convection. HF refers to the provision of either pre- or post-filter replacement fluid into the extra-corporeal circuit. In hemodiafiltration, a combination of diffusive clearance (hemodialysis) and convective clear-ance (hemofiltration) is used in close to equal propor-tion for the purpose of solute removal.

Ultrafiltration

Ultrafiltration (UF) refers to the process of movement of fluids through a membrane caused by a pressure gradient. The pressure gradient in the extracorporeal circuit is created by positive or negative hydrostatic pressure using pumps, or by oncotic pressure generated from non-permeable solutes.

Ultrafiltration results in removal of fluid (plasma water) from the patient's blood. The fluid that is removed is referred to as the ultrafiltrate.

Adsorption

Adsorption refers to the adherence of molecules to the membrane surface or interior. Convection also drives the adsorption of molecules. Adsorption can be either surface adsorption onto the membrane, or bulk adsorption within the membrane when the molecules can permeate it. Solute adsorption onto a membrane results from the chemical properties of the membrane. These adsorptive properties may be influenced by elec-trical charge or the affinity of the membrane to attract and be retained in the membrane surface.

Sieving Coefficient

The sieving coefficient is the ratio between the filtrate concentration and plasma concentration for a given molecule. Molecules which filter freely (e.g., elec-trolytes, urea, glucose) have a sieving coefficient of 1.0. Large molecules (e.g., some drugs) may have a lower sieving coefficient because the relatively small filter pores retard the passage of large molecules. The sieving coefficient for very large molecules (>20,000 Da) such as albumin is zero.

Slow Continuous Ultrafiltration (SCUF)

SCUF is a form of CRRT that is not associated with fluid replacement and is often used in the manage-ment of refractory edema with or without renal failure (Figure 35-1A). The primary aim of SCUF is to achieve safe and effective treatment of fluid overload.

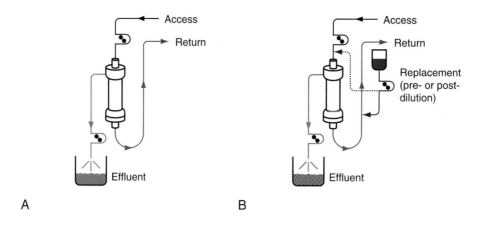

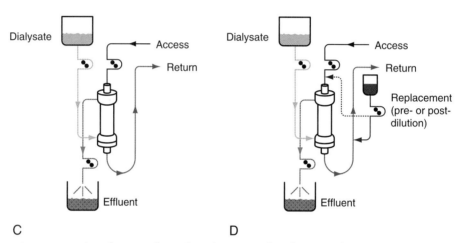

Figure 35-1   Schematic representation of commonly used continuous renal replacement therapy (CRRT) techniques. (A) Slow continuous ultrafiltration technique (SCUF). (B) Continuous venovenous hemofiltration (CVVH) technique. As shown in the figure, the replacement fluid is run either pre- or post-filter. (C) Continuous venovenous hemodialysis (CVVHD) technique. As shown in the figure, this procedure is characterized by slow countercurrent dialysate flow into the ultrafiltrate-dialysate compartment of the membrane. (D) Continuous venovenous hemodiafiltration (CVVHDF) technique. This method uses both slow countercurrent dialysate flow into the ultrafiltrate-dialysate compartment of the membrane and replacement fluid (either pre- or post-dilution). (These figures are adapted with permission from Gambro/Prisma Education Program CD.)

Continuous Arteriovenous Hemofiltration (CAVH)

In CAVH, patient perfusion pressure determines the blood flow through the filter. Two access sites are required: an arterial site to generate blood flow, and a venous site for blood return. UF generation is blood flow-dependent so that patients with poor perfusion pressure will have low UF generation. Continuous anticoagulation is administered through a prefilter tubing connection. However, problems in the control of blood flow and ultrafiltration, the increased propensity for filter clotting, and the potential for arterial complications such

as thrombosis associated with prolonged catheter placement, all weigh against CAVH as a routine procedure in the intensive care unit.

Continuous Arteriovenous Hemodialysis (CAVHD)

In CAVHD, a diffusive component is added to CAVH in order to enhance urea clearance. The circuit is the same as that used for CAVH but with the addition of a constant infusion of dialysate passing through the filtrate compartment of the filter.

Continuous Venovenous Hemofiltration (CVVH)

The CVVH circuit requires a blood pump and an air detector, and is often equipped with arterial and venous pressure monitors. In this case, the ultrafiltrate produced is replaced completely or in part by sterile filter replacement fluid (Figure 35-1B). This technique has the clear advantage of avoiding the potential complications of arterial access, and is capable of providing a substantial amount of convection-based clearance. Solute clearance is dependent on blood flow rate and the surface area of the membrane used.

Continuous Venovenous Hemodialysis (CVVHD)

CVVHD is a technique whereby the extracorporeal circuit is characterized by slow countercurrent dialysate flow into the ultrafiltrate-dialysate compartment of the membrane (Figure 35-1C). Fluid replacement is not administered, and solute clearance is mostly diffusive. The pump from the filter controls not only the dialysate flow rate but also the UF volume.

Continuous Venovenous Hemodiafiltration (CVVHDF)

CVVHDF is a technique whereby solute removal occurs via both diffusive and convective molecular transport mechanisms. Diffusive clearance is accomplished by the addition of a slow countercurrent dialysate flow to the ultrafiltrate-dialysate compartment of the membrane and the convective clearance achieved by the use of replacement fluid (Figure 35-1D). Combinations of both hemofiltration and diafiltration lead to enhanced solute clearance.[8,10] Some data suggest that convective clearance may enhance the removal of larger molecules compared to diffusive clearance.

CRRT EQUIPMENT

Machines

Several CRRT machines suitable for pediatric use are available, and these are listed in Table 35-1. Membranes used in hemofiltration are designed with high hydraulic permeability to promote UF. Membranes are manufactured from polymeric thermoplastics such as polysulfone, polyamide, polyacrylonitrile, and polymethylmethacrylate. The hemofiltration membrane is a composite structure consisting of an inner thin layer adjacent to the blood path surrounded by a supporting superstructure that

Table 35-1 CRRT Machines	
Company	**Machine**
Edwards Lifesciences	Aquarius®
Gambro	Prisma®
Baxter	BM 11[*]
	BM 11a[*]
	BM 25®
	Accura®
Fresenius	2008®
B Braun	Diapact®

[*]Blood pump only; addition of the BM14 is needed to make the total of a BM25 for the blood and ultrafiltration combined.

provides mechanical integrity without restricting the passage of water or any solutes small enough to pass through the pores of the inner layer. Hemodialysis membranes contain long, tortuous interconnecting channels that result in a higher resistance to fluid flow. The hemofiltration membrane consists of straight channels of increasing diameter that offer lower resistance to fluid flow.

All HF machines currently available commercially can provide circuit volumes that offer the adaptability to sustain therapy for smaller and larger size individuals. The Baxter, Braun and the Fresenius machines allow for individual choice of hemofilter membrane, while the Gambro machine uses a single membrane (AN-69) incorporated into a cassette containing blood tubing and pressure pods. The properties of the different hemofilters are listed in Table 35-2.

Table 35-2 CRRT Hemofilters		
Hemofilter	**Properties/ Surface Area (m²)**	**Priming Volume (ml)**
Amicon Minifilter Plus	Polysulfone/0.07	15
Renaflo II	Polysulfone	
HF 400	0.3	28
HF 700	0.7	53
HF 1200	1.25	83
Gambro		
Multiflow 100	AN-69/0.8	107
Multiflow 60	AN-69/0.6	84
Multiflow 10	AN-69/0.3	50
HF 1000	Polysulfone/1.16	128
Asahi PAN	Polyacrylonitrile	
0.3	0.3	33
0.6	0.6	63
1.0	1.0	78

Vascular Access

CRRT dialysis treatment efficiency depends on a properly functioning vascular access. Blood flow is related to resistance within a circuit. Vascular access resistance depends upon both the internal diameter and length of the catheter. Catheters with smaller internal diameters or longer lengths produce a higher resistance to blood flow, which can predispose to circuit clotting. Due to the relatively low blood flow rate (BFR) used in CRRT (3–5 ml/kg/min), as well as the smaller size of blood vessels in infants and children, access appropriate for size and BFR is needed for this population. Catheters should be small enough to avoid vascular injury, yet should allow for adequate BFR.

The use of double-lumen catheters (DLC) has simplified CVVHD vascular access. DLCs are designed to withdraw blood from a large vein through holes in the side of the catheter that enter the outside lumen ('arterial' lumen). Blood is returned down the central venous lumen and delivered through a single hole in the tip of the catheter that extends a short distance further into the vessel, beyond the arterial holes on the side of the catheter. This design is intended to reduce recirculation of the blood by withdrawing from a site that is more distal and returning to a more proximal location within the same large vein. When the catheter's overall diameter is too large and closely resembles the internal diameter of the vessel, poor arterial flow may result from collapse of the vein against the side holes of the catheter. This problem may be resolved by reversing flow (i.e., withdrawing from the venous and returning through the arterial lumen).

Depending upon the size of the patient, the access site and size may vary as listed in Table 35-3. Due to the potential long-term complication of subclavian vein stenosis, use of either internal jugular or femoral vein is preferred for catheter placement.

Blood Pump and Extracorporeal Circuit

CRRT pumps typically have devices to monitor pressures in the arterial and venous limbs of the circuit, which stops blood flow and alarms automatically when the pressures are outside acceptable ranges. If pressure in the arterial limb is too negative, blood flow from the patient is inadequate, usually because of clotted vascular access or a vein collapsing around the catheter. If the pressure in the venous limb is too high, blood return to the patient is inadequate, usually because of catheter occlusion or a clot in the venous drip chamber. If the catheter has been present for some time, tissue plasminogen activator (t-PA) treatment may remove clots obstructing the catheter. If the venous pressure is too low when the arterial pressure is adequate, there may be leak or disconnection in the circuit, or the pump speed may be too slow for the size of the catheter.

The volume of the tubing for the typical hemofiltration circuit and the hemofilter often exceeds 10% of the estimated blood volume of a child weighing less than 10 kg. To prevent hemodynamic instability, CRRT circuit priming with colloid is often employed in situations where the extracorporeal circuit volume exceeds 10–15% of the patient's blood volume.

Prescription

CRRT prescriptions vary from center to center. The main components of the prescription are the circuit priming solution, type of dialysate used, type of anticoagulation used to prevent circuit clotting, replacement fluid used for hemofiltration, blood pump speed, dialysate rate, and UF rate. Most circuits can be primed safely with saline. If the extracorporeal volume is >10–15% of the patient's estimated blood volume, priming with blood often becomes necessary. Since stored blood has a low pH and is anticoagulated with citrate, rapid infusion of a blood prime into an unstable patient can cause acute acidosis and hypocalcemia – leading to hypotension. Simultaneous infusion of sodium bicarbonate and calcium gluconate with the blood prime prevents this phenomenon.[5]

The blood pump speed (Qb) may vary from 2 to 10 ml/kg/minute, and should be optimized to the patient's hemodynamic stability. While no definitive data

Table 35-3 Suggested Size and Selection of Hemofiltration Vascular Access for Pediatric Patients

Patient Size (kg)	Catheter Size and Source	Site of Insertion
Neonate	Single-lumen 5 Fr (Cook)	Femoral artery or vein
	Dual-lumen 7 Fr (Cook/Medcomp)	Femoral vein
3–6	Dual-lumen 7 Fr (Cook/Medcomp)	Internal/external-jugular, subclavian or femoral vein
	Triple-lumen 7 Fr (Medcomp)	Internal/external-jugular, subclavian or femoral vein
6–30	Dual-lumen 8 Fr (Kendall, Arrow)	Internal/external-jugular, subclavian or femoral vein
>15	Dual-lumen 9 Fr (Medcomp)	Internal/external-jugular, subclavian or femoral vein
>30	Dual-lumen 10 Fr (Arrow, Kendall)	Internal/external-jugular, subclavian or femoral vein
>30	Triple-lumen 12.5 Fr (Arrow, Kendall)	Internal/external-jugular, subclavian or femoral vein

exist which describe the optimal clearance rates for CRRT, initial studies suggest use of a dialysate rate (Qd) or replacement fluid at 2000 ml/h/1.73 m^2 are associated with improved patient survival.[21]

Ultrafiltration rates (UFR) should be prescribed depending on the patient's hemodynamic and fluid status. Ideally, the UFR should be ≤5% of the blood flow rate in order to prevent hemoconcentration in the filter, while the net patient UF (i.e., the total intravenous input minus the total patient UF) can be safely targeted at 1–3% of the patient's blood volume per hour.

Solutions

A list of CRRT replacement and dialysate solutions is provided in Table 35-4. Replacement solutions can be infused either pre- or post-hemofilter. Most centers use saline or Ringer's lactate as a relatively inexpensive form of replacement fluid. Extemporaneously pharmacy-prepared solutions can be custom-made according to the patient's needs. The decision to use replacement fluid is often based on the overall solute and UF clearance requirements of the patient, as well as the local standard of care.

FDA-approved dialysis solutions are available both in lactate (Baxter, Deerfield, Illinois, USA) and bicarbonate form (Dialysis Solutions Inc, Richmond Hill, Ontario, Canada). Pharmacy-made customized solutions (usually bicarbonate-based) are also available. All of these solutions appear to be effective for overall urea clearance. An adult cross-over study by Zimmerman et al.[25] demonstrated that a bicarbonate-buffered dialysis solution provided equal acid–base control, but maintained more normal lactate levels than a lactate-buffered dialysis solution. Moreover, patients with hepatic failure may not be able to convert lactate to bicarbonate, and use of lactate-based dialysis solution may produce or exacerbate lactic acidosis. Hence, bicarbonate-based dialysis solutions are preferred for patients with hepatic failure.

Anticoagulation

Optimal extracorporeal circuit anticoagulation balances the maintenance of circuit patency while minimizing patient complications of anticoagulation therapy. A patient's clotting system is activated in CRRT circuits because of the circulating blood's contact with artificial surfaces.[17] Low blood flow rates and a high patient hematocrit enhance this effect. Individual circumstances dictate anticoagulation requirements, and patients with disseminated intravascular coagulation (DIC) or hepatic failure may not require pharmacological anticoagulation. While various methods of anticoagulation have been used in CRRT, randomized controlled studies comparing different methods are lacking. Currently available anticoagulation choices are a no anticoagulant (saline-flush) method, controlled dose (low-dose) heparin,[14] low molecular-weight (LMW) heparin, regional citrate, prostacyclin, and nafamostat mesylate.

One of the major disadvantages of CRRT is the ongoing necessity for anticoagulation, which increases the risk of bleeding and thrombocytopenia. In addition, turbulent blood flow, shear stress, and platelet–membrane interaction may cause platelet dysfunction, which further enhances the risk of bleeding. The most commonly used anticoagulation method employs continuous administration of heparin in the arterial line of the extracorporeal circuit. A common method for extracorporeal circuit priming is using 1–2 l of saline containing 1000–2000 U of heparin. Monitoring the activated clotting time (ACT) ensures the adequacy of heparin administration to prevent circuit clotting. The initial heparin bolus and the subsequent continuous heparin administration should be individualized for each patient according to the bleeding/clotting risk. Most centers aim to maintain ACT in the range of 180–240 seconds. ACT monitoring can be performed at 1- to 4-hour intervals.

Table 35-4 Commercially Available CRRT Solutions

Additives	PrismaSate® BK0/3.5	PrismaSate® BK2/0	Normocarb®	Hemofiltration Solution
Na (mEq/L)	130	130	140	140
K (mEq/L)	0	2	0	2
Cl (mEq/L)	109.5	108	105	117
HCO$_3$ (mEq/L)	32	32	35	0
Lactate (mEq/L)	3	3	0	30
Ca (mEq/L)	3.5	0	0	3.5
PO$_4$ (mEq/L)	0	0	0	0
Mg (mEq/L)	1	1	1.5	1.5
Glucose (mg/dL)	0	110	0	1

Of the other anticoagulation modalities available, regional citrate anticoagulation has gained much recent attention and has been increasingly used in many pediatric centers.[9] Regional citrate anticoagulation works via chelation of ionized calcium in the CRRT circuit, which prevents calcium-dependent clotting factor activation and thereby inhibits the intrinsic and extrinsic coagulation cascades.[20] In the patient, citrate is metabolized to bicarbonate, thereby releasing the ionized calcium, and a calcium chloride solution is infused into a central venous line, which normalizes the patient's ionized calcium and prevents anticoagulation of the patient. Citrate is infused into the arterial limb of the CRRT circuit, with the aim of keeping the ionized Ca^{2+} concentration at <0.5 mmol/l. Commonly used citrate solutions include trisodium citrate and anticoagulant citrate dextrose-formula A (ACD-A) solution. To prevent hypocalcemia in the patient (the aim being to keep the patient's ionized Ca^{2+} >1.1 mmol/l), calcium chloride is infused via a different central line. Both the patient and circuit ionized Ca^{2+} levels are monitored at regular intervals. Possible side effects of regional citrate anticoagulation are hypernatremia, hypocalcemia, and metabolic alkalosis. Furthermore, the development of a citrate buffer for calcium can occur in the patient, which leads to increasing total calcium levels with decreasing ionized calcium levels. This phenomenon is termed 'citrate lock,' and is easily reversed by stopping the citrate infusion for 4 hours.[9]

NUTRITION AND CRRT

Protein malnutrition is an inevitable consequence of a low-protein nutritional regimen in critically ill patients with ARF.[11,18,19] Protein depletion and a persistent and markedly negative nitrogen balance are highly undesirable, and result in respiratory muscle wasting and, possibly, immunological dysfunction and delayed renal recovery. The advent of CRRT now permits the virtually unrestricted administration of nutrition and proteins to patients with ARF and critical illness, but may also contribute to the development of a negative nitrogen balance through loss of free amino acids and peptides across hemofilters. Studies recently conducted demonstrate significantly improved nitrogen balance when patients are provided higher protein intake in combination with increasing CRRT clearance to control resultant azotemia. In a non-dialytic setting of ARF the standard recommendation for protein requirements is in the range of 1.5 g/kg per day. In patients receiving CRRT, protein requirements may be in the range of 3–4 g/kg per day or greater in order to maintain a positive nitrogen balance.[18,19]

INDICATIONS FOR CRRT

CRRT is generally prescribed for patients with ARF and fluid overload who do not respond to conservative medical management (pressors and diuretics) and who are hemodynamically unstable to tolerate conventional hemodialysis. CRRT is ideally suited to subgroups of patients, including bone marrow transplant patients with ARF and fluid overload, patients with septic shock and multi-organ failure, and liver transplant and heart transplant patients with ARF and fluid overload.

Sepsis with systemic inflammatory response syndrome (SIRS) and its late sequela, multi-organ failure, are caused by an uncontrolled immune response, leading to the generation of pro-inflammatory mediators of sepsis. Several investigators have contributed to the idea that at least part of this mediator load could be removed by hemofiltration. Grootendorst et al.[16] demonstrated significant differences between the clearances of interleukin (IL)-6, IL-8 and IL-10 with CRRT. It was found that the efficacy of IL-6 removal with polyamide is low, and the ultrafiltrate IL-10 concentration is below detection level, while IL-8 is cleared more effectively. Since the sizes of the interleukins are roughly equal, hemofiltration interleukin removal efficacy cannot be predicted from molecular weight alone. Bellomo and colleagues[2,3] showed that CVVHD using a polyacrylonitrile membrane is associated with the extraction of IL-6 and IL-8 from the circulation of patients with septic multi-organ and renal failure. However, no study to date has demonstrated that improved SIRS mediator removal is associated with improved patient outcome. This lack of association likely results from the relative non-selectivity of CRRT membrane in the removal of anti-inflammatory as well as pro-inflammatory cytokines. Further investigation into more selective removal techniques using CRRT is needed to determine whether specific cytokine removal can lead to improved patient outcome.

NON-RENAL INDICATIONS OF CRRT

When CRRT is used for the non-renal indications described below, efficient clearance of potassium and phosphorus may result. However, frequent monitoring of serum potassium and phosphorus levels is warranted, and replacement may be needed through TPN or as a separate infusion.

Inborn Errors of Metabolism

The use of CRRT in the treatment of inborn errors of metabolism, such as urea cycle defects, is becoming standard practice.[12] In infants and children with very high ammonia levels, a standard HD treatment may be used first to rapidly lower the ammonia level. CRRT can then be initiated upon HD treatment termination, in order to prevent the usual ammonia level rebound associated with intermittent HD.

Lactic Acidosis

As CRRT allows for infusion of bicarbonate without the risk of hypernatremia or fluid overload, these techniques are used for management of lactic acidosis secondary to inborn errors of metabolism.

Intoxications

CRRT can be useful in the treatment of intoxication by lithium, carbamazepam, phenytoin and *N*-acetyl procainamide. The clearance of intoxicants with significant protein binding may be improved by the addition of albumin to the dialysate.

Tumor Lysis Syndrome

CRRT has been employed in the prevention and treatment of hyperphosphatemia, hyperuricemia, and ARF associated with tumor lysis syndrome.

DRUG MANAGEMENT DURING CRRT

Drug elimination by hemofiltration depends mainly on the rate of UF, the drug protein binding, and the sieving coefficient for a particular drug.[4] Because patients undergoing continuous hemofiltration have impaired renal function, dosage reduction is often recommended so that adverse drug reactions are avoided. In contrast, if drug removal by hemofiltration is significant, then dosage supplementation may be required to ensure therapeutic efficacy. Therefore, knowledge of the impact of CRRT on drug elimination and the pharmacokinetic profile of drugs is essential for good clinical management. Unfortunately, few pediatric data exist to describe CRRT clearance characteristics for many commonly used medications. Factors that complicate the generalization of pharmacokinetic data from one study to a particular patient include the use of different modality, filter, blood flow rate, ultrafiltrate flow rate, dialysate flow rate, and patient population.

Drugs cleared primarily via the non-renal route usually do not require CRRT dose adjustments. Drugs cleared primarily via the renal route need CRRT dose adjustment, and drugs that have some renal clearance potentially require some dose adjustment. CRRT medication clearance varies markedly from drug to drug, and depends on the pharmacokinetic properties of the drug, the rate of CRRT, and the type of filter used.

For drugs with a wide therapeutic window, standard dosing guidelines for ARF and dialysis removal are probably adequate. For drugs with narrow therapeutic window, starting with the recommended initial dose for patients with ARF receiving dialysis dose is reasonable, and frequent serum drug level monitoring should be performed if possible.

COMPLICATIONS

Filter Clotting

Clotting of the hemofilter is the most common complication of CRRT. Factors that predispose the filter to clotting include interrupted blood flow, high resistance anywhere in the circuit (especially in the venous limb of the access), high filtration fraction, air pockets within the filter fibers, and inadequate anticoagulation. Among these factors, inadequate anticoagulation and vascular access malfunction are most commonly encountered. Thromboembolic and infectious complications are also more likely to occur in patients with frequent filter clotting.

The average filter lifespan varies widely among patients, and may also change as conditions change in the individual patient. For instance, patients recovering from sepsis may demonstrate resolution of DIC and may have increased pharmacological anticoagulation requirements. The present authors' practice indicates average filter lifespans to range from 48 to 60 hours. Most manufacturers recommend scheduled filter changing at 72 hours of filter life.

Membrane Reactions

One of the more biocompatible membranes (PAN, AN-69) has been shown to cause a bradykinin release syndrome in patients who are acidotic at the onset of HF or in children who require a 'blood prime' in the setting of one of these membranes.[5] These membranes, in the face of interacting with an acidotic plasma environment, generate bradykinin, which may result in reactions from minor nausea to clinical anaphylaxis. In those patients who require blood priming, transfusing the post hemofilter with a generous administration of sodium bicarbonate, or using a priming mixture of 100 ml packed red blood cells, 100 mmol of sodium bicarbonate and 400 mg of calcium gluconate, makes this reaction virtually non-existent.

Temperature Control

Hypothermia can be a potential problem especially in infants, as the heat can be lost from the extracorporeal circuit. However, with the advent of thermic controllers this has become less of a clinical problem. The Hot Line® is one such thermic controller comprised of a segment of intravenous tubing surrounded by a second tube that contains circulating water warmed to body temperature. The Hot Line® is added to the venous limb of the circuit (the volume of the Hot Line® is 17.5 ml, which increases the extracorporeal circuit volume), thus warming the blood as it is returned to the patient. In the smaller child, CRRT using one of the thermic controllers will result in euthermia and may mask a fever, so the clinician must remain vigilant for a new or ongoing infection, even in the absence of fever.

Nutrient and Electrolyte Losses

Protein losses during high-volume CRRT are substantially lower than previously reported, and range between 1.2 and 7.5 g per day.[19] Amino acid losses represent a far greater loss of protein nitrogen, estimated to be between 7 and 50 g per day.[19] The critically ill patient is often severely catabolic, so when estimating adequate protein and energy intake, these losses should be considered. Vitamin losses have been reported in continuous hemofiltration, although a real depletion syndrome is not commonly observed.[22]

Continuous loss of phosphate amounting to about 200–800 mg per day occurs with CRRT, especially in patients receiving parenteral nutrition. Severe phosphate depletion impairs the energy supply and also increases the risk of bacterial and fungal infection. As these losses are difficult to manage, phosphate administration is rapidly necessary and the blood phosphate concentration should be regularly assessed.

Electrolytes such as sodium, potassium, and magnesium are also lost in proportion to the serum concentrations, but these can be easily replaced.

OUTCOME

No prospective randomized controlled trials have been conducted to assess outcome in children with ARF after renal replacement therapy. In fact, few such studies exist for adult patients. Ronco et al.[21] conducted a prospective randomized study of the impact of different hemofiltration doses on patient survival. The results showed that critically ill patients who received CRRT with a lower clearance (20 ml/kg/h) had worse survival (41%) compared to those who received a higher clearance (35 ml/kg/h; survival 57%, p = 0.0007 versus 45 ml/kg/h; survival 58%, p = 0.0013).[23] In addition, an increased APACHE II score, increased blood urea nitrogen (BUN) concentration at the start of CRRT, and the presence of sepsis were also significantly associated with mortality.

As no single pediatric center cares for enough patients to make statistically valid conclusions, pediatric data,[7,15,24] which solely represent single-center studies can only describe trends of practice and related outcome. Goldstein et al.[15] examined outcome in 21 critically ill pediatric patients who received CVVHD using the pediatric risk of mortality (PRISM) score to control for patient severity of illness.[13] The mean patient weight, age, PRISM score at ICU admission and at CVVHD initiation, maximum pressor number, estimated glomerular filtration rate at CVVHD initiation, and change in mean airway pressure did not differ between survivors and non-survivors. However, the degree of fluid overload at CVVHD initiation was significantly lower in survivors (16.4 ± 13.8%) compared with non-survivors (34.0 ± 21.0%, p = 0.03), even when the severity of illness was controlled by the PRISM score in a multiple regression analysis. These data suggest that, in some cases, earlier CRRT at lesser degrees of fluid overload may be beneficial to allow blood product and intravenous nutrition administration while preventing increasing fluid overload.

Bunchman et al.[7] retrospectively examined 226 children with ARF treated with renal replacement therapy (HF, n = 106; HD, n = 61; and PD, n = 59), looking for predictors of outcome. The diagnoses in these groups varied from sepsis to inborn error of metabolism to intoxications. The authors concluded that, of the clinical variables reviewed (age, low blood pressure, diagnosis, CRRT modality and pressor use), increased pressor number was most strongly associated with worse survival.

Currently, a multi-center prospective pediatric CRRT registry is collecting data regarding numerous clinical variables, including nutrition provision, CRRT modality, clearance prescriptions, and pre-CRRT fluid management, which could potentially effect survival in children receiving CRRT. In addition, the registry is assessing the effect of different anticoagulation methods on the CRRT circuit lifespan and initiating a study of CRRT clearance of cytokines in children.

REFERENCES

1. Bellomo R, Ronco C, Mehta RL. Nomenclature for continuous renal replacement therapies. Am J Kid Dis 1996; 26:S2-S7.

2. Bellomo R, Tipping P, Boyce N. Interleukin-6 and interleukin-8 extraction during continuous venovenous hemodiafiltration in septic acute renal failure. Renal Failure 1995;17:457-466.

3. Bellomo R, Teede HN. Anticoagulant regimens in acute continuous hemodiafiltration: a comparative study. Int Care Med 1993;19:329-332.

4. Bressolle F, Kinowski JM, Coussaye JE, et al. Clinical pharmacokinetics during continuous hemofiltration. Clin Pharmacokinet 1994;26:457-471.

5. Brophy PD, Mottes TA, Kudelka TL, et al. AN-69 membrane reactions are pH-dependent and preventable. Am J Kidney Dis 2001;38:173-178.

6. Brunet S, Leblanc M, Geadah D, et al. Diffusive and convective solute clearances during continuous renal replacement therapy at various dialysate and ultrafiltration flow rates. Am J Kidney Dis 1999;34:486-492.

7. Bunchman TE, McBryde KD, Mottes TE, et al. Pediatric acute renal failure: outcome by modality and disease. Pediatr Nephrol 2001;16:1067-1071.

8. Bunchman TE, Donckerwolcke RA. Continuous arterial-venous diahemofiltration and continuous veno-venous diahemofiltration in infants and children. Pediatr Nephrol 1994;8:96-102.

9. Bunchman TE, Maxvold NJ, Barnett J, et al. Pediatric hemofiltration: Normocarb dialysate solution with citrate anticoagulation. Pediatr Nephrol 2002;17:150-154.

10. Bunchman TE, Maxvold NJ, Kershaw DB, et al. Continuous venovenous hemodiafiltration in infants and children. Am J Kidney Dis 1995;25:17-21.

11. Davies SP, Reaveley DA, Brown EA, et al. Amino acid clearances and daily losses in patients with acute renal failure treated by continuous arteriovenous hemodialysis. Crit Care Med 1991;19:1510-1515.

12. Falk MC, Knight JF, Roy LP, et al. Continuous venovenous hemofiltration in the acute treatment of inborn errors of metabolism. Pediatr Nephrol 1994;8:330-333.

13. Fargason CA, Langman CB. Limitations of pediatric risk mortality score in assessing children with acute renal failure. Pediatr Nephrol 1994;7:703-707.

14. Geary DF, Gajaria M, Fryer-Keene S, et al. Low-dose and heparin-free hemodialysis in children. Pediatr Nephrol 1991;5:220-224.

15. Goldstein SL, Currier H, Graf JM, et al. Outcome in children receiving continuous hemofiltration. Pediatrics 2001;107:1309-1312.

16. Grootendorst AF, Bouman CSC, Hoeben KHN, et al. The role of continuous renal replacement therapy in sepsis and multiorgan failure. Am J Kidney Dis 1996;28:S50-S57.

17. Manns M, Sigler MH, Teehan BP. Continuous renal replacement therapies: an update. Am J Kidney Dis 1998;32:185-207.

18. Maxvold NJ, Smoyer WE, Custer JR, et al. Amino acid loss and nitrogen balance in critically ill children with acute renal failure: a prospective comparison between classic hemofiltration and hemofiltration with dialysis. Crit Care Med 2000;28:1161-1165.

19. Mokrzycki MH, Kaplan AA. Protein losses in continuous renal replacement therapies. J Am Soc Nephrol 1996;7:2259-2263.

20. Palsson R, Niles JL. Regional citrate anticoagulation in continuous venovenous hemofiltration in critically ill patients with a high risk of bleeding. Kidney Int 1999;55:1991-1997.

21. Ronco C, Bellomo R, Homel P, et al. Effects of different doses in continuous veno-venous hemofiltration on outcomes of acute renal failure: a prospective randomized trial. Lancet 2000;356:26-30.

22. Ronco C, Bellomo R. Complications with continuous renal replacement therapy. Am J Kidney Dis 1996;28:S100-S104.

23. Roy D, Hogg RJ, Wilby PA, et al. Continuous veno-venous hemofiltration using bicarbonate dialysate. Pediatr Nephrol 1997;11:680-683.

24. Smoyer WE, McAdams C, Kaplan BS, et al. Determinants of survival in pediatric continuous hemofiltration. J Am Soc Nephrol 1995;6:1401-1409.

25. Zimmerman D, Cotman P, Ting R, et al. Continuous venovenous hemodialysis with a novel bicarbonate dialysis solution: prospective crossover comparison with a lactate buffered solution. Nephrol Dial Transplant 1999;14:2387-2391.

CHAPTER 36

Evaluation for Pediatric Renal Transplantation

H. JORGE BALUARTE, M.D.,

JO-ANN PALMER, C.R.N.P., AND

JULIE PETRO MONGIELLO, C.R.N.P.

INTRODUCTION

Renal transplantation is accepted as the therapy of choice for children with end-stage renal disease (ESRD). This is based upon the belief that successful transplantation not only ameliorates uremic symptoms but also allows for significant improvement, and often correction of, delayed skeletal growth, sexual maturation, cognitive performance, and psychosocial functioning.[2] The child with a functional allograft can lead a life of superior quality when compared with that achieved with available dialysis.

Success in pediatric renal transplantation remains a challenging undertaking. Children and adolescents are constantly growing, developing, and changing. Therefore, each developmental stage represents a series of medical, biological, and psychological challenges. Improvements in pediatric renal transplantation are attributed to contributions of better age-appropriate clinical care, histocompatibility matching, and newer immunosuppressive therapy.

EPIDEMIOLOGY OF END-STAGE RENAL DISEASE IN CHILDREN

Incidence

The incidence of ESRD in children aged less than 19 years is 15 per million population per year [2002 USRDS Annual Data Report]. The highest incidence of ESRD in children occurs between the ages of 15 and 19 years, with adolescents comprising 47% of pediatric ESRD patients. The incidence is higher in blacks across all age groups, but is most prominent in the 15- to 19-year-old age group (60 per million blacks versus 20 per million whites). Boys have a higher incidence than girls in all age groups because of a higher incidence of congenital disorders.

Etiology

Primary glomerulonephritis is the largest single disease category causing ESRD in children (Table 36-1). The etiology of ESRD varies significantly with age. Congenital, hereditary, and cystic diseases cause ESRD in over 52% of children prior to the age of 6 years, whereas glomerulonephritis and focal segmental glomerulosclerosis account for 38% of cases of ESRD in patients aged 10 to 19 years.

Table 36-1 Incidence of Treated End-Stage Renal Disease in Pediatric Patients according to Primary Disease*

Primary Renal Disease	Incidence (%)
Obstructive uropathy	16.2
Aplastic/hypoplastic/dysplastic kidney	15.9
Focal segmental glomerulosclerosis	11.4
Reflux nephropathy	5.3
Chronic glomerulonephritis (GN)	3.8
Polycystic disease	2.8
Medullary cystic disease	2.8
Hemolytic uremic syndrome	2.7
Prune belly syndrome	2.6
Congenital nephrotic syndrome	2.5
Familial nephritis	2.4
Cystinosis	2.1
Membranoproliferative GN – type I	2.0
Interstitial nephritis/pyelonephritis	2.0
Idiopathic crescentic GN	1.9
SLE nephritis	1.6
Renal infarct	1.6
Henoch–Schönlein nephritis	1.3
IgA nephritis (Berger)	1.3
Membranoproliferative GN – type II	0.9
Oxalosis	0.6
Wilms' tumor	0.6
Denys–Drash syndrome	0.6
Wegener's granulomatosis	0.6
Membranous nephropathy	0.5
Other systemic immunologic disease	0.4
Sickle cell nephropathy	0.2
Diabetic GN	0.1
Other	7.6
Unknown	5.6

Data from NAPRTCS: Transplant patient characteristics, p. 21. Annual Report of the North American Pediatric Renal Transplant Cooperative Study (NAPRTCS), 2002.

Access to Transplantation

About 5% of kidney transplants performed in the United States are in children. The absolute numbers of pediatric kidney transplants has remained relatively constant. Between 1987 and 2001, a total of 7247 children received 7951 transplants [North American Pediatric Renal Transplant Cooperative Study (NAPRTCS) 2002 annual report]. The mean age of transplant is 10.9 years; about 46% of pediatric recipients are aged over 12 years, 34% are aged 6–12 years, 15% are aged between 2 and 5 years, and only about 5% are aged less than 2 years. Among these recipients, 60% are male, 62% are white, 16% are black, and 16% are Hispanic.

Living donation (LD) now accounts for 55% of all pediatric kidneys transplanted. This trend results from a heightened awareness that transplantation is the best therapeutic option for children with ESRD, combined with increased waiting times for cadaver donor (CD) organs.

INDICATIONS FOR, AND TIMING OF, RENAL TRANSPLANTATION

All children reaching ESRD are considered as candidates for renal transplantation. Indeed, renal transplantation should always be considered when renal replacement therapy is indicated. Dialysis may be required before transplantation in order to optimize nutritional and metabolic conditions, to achieve an appropriate size in small children, or to keep a patient stable until a suitable donor is available. Most centers try to achieve a recipient patient weight of at least 8–10 kg, as this minimizes the risk of vascular thrombosis and the child can accommodate an adult-sized kidney. This target weight of 10 kg may not be achieved until 12 to 24 months of age.

Preemptive transplantation is transplantation without prior dialysis, and this accounts for 24% of pediatric renal transplants. Most kidneys for preemptive transplant recipients are from LD. Candidates for preemptive transplantation need careful pre-transplant psychological assessment because there may be an increased tendency for non-adherence in this group of recipients. Nevertheless, there appears to be no impairment in graft outcome in pediatric recipients who have undergone preemptive transplantation when compared with those who have dialysis before transplantation (Box 36-1).

Box 36-1 Contraindications to Transplantation in Children

ABSOLUTE
- Human immunodeficiency virus (HIV) disease (may become a relative contraindication)
- Active or untreated malignancy
- Severe multi-organ failure
- Chronic active infection with hepatitis B virus
- Debilitating, irreversible brain injury
- Current positive direct cross-match

RELATIVE
- ABO incompatibility with the donor
- Chronic infection with hepatitis C virus
- Active autoimmune disease (systemic lupus erythematosus or antiglomerular basement membrane (GBM) disease with high levels of anti-GBM antibodies)
- Severe psychomotor retardation or psychiatric illness that requires custodial care
- Serious long-standing non-compliance with medical management
- Lack of family support or adequate home supervision

THE ORGAN DONATION PROCESS

Living Kidney Donation

Living donors may be parents, aunts, uncles or grandparents; living-unrelated donors may be step-parents, adoptive parents, or close family friends; altruistic donors are those who are strangers. Living donors undergo extensive evaluations that include a detailed history, physical examination, laboratory, and radiology evaluations, and a psychological evaluation. Donor kidney function, cardiovascular and pulmonary status, and the potential for infectious disease are fully examined. Great care is taken during the evaluation to ensure that not only is the kidney suitable for the potential recipient, but also that there is low risk to the potential donor. During the donor's psychological evaluation, the mental health of the donor, motivation for donation, elements of coercion and social supports are explored. The National Organ Transplant Act, passed by Congress in 1984, outlawed the sale of human organs. As a result, any exchange of money or gifts is strictly prohibited.

Cadaveric Kidney Donation

For many children, LD transplant is not an option, most often due to the lack of a compatible or medically acceptable donor. Occasionally, the patient's disease is such that an unrelated kidney may be a better option in order to decrease the risk of recurrent disease following transplant. For these patients, the CD list is the best option.

As of November 2002, there were 85,879 people in the United States awaiting a solid organ transplant. During the past 10 years this number has *tripled*. More than 50,000 of those patients are awaiting a kidney transplant; however, less than 3% are under the age of 17 years. All patients awaiting a CD transplant are listed on a national transplant waiting list through the United Network for Organ Sharing (UNOS), a private, non-profit organization that maintains the organ transplant waiting list under contract with the Health Resources and Services Administration of the U.S. Department of Health and Human Services. UNOS oversees the 59 local organ procurement organizations (OPO) located in 11 federally designated regions throughout the United States. The OPO provide the link between the patients awaiting transplant at the area transplant centers and the potential organ donors at area hospitals. Organ procurement coordinators from area OPO are responsible for the identification of suitable donors, allocation, and the retrieval, preservation and transportation of organs for transplantation. They are also involved in data follow-up regarding CD. In addition, they engage in public education on the critical need for organ donation throughout their communities.

The goal of local OPO is that all potential organ donors are referred to their organization, regardless of disease or organ function, prior to the withdrawal of support. Patients that have suffered cardiovascular death are suitable only for tissue donation. Only the very small percentage of patients that have sustained an irreversible and devastating neurological event may be suitable for donating a kidney. A potential organ donor, in most cases, meets the criteria for brain death. A very small number of organ donors have suffered cardiovascular death prior to organ recovery; however, that topic is beyond the scope of this chapter. It is critical that brain-dead patients or those who are approaching brain death be referred to the local OPO prior to withdrawal of ventilator and cardiovascular support in order to preserve optimal organ function for transplantation, thereby ensuring the option of donation for families. In this way, the number of organs available for transplant is maximized. It is the responsibility of the OPO to determine suitability for donation and approach families regarding the option of organ donation.

Kidneys are allocated to candidates on the national waiting list through an intricate computer 'point' system that strives to distribute organs in as equitable manner possible. Organs are allocated according to the characteristics of each organ donor. Therefore, with every donor, a new list is created with a completely different order of potential candidates (Box 36-2).

Box 36-2 Factors Influencing Kidney Allocation

DONOR

Blood type
- Only patients who are blood type-compatible with the donor will 'print out'
- Organs are first allocated to ABO identical recipients

Human leukocyte antigen (HLA)
- HLA match is taken into account to improve the survival of the graft

Location of the procurement
- Kidneys are given to recipients in the same local area as the donor to decrease the cold ischemia time, thereby improving graft function

RECIPIENT

Panel of reactive antibody (PRA)
- The higher the PRA, the more likely the patient will have a positive cross-match
- This indicates a very high likelihood of hyperacute reaction

Waiting time
- An unusual HLA type does not penalize candidates because length of time on the waiting list is heavily weighted

Box 36-3 Pediatric Kidney Policy

- Patients not transplanted within specified time goals receive added priority
- Children aged under 5 years should receive an allograft in 6 months
- Children aged 6–10 years should receive an allograft in 12 months
- Children aged 11–17 years should receive an allograft in 18 months
- Exceptions are O-antigen mismatch allocation and highly sensitized (>80% PRA) patients

Box 36-4 Prospective Donor Evaluation

- ABO compatibility
- Negative lymphocytotoxic cross-match with recipient sera
- Histocompatibility matching
- Psychosocial evaluation
- Chest radiograph, KUB, and electrocardiogram
- Urinalysis, urine culture, and two 24-hour collections for protein and creatinine measurement
- Hepatitis profile, CMV titer, EBV titer, and antibody for HIV
- Renal angiogram or computed tomography angiogram
- A repeat cross-match is performed immediately before transplant

A pediatric kidney policy is ethically appropriate because young children and adolescents experience poor growth and have difficulties with dialysis access issues (Box 36-3). Rapid restoration of normal renal function is the best way of preventing long-term deficits. While kidneys are allocated through UNOS and the local OPO, the final decision to transplant a particular recipient is left to the transplant surgeon. In this way, the philosophy of the program is maintained and the suitability for individual recipients is taken into consideration. For example, a kidney that may be an O-antigen mismatch for a recipient may not be the best choice if the donor history, donor location or the current medical status of the donor is not optimal for the individual recipient.

PRE-TRANSPLANT EVALUATION

Evaluation of the Living Donor

Almost half of all kidney transplants performed in children are from LD. The first LD for a child is most frequently a one-haplotype-matched parent. As a general rule, it is possible to consider an adult donor of almost any size for a child, no matter how young. LD from siblings is usually restricted to donors who have reached 18 years of age. The extremely low mortality, as well as the fact that the long-term morbidity for donation is also small and the outcome of LD kidneys is superior to that of CD kidneys, has made LD acceptable in many different cultures. LD candidates with systemic disease such as diabetes or hypertension are excluded by an initial medical history (Box 36-4)

Children needing a kidney transplant are affected by the limited number of cadaver donors. This has resulted in the LD pool being expanded to include donors outside of the immediate family, so that there has been an increase in the percentage of unrelated living kidney donors, from 2.5% in 1991 to 10.6% in 2000 (UNOS 2001 Annual Report). Unrelated kidney donors are usually emotionally related, such as an adoptive parent or a close friend of the family. The use of altruistic kidney donors is controversial.[1]

Evaluation of the Recipient

The precise cause of ESRD should be established if possible, because of the possibility of post-transplantation recurrence. Surgical correction may be required for structural abnormalities. The preparation of recipients is shown in Box 36-5.

MEDICAL, SURGICAL, AND PSYCHIATRIC ISSUES IN PEDIATRIC TRANSPLANT CANDIDATES

Neurological Development

Infants with onset of ESRD during the first year of life frequently have neurological abnormalities. These may include alterations in mental function, microcephaly, myoclonus, cerebellar ataxia, tremors, seizures, and hypotonia. Preemptive kidney transplantation or the institution of dialysis at the earliest sign of head-circumference growth rate reduction or developmental delay may ameliorate the problem. Successful transplantation in infants has been accompanied by an improvement in psychomotor development, with many regaining normal developmental milestones.

It is often difficult to assess to what extent uremia contributes to cognitive delay and impairment in older children. Uremia has an adverse, but often-reversible effect on a child's mental functioning, and it may cause psychological depression. Initiation of dialysis improves

Box 36-5 Standard Preparation of Pediatric Renal Transplant Candidates

Complete history and physical examination

- Height, weight, blood pressure
- Blood transfusion and/or erythropoietin therapy
- Previous transplantation (type of donor, HLA, induction therapy, rejection)
- Dialysis (modality and history)
- Urologic abnormalities

Laboratory tests

- Hematology (CBC, differential, platelets)
- Coagulation (PT, PTT, bleeding time)
- Chemistry (comprehensive metabolic panel, lipid profile, intact PTH)
- Urine volume, culture, and urinalysis

Blood bank (histocompatibility)

- ABO blood type
- ABO antibody specificities
- HLA type
- Preliminary and final cross match with potential donors
- Mixed lymphocyte culture (if available and applicable)
- Panel-reactive antibodies (PRA) for potential cadaver recipients

Immunology/infectious disease – serologic status

- CMV, EBV, herpes simplex virus, varicella (VZV), hepatitis A, B, and C virus
- HIV, toxoplasma (if indicated clinically), polyoma virus (BK virus)

Imaging studies

- Chest X-radiography, bone age, VCUG

Baseline health and functional status

- Vision, dental health, purified protein derivative (PPD) (tuberculin testing), age-appropriate Pap smear and pregnancy test, audiometry, cardiovascular status (ECG, echocardiogram), urologic status

Consultations: social worker, psychologist, nutritionist

Immunization status

- DPT/OPV, MMR, HIB, pneumococcal, Varivax®, influenza

the uremic symptoms, making possible a more precise assessment of the child's mental function. This may often permit progression to transplantation in situations in which this might otherwise have not seemed feasible. On the other hand, severely retarded children respond poorly to the constraints of ESRD care, and cannot comprehend the need for procedures that are often confusing and uncomfortable. This does not preclude ESRD care, but the family must be informed, involved and supported in any decision they take on whether or not to include chronic dialysis or transplantation.

A seizure disorder requiring anticonvulsant medication may be present in up to 10% of young pediatric transplant candidates. Before transplantation, seizures should be controlled, whenever possible, with drugs that do not interfere with calcineurin inhibitors or prednisone metabolism. Benzodiazepines are a good choice when circumstances permit. Carbamazepine (Tegretol®) reduces calcineurin inhibitor and prednisone levels, but its effect is not as great as that of phenytoin or barbiturates.

Psycho-Emotional Status

Psychiatric and emotional disorders are not by themselves contraindications to dialysis and transplantation. However, the involvement of healthcare professionals skilled in the care of affected children is mandatory. Primary psychiatric problems – including depression – may be amenable to therapy and should not exclude children from consideration for transplantation. Non-adherence is a problem in adolescent transplant recipients. Patterns of medication and dialysis compliance should be established as part of the transplant evaluation. Psychiatric evaluation should be performed in high-risk cases. If non-adherence is identified or anticipated, behavioral modification and other programs should be instituted prior to transplantation.

Cardiovascular Disease

Hypertension and chronic fluid overload during dialysis may predispose to left ventricular hypertrophy, and hypertensive cardiomyopathy and congestive heart failure may supervene. Hypertension control in children with ESRD cannot be overemphasized, and may reduce long-term morbidity and mortality. Bilateral nephrectomy is occasionally required during the pre- or post-transplant period.

Infection

Urinary tract infections and infections related to dialysis access are common sources of bacterial infections in children with ESRD. Aggressive antibiotic therapy and prophylaxis may effectively suppress infection, although nephrectomy is occasionally required for recalcitrant infections with obstructive uropathy and vesicoureteral reflux.

The incidence of cytomegalovirus (CMV) and Epstein–Barr virus (EBV) infection increases with age. Young children are unlikely to be seropositive for CMV or EBV.

Primary EBV infection, in the context of potent immuno-suppression, may predispose to an aggressive type of post-transplantation lymphoproliferative disorder (PTLD).

Immunizations should be brought up to date if possible. Live viral vaccines are contraindicated in immuno-suppressed patients; therefore, every effort should be made to complete these vaccinations, including varicella vaccination, before transplantation. Diphtheria, tetanus, and hepatitis B vaccine can be given safely after transplantation, although pre-transplantation administration is preferred. Influenza and pneumococcal vaccines are recommended.

Urologic Problems

Children with structural abnormalities often require multiple corrective procedures to improve urinary tract anatomy, and this is best done before transplantation. Procedures include ureteric reimplantation, bladder augmentation, creation of a vesicocutaneous fistula using the appendix to provide a simple and cosmetically acceptable way for intermittent catheterization (Mitrofanoff procedure), and the excision of duplicated systems or ectopic ureteroceles that may cause recurrent infections. Intractable urinary infection, in the presence of hydronephrosis or severe reflux, may require nephrectomy before transplantation. An abnormal lower urinary tract is not a contraindication to transplantation. Bladders that are dysfunctional because of a previous urinary diversion can be hydrodilated and assessed for adequacy for use after transplantation. Malformations and voiding abnormalities such as neurogenic bladder, bladder dyssynergia, remnant posterior urethral valves, and urethral strictures should be identified and repaired, and it may be possible to teach self-catheterization safely and successfully.

Renal Osteodystrophy

Aggressive diagnosis and treatment of hyperparathyroidism, osteomalacia, and aluminum bone disease are important during the pre-transplantation period. Control of hyperparathyroidism with vitamin D analogues (or even parathyroidectomy) may be required, because failure to do so may predispose to post-transplantation hypercalcemia, hypophosphatemia and also limit the growth potential of a successful transplant recipient.

Peritoneal Dialysis

The extra-peritoneal placement of the allograft may allow for continued peritoneal dialysis after transplantation in the event of delayed graft function. Intra-peritoneal graft placement is not an absolute contraindication to

peritoneal dialysis. Potential transplant recipients with an episode of acute peritonitis should be treated for 10–14 days and have a negative peritoneal fluid culture off antibiotic treatment before contemplating transplantation. If a chronic exit-site infection is present at the time of surgery, the catheter should be removed and appropriate parenteral antibiotics administered. Overt tunnel infections should be treated before transplantation. The incidence of post-transplantation peritoneal dialysis-related infections is low, and such infections typically respond to appropriate antibiotic therapy, although catheter removal may be necessary for recurrent infections. In the absence of infections, the peritoneal catheter is usually removed at the time of transplantation in cases of living related transplantation. On the other hand, it may be left in place until good graft function has been established for 2–3 weeks, particularly in cases of cadaveric transplantation.

Nephrotic Syndrome

In children with glomerular diseases, proteinuria usually diminishes as kidney function deteriorates and ESRD ensues. Occasionally, a florid nephrotic syndrome may persist, particularly with focal glomerulosclerosis. Control of heavy proteinuria prior to transplantation is important, and can sometimes be achieved with prostaglandin inhibitors such as meclofenamate; renal embolization or bilateral nephrectomy may be required. In congenital nephrotic syndrome of the Finnish type, unilateral or bilateral nephrectomy is usually performed early in the course of the disease to allow for better growth while on dialysis. Congenital nephrotic syndrome due to diffuse mesangial sclerosis with Denys–Drash syndrome usually requires bilateral nephrectomy as part of the treatment or prevention of Wilms' tumor.

Portal Hypertension

Portal hypertension occurs in children with autosomal recessive polycystic kidney disease (ARPKD). Esophageal varices require sclerotherapy or portosystemic shunting. If severe neutropenia and thrombocytopenia are present as a result of hypersplenism, then partial splenectomy or splenic embolization may be required.

Prior Malignancy

Wilms' tumor is the main malignancy that produces ESRD in children because of bilateral nephrectomies. A disease-free period of 1–2 years is required before transplantation, because earlier transplantation has been associated with the development of recurrent or metastases in almost half of the cases. Premature transplantation in this setting has also been associated with overwhelming sepsis, which may be related to chemotherapy. The presence of a primary non-renal malignancy is not an absolute contraindication to transplantation, although an 'appropriate' waiting time is needed between tumor extirpation and transplantation.

Nutrition

Poor feeding and malnutrition are prominent features of uremia. Aggressive nutritional support is essential. Nasogastric or gastric tube feeding is often used to improve caloric intake and promote growth. A target weight of 8–10 kg should be reached, because of technical difficulties, before transplantation.

REFERENCES

1. Kaplan BS, Polise K. In defense of altruistic kidney donation by strangers Pediatr Nephrol 2000;14:518–522.

2. Salvatierra O, Tanney D, Mak R, et al. Pediatric renal transplantation and its changes. Transplant Rev 1997;11:51–69.

CHAPTER 37

Complications after Renal Transplantation

H. JORGE BALUARTE, M.D.,

JO-ANN PALMER, C.R.N.P., AND

JULIE PETRO MONGIELLO, C.R.N.P.

Recurrence of the Primary Disease
  and De-novo Disease
  Glomerular Diseases
    Focal Segmental Glomerulosclerosis (FSGS)
    Membranoproliferative Glomerulonephritis (MPGN)
    IgA Nephropathy (IgA N) and Henoch–Schönlein
      Purpura (HSP)
    Anti-Glomerular Basement Membrane (GBM) Disease
    Membranous Nephropathy (MN)
    Alport Syndrome
    Hemolytic Uremic Syndrome (HUS)
    Congenital Nephrotic Syndrome, Finnish Type (CNF)
    Other Glomerular Diseases
  Metabolic Diseases
    Primary Hyperoxaluria Type I
    Nephropathic Cystinosis
Growth after Transplantation
  Age at Transplantation
  Corticosteroid Dose
  Growth Hormone
Infections
  Cytomegalovirus (CMV)
  Varicella
  Epstein–Barr virus (EBV)
  Herpes Simplex Virus
Hypertension
Hyperlipidemia
Malignancy and PTLD

RECURRENCE OF THE PRIMARY DISEASE AND DE-NOVO DISEASE

Recurrent or de-novo disease accounts for 5% of graft loss of primary transplants and for 10% of repeat transplants in pediatrics. With improving outcomes and decreasing incidence of irreversible rejection, the recurrence of disease in the allograft takes on greater significance. Although glomerular and metabolic diseases can recur, most recurrences are due to glomerular diseases.

Glomerular Diseases

Focal Segmental Glomerulosclerosis (FSGS)

FSGS is the most common cause of graft loss from recurrent disease. It recurs in 50–80% of patients, with graft failure occurring in about half of them. FSGS may recur either immediately, or months later. Recurrence is usually characterized by massive proteinuria, and nephrotic syndrome. Factors that predict a recurrence of FSGS are rapid progression to end-stage renal failure within 3 years, poor response to therapy, mesangial proliferation, and onset under the age of 6 years. Although the incidence and severity of FSGS is higher in blacks, as children they have a lower risk of post-transplant recurrence. Recurrence post-transplant is rare in inherited cases of FSGS. The concentration of serum protein permeability factor(s) isolated from patients with FSGS correlates with the recurrence and severity of disease in the transplanted kidney. Early post-transplant recognition of recurrent FSGS is important, because plasmapheresis may decrease serum levels of the protein permeability factor(s) and significantly reduce graft loss. High doses of cyclosporine A (CsA) and in some cases, cyclophosphamide, may induce remission of the nephrotic syndrome. Angiotensin-converting enzyme (ACE) inhibitors and/or receptor blockers are given for their antiproteinuric and antifibrotic benefits. The potential for recurrence of FSGS is not generally regarded as a contraindication to living donor (LD) transplantation, although if a primary transplant has been lost to rapid recurrence, the use of a LD for repeat transplantation is not recommended.

Membranoproliferative Glomerulonephritis (MPGN)

There are no clinical features that may predict the risk of a recurrence of MPGN in an allograft. Histological evidence of recurrence of MPGN type 1 is found in up to 75% of cases, and graft loss occurs in up to 30% of cases. Histological recurrence of MPGN type II is seen in 85% of recipients, but most do not cause graft dysfunction or loss. Serum complement concentrations do not correlate with recurrences. Plasmapheresis and high doses of corticosteroids may be beneficial in some cases of crescentic MPGN type II.

IgA Nephropathy (IgA N) and Henoch–Schönlein Purpura (HSP)

Histological recurrence of mesangial IgA deposits occurs in 45% of patients with IgA N nephropathy and 25% of patients with HSP. Most patients are asymptomatic, but graft loss may occur.

Anti-Glomerular Basement Membrane (GBM) Disease

Anti-GBM disease is rare in children. Circulating anti-GBM antibodies prior to transplantation are thought to be associated with a risk of recurrence. Therefore, before transplantation is performed, there must be a waiting period of 6–12 months, and titers of anti-GM antibodies must be undetectable. Histological recurrence occurs in 50% of cases, with clinical manifestations of nephritis in 25% of these. Spontaneous resolution may occur, and graft loss is uncommon.

Membranous Nephropathy (MN)

Recurrence of MN is rare in children. De-novo MN occurs in fewer than 10% of transplanted children. This usually presents between 4 months and 6 years after transplant, whereas recurrent MN usually manifests within 2 years. The recurrence rate of MN is 29% at 3 years post-transplantation, and graft loss is 52% at 10 years.

Alport Syndrome

Alport syndrome does not recur after transplantation. Most patients develop anti-anti-GBM antibodies, but fewer than 5% have clinical glomerulonephritis. This usually occurs in hemizygous males because of a complete absence of the non-collagenous domain of the $\alpha3$ chain of type IV collagen in the GBM. However, this may also occur rarely in heterozygous females with Alport syndrome. Anti-GBM glomerulonephritis is a rapidly progressive crescentic glomerulonephritis with linear deposits of IgG along the basement membrane. This often leads to graft loss.

Hemolytic Uremic Syndrome (HUS)

HUS associated with diarrhea (Stx-HUS, D+ HUS) does not recur after transplantation. Recurrent HUS occurs in half of the patients with atypical and/inherited types of the syndrome. Factors that may favor a recurrence are transplantation within 6–12 months of the acute episode, and the use of a LD. The use of CsA, tacrolimus, or antithymocyte globulin is also associated with recurrent episodes. A renal biopsy should be performed as soon as possible to confirm the diagnosis. It is important to initiate plasmapheresis and to discontinue the calcineurin inhibitor.

Congenital Nephrotic Syndrome, Finnish Type (CNF)

The outcome of CNF is optimized by bilateral nephrectomy, followed by dialysis and transplant. De-novo nephrotic syndrome occurs in 24% of cases, and is associated with anti-nephrin autoantibodies. The recurrence may be immediate, or up to 3 years after transplant. There is no specific treatment, despite the finding of histological lesions resembling minimal-change disease. Graft loss occurs in 60% of cases. In addition, vascular thrombosis and death with a functioning graft (mostly due to infectious complications) occur in 26% and 23% of cases, respectively, and account for higher rates of graft failure in patients with CNF.

Other Glomerular Diseases

Recurrence of lupus nephritis and Wegener's granulomatosis is uncommon.

Metabolic Diseases

Primary Hyperoxaluria Type I

Type I primary hyperoxaluria results from a deficiency of the hepatic enzyme alanine:glyoxylate aminotransferase, and this results in the deposition of oxalate in all body tissues, including the kidneys. Renal transplantation does not correct the enzyme deficiency, and therefore graft loss is inevitable. However, a combined liver and kidney transplantation leads to higher success rates.

Nephropathic Cystinosis

Cystinosis is an inherited metabolic disease characterized by intracellular accumulation of free cystine in many organs, including the kidneys. Renal transplantation gives comparable results to those in children with other renal diseases. Cystinosis does not recur, although cystine, from the host macrophages, may accumulate in the renal interstitium.

GROWTH AFTER TRANSPLANTATION

Growth failure is common in children with chronic renal insufficiency. Achieving adequate growth is a challenge because diminished growth rates may develop when the glomerular filtration rate (GFR) decreases below 75 ml/min/1.73 m^2. The severity of growth retardation is directly related to the age of onset of renal failure, and correlates with the presence of renal osteodystrophy, metabolic acidosis, electrolyte disturbances, anemia, protein and calorie malnutrition, delayed sexual maturation, and accumulation of uremic toxins.

A successful renal transplant is the best treatment for infants, children, and adolescents with end-stage renal disease (ESRD).[6] One measurement of the long-term success of the procedure is the attainment of targeted (genetic potential) adult height. Unfortunately, growth retardation may persist despite successful transplantation, and therefore growth retardation continues to be a major concern for both patients and families after transplantation.

Multiple factors have been implicated for the failure to achieve normal or accelerated growth following renal transplantation; perturbations of the growth hormone (GH)/insulin-like growth factor (IGF) axis resulting from corticosteroid therapy and/or suboptimal allograft function play a pivotal role.

Age at Transplantation

The finding that the youngest children benefit the most in linear growth from early transplantation provides a strong argument for expedited transplantation in an attempt to optimize the attainment of normal stature. In addition, earlier transplantation allows less time for ongoing growth failure while on dialysis.

Corticosteroid Dose

Corticosteroids can inhibit GH release, reduce IGF activity, directly impair cartilage growth, decrease calcium absorption, or increase renal phosphate wasting. Strategies to reduce the impact of corticosteroid therapy on growth are to use lower daily doses, to switch to an alternate-day regimen, and to attempt to stop corticosteroid treatment.

By 5 years after transplantation, alternate-day corticosteroids is the regimen used in 32% of patients. This improves linear growth significantly, without increased rates of rejection or graft loss. Conversion to alternate-day dosing is for selected, stable patients who are compliant. In tacrolimus-based immunosuppressive regimens, the withdrawal of steroids has been successfully performed in more than 70% of patients, usually by 5 months after transplantation. The effect of this approach on growth has been remarkable, with improvement in the SDs at 2 years after transplantation in children aged less than 13 years of 3.62 SD in the withdrawn group compared with 1.48 SD in the control group.

The rates of acute rejection in the withdrawn group, however, were high, and this could adversely affect growth by virtue of a decline in graft function and the need for high-dose corticosteroids to treat rejection.

Growth Hormone

Use of recombinant GH (rhGH) in growth-retarded pediatric renal-allograft recipients results in impressive improvements in growth, without any increase in allogenic immune responsiveness.[3] rhGH therapy is usually started in prepubertal children at least 1 year after transplantation, and continued until catch-up growth is achieved or until puberty ensues.

INFECTIONS

Infections account for most of the complications after transplant, are the main cause of morbidity and mortality, and account for 34% of all post-transplant deaths. Immunosuppression renders the recipient susceptible to numerous viral and bacterial infections. Pneumonia and urinary tract infections are the most common post-transplantation bacterial infections. Urinary tract infections due to *Staphylococcus aureus* or *Escherichia coli* may be seen in as many as 50% of patients during the first 3 months, and at times can progress rapidly to urosepsis and may be confused with acute rejection. Trimethoprim-sulfamethoxazole (TMP/SMZ) chemoprophylaxis for *Pneumocystis carinii* should be provided for all patients, and may be continued up to 1 year in patients whose original disease was urologic in origin. *Pneumocystis carinii* pneumonia (PCP) occurs in about 3% of renal allograft recipients. The clinical features of a diffuse pneumonia are dyspnea and hypoxemia. The risk is highest during the first month, and if diagnosed quickly can be treated effectively; however, delay can be fatal, and therefore prophylaxis is standard.

Most centers prescribe an intravenous cephalosporin for the first 48 hours after transplantation to reduce infection from graft contamination and via the transplant incision. Nightly TMP/SMZ for the first 3 to 6 months after transplantation serves as prophylaxis against *Pneumocystis carinii* pneumonia and urinary tract infections. Prophylactic oral nystatin (Mycostatin®) minimizes oral and gastrointestinal fungal infections. Splenectomized patients must be given pneumococcal vaccine and postoperative prophylaxis for Gram-positive and Gram-negative organisms.

Many young children have not been exposed to herpetic viruses (cytomegalovirus, herpes virus, varicella zoster, and Epstein–Barr virus), and because they lack protective immunity, they are at increased risk for serious primary infections. The incidence of these infections is higher in children treated with antibody induction therapy and after treatment of acute rejection.

Cytomegalovirus (CMV)

This is an important infection in transplant recipients. The incidence of CMV seropositivity is about 30% in children aged over 5 years, and increases to about 60% in teenagers. Therefore, the younger the child, the greater is the potential for serious infection with a CMV-seropositive donor kidney. CMV infection may be asymptomatic, or it may present with fever, a mononucleosis-like syndrome, leucopenia, thrombocytopenia, pneumonitis, hepatitis, enteric ulceration, chorioretinitis, and allograft dysfunction. Evaluation for CMV infection may be made with an antigenemia assay, by rapid viral isolation, or with a polymerase chain reaction (PCR). A new CMV detection assay, hybrid capture, involves the specific hybridization of a CMV-specific probe to CMV nucleic acid sequences inside white blood cells. This technique appears to be as sensitive as the CMV culture, but has a much shorter turn-around time (<24 hours). Various strategies have been proposed to prevent CMV disease or minimize its impact. CMV hyperimmune globulin, high-dose standard immune globulin, oral acyclovir, and high-dose oral ganciclovir are valuable therapeutic options.[1] Reduction of immunosuppression is an important adjunct to antiviral therapy. Paradoxically, CMV may contribute to allograft immunogenicity and is associated with both acute and chronic rejection. It has been suggested that seronegative children receive only kidneys from seronegative donors; however, given the frequency of seropositivity in the adult population, this restriction would penalize seronegative children by prolonging the wait for a transplant at a critical growing period.

Varicella

This is a constant concern because exposure in the pediatric age range is extremely high. Varicella zoster infection in older pediatric transplant recipients is localized along a dermatomal distribution. In younger children, primary varicella infection (chickenpox) can result in a rapidly progressive and overwhelming infection, with encephalitis, pneumonitis, hepatic failure, pancreatitis, and disseminated intravascular coagulation. It is important to know the varicella zoster antibody status of the child, because seronegative children require prophylactic varicella zoster immune globulin (VZIG) within 72 hours of accidental exposure. VZIG favorably modifies the disease in 75% of cases. Administration of varicella vaccine before transplantation is recommended for seronegative patients. The safety and efficacy of varicella vaccine after transplantation are unknown. A child with a kidney transplant who develops chickenpox must be given parenteral acyclovir without delay. Varicella zoster infection poses less danger of dissemination, but acyclovir should be given. In both situations, it is wise to discontinue azathioprine or mycophenolate mofetil (MMF) until 2 days after the last new crop of vesicles has dried. The doses of other immunosuppressive agents will depend on the clinical situation and response to therapy.

Epstein–Barr Virus (EBV)

EBV infection is problematic in a seronegative patient who receives an organ from a seropositive donor. Approximately half of children are seronegative for EBV, and infection will occur in about 75% of these patients. Most EBV infections are clinically silent; however, there may be an infectious mononucleosis syndrome, hepatitis, and post-transplant lymphoproliferative disease (PTLD). Surveillance for EBV infection is most expeditiously performed with PCR. PTLD in children, as in adults, may be related to EBV infection in the presence of vigorous immunosuppression. Some transplant centers adjust the level of immunosuppression based on the degree of EBV expression as detected and quantified by PCR.

Herpes Simplex Virus

Typical perioral herpetic ulcerations are common in immunosuppressed children, and usually respond to oral acyclovir therapy. Disseminated herpes infection is rare.

HYPERTENSION

Hypertension is common immediately after renal transplantation, and at 1 month after transplantation 70% of patients require antihypertensive medication; however, the incidence decreases to 59% at 24 months.[2] The causes and pathogenesis of post-transplant hypertension are multifactorial and primarily related to the side effects of corticosteroid and calcineurin inhibitor therapy (Box 37-1). Corticosteroid-induced hypertension occurs through multiple mechanisms, including salt and water retention, often with a significant reduction in blood pressure in patients in whom total steroid withdrawal is possible. The blood pressure rises again if corticosteroid therapy has to be restarted in the same patients. Calcineurin inhibitors may cause hypertension by inhibiting prostaglandin production and increasing the production of thromboxane. Calcium-channel blockers, such as nifedipine, counteract the intrarenal vasoconstriction associated with calcineurin inhibitors.[5]

Box 37-1 Causes of Hypertension after Renal Transplantation

- Hypertension prior to the transplant
- Corticosteroids
- Calcineurin inhibitors
- Acute and chronic rejection
- Renal artery stenosis
- High renin output from native kidneys
- De-novo or recurrent disease in the allograft
- Urinary tract obstruction

ACE inhibitors are an attractive alternative for the treatment of hypertension. The 'renoprotective' effect of ACE inhibitors is attributed to a reduction in intraglomerular pressure. In addition, they may inhibit the activation of transforming growth factor-β (TGF-β), one of the growth factors involved in the pathogenesis of chronic allograft fibrosis. Clonidine, delivered via a transdermal patch, is valuable in non-compliant adolescents.

HYPERLIPIDEMIA

Lipid abnormalities frequently occur after transplantation, despite normal allograft function. At 1 year after transplant, pediatric patients have significantly elevated levels of plasma cholesterol and VLDL cholesterol compared to normal controls; however, the elevated cholesterol levels (mean 213 mg/dl) were not high enough to require lipid-lowering agents (NAPRTCS). Corticosteroids, calcineurin inhibitors and sirolimus may induce hyperlipidemia. Patients should be screened at least once during the first 6 months, and again at 1 year after transplantation, with fasting total cholesterol, LDL, HDL, and triglyceride measurements. Long-term studies of hyperlipidemia and its treatment in children are needed to provide evidence for recommendations. Although no prospective clinical studies to date have shown that lipid-lowering therapy improves long-term outcomes, this lack of clinical data should not be used as justification to neglect the importance of hyperlipidemia. Dietary measures should be implemented and, if insufficient, statins can be added. There are, however, insufficient data to make firm recommendations for the use of pharmacologic measures in children. However, in children with serum cholesterol levels above 250 mg/dl, 3-hydroxy-3-methylglutaryl (HMG)-Coenzyme A reductase inhibitors are generally effective and safe. Corticosteroid withdrawal after transplantation significantly reduces serum cholesterol and LDL cholesterol levels, but may also reduce HDL cholesterol.

MALIGNANCY AND PTLD

An increased incidence of cancer is a well-recognized complication of organ transplantation in children. These tumors likely are the result of a complex interplay of numerous factors. These include the immunocompromised state *per se*, immunosuppressive agents, oncogenic viruses, and possible synergistic effects of immunosuppressive agents with carcinogens such as sunlight, viruses, infections, and hormonal factors. Sufficient experience has been gained to analyze separately those tumors that occur in patients who received organ transplants during childhood. The pattern of malignancies in pediatric transplant recipients differs significantly from that in adult renal allograft recipients and the general population. According to the Cincinnati Transplant Tumor Registry, PTLD is the most common neoplasm in pediatric transplant recipients. This occurs on average about 36 months after transplantation. Skin carcinomas (squamous cell and basal cell carcinomas) are the second most common malignancy.

The incidence of PTLD is higher after heart, lung, liver, and intestinal transplantation. The number of published reports seems to be increasing, perhaps as a result of new immunosuppressive agents. Treatment with antilymphocyte antibodies may increase the risk of developing PTLD. After the introduction of CsA there was a high incidence of PTLD, but this markedly decreased after CsA levels were monitored, permitting the use of smaller doses. Suppression of natural cytotoxic T-cell activity may be the cause of an uncontrolled EBV-driven proliferation of B-cells. The clinical presentation of PTLD is heterogeneous, but most cases can be divided into several syndromes (see Box 37-2). Pediatric transplant recipients are at increased risk for lymphotropic virus-associated disorders. Primary infection with EBV increases the risk of PTLD, so determination of pre-transplant antibody status in recipients, rapid detection of EBV infection in seronegative symptomatic recipients, and regular screening for persistent EBV DNA viral load in patients at risk for developing PTLD are recommended; measurement of viral load appears to be of little value in predicting PTLD.[4]

The treatment of PTLD depends on the extent of involvement. The mainstay of management of PTLD is the drastic reduction or cessation of immunosuppressive treatment to allow recovery of the recipient's cytotoxic T-cell-directed EBV surveillance mechanism. It is advisable to withdraw azathioprine or MMF, and to reduce prednisolone to about 10 mg per day. CsA or tacrolimus are reduced in a step-wise fashion by about one-fifth every 2 weeks, and it is common to stop the reduction when approximately 30% of the initial dose is reached. Of interest, in many of these cases, the graft is not rejected despite the significant lowering or discontinuation of immunosuppressive medications. Antiviral drug therapy has at present only been shown to be of limited therapeutic benefit. However, intravenous ganciclovir given during antilymphocyte therapy and followed by 3 months of high-dose oral acyclovir may decrease the occurrence of PTLD, especially in EBV-seronegative patients (Box 37-2).

REFERENCES

1. Ahsan N, Holman MJ, Yang HC. Efficacy of oral gancyclovir in prevention of cytomegalovirus infection in post-transplant patients. Clin Transplant 1997;11:633–639.

2. Baluarte HJ, Gruskin AB, Ingelfinger JR, et al. Analysis of hypertension in children post renal transplantation – A report of the North American Pediatric Renal Transplant Cooperative Study (NAPRTCS). Pediatr Nephrol 1994;8:570–573.

3. Fine RN, Stablein D, Cohen AH, et al. Recombinant human growth hormone post-renal transplantation in children: a randomized controlled study of the NAPRTCS. Kidney Int 2002;62:688–696.

4. Green M. Management of Epstein–Barr virus-induced post-transplant lymphoproliferative disease in recipients of solid organ transplantation. Am J Transplant 2001;1:103–108.

5. Midtvedt K, Hartman A, Holdaas H, et al. Efficacy of nifedipine or lisinopril in the treatment of hypertension after renal transplantation: a double-blind randomized comparative study. Clin Transplant 2001;15:426–431.

6. Tejani A, Cortes L, Sullivan EK. A longitudinal study of the natural history of growth post-transplantation. Kidney Int Suppl 1996;53:103–108.

Box 37-2   Clinical Presentations of PTLD

ACUTE INFECTIOUS MONONUCLEOSIS-LIKE DISEASE
- Marked constitutional symptoms, rapid enlargement of tonsils and cervical nodes
- Typical pattern in the first year after transplantation

A FULMINANT PRESENTATION
- Within weeks of transplantation
- Widespread infiltrative disease with multi-organ involvement, grave prognosis

CENTRAL NERVOUS SYSTEM PTLD
- Often devastating, and rapidly fatal

ISOLATED OR MULTIPLE TUMORS
- Multiple tumors often involve the allograft
- May be mistaken for rejection
- Usually an indolent disease with visceral, nodal, and extra-nodal tumors
- Gastrointestinal involvement and pulmonary nodules are relatively frequent

CHAPTER 38

Management of the Pediatric Renal Transplant Recipient

H. JORGE BALUARTE, M.D.,

JO-ANN PALMER, C.R.N.P., AND

JULIE PETRO MONGIELLO, C.R.N.P.

PERIOPERATIVE MANAGEMENT

Preparation for Transplantation

Recipients are admitted within 24 hours of transplantation. A final cross-match is performed within 48 hours of the transplantation date. A detailed history and physical examination are performed to identify any risk factors, especially the presence of active or recent infection. A set of laboratory tests is obtained to detect any metabolic abnormalities that require correction by dialysis. Aggressive fluid removal is discouraged in the immediate preoperative period to reduce the risk of delayed graft function (DGF). Plasmapheresis is carried out when recurrent FSGS is anticipated. Living donor (LD) transplantation permits commencement of an immune-conditioning regimen with mycophenolate mofetil (MMF) and prednisone for 3–7 days before the transplantation date. Immediate preoperative immunosuppressive therapy with basiliximab (Simulect®) or Daclizumab (Zenapax®) by intravenous infusion is common practice in some transplant centers for cadaveric donor (CD) transplant recipients. Preoperative immunotherapy was employed in 54% of LD transplants (2002 NAPRTCS annual report).

Intraoperative Management

Immunosuppression is continued intraoperatively with methylprednisolone (Solu-Medrol®), with 10 mg/kg given intravenously at the beginning of the operation. At the Children's Hospital of Philadelphia, induction therapy with a polyclonal antibody (Thymoglobulin®) is given through a central catheter intraoperatively. A central venous catheter is inserted to monitor the central venous pressure (CVP) throughout the operation.

Close attention is paid to blood pressure and hydration status to reduce the incidence of DGF. Hydration should be optimized to achieve adequate renal perfusion. A CVP of 12–15 cmH$_2$O should be achieved before removal of the vascular clamps, but a higher CVP is desirable in the case of a small infant receiving an adult-sized kidney. Additionally, the mean arterial blood pressure is kept above 65–70 mmHg by adequate hydration with a crystalloid solution or 5% albumin, and if necessary, the use of dopamine. Dopamine is usually started at 2–3 µg/kg/min and increased as required; it is then continued for 24–48 hours postoperatively to assure adequate renal perfusion. Blood transfusion with packed red blood cells is often required in very small recipients because the hemoglobin may decrease as a result of sequestration of about 150–250 ml of blood in the transplanted kidney. Mannitol and furosemide are given before removal of the vascular clamps in order to increase the effective circulatory volume and facilitate diuresis. After the transplanted kidney starts to produce urine, volume replacement should be commenced immediately with 0.45% saline solution and 22 mEq/l of sodium bicarbonate.

Postoperative Management[1]

Urine output replacement with 0.45% saline solution and 22 mEq/l of sodium bicarbonate is started in the recovery room and continued in the intensive care unit for 24–48 hours, in addition to replacement of insensible water losses. Dextrose is not added to the replacement solution to prevent osmotic diuresis, and is only used as part of the insensible water loss replacement solution. The lack of concentrating ability of the newly transplanted kidney accounts for the obligatory high urine output that may be observed in the first few post-transplantation days. As the kidney function improves gradually and the serum creatinine concentration decreases, the urine-concentrating capacity recovers, and volume per volume urine output replacement can be stopped. The daily fluid intake is usually set to provide about 150% to 200% of the maintenance daily intake, initially as IV plus oral intake and then administered orally.

Hypertension is commonly observed, but aggressive use of antihypertensive therapy is discouraged to avoid sudden swings in blood pressure that may impair renal perfusion. If hypertension persists, a calcium-channel blocker (nifedipine) is usually the first drug of choice, especially when cyclosporine or tacrolimus is used as part of the immunosuppressive regimen. Common electrolyte disorders encountered early in the postoperative course include hyperchloremic metabolic acidosis, hyperkalemia, hypophosphatemia, hypo- or hypercalcemia, and hypomagnesemia (Figure 38-1).

IMMUNOSUPPRESSIVE DRUGS AND PROTOCOLS

Immunosuppressive protocols for pediatric renal transplant recipients are based on the same principles as those for adults.[6] In the search for new drugs, three essential criteria needed for safe clinical use have emerged: specificity to cells of the immune system; weak potency against memory responses; and minimal side effects. Central to all current immunosuppressive regimens is a calcineurin inhibitor (tacrolimus or cyclosporine) in combination with steroids and an adjunctive antiproliferative agent (mycophenolate mofetil or azathioprine). According to the 2002 NAPRTCS annual report, approximately 80% of patients receive triple therapy at 1 year post transplant. Corticosteroids continue to be used in more than 95% of transplant recipients, with many children treated with alternate-day steroid regimens. Cyclosporine is used in about 45%, tacrolimus in 50%, and azathioprine has been replaced by MMF in most of the pediatric transplant recipients. Antibody induction therapy is used in 65% of pediatric transplant recipients. Pediatric experience with sirolimus is limited.

The choice of the immunosuppressive regimen employed is mostly center-specific, but modifications are often made to address the clinical circumstances. For example, when transplantation is contemplated in a child with prior malignancy, a two-drug regimen (including sirolimus) or even monotherapy may be considered, the use of antibody induction is generally avoided, and living donation is encouraged to provide the best HLA match. Children with prior transplants that failed because of repeated episodes of acute rejection may be highly sensitized, and therefore may require a more intensified immunosuppressive regimen. Tacrolimus may be preferred to cyclosporine when there is particular concern about non-adherence because of cosmetic side effects of cyclosporine. The Children's Hospital of Philadelphia pediatric renal transplant program immunosuppressive protocol is detailed in Figure 38-1.

Maintenance Immunosuppression

Calcineurin Inhibitors

Cyclosporine (CsA)

Children require higher doses of CsA than adults when calculated on a milligram per kilogram body weight basis. This is especially true when CsA is used in children aged under 2 years, particularly in the early postoperative period. The requirement for higher doses is believed to be due to an increased rate of metabolism by the hepatic cytochrome P-450 3A4 isoenzymes. Dosing based on surface area, or thrice-daily dosing, appears to provide better therapeutic levels in smaller

	< 20 kg	> 20 kg	Max dose
Week 1	2 mg/kg	1.5 mg/kg	80 mg
Week 2	1.5 mg/kg	1.0 mg/kg	60 mg
Week 3	1 mg/kg	0.75 mg/kg	45 mg
Week 4	0.75 mg/kg	0.5 mg/kg	40 mg
Week 5	0.6 mg/kg	0.4 mg/kg	30–35 mg
Week 6	0.5 mg/kg	0.3 mg/kg	20–25 mg
Week 7	0.4 mg/kg	0.25 mg/kg	15–20 mg
Week 8	0.3 mg/kg	0.2 mg/kg	12.5 mg
Month 3	0.2 mg/kg	0.2–0.15 mg/kg	10 mg

PRE-OP STUDIES FOR RENAL TRANSPLANT

- ☐ Comprehensive metabolic panel
- ☐ CBC with differential
- ☐ PT/PTT
- ☐ Type and cross for 2 U PRBCs
- ☐ Urine culture and urinalysis
- ☐ Repeat CMV, EBV
- ☐ Chest X-Ray

INTRA-OP FLUID MANAGEMENT

- ☐ Pre clamp: Assure CVP is at least 15
- ☐ During clamp: Increase CVP to 20
- ☐ Post clamp: CVP 12–15

ADDITIONAL INTRA-OP MEDS:

- ☐ Mannitol (0.25 g/kg) – during clamp
- ☐ Lasix (1 mg/kg) – during clamp

POST-OP FLUID MANAGEMENT

- ☐ D5W @ insensible losses: 35 ml/100 calories
- ☐ Urine replacement: 0.45% NS + 22 mEq NaHCO$_3$/L at ml/ml replacement. After initial post-operative period (24–48 h), change to fixed rate (PO + IV): 1.5 times maintenance
- ☐ Indication for bolus in the initial post-op period: reduced urine output and CVP 3

BLOOD PRESSURE MANAGEMENT

Initial treatment for persistent SBP > and/or DBP >

- ☐ Hydralazine (0.1–0.2 mg/kg) IV prn q. 4–6 h
- ☐ Nifedipine (~0.25 mg/kg) p.o. prn q. 4–6 h

IMMUNOSUPPRESSION

- ☐ Thymoglobulin induction

First dose intra-op after receiving solumedrol as premed (no test dose needed). Thymoblobulin IVSS (1.5 mg/kg) over 6 hours to start intra-op. Subsequent doses to be given over 4 hours. Premedicate with A.M. dose of solumedrol, acetaminophen (15 mg/kg), benadryl (1 mg/kg). Usually plan to treat for 7 days. The treatment time will be on the cyclosporine/FK level and the graft function.

MUST BE ADMINISTERED THROUGH A CENTRAL LINE AND IN-LINE (HAL) FILTER

- ☐ Simulect (Basiliximab) (12 mg/m^2)

It can be administered through a central or peripheral line. The first dose should be given within 2 hours prior to transplant. The reconstituted Simulect (20 mg in 5 ml) should be further diluted in 50 ml of saline or 5% dextrose, and infused over 20 –30 minutes. The second dose should be given 4 days after transplantation.

- ☐ Mycophenolate mofetil (Cellcept®) or Azathioprine

Initial post-transplant period: Azathioprine (2 mg/kg) IV, once taking PO, initiate treatment with Cellcept (600 mg/m^2/dose) p.o. q. 12 h

- ☐ Tacrolimus

(0.15 mg/kg/dose) q 12 h to begin when graft function stable. Target trough levels: 10–15 ng/ml

- ☐ Solumedrol/prednisone

Intra-op: Medrol (15 mg/kg) — preclamp
Post-op: Medrol (1.5 or 2 mg/kg) IV daily (AM) until on PO's then change to oral prednisone at same dose. Steroid taper (IV solumedrol or PO prednisone). Total dose given in the morning (as premedication for Thymoglobulin).

PROPHYLAXIS

- ☐ Cefazolin (50 mg/kg/day divided q 8 h) first dose in OR, then × 3 doses post-op
- ☐ Gentamicin (2–2.5 mg/kg) × 1 dose in OR
- ☐ Ganciclovir IV (to be given unless the donor and the recipient are CMV-negative). It should be started on the first post-op day and continued for at least 7 days.

5 mg/kg/q. 12 h	GFR > 75 ml/min/1.73 m^2
5 mg/kg/q. 24 hr	GFR 50–75
2.5 mg/kg/q. 24 hr	GFR 25–50
1.25 mg/kg/q. 24 h	GFR 10–25
1.25 mg/kg/q. 48 h	GFR <10

Change to PO ganciclovir through the 5th month
> 70 kg (normal GFR) give 1g q. 8 h
< 70 kg (normal GFR) give 40 mg/kg q. 8 h (up to 1 g q. 8 h)
GFR 50–70 ml/min/1.73 m^2 give 20–30 mg/kg/day, divided BID
GFR 25–50 to 10–15 mg/kg/day, once or BID

- ☐ Acyclovir
- ☐ Nystatin 2–5 ml (100,000 units/ml) TID/QID
- ☐ Cotrimoxazole 2 mg (TMP)/kg/q. Hs
- ☐ Ranitidine 2–4 mg/kg/day ÷ q 8 h, then 4–5 mg/kg/day ÷ q 12 h

Figure 38-1   Transplant protocol at the Children's Hospital of Philadelphia.

children and in children in whom metabolism is accelerated (e.g., patients receiving certain anticonvulsant medications). Dosage adjustments are constantly necessary because of irregular absorption and inherent nephrotoxicity. The introduction of the microemulsion formulation of CsA (Neoral®) addressed the highly variable, partial, and bile-dependent gastrointestinal absorption of the previous oil-based drug preparation (Sandimmune®), resulting in a further significant reduction in the incidence of acute rejection episodes. The median initial dose is 8.3 mg/dl, and at 5 years post-transplant the median dose is 5 mg/kg per day.

Nephrotoxicity is the primary concern with the use of CsA. Clinically, three kinds of nephrotoxicity are observed. The first occurs immediately after transplantation, particularly if CsA is used intravenously for induction purposes and is seen in association with prolonged ischemia. The second type is seen after the first few weeks, and manifests clinically as deteriorating renal function and high CsA levels; lowering the CsA dosage reverses the effect on serum creatinine. Chronic nephrotoxicity is most worrisome as it manifests as a slow but steady decline in renal function, and may be associated with interstitial fibrosis. The mechanism of this nephrotoxicity appears to be a decrease in blood flow with an increase in renal vascular resistance in the afferent arteriole. Treatment with calcium-channel blockers seems to ameliorate the toxicity in both the short and long term.

Hyperkalemia, hyperuricemia, and hypomagnesemia are also observed as a result of altered tubular function. Other side effects that are a major concern to the children are hirsutism, gingival hyperplasia, and facial dysmorphism or coarsening facial features. These side effects in adolescents, especially girls, may be devastating. They may cause severe emotional distress and may result in non-adherence. Tremors, seizures, paraesthesias, hypercholesterolemia, and hypertriglyceridemia may occur. Hyperglycemia and overt diabetes mellitus occur in less than 5% of children.

Tacrolimus

Trials in adult and pediatric renal transplant recipients comparing the clinical efficacy and safety of tacrolimus (Prograf®) a macrocyclic lactone, with CsA showed that acute rejection was significantly reduced with tacrolimus.[2,13] These advantages may have important clinical implications for long-term graft survival. The recommended initial oral daily tacrolimus dose is 0.3 mg/kg, administered in two divided doses; subsequent doses are adjusted on the basis of clinical evidence of efficacy and occurrence of adverse events, and to maintain the target whole-blood trough levels within the range of 10–20 ng/ml for the first month and 5–10 ng/ml from day 30 onwards.

The nephrotoxicity profiles of tacrolimus and CsA are the same. Hypertension, gingival hypertrophy, and hirsutism are less prevalent and less severe with tacrolimus. Post-transplant lymphoproliferative disease (PTLD) and post-transplantation glucose intolerance are more common; recent data indicate that diabetes occurs less frequently with lower doses than are currently used. Neurotoxicity with tacrolimus is more serious, with more marked tremor and a higher incidence of seizures. CsA and tacrolimus, although chemically distinct, have a similar mechanism of immunosuppressive action.

Corticosteroids

The most important concern of corticosteroid treatment in children is retarded skeletal growth. Other side effects include increased susceptibility to infection, impaired wound healing, and aseptic necrosis of the bone, osteopenia, cataracts, glucose intolerance, hypertension, cushingoid faces, acne, obesity, and hyperlipidemia. The dosage is usually high in the immediate post-transplant period (1.5–2 mg/kg/day), with a gradual reduction to about 0.2–0.3 mg/kg per day within 6 months to 1 year. Newer, less-toxic steroid preparations have been used successfully in the treatment of pediatric nephrotic syndrome and in renal transplantation. Preliminary studies with deflazacort (DFZ, an oxazolone derivative of prednisone) in combination with a standard immunosuppressive regimen suggest that it is an effective immunosuppressive agent with fewer side effects. Growth velocity and growth hormone secretion were improved in patients who received DFZ as part of their therapy. DFZ also improved the cushingoid features and significantly decreased the weight-to-height ratio of pediatric recipients. The precise mechanism of action of corticosteroids remains unclear.

The emergence of more powerful immunosuppressive agents has led to an improvement in acute rejection rates, and has allowed the use of lower daily doses of corticosteroids. Many attempts have been made to withdraw steroids, with variable degrees of success. Corticosteroids, therefore, continue to be used in most regimens, with an increased tendency toward using lower daily maintenance and particularly alternate-day dosing, which appears to reduce the growth-inhibiting effect without unduly increasing rejection episodes.[7]

Adjunctive Immunosuppressive Agents

Azathioprine (Imuran®)

The NAPRTCS 2002 annual report showed that the use of azathioprine has decreased considerably (from 50% in 1996 to 8% in 2001) as an indication of increased familiarity with MMF. Azathioprine is a competitive inhibitor of both de-novo and salvage enzyme pathways on nucleotide synthesis.

Mycophenolate Mofetil (MMF; CellCept®)

Mycophenolate mofetil, the morpholino ethyl ester of mycophenolic acid, is a prodrug and is rapidly converted by plasma esterases into mycophenolic acid after oral administration. MMF inhibits the proliferation of T cells and B cells, as well as the production of antibodies by B cells. Three clinical trials compared MMF with azathioprine or placebo in recipients of renal allografts who were also receiving CsA and corticosteroids. These trials showed that MMF lowers the incidence of acute rejection at 6 months by approximately 50%; however, extended studies failed to demonstrate a better graft survival compared to azathioprine. The recommended dose of MMF for pediatric patients is 1200 mg/m^2 per day, divided into two doses.[4] In the NAPRTCS database, cadaveric transplant recipients appeared to benefit the most from MMF, with acute rejection rates of 18%, compared with 60% for historical controls taking azathioprine. For LD transplant recipients, the relative benefits of MMF were small. Gastrointestinal and hematologic side effects can be troublesome and may respond to dose reduction. Nausea, vomiting, esophagitis, gastritis, and bleeding are common, as well as susceptibility to invasive forms of cytomegalovirus (CMV). In some patients the drug has had to be withdrawn because of intolerable diarrhea.

Biological Immunosuppressive Agents

Antibody-induction therapy refers to the use of OKT3 or the polyclonal antibody (equine Atgam and rabbit Thymoglobulin) in the first 7–10 days after transplantation. The calcineurin inhibitor is withheld, or its dose is kept to a minimum until 2–3 days before the antibody course is completed. In sequential therapy, the OKT3 or the polyclonal antibody is administered and the calcineurin inhibitor is introduced only when renal function has reached a predetermined level (calculated GFR of 20–30 ml/min/1.73 m^2). The antibody is discontinued as soon as adequate calcineurin inhibitor levels are achieved. Polyclonal antibodies bind to cell surface receptors, thereby opsonizing lymphocytes for complement-mediated lysis or reticuloendothelial cell-dependent phagocytosis. In pediatric cadaver transplantation, there is a 10% advantage in the 5-year graft survival rate using antibody induction. Acute rejection episodes are 30% less frequent, and tend to occur later. The side-effect profiles of these agents are similar. The potential advantages of antibody induction therapy are: shortening of a period of delayed graft function, obviating early use of calcineurin inhibitor; delaying the onset of rejection; and permitting a less aggressive maintenance regimen. The disadvantages are a central line for administration, greater cost, prolonging the length of stay, higher incidence of CMV infection, risk for first-dose reaction (OKT3), and occasional limitation of future treatment options. Antibody induction in some centers is reserved for immunologically high-risk recipients, patients with delayed graft function, and patients requiring anticonvulsant drugs.

The interleukin (IL)-2 receptor monoclonal antibodies (IL-2R mAb) basiliximab (Simulect®) and Daclizumab (Zenapax®) are effective, easy to administer, and have few side effects. These antibodies bind to the alpha chain (CD25) of the IL-2R that cannot trigger cellular activation; thus these antibodies do not elicit the cytokine release syndrome. Basiliximab has a 10-fold greater avidity for IL-2R than daclizumab; therefore it is given intravenously on the day of surgery and on the fourth day post-transplant. Daclizumab is administered at 1 mg/kg per day intravenously within 24 hours of surgery, followed by equal doses every 14 days for a total of five doses. With daclizumab used in addition to a triple-drug regimen with either CsA or tacrolimus with MMF and prednisone, the rate of acute rejection was only 7% at 6 months and 16% at 1 year. Rejections were mild and steroid-responsive. No first-dose or cytokine-release effect or anaphylactic reactions were observed. The rates of opportunistic infections were not increased.

Newer Immunosuppressives
Sirolimus

Sirolimus (Rapamune®, SRL, Rapamycin) and tacrolimus are macrolides that bind to the same cytoplasmic protein (FKBP), but sirolimus does not inhibit calcineurin phosphatase or cytokine transcription.[12] Sirolimus has a long half-life (approximately 63 hours), justifying both a loading dose to rapidly attain steady-state concentrations and once-daily dosing. A good correlation exists between sirolimus trough levels and the area under the concentration-time curve; therefore, the recommendation for its monitoring is based on trough levels. Sirolimus is available in liquid and solid formulations, with comparable bioavailability. The recommended initial dose when used in combination with a calcineurin inhibitor and corticosteroids is 6 mg or 3 mg/m^2 once a day, and the maintenance dose is 3 mg or 1 mg/m^2 once a day. Dosing for children has not been established. The use of sirolimus in place of azathioprine in CsA-based regimens lowers the incidence of acute rejection. However, impaired renal function and hypertension in the sirolimus group seems to be due to an interaction between sirolimus and CsA that potentiates the nephrotoxic effects of CsA. Preliminary clinical data suggest that combining sirolimus with tacrolimus (instead of cyclosporine) may even be more effective. The side effects of sirolimus therapy include headaches, polyarthralgia, mild stomatitis, epistaxis, diarrhea, and mild acne; however, thrombocytopenia, leukopenia, hyperlipidemia, and problems related to over-immunosuppression remain the major concern.

RENAL ALLOGRAFT REJECTION

Acute Rejection

Rejection is an anti-allograft response mounted by the recipient's T cells. The activation of the T cells is initiated upon recognition of antigen-presenting cells.

Antigen recognition stimulates a redistribution of cell-surface proteins, leading to a clustering of the T-cell receptor (TCR) and the CD3 complex with the CD4 or CD8 antigens. The TCR-CD3 complex is associated with intracellular tyrosine kinases. Activation of protein kinase C (PKC) promotes the expression of several nuclear regulatory proteins, and the transcription and expression of genes essential to T-cell growth such as IL-2 and receptors for IL-2. In addition to antigenic signaling, a co-stimulatory signal is essential for full activation. The net consequence of cytokine production is the emergence of antigen-specific and graft-destructive T cells. The cytokines involved in cellular immunity also facilitate the humoral arm of immunity by stimulating the production of antibodies that damage the renal allograft via antibody-dependent cell-mediated cytotoxicity mechanisms (Box 38-1).

Hyperacute Rejection

This occurs as a result of preformed anti-HLA antibodies that bind to vascular endothelial cells and activate the complement cascade. The incidence is less than 0.25%. The only treatment is surgical removal of the graft. Glomerular thrombosis, fibrinoid necrosis, and polymorphonuclear leukocyte infiltration are seen histologically.

Acute Cellular Rejection

This is an important risk for pediatric renal transplant recipients, despite advances in transplant pharmacotherapy. The first rejection episode occurs within the first 3 months after transplantation in about half of the patients, with higher frequency and earlier recurrence in recipients of cadaveric transplants. Black race, DGF, and poor HLA matching may predispose to rejection.

Acute rejection is the single most important predictor of chronic rejection, and precedes graft failure from chronic rejection in over 90% of cases.[8]

Any increase in serum creatinine concentration, especially with hypertension, should be considered a result of acute rejection until proven otherwise. Fever and graft tenderness – the classical signs of acute rejection – are rarely seen in this era of calcineurin inhibitors and prophylactic T-cell antibody therapy. In very young transplant recipients acute rejection is not always straightforward, and requires a high index of suspicion. Because most small children are transplanted with adult-sized kidneys, the elevation in serum creatinine concentration may be a late sign of rejection as a result of the large renal reserve compared with the body mass. Therefore, significant allograft dysfunction may be present, with little or no increase in the serum creatinine concentration. One of the earliest and most sensitive signs of rejection is the development of hypertension along with low-grade fever. Late diagnosis and treatment of rejection are associated with higher incidence of resistant rejections and graft loss (Box 38-2).

The incidence of DGF ranges from 10% to 50%. Evaluation includes a urinalysis and urine culture, an ultrasound to rule out anatomic obstruction, and a radionuclide renal scan. None of these tests can distinguish among the various causes of graft dysfunction, such as rejection, CsA toxicity, and acute tubular necrosis (ATN), and therefore, a definitive diagnosis requires a transplant biopsy. The biopsy procedure is easy and safe when conscious sedation, ultrasound guidance, and an automated biopsy 'gun' is used. Glomerular changes are restricted to increased prominence of the mesangial stalk. A tubulitis is the hallmark of acute rejection. Semi-quantitative analysis and grading of acute rejection biopsy findings is performed using the Banff criteria (Box 38-3).

The standard treatment of an episode of acute rejection is intravenous methylprednisolone in doses from 5 to 10 mg/kg per day (up to 1 g per dose) for 3–5 days. Maintenance corticosteroid doses are then either

---

Box 38-1 Types of Rejection after Renal Transplantation

HYPERACUTE REJECTION

- This occurs within the first few minutes following reperfusion of the graft

ACCELERATED ACUTE REJECTION

- This occurs within the first week after transplantation

ACUTE REJECTION

- This generally occurs within the first year of transplantation

LATE ACUTE REJECTION

- This occurs after the first year

CHRONIC REJECTION – 'CHRONIC ALLOGRAFT NEPHROPATHY'

- This may occur as early as 3 months or years later

Box 38-2 Differential Diagnosis of Acute Allograft Dysfunction or Delayed Graft Function

- Acute tubular necrosis
- Ureteral obstruction – perirenal fluid collection, lymphocele, hematoma, abscess
- Urinary leak
- Renal arterial occlusion or venous thrombosis
- Intravascular volume contraction
- Nephrotoxicity
- Acute rejection
- Infection

<table>
<tr><td colspan="2">Box 38-3 Banff Criteria for Acute Rejection</td></tr>
<tr><td>Grade I</td><td>Focal interstitial lymphocyte infiltrate; mild tubulitis; normal vessels</td></tr>
<tr><td>Grade II</td><td>Extensive interstitial infiltrate; tubulitis; vacuolization in arterial vessels</td></tr>
<tr><td>Grade III</td><td>Extensive interstitial infiltration; tubulitis; lymphocyte infiltration of arterial walls; occasional fibrinoid changes</td></tr>
</table>

Box 38-4 Chronic Allograft Nephropathy

CLINICAL PICTURE
- Gradually declining renal function with proteinuria and hypertension
- Usually months or years after transplantation

HISTOPATHOLOGY
- Obliterative intimal fibrosis in the arteries (transplant arteriopathy)
- Duplication of glomerular basement membrane (chronic transplant glomerulopathy)
- Increased lobularity of the tuft (similar to membranoproliferative
- Glomerulonephritis
- Tubular atrophy
- Interstitial fibrosis with foci of lymphocytes and plasma cells

resumed at the pre-rejection levels or increased and tapered to baseline levels over a few days. The serum creatinine concentration may rise slightly during therapy, and may not return to baseline until 3–5 days after therapy is completed. Complete reversal of acute rejection – as judged by a return of the serum creatinine concentration to baseline – is achieved in about half of the children; 40–45% achieve partial reversal, and graft loss occurs in the remainder. Complete reversal from acute rejection is less likely with subsequent rejection episodes. Younger transplant recipients are at a higher risk for graft loss from acute rejection. Steroid-resistant rejection episodes are treated with one of the T-cell antibodies.

Refractory rejection usually refers to episodes of acute rejections that do not respond to, or reoccur after, treatment with methylprednisone and T-cell antibody therapy. Conversion from CsA to tacrolimus, or the addition of MMF, may reverse or stabilize a rejection episode. The risks for opportunistic infections and PTLD increase whenever such aggressive immunosuppressive therapy is used, and therefore viral prophylaxis and infection surveillance are necessary.

Chronic Rejection (Chronic Allograft Nephropathy)

Chronic rejection is the most common cause of graft loss. In pediatrics, 33% of graft failures are caused by chronic rejection (NAPRTCS 2002 annual report). A single episode of acute rejection imposed a relative risk for chronic rejection of 3.1, while multiple rejection episodes increased the relative risk to 4.3. The more inclusive term 'chronic allograft nephropathy' is used because, in addition to the critical role of acute rejection, many other factors play a part in chronic rejection (Box 38-4).

The pathogenesis of chronic allograft nephropathy involves complex interacting factors including: antigen-specific cellular and humoral immune mechanisms; number of HLA mismatches; production of alloantibodies against donor HLA class I or II antigens; and C4d deposits in peritubular capillaries suggesting an ongoing immunologic process. Non-immune factors that play a role are

delayed graft function, hypertension, hyperlipidemia, and long-term treatment with calcineurin inhibitors.

Maneuvers with the potential to reduce initial ischemic injury to the allograft are new preservation techniques, optimal selection and treatment of donors before recovery of the organ, shortening the duration of cold ischemia, and preferential use of living donors. There is no specific treatment for established chronic allograft nephropathy. Hypertension must be controlled; ACE inhibitors and angiotensin-II receptor blockers in stable allografts are renoprotective.[11] It is believed that because appropriate blood pressure control and reduction of hyperlipidemia are cardioprotective and renoprotective, this will improve long-term outcomes.

GRAFT SURVIVAL

The results of outcomes in renal transplantation from pediatric renal centers vary, usually because the number of patients at any one center is small. The main sources of data on pediatric renal transplantation are the NAPRTCS, the USRDS, and the UNOS registries. The NAPRTCS – a dedicated pediatric renal transplant registry established in 1987 – has collected data from more than 7000 patients representing more than 150 pediatric transplant centers.[3] Some of the data presented are extracted from the 2002 NAPRTCS Annual Report, which analyzes data on 7951 transplants performed in 7247 patients from 1987 through 2001. A total of 1968 graft failures among 7951 (25%) transplants has occurred. Chronic rejection is the leading cause of graft failure, and accounts for 33% of graft failures. Other causes include acute rejection (15%), vascular thrombosis (12%), and recurrence of original disease (7%), patient non-compliance

(4.4%), primary non-function (2.6%), infection (2%), and malignancy (1.4%). Although some causes of graft failure, such as graft thrombosis and recurrence of the original disease, have remained constant during the past 10 years, loss from acute rejection has decreased dramatically. LD graft survival rates at 1, 3, and 5 years are 92%, 86% and 81%, respectively. By comparison, CD graft survival rates at 1, 3, and 5 years are 84%, 75% and 67%, respectively. The more recent CD graft transplants have a survival of 92% that is similar to that of LD transplants from 1987 to 1995. These results may be related to temporal trends in immunosuppressive drugs and dosages, decreased transfusion requirements, and the decreased use of young cadaver donors.[9]

PROGNOSTIC FACTORS INFLUENCING GRAFT SURVIVAL

Donor Source

Short- and long-term graft and patient survival rates are better in recipients of LD transplants in all pediatric age groups. Registry data show that recipients of kidneys from living donors have a 10–20% advantage in graft survival at 1, 3, and 5 years. Younger transplant recipients benefit the most from LD transplantation, and have a 20–30% better graft survival rate at 5 years after transplantation. A shorter cold ischemia time, better human leukocyte antigen (HLA) matches, lower acute rejection rates, and better preoperative preparation all help to account for the better outcome in recipients of LD kidneys.

Recipient Age

Children under 6 years of age, and especially those under 2 years of age, have lower graft survival rates than older children, especially with CD kidneys. The 5-year graft survival rates in recipients aged less than 2 years are 80% and 52% for LD and CD transplants, respectively. This is primarily due to early graft losses within the first 6 months after transplantation. Higher rates of vascular thrombosis and irreversible acute rejection help to account for this early graft loss. In infants with a CD graft, 14% of acute rejection episodes result in transplant failure or death, compared with rates of 6–7% in older children. In recipients of LD transplants, the results are not as extreme: 8% of acute rejections in infants eventuate in graft loss or death, compared with 4–5% in older children. The 5-year graft survival rates in recipients aged over 12 years are 5–10% lower than those in recipients aged between 2 and 12 years.

Donor Age

Kidneys from donors aged from 16 to 40 years provide optimal graft survival and function. Although transplanted kidneys grow in size with the growth of the recipient, transplantation with cadaver kidneys from donors aged less than 6 years is associated with markedly decreased graft survival. The 5-year survival rate for recipients of cadaver kidneys from donors younger than 1 year of age is about 50%, compared to 60% and 70% for recipients of grafts from donors 2–5 years of age and older than 6 years of age, respectively. Children aged less than 5 years who receive a kidney from a donor aged less than 6 years have the highest relative risk of graft failure. CD kidneys older than 50 years of age are most likely to result in suboptimal long-term outcomes.

Race

Black race is the most significant factor associated with poor outcome among recipients of LD kidneys. Graft survival rates in black children are lower by 10% and 25% at 1 and 5 years after transplantation, respectively, for recipients of LD kidneys. For CD transplants, the 5-year graft survival in black recipients is lower than that in white recipients, by about 20%.

Tissue Type

Long-term graft survival is best when the graft is from an HLA-identical sibling. Transplants from HLA haploidentical sibling donors have a half-life (time to failure of 50% of grafts) of 12–14 years, compared with 25 years in transplant recipients from HLA-identical siblings.

Pre-sensitization

Repeated blood transfusions expose the recipient to a range of HLA antigens, and may result in sensitization to these antigens, leading to higher rates of rejection and graft failures. The graft failure rate almost doubles in LD transplant recipients with more than five blood transfusions before transplantation, compared with those who had five or fewer transfusions (30% versus 15%, respectively, at 5 years after transplantation). The figures for CD transplant recipients are 45% in those with a prior history of more than five blood transfusions, and 30% in those who had five or fewer transfusions. Fortunately, blood transfusions have become less common since human recombinant erythropoietin became an integral part of end-stage renal disease (ESRD) therapy. Similarly, sensitization may result from the rejection of a previous transplant, and the 5-year graft survival for repeat cadaveric transplantations is about 20% lower.

Immunologic Factors

Immunologic parameters in younger children are different from those in adults and older children. Such differences include higher numbers of T and B cells, a higher CD4+ to CD8+ T-cell ratio, and increased blastogenic responses. These differences may account for increased immune responsiveness to HLA antigens, and may be partly responsible for the higher rates of rejection observed in children.

Technical Factors and Delayed Graft Function (DGF)

Small children present a difficult challenge in the operating room. The relatively large size of the graft may result in longer anastomosis times, a longer ischemia time, and subsequently higher rates of early graft dysfunction. DGF (defined by the requirement for dialysis within the first week of transplantation) occurs in about 5% of LD and 20% of CD transplantations, and is associated with a reduced graft survival. In children with DGF, the 3-year graft survival rates are reduced by about 20% and 30% in recipients of CD and LD donor kidneys, respectively. Risk factors for DGF are more than five prior transfusions, prior transplantation, native nephrectomy, and black race.

The transplanted kidney is usually placed in an extraperitoneal location to allow easier clinical monitoring and access to the graft. Occasionally, native kidney nephrectomy is necessary at the time of transplantation to make room for the transplanted kidney, especially in a very small child. The aorta and inferior vena cava are usually used for anastomosis to ensure adequate blood flow, but smaller vessels may be used. Vascular anastomosis may be problematic in a child with previous hemodialysis accesses placed in the lower extremities. Children should be evaluated thoroughly before transplantation to identify any potential anastomotic difficulties. Unidentified vascular anomalies may lead to prolonged anastomosis times and subsequently to higher rates of DGF and graft thrombosis.

Antibody Induction

Antibody induction with polyclonal antibodies or OKT3 is used either for prophylaxis against rejection or in a sequential manner to avoid nephrotoxicity resulting from early use of calcineurin inhibitors. In cadaveric transplantation, antibody induction is associated with about a 10% advantage in the 5-year graft survival rate. First acute rejection episodes tend to be more frequent and to occur earlier in patients not treated with an antilymphocyte preparation.

Transplant Center Volume Effect

Transplant outcomes in high-volume pediatric renal transplant centers are superior to those in lower-volume centers. High-volume centers (defined as the performance of more than 100 pediatric transplants between 1987 and 1995) reported a lower incidence of graft thrombosis, DGF, improved long-term graft survival, and more frequent use of antibody induction.

Cohort Year

The results of pediatric renal transplantation are dramatically improving. CD transplants performed between 1987 and 1989 had a 1-year graft survival rate of 73.4%, whereas LD transplants had a 1-year rate of 89.7%. In 1999 to 2001, the 1-year graft survival rates for LD and CD transplants were 92.4% and 95.7%, respectively. These results may be related to temporal trends in immunosuppressive drugs and dosages, decreased transfusion requirements, and the decreased use of young cadaver donors.

Non-adherence in Pediatric Transplantation[5]

Non-adherence is the principal cause of graft loss in at least 15% of all pediatric kidney transplant recipients, and for retransplanted patients, this figure may exceed 25% (see Chapter 9).

LONG-TERM OUTCOME

Morbidity

The NAPRTCS measures morbidity by the number of hospitalization days. The median duration (to initial discharge) of hospitalization at the time of transplant is 13 days, with longer stays required for younger patients and for recipients of CD grafts. Most children require re-hospitalization at least once after initial discharge following transplantation. During months 1 to 5, 50% of LD-graft recipients were re-hospitalized compared to 58% of CD-graft recipients. The hospitalization rate falls with increasing time after transplantation. The most common reason for hospitalization in this interval is diagnosis and treatment of rejection, which occurred in 30% and 21% of CD and LD patients, respectively. Treatment of viral (16% versus 13%) and bacterial (14% versus 12%) infections, and treatment of hypertension (6% versus 4%) are the next most common reasons for hospitalization. The most common bacterial infection in children under the age of 5 years is *Clostridium difficile* diarrhea, and urinary tract infection is the most common in those aged over 5 years.

Mortality

Patient survival after transplantation is superior to that achieved by dialysis for all pediatric age groups. In order to assess post-transplant survival, 6668 transplants (3704 LD and 2964 CD) were considered. The percentage patient survival for all patients at 12, 24, and 60 months post transplant is 97%, 96%, and 94%, respectively. Percentage patient survival for recipients of primary living donor kidneys are 98%, 97%, and 95%, at 12, 24, and 60 months post transplant, respectively. Comparable values for recipients of primary CD allografts are 97%, 96%, and 93%. Post-transplant survival is markedly lower for infants (<24 months old at transplant), particularly for recipients of CD grafts. The 3-year patient survival of cadaver source grafts has increased from 78% in 1987–1994 to 94% in 1995 and later. For infants receiving LD grafts, their 3-year survival also improved from 88% in 1987–1994 to 95% in 1995 and beyond.

According to the 2002 NAPRTCS data, reports of death have been received for 365 of the 6668 patients (5.5%). Crude donor source-specific mortality rates are 4.6% for recipients of LD primary transplants, and 6.6% for recipients of CD primary transplants. Infection was the cause of death in 118 patients (32.3% of deaths). Other major causes include malignancy (45; 12.3%), cardiopulmonary (55; 15.1%), and dialysis-related complications (11; 3%). Risk factors for excess mortality include young recipient age, DGF at day 30 after transplant, and certain underlying renal diseases (oxalosis, congenital nephrotic syndrome, Denys–Drash syndrome). Mortality more than 10 years after transplantation seems to be related primarily to cardiovascular causes, which may be linked to dyslipidemia and hypertension.

Rehabilitation and Quality of Life

Organ transplantation usually results in a dramatic improvement of all aspects of physical, emotional, and social functioning.[10] Cognitive skills improve after successful renal transplantation, suggesting stabilization of neuropsychologic functioning. Successful re-entry into school after transplantation requires coordinated preparation of the child, family or caregivers, classmates, and school personnel (see Chapter 11). Medication side effects, social and emotional difficulties, academic difficulties, school resources, and care-giver attitudes all play a role, and should be addressed. The health-related quality of life measures are generally good, especially in older children and adolescents, although all ages report some problems with usual activities.

Within a year of successful transplantation, the social and emotional functioning of the child and the child's family appears to return to pre-illness levels. Pre-transplantation personality disorders, however, continue to manifest themselves. Within a year after transplantation, more than 90% of children attend school; fewer than 10% are not involved in any vocational or education programs. By the 3-year follow-up, almost 90% of children are in an appropriate school or job placement.

Surveys of 10-year survivors of pediatric kidney transplants report that most patients consider their health to be good; they engage in appropriate social, educational, and sexual activities; and they experience a very good or excellent quality of life.

REFERENCES

1. Baluarte HJ, Braas C, Kaiser AB, et al. postoperative management of pediatric transplant patient. In: Tejani AH, Fine RN (eds), *Pediatric Renal Transplantation.* Wiley-Liss, Inc., New York, 1994, pp. 239–255.

2. Ellis D. Clinical use of tacrolimus (FK-506) in infants and children with renal transplants. Pediatr Nephrol 1995;9:487–494.

3. Elshihabi I, Chavers BM, Donaldson L, et al. Continuing improvement in cadaver donor graft survival in North American children: the 1998 Annual report of the North American Renal Transplant Cooperative Study (NAPRTCS) 2000;4:235–246.

4. Ettenger R, Cohen A, Nast C, et al. Mycophenolate mofetil as maintenance immunosuppression in pediatric renal transplantation. Transplant Proc 1997;29:340–341.

5. Fennell RS, Foulkes LM, Boggs SR. Family-based program to promote medication compliance in renal transplant children. Transplant Proc 1994;26:102–103.

6. Hong C, Kahan BD. Immunosuppressive agents in organ transplantation: past, present and future. Semin Nephrol 2000;20:108–125.

7. Jabs K, Sullivan EK, Avner ED, et al. Alternate-day steroid dosing improves growth without adversely affecting graft survival or long-term graft function. A report of the North American Pediatric Renal Transplant Cooperative Study. Transplantation 1996;61:31–36.

8. Matas AJ. Impact of acute rejection on the development of chronic rejection in pediatric renal transplant recipients. Pediatr Transplant 2000;4:92–99.

9. McDonald R, Donaldson L, Emmett L, et al. A decade of living donor transplantation in North American children: the 1998 Annual Report of the North American Pediatric Renal Transplant Cooperative Study (NAPRTCS). Pediatr Transplant 2000;4:221–234.

10. Morel P, Almond PS, Matas AJ, et al. Long-term quality of life after kidney transplantation in childhood. Transplantation 1991;52:47–53.

11. Pascual M, Theruvath T, Kawai T, et al. Strategies to improve long-term outcomes after renal transplantation. N Engl J Med 2002;346:580–590.

12. Saunders RN, Metcalfe MS, Nicholson ML. Rapamycin in transplantation: a review of the evidence. Kidney Int 2001;59:3–16.

13. Trompeter R, Filler G, Webb N, et al. Randomized trial of tacrolimus versus cyclosporin microemulsion in renal transplantation. Pediatr Nephrol 2002;17:141–149.

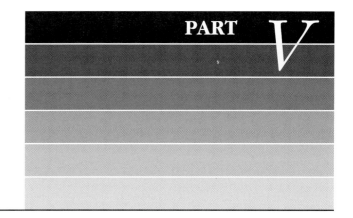

PART *V*

CHAPTER 39

Voiding Problems in Children

SETH L. SCHULMAN, M.D.

INTRODUCTION

Children who continue to wet beyond the expected age where control is expected are a vexing problem for their parents, primary care providers, teachers and, of course, the children themselves, who often suffer from low self-esteem. The vast majority of these children do not wet because they have an organic pathology; rather, this is felt to represent a maturational lag for which a specific etiology may not always be evident. Health professionals can usually reassure parents and start treatment after taking a detailed history, obtaining a physical examination, and performing a limited selection of laboratory and radiographic studies. This chapter will assist individuals caring for such children to perform a proper evaluation and to identify deviations from normal that may be uncovered after data gathering. It will review the etiology of wetting in children, and present treatment options.

DEFINITIONS

The International Continence in Children Society has provided standard definitions of lower-tract dysfunction in children:

- *Incontinence* implies urinary leakage, rather than soaking, and can occur during the daytime or at night.
- *Enuresis* is defined as complete expulsion of urinary contents after a period where urinary control is anticipated. Generally, children are expected to be dry during the day by age of 4 years, and at night by the age of 5.
- *Nocturnal enuresis* is wetting at night, and *diurnal enuresis* is wetting during the day.
- A condition is *primary* if there has been no dry period longer than six consecutive months, and *secondary* if a previous dry period lasted at least 6 months.
- *Monosymptomatic nocturnal enuresis* describes bedwetting exclusively with no daytime concerns, as opposed to *polysymptomatic nocturnal enuresis* where complaints such as urinary tract infection, urinary urgency, frequency, or wetting may coexist. The latter condition is usually more difficult to treat.

EPIDEMIOLOGY

Because toileting is a maturational process, the prevalence of both day and night wetting decreases with age. The prevalence of night wetting by age is

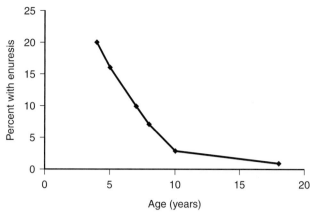

Figure 39-1 Prevalence of nocturnal enuresis by child's age.

shown in Figure 39-1. Key points to note are that 20% of 5 year-old children still wet at night, and that the rate of spontaneous resolution of nocturnal enuresis is 15% per year.[10] Boys are affected more frequently than girls, until puberty. It is estimated that about 1% of adults wet at night, albeit less frequently than children.

Data on the prevalence of daytime wetting suggest that this is a more common phenomenon than most practitioners think, with 5–10% of children aged between 5 and 10 years being affected. Daytime wetting is two to three times more common in girls than in boys. Long-term follow-up of children presenting with daytime wetting reveals that the vast majority (94%) improve by adolescence.[19]

Behavioral Issues

The origins of wetting were initially believed to be strictly behavioral. However, children wetting at night have not been shown to experience unusually stressful events, and there seems to be no difference in the prevalence of enuresis in children with or without psychosocial problems.[6] Studies show differences among some children who wet during the day that may relate to attention-deficit hyperactivity disorder.[8]

Children who wet suffer from shame and low self-esteem compared with dry children; these differences no longer exist when the wetting resolves.[4] In one study in which children were asked to grade stressful events, wetting was found to be third behind losing a parent and going blind. These children hide their wet clothing and, if they wet at night, may refuse to attend sleepovers or camping trips. In some cases these feelings are a result of parental pressure or even punishment. Teasing by siblings can also exacerbate the situation. Parents are often frustrated by the cost of laundry and continence aids, and can become sleep-deprived if they awaken their child at night. Thus, it is imperative that healthcare

providers identify and discuss the child's situation with the family, and offer appropriate treatment and explanation of the reasons for delaying treatment in very young children. There is an entire industry dedicated to keeping children dry – these programs may cost over $1800 and they often prey on the families of enuretic children.

DEVELOPMENTAL ASPECTS OF BLADDER CONTROL

Children follow a predictable course of continence for both bowel and bladder. First, bowel control is established at night, followed by bowel control during the day. Soon afterwards, bladder control is achieved during the day – usually after 24 months and before 4 years. Finally, children remain dry at night.

Voiding in infancy has traditionally been thought to be reflexive in nature, with the brain having a passive role coordinating the flow. Recent studies have shown that the cortex is stimulated in infants and, in fact, that infants awaken when they void at night. It has also been shown that infants do not always void in a coordinated fashion, which suggests that they contract their pelvic floor musculature.

Three important accomplishments occur during toilet training. First, the toddler develops the ability to sense bladder fullness and inhibit bladder contractions. Second, the ability to void volitionally develops as the toddler relaxes the pelvic floor and the bladder contracts. Finally, children are able willfully to contract their sphincter during voiding, if they so choose, and stop voiding. Infants void approximately 20 times per day.[1] The frequency of voiding decreases with age, such that 6-year-old children void about six times per day. This is attributable largely to a bladder capacity that increases with age, in combination with decreased fluid intake as the child relies on table food for nutrition. The normal bladder capacity can be approximated in ounces by adding 2 to the child's age (Table 39-1).

Table 39-1	Bladder Capacity
Age (years)	**Volume**
1	3 oz/90 ml
2	4 oz/120 ml
3	5 oz/150 ml
4	6 oz/180 ml
5	7 oz/210 ml
6	8 oz/240 ml

ETIOLOGIES AND CLASSIFICATIONS OF DAY AND NIGHT WETTING

Physicians caring for children who wet must consider the organic causes of incontinence or enuresis (Table 39-2). Some of these conditions can be corrected, thereby alleviating symptoms. In some cases parental concern is primarily based on a fear that the child has a serious problem.

Since toilet training is a developmental milestone, it is not surprising that children with developmental delays will take longer to accomplish this task. Secondarily, perturbations that arise during toileting may explain why some children develop functional voiding difficulties during the day. Chronic urethritis caused by chemical irritation, recurrent urinary tract infections and constipation can cause children inappropriately to contract their external sphincter secondary to the fear of pain and/or increase the bladder's likelihood to contract without central inhibition.[1] Both of these actions will decrease the functional bladder capacity and increase the chances of wetting and, in some cases, urinary tract infection. Infections perpetuate this cycle by reinforcing the child's fear of urinating – just like constipation inhibits effective defecation.

Table 39-2 Organic Causes of Incontinence

Cause	Historical, Physical, Laboratory, and Radiographic Clues
Urinary tract infection	• Dysuria, fever, foul-smelling urine • Nitrituria, pyuria
Ectopic ureter	• Constant wetting with no dry interval • No urgency, frequency • Renal duplication anomaly with upper pole dilation
Posterior urethral valves	• Dribbling, weak urinary stream • Distended bladder • Thick-walled bladder • Hydroureteronephrosis
Ureterocele	• Prolonged stream • Distended bladder • Presence of ureterocele on bladder ultrasound
Diabetes mellitus	• Polyuria, polydipsia • Glycosuria
Diabetes insipidus	• Polyuria, polydipsia • Hyposthenuria
Tethered spinal cord (neuropathic bladder)	• Abnormal gait • Back pain • Abnormal spine (dimple, hairy tuft) • Abnormal gluteal crease • Abnormal neurologic examination (rectal tone, perineal sensation, bulbocavernosus reflex)

The role of constipation must be accentuated in children with day and night wetting; its importance has caused some to view the entire condition as a 'dysfunctional elimination syndrome.' Constipation may interfere with central inhibition causing detrusor instability, it may compress the bladder decreasing its maximum capacity, and it may result in incomplete relaxation, leading to post-void residual urine. Studies show that aggressive treatment of constipation may result in the resolution of day and night wetting.[11]

Benign Urinary Frequency (Pollakiuria)

Children with this condition suddenly need to void excessively frequently, as often as 30 times per day. They do not complain of dysuria, and rarely wet during the day. At night, once asleep these children do not awaken and do not wet their bed. Urinary tract infection should be excluded. This condition is self-limited, is felt to be related to stress, and responds to reassurance. Recent studies suggest a relationship between this behavior and PANDAS (Pediatric Autoimmune Neuropsychiatric Disorders Associated with Streptococcal infections) in some children.[2]

Post-Void Dribbling

Girls with this condition actually leak after standing, or complain of incomplete emptying and a need to void again. They often wipe themselves excessively, thereby irritating the perineum. This condition is related either to vaginal pooling of urine or detrusor contractions after voiding. Advising these girls to void with their legs straddling the toilet may be helpful. Labial fusion should be excluded on examination.

Giggle Enuresis

Almost exclusively seen in girls, this condition is associated with complete expulsion of the bladder contents on laughing. This embarrassing condition is often confused with urge incontinence (see below) or stress incontinence, which is uncommon in children. It may be functionally related to cataplexy and, in uncontrolled studies, has been found to respond to stimulants such as methylphenidate.

Diurnal Enuresis

Children with this condition put off voiding until the last minute. They void infrequently, and are often easily distracted. They respond well to voiding schedules that are structured, and are often suspected to have attention-deficit disorder. Although urgency is seen in these children, this should not be confused with urge syndrome, where children often need to void frequently due to detrusor instability.

Urge Syndrome

Also known as unstable or immature bladder syndrome, children with this common condition complain of increased urinary urgency, frequency, and wetting. In many cases these children will utilize maneuvers to prevent leakage such as Vincent's curtsy, where girls squat with their heel compressing their perineum. Urodynamically, the detrusor is contracting during filling without cortical inhibition. Concomitantly the pelvic floor is contracting to prevent leakage.

Dysfunctional Voiding

In this condition the child may fill their bladder normally, but empty poorly. The urinary stream is abnormally prolonged and may be interrupted due to poor relaxation of the pelvic floor. The most frequent symptom noted, primarily in girls, is recurrent urinary tract infections. Incontinence may develop due to decreased functional capacity secondary to post-void residual. In rare cases the bladder becomes enlarged, voiding is less frequent, and overflow incontinence can develop.

Hinman Syndrome

This rare syndrome represents the extreme spectrum of voiding dysfunction. First described in boys, this condition appears to resemble a neurogenic bladder and has been termed 'non-neurogenic neurogenic bladder.' Urinary tract infections occur frequently. Functional obstruction is so marked that dilation of the upper tracts develops and kidney damage may be seen. Severe constipation and encopresis are commonly associated with this syndrome. A multidisciplinary approach (medical, surgical and psychosocial) is necessary to effectively manage these children.

Nocturnal Enuresis

The etiologies of monosymptomatic nocturnal enuresis are multifactorial. Clearly, genetic predisposition is an important factor associated with this condition. If one parent wetted the bed as a child, then the likelihood of offspring wetting is over 40%. The chances increase to nearly 80% if both parents wetted. The search for a gene responsible for enuresis has proven to be elusive. Genes on chromosomes 8, 12, 13, and 22 have all been implicated in various reports.[12] There does not appear to be a correlation between phenotype and genotype.

The specific pathogenesis of nocturnal enuresis has centered on three hypotheses. Children who wet at night sleep deeply, have small bladder capacities, and/or have nocturnal polyuria secondary to a lack of the physiological nocturnal peak of vasopressin.

Many parents claim that their child sleeps deeply, based on their experience attempting to wake the child to get them to void. Wetting appears to occur throughout all stages of sleep. Recent studies have emphasized that enuretic children have abnormal arousal from sleep.[20] By using earphones that emit noise during sleep, one investigator found that 8.5% of enuretic children awakened, compared to 40% of controls. The problem with this hypothesis is that one wonders why these children need to awaken in the first place. Most children who stay dry and sleep through the night do not need to awaken. In addition, one only chooses to awaken children who wet. We do not know whether some dry children who sleep through the night are just as difficult to arouse as those who wet. One correctable sleep disturbance associated with nocturnal enuresis is obstructive sleep apnea. Reports have documented the resolution of enuresis after the treatment of obstructive sleep apnea.

Bladder instability is also a cause of wetting. Several studies have shown that children who wet at night also have urodynamic abnormalities, even in the absence of daytime symptoms.[15] These abnormalities create a functionally small bladder. This hypothesis as the sole etiology of nocturnal enuresis is also flawed when one considers that not all children with daytime wetting have this problem at night.

Some children with primary nocturnal enuresis do not secrete adequate amounts of antidiuretic hormone (ADH) at night.[13] This relative deficiency of ADH is thought to cause nocturnal polyuria exceeding the night-time storage capacity of the bladder. Subsequent studies have not confirmed this observation, suggesting some patients may have resistance to ADH. Many – but not all – children with diseases associated with resistance to ADH such as sickle cell disease wet the bed, confirming that nocturnal polyuria alone does not explain bedwetting in all children.

By combining all three theories (Figure 39-2), it is possible to understand why children are likely to wet.

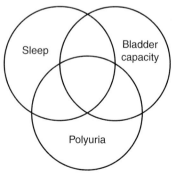

Figure 39-2   Etiologies of nocturnal enuresis.

Children falling into the intersection of two or three of the etiologies are probably enuretic. Despite the research supporting these theories, most patients are not usually tested to determine if they have a sleep abnormality (unless apnea is suspected), bladder instability, or a relative deficiency of ADH.

Previous recommendations were that secondary nocturnal enuresis was caused by pathology that mandated a more extensive evaluation. Stress either due to psychosocial issues (e.g., moving to a new home) or trauma (e.g., child abuse) should be considered. However, in the majority of cases no specific etiology is found and usually the evaluation does not need to be more comprehensive than the evaluation performed for children with primary nocturnal enuresis.[14]

Voiding Dysfunction and Vesicoureteral Reflux

Increased intravesical pressure can promote reflux through a marginally competent vesicoureteral junction. Reflux may be identified prior to the knowledge of voiding dysfunction as part of the evaluation for urinary tract infection.[9] It is important, therefore, to obtain a history that includes questions that focus on voiding behavior. In many cases reflux resolves with treatment of voiding dysfunction, without the need for surgery. Theoretically, surgical treatment alone does nothing to help children for their voiding problems. Surgical complications may develop, especially if the intravesical pressures are high and the bladder wall is thickened.

DATA GATHERING

The history should emphasize the child's voiding and defecation habits (Table 39-3). Unfortunately, many parents lack knowledge about their child's urinary habits, including the frequency and the character of the urinary stream, nor do they know the consistency of their stool. Ultimately, the healthcare provider needs to distinguish key elements that suggest organic pathology. For example, constant wetting without any dry period suggests the presence of an ectopic ureter draining below the sphincter or elsewhere in the perineum. Wetting that occurs after voiding suggests pooling in the vagina that can be seen in girls with labial fusion. Dysuria, urgency, and foul-smelling urine are seen with acute cystitis. A weak urinary stream in boys can be seen in posterior urethral valves. Both diabetes mellitus and diabetes insipidus cause polyuria and polydipsia. A history of urinary tract infections, especially if associated with fevers, may indicate the presence of vesicoureteral reflux. A change in gait in conjunction with the secondary onset of wetting implies tethering of the

Table 39-3   Patient History

Day wetting	• How long has your child been wetting? • How often does your child wet per day (week)? • Does your child dampen their undergarments or soak their clothing? • How have you managed this problem so far?
Night wetting	• Has your child been wetting regularly at night since toilet training? • How many nights per week does your child wet? • Does your child dampen or soak the bed sheets or saturate a continence aid? • Does your child snore heavily or have periods of holding his or her breath? • How have you managed this problem so far?
Urinary tract infection	• Has your child ever had a urinary tract infection? • If so, what symptoms did your child have? Did your child have a fever? • Does your child complain of burning on urination?
Voiding behavior	• How often does your child urinate? • Does your child indicate that he or she needs to void immediately? • Does your child hold him or herself or squat to prevent leakage? • Does your child strain to void? • Does it appear that your child voids in a continuous or interrupted pattern?
Bowel habits	• How often does your child defecate? • Are your child's bowel movements large or hard? • Does your child complain of discomfort when defecating? • Does your child have bowel accidents (soil)?
Psychological history	• How upset does your child get about this problem? • Does your child refuse to attend school functions or sleepovers? • How is your child doing academically and socially in school? • Have your child's teachers advised you that your child may have issues with attentiveness?
Diet history	• How much fluid does your child drink? • What fluids does your child drink?
Miscellaneous	• Are there family members who had similar problems when they were growing up? • What medications is your child taking?

spinal cord. A history of snoring suggests an increased risk of obstructive sleep apnea.

A normal physical examination excludes organic diseases that are associated with wetting. Emphasis should be placed on the abdominal examination to identify masses such as a dilated bladder or severe obstipation. The lower back should be examined for the presence of a lipoma, sinus, tufts of hair or abnormal gluteal crease, which suggests an occult neurologic disorder. Abnormal tone on rectal examination, absent perineal sensation and an absent bulbocavernosus reflex can be confirmatory of a neurogenic etiology for wetting. Inspection of the genitalia for meatal stenosis in boys and labial fusion in girls should be performed.

Diagnostic testing in children with primary, monosymptomatic nocturnal enuresis is limited to obtaining a first morning specimen of urine for a chemical and microscopic urinalysis. A concentrated specimen with no abnormal elements can safely exclude diabetes mellitus, diabetes insipidus, renal insufficiency and, in most cases, urinary tract infection. Imaging of the urinary tract is usually not necessary.

In children with daytime symptoms a urine culture should be obtained. A renal and bladder ultrasound performed both before and after voiding will help to diagnose obstructive uropathy, and will establish the functional bladder capacity. Children with recurrent afebrile urinary tract infections or a single episode of a febrile urinary tract infection, as well as boys with thick-walled bladder and poor stream, should have a voiding cystourethrogram to identify vesicoureteral reflux and posterior urethral valves. A scout film of the abdomen can determine if there are bony abnormalities of the spine or severe constipation. In some cases, magnetic resonance imaging of the lumbosacral spine is indicated to exclude spinal cord anomalies.

Urodynamic testing is reserved for children who do not respond to conservative treatment.[17] This study can be done in children of any age, although it is easier to interpret results when the patient is cooperative. A double-lumen catheter is placed transurethrally to simultaneously fill and measure bladder pressure. A rectal catheter measures abdominal pressure. Patch electrodes placed perianally measure the electromyogram activity of the pelvic floor. Finally, a uroflow determines the voiding profile, including the velocity and flow time. The composite data derived from the history, physical examination, radiographic studies and urodynamic studies assigns patients into the broad classifications of voiding abnormalities described previously.

TREATMENT

The fundamental elements of therapy require that patients understand their behavior, and that the caregiver is willing to spend time working with the families. Diaries are utilized to identify the frequency of the child's voiding, wetting, and defecation. Children are instructed to drink at least three glasses of water daily that they log in their diary, and are instructed to avoid known bladder irritants such as caffeine. Specific treatment hinges on the data accumulated on the diary. Problems related to the bowel (constipation and encopresis) are managed

first and daytime wetting is managed second, leaving treatment for nocturnal enuresis to last. The rationale for this approach is that it approximates the normal maturational process, and it does not make sense trying to keep a child dry while they are asleep if they still wet during the day.

Bowel Program

Combined behavioral, dietary, and pharmacologic treatments are instituted. The goal is to ensure that the child can sense he or she needs to defecate, and can do so painlessly. Behavioral measures include timed seating at least twice a day for 5–10 minutes after meals to take advantage of the gastrocolic reflex. Dietary changes may be necessary so that the intake of water and fiber is increased. Medications such as mineral oil and lactulose to aid the child in defecating effectively should be prescribed. Recalcitrant cases may require polyethylene glycol 3350 (MiraLax™). Psychological counseling is often necessary to maintain the treatment regimen.

Daytime Wetting

Specific therapy depends on the etiology of the daytime wetting. In all children, voiding diaries can serve as a barometer of a family's interest and motivation. Children are informed that their bladders are acting 'bossy' when they need to void, but that their brains are the boss when they choose to void. By increasing (or simply documenting) voiding frequency six or seven times per day or approximately every 2 hours, patients will fall into one of three categories.

Some children improve due to the structure that scheduled voiding provides and do not require additional assistance. Other children resist adhering to a schedule. These families may benefit from the additional support that psychological counseling can provide. The counselor can delve into the causes for the resistance and optimize motivation in the setting specific to the family.[17] In cases where children are sufficiently motivated yet unable to remain dry despite voiding regularly, adhering to a bowel program, and increasing their intake of water, definitive treatment is required. Children with urge syndrome and difficulty with bladder storage may improve with the addition of an anticholinergic medication such as oxybutynin, tolterodine, or hyoscyamine. These medications decrease detrusor instability, thereby allowing the patient to increase bladder capacity. Side effects such as lethargy and difficulty in reading secondary to poor accommodation of the eyes may limit their use. Long-acting preparations may reduce adverse effects and improve compliance. Children should continue to void regularly, even if positive effects of the medication are noted.

Biofeedback can be employed in children with dysfunctional voiding where bladder emptying is incomplete. Although different methods are utilized, the primary objective is to teach the child to recognize how to control their pelvic floor so that they can completely relax when they void. This form of treatment is benign, but the child needs to understand what is being asked, and also practice between sessions. Making a game of biofeedback training has been shown to optimize motivation.[5]

Children with recurrent urinary tract infections who have vesicoureteral reflux should be placed on antibiotic prophylaxis until the reflux resolves. Short-term prophylaxis may be useful in patients without reflux in order to break the cycle of dysuria causing poor relaxation, which increases the risk of further infection until biofeedback can be started.

Nocturnal Enuresis

Treatment for nocturnal enuresis should commence when the child and family begin to feel that bedwetting is at risk of affecting the child's self-esteem. This usually correlates with the time when children are invited to sleepovers or camping trips, but it can occur earlier if the family's approach to dealing with enuresis involves punishment. Parents of younger children are educated that this is a developmental problem and are reassured that treatment will ensue if the problem persists. Regardless of the specific treatment chosen, the children and parents need to work together as a team to maximize response while minimizing the child's sense of shame. Initial measures such as voiding before bedtime,

limiting excessive fluid intake, establishing a first morning routine that involves the child, and monitoring progress on a chart are often helpful.

The primary behavioral therapy used to treat bedwetting is an enuresis alarm. The alarms that are currently available are compact and portable. Healthcare providers should keep an alarm in the office to demonstrate its use to families. A sensor is worn in the undergarment that is attached to or part of an audio and/or vibratory alarm. As the child wets, an alarm signals to awaken them. Eventually the child is conditioned to awaken prior to the signal from the alarm, and remains dry either because they awaken with nocturia or sleep through the night.

The advantages of an alarm include its cost, safety, efficacy and, most importantly, its ability to teach and therefore cure the child. Long-term cure rates using the alarm range from 50 to 80% with low rates of relapse, which are superior to rates seen using pharmacologic treatment.[18] The disadvantage of the alarm is that they are time-intensive and require considerable motivation both from the child and family. The alarm should be used every night, and the family enlisted to help the child totally awaken. Only the child should disconnect the alarm. Failures occur when either the parents or child are not sufficiently motivated, the alarm signals more frequently than once per night, or when the family cannot awaken the child. Success is more likely to occur if the family understands how the alarm works, and recognizes ways to avoid pitfalls that frequently develop.[16]

Medications used to treat nocturnal enuresis are shown in Table 39-4. Desmopressin is a synthetic analogue of vasopressin. Available as a spray administered intranasally

Table 39-4 Medications for Nocturnal Enuresis

Medication	Dose	Adverse Events	Comments
Desmopressin acetate			May combine with alarm or anticholinergics Expensive
Intranasal	20–40 µg 1 h before bedtime	Headache, epistaxis	Limit fluids 2 h before bedtime May be less effective if patient has nasal congestion
Oral	0.2–0.4 mg 1 hour before bedtime	Headache	Limit fluids as above
Imipramine	Start 25 mg nightly Maximum dose: 8–12 years: 50 mg >12 years: 75 mg	Irritability, dry mouth, headaches, decreased appetite	Counsel family about toxicity of accidental overdose May combine with alarm
Anticholinergics			May combine with alarm or desmopressin acetate Not FDA-approved for treatment of nocturnal enuresis
Oxybutynin	5–10 mg nightly (0.1 mg/kg)	Dry mouth, flushing, blurry vision, constipation	Short-acting preparation, may intensify side effects and not last as long as needed
Ditropan XL®	5–10 mg nightly	Same as above	Long-acting preparation, expensive
Detrol LA®	2–4 mg nightly	Same as above	Same as above
Levbid®	0.375 mg nightly	Same as above	Same as above

and as tablets taken orally, desmopressin binds to V2 receptors in the collecting duct that increases the permeability of water, in turn decreasing urine output. Success rates range from 40 to 80%, but the rate of relapse after discontinuing the medication is high. The medication is well tolerated with few side effects, even when used on a long-term basis (>6 months),[7] but it is expensive. Fluid intake must be limited at night in order to avoid the risk of symptomatic hyponatremia.

Imipramine, a tricyclic antidepressant, is approved for the treatment of children with primary nocturnal enuresis. It has an anticholinergic effect that increases functional bladder capacity, as well as a central effect that may increase the child's ability to arouse at night. Approximately 50% of children benefit from the use of imipramine, although the relapse rate is high. Between 10 and 20% of children experience side effects such as nausea, constipation, and personality changes. Overdoses can cause fatal arrhythmias and families must be warned to keep the medication out of the reach of small children, preferably in a locked cabinet.

Anticholinergic medications are especially effective in children with polysymptomatic nocturnal enuresis. However, they have limited effect when used alone, and they should be given with desmopressin or used with an alarm. Other combinations such as an alarm with desmopressin or an alarm with imipramine are also useful.[3]

CONCLUSION

Healthcare providers need to ask about their patient's toileting behavior to identify those with voiding problems. Although the risk of anatomic or neuropathic pathology is small, a comprehensive history with emphasis on bowel and bladder function and physical examination supported by specific radiographic and laboratory studies will identify organic causes. Parental education aimed at explaining the putative causes of wetting, followed by a therapeutic plan that is primarily behavioral, may be sufficient for some patients. Other patients may require more intensive, multidisciplinary management, including referral to an experienced specialist. Regardless of the specific therapy offered, patients and their families deserve more than an empty reassurance that the child will simply "outgrow" the problem.

REFERENCES

1. Austin PF, Ritchey ML. Dysfunctional voiding. Pediatr Rev 2000;21:336–341.

2. Bottas A, Richter MA. Pediatric autoimmune neuropsychiatric disorders associated with streptococcal infections (PANDAS). Pediatr Infect Dis J 2002;21:67–71.

3. Butler RJ. Combination therapy for nocturnal enuresis. Scand J Urol Nephrol 2001;35:364–369.

4. Hägglöf B, Andrén O, Bergström E, et al. Self-esteem before and after treatment in children with nocturnal enuresis and urinary incontinence. Scand J Urol Nephrol 1997; 31(Suppl. 183):79–82.

5. Herndon CD, Decambre M, McKenna PH. Interactive computer games for treatment of pelvic floor dysfunction. J Urol 2001;166:1893–1898.

6. Hirasing RA, van Leerdam FJM, Bolk-Bennink LB, et al. Bedwetting and behavioural and/or emotional problems. Acta Paediatr 1997;86:1131–1134.

7. van Kerrebroeck PEV. Experience with the long-term use of desmopressin for nocturnal enuresis in children and adolescents. Br J Urol 2002;89:420–425.

8. Kodman-Jones CK, Hawkins, L, Schulman, SL. Behavioral characteristics of children with daytime wetting, J Urol 2001;166:2392–2395.

9. Koff SA, Wagner TT, Jayanthi VR. The relationship among dysfunctional elimination syndromes, primary vesicoureteral reflux and urinary tract infections in children. J Urol 1998;160:1019–1022.

10. Lawless MR, McElderry DH. Nocturnal enuresis: current concepts. Pediatr Rev 2001;22:399–406.

11. Loening-Baucke V. Urinary incontinence and urinary tract infection and their resolution with treatment of chronic constipation of childhood. Pediatrics 1997;100: 228–232.

12. Nevéus T, Läckgren G, Tuvemo T, et al. Enuresis – Background and treatment. Scand J Urol Nephrol 2000; Suppl. 206:1–44.

13. Rittig S, Knudson UB, Norgaard JR, et al. Abnormal diurnal rhythm of plasma vasopressin and urinary output in patients with enuresis. Am J Physiol 1989;256:F664–F671.

14. Robson WL, Leung AK. Secondary nocturnal enuresis. Clin Pediatr (Phila) 2000;39:379–385.

15. Rushton HG, Belman AB, Zaontz MR. The influence of small functional bladder capacity and other predictors on the response to desmopressin in the management of monosymptomatic nocturnal enuresis. J Urol 1996;156: 651–655.

16. Schmitt BD. Nocturnal enuresis. Pediatr Rev 1997; 18:183–191.

17. Schulman SL, Quinn CK, Plachter N, Kodman-Jones C. Comprehensive management of dysfunctional voiding. Pediatrics 1999;103:e31.

18. Schulman SL, Colish Y, von Zubin FC. Effectiveness of treatments of nocturnal enuresis in a heterogenous population. Clin Pediatr (Phila) 2000;39:359–364.

19. Saedi N, Schulman SL. Natural history of voiding dysfunction. Pediatr Nephrol 2003;18:894–897.

20. Wolfish NM, Pivik RT, Busby KA. Elevated sleep arousal thresholds in enuretic boys. Acta Pediatr 1997;86:381–384.

CHAPTER 4

Urinary Tract Infection in Childhood

ANNE METTE CHRISTENSEN, M.D. AND

KATHY SHAW, M.D.

INTRODUCTION

Urinary tract infections (UTIs) are relatively common in infants and young children. In the evaluation of febrile infants for serious bacterial illness, UTI is the most commonly identified bacterial source of infection. Nuclear renal scans demonstrate that most febrile young children with a positive urine culture have pyelonephritis; this puts them at risk for renal scarring.[25] Therefore, early diagnosis and prompt treatment of UTI in febrile young infants and young children is important in preventing progressive renal damage and the long-term sequelae of hypertension and reduced renal function.[15] Prevention of further UTIs is essential. This requires further testing to identify urological and renal anomalies or dysfunctional voiding. Children at risk for recurrent UTIs must be monitored or treated with prophylaxis.

PATHOGENESIS OF UTI

The urine and the urinary tract are normally sterile. UTI occurs when bacteria ascend from the periurethral area. Colonization of the perineum and periurethral area with *Escherichia coli*, Enterobacteriaceae and *Enterococcus* sp. is normal in young infants and children.[21] In addition, young uncircumcised boys have a reservoir for various *Proteus* species beneath the prepuce. Periurethral colonization decreases beyond 1 year of age, and intestinal bacteria are rarely found beyond 5 years of age. Periodic temporary entry of bacteria into the urethra and bladder does occur. The bacteria are usually cleared spontaneously without producing symptomatic urinary tract infection.[21] Patients with anatomical abnormalities in the urinary tract, functional bladder problems, urinary stasis, and/or presence of specific bacterial virulence factors have an increased risk of developing symptomatic UTI.

At least 80% of community-acquired first-time UTIs in the pediatric age group are caused by uropathogenic *E. coli* (UPEC).[21] Other causative bacteria are listed in Table 40-1.

Table 40-1 Bacteria that Cause UTI in Childhood

Common, More Virulent	Rare, Less Virulent
E. coli	*Pseudomonas*
Proteus	Group B *Streptococcus*
Klebsiella	*Staphylococcus aureus* and
Staphylococcus saprophyticus	*Staph. epidermidis*
Enterococcus	*Haemophilus influenzae*
Enterobacter	

Common contaminants include: *Lactobacillus* sp., *Corynebacterium* sp., coagulase-negative *Staphylococcus* sp. and α-hemolytic *Streptococcus*.

Bacterial Properties and Host Defense Mechanisms

All *E. coli* isolated from patients with febrile UTIs have virulence factors that facilitate their survival in the urinary tract, despite hostile local defense mechanisms. Without these factors, UPEC are unable to ascend the urinary tract against the flow of urine.[18]

Pili (S, P, and type 1) are adhesive molecules expressed on the surface of UPEC. S- and P-pili promote adherence to urinary epithelium in the upper tract and kidney cells. Type 1 pili increase adherence to bladder epithelium and mediate epithelial internalization of UPEC. These bacteria are protected from the host defense system and the actions of antibacterial drugs, and can remain dormant in the urinary epithelium.[18] It is not understood what stimuli reactivate them.

Most normal bladder defense against bacterial invasion is accomplished through voiding. Urinary stasis increases the risk of bacterial invasion. Obstruction of the urinary tract or incomplete bladder emptying prevents individuals from efficiently clearing contaminated urine or weakly adherent bacteria.[18,21] Normal urinary composition and high osmolality have an inhibitory effect on bacterial growth and survival. The presence of bacteria that survive in the urinary tract initiates either a local (cystitis) or generalized (pyelonephritis) inflammatory reaction. Pro-inflammatory cytokines initiate infiltration of phagocytic neutrophils into the bladder and urine to combat the infection. Exfoliation of the infected bladder epithelium may occur, leading to a large reduction in the number of adherent bacteria in the bladder. The mechanisms of this immune response are not completely understood. UPEC often stimulate a more aggressive immune response when compared with bacteria with less virulence factors; this is consistent with the occurrence of more invasive disease with UPEC. Interleukins 6 (IL-6) and 8 (IL-8) are produced by the bladder, help to modulate disease, and are excreted in the urine. The concentration of these cytokines correlates with the severity of the disease.[18]

DEFINITION OF UTI

Urine is normally sterile, and ideally any growth of bacteria should be considered an infection. However, most methods of obtaining urine specimens introduce a risk of contamination, thereby making it difficult to interpret urine culture results. The 'gold standard' for obtaining urine in an infant is by suprapubic aspiration. Without the use of ultrasonography, however, this method is often not successful in clinical practice. Urinary catheterization is the next best method to obtain

urine without significant contamination. Although some parents, nurses, and physicians may be reluctant to perform urethral catheterization for fear of causing pain or discomfort, the unacceptably high contamination rate from using a urine specimen collected by a non-invasive 'bag' technique is associated with greater risk and morbidity. In a study of over 7500 urine cultures obtained from children aged <24 months, the contamination rate was 62.8% in urine obtained by bags and 9.1% in catheter specimens. Infants whose urine was obtained by bag versus catheter, were four- to five-fold more likely to have unnecessary treatment and radiological investigation, 12-fold more likely to have unnecessary hospitalization, and were more likely to have delayed diagnosis and treatment.[2] The use of a small-diameter, lubricated feeding tube using slow gentle pressure is the method of choice for obtaining urine in most infants. Clean-catch, mid-stream urine specimens can be collected in older, toilet-trained children while closely supervised by a healthcare provider. A second specimen, preferably obtained by urethral catheterization, should be obtained prior to starting treatment because contamination rates from clean-catch urines remain high in children aged between 2 and 5 years.

The interpretation of bacterial growth is dependent on the method of urine collection; higher colony counts are required for urine to be considered infected with methods more prone to contamination (Table 40-2). The bacterial growth should be that of a single known urinary tract pathogen (see Table 40-1). No absolute cut-off can perfectly predict the presence or absence of a UTI. Low bacterial counts are not uncommon in infants with symptomatic UTIs. Growth of a lesser amount of a pure pathogen, a culture with two pathogens, or a mixed culture with a predominant pathogen, is suspicious or indeterminate and should be repeated. The growth of non-pathogenic bacteria or lesser amounts of colonies

Table 40-2   Definition of a Positive and Negative Urine Culture Result by Method of Obtaining Specimen

Method	Positive[*]	Negative
Suprapubic	$\geq 10^2$ CFU/ml, one pathogen	No growth
Catheterization	$\geq 10^3$ CFU/ml, one pathogen	<500 CFU/ml, any organisms
Clean catch	$\geq 10^5$ CFU/ml, one pathogen	<5000 CFU/ml, any organisms

[*]The following are indeterminate and should be repeated:
- Significant growth of two pathogens
- A predominant pathogen with a contaminant
- Intermediate growth of a single pathogen

are considered contaminated specimens. Common contaminants are *Lactobacillus* sp., *Corynebacterium* sp., coagulase-negative *Staphylococcus*, and α-hemolytic *Streptococcus*. The interpretation of the urine culture result should take into account the clinical presentation, past history of UTI, urinary tract anomalies, antibiotic use, and examination of the urine for pyuria and bacteriuria. Although pyuria is usually present in children with UTI, its absence does not exclude a UTI. Approximately 20% of young febrile infants with positive urine cultures and documented pyelonephritis by nuclear scan do not have pyuria on initial urinalysis.[7,13,23] Older children usually have classic symptoms of UTI and pyuria or bacteriuria.

MAKING THE DIAGNOSIS OF UTI

Clinical Signs and Symptoms of UTI in Children

Identifying young children with UTI is the first and most important step in preventing renal damage. Infants do not have the common signs of UTI that are seen in older children and adults. Fever is the most frequent symptom of a UTI in young children. In a prospective study of over 2000 febrile infants presenting to an emergency department, 64% of those diagnosed with UTI were thought by the examining physician to have other sources for their fevers.[22] Symptoms of UTI in infants are not specific, and include irritability and poor feeding that may mimic other infections (Table 40-3). Jaundice, failure to thrive, and abdominal pain or discomfort may also be diagnostic signs in infants with UTI. Few parents report dysuria or malodorous urine.

In older children and adolescents, the characteristic findings of dysuria, frequency, urgency enuresis, hesitancy, and suprapubic discomfort are associated with lower-tract infections. Chills, nausea, and flank pain may indicate pyelonephritis. Young children may present with new onset of bed-wetting or loss of toilet training skills. In some older children nausea, vomiting and abdominal pain may be the only indicator of pyelonephritis (Box 40-1).

The discomfort from pyelonephritis must be differentiated from other causes of abdominal pain such as appendicitis, gastroenteritis, or constipation. Fever and irritability may also be due to meningitis, sepsis, or pneumonia in infants (see Table 40-3).

PREVALENCE AND RISK FACTORS FOR UTI

The incidence of febrile UTI or pyelonephritis is greatest in infants under 1 year of age, and gradually decreases approaching school age. The prevalence of UTI in young febrile infants aged less than 24 months is 3–5%, even amongst those thought to have another potential reason for their fever such as an upper respiratory tract infection, otitis media, or gastroenteritis.[9,22] Therefore, UTI should be considered in any infant aged less than 2 years with unexplained fever.[3] The prevalence of UTI varies with age, sex, race, severity and duration of fever.[3,9,19,22]

Even after the first year of age, UTI should be considered in any febrile, uncircumcised male infant who is not toilet trained. Female infants are at twice the risk of having a UTI compared to circumcised male infants. Risk factors for UTI in febrile female infants aged <24 months include age less than 1 year, white race, temperature >39°C, fever for 2 days or more, and absence of another source of fever on examination.[8,9,19,22] Risk factors in older children include dysfunctional voiding, previous UTI, poor hygiene, and sexual activity in adolescents.

Table 40-3 Differential Diagnosis of UTI in Childhood

Fever and Irritability	Abdominal Pain ± Fever	Dysuria	Change in Voiding	Change in Urine Color
Meningitis	Appendicitis	Foreign body (vagina or urethra)	Diabetes	Dehydration
Osteomyelitis	Constipation		Dysfunctional voiding	Food color
Otitis media	Lower lobe pneumonia	Local irritants		Hematuria or hemoglobin
Pneumonia	Ovarian or testicular syndrome	Pinworms	Excessive fluid intake	Myoglobinuria
Sepsis		Urethritis		
Viral illness	PID	Sexual abuse	Mass adjacent to bladder	
	Gastroenteritis	Vaginitis		
	Renal calculus			

PID = pelvic inflammatory disease.

Box 40-1   The Differential Diagnosis of Cystitis of Lower Urinary Tract Infection

- Vaginitis
- Vaginal foreign body
- Urethral foreign body
- Pinworms
- Local irritants – bubble baths, swimsuits
- Sexual abuse

LABORATORY SCREENING FOR UTI

Rapid screening tests for UTI (Table 40-4) look for evidence of bacteriuria (Gram stain, bacteria by microscopy; positive nitrite on dipstick) or pyuria (white blood cells [WBCs] per high-power field [HPF], WBCs per mm^3; leukocyte esterase on dipstick). Although rapid screening tests are sometimes used to determine which children should have urine cultures, they miss 20% of infants with UTI who would have a positive culture without pyuria or bacteriuria. Some practitioners use the results of rapid screening on urine obtained by 'non-invasive bag' technique to determine when to get a culture. Treatment of infants, however, should not be started on the basis of a rapid screening test without first obtaining a urine culture by urethral catheterization or suprapubic bladder tap.[2]

The 'gold standard' for the diagnosis of UTI is the urine culture, but the results are not available for 24–48 hours. Early detection and treatment, however, are essential in preventing morbidity from UTI in children. Therefore, rapid screening tests are used to determine which children should be treated empirically for UTI.

The dipstick urinalysis can be performed at the bedside, is inexpensive, does not require Clinical Laboratory Improvement Amendments Certification, and has great sensitivity and specificity for UTI. The standard microscopic urinalysis provides no additional benefit over the dipstick for detection of UTI, but adds cost and may delay appropriate clinical care.[23] The urine Gram stain is an excellent test, with good sensitivity and specificity, but it requires a laboratory and training to perform. The enhanced urinalysis, that is, determination of the number of WBCs/mm^3 by hemocytometer of dilute urine plus the Gram stain, is the most sensitive method for detecting UTI in young infants, but has poor specificity. This test is often reserved for use in neonates with fever for whom early detection and treatment of a serious bacterial illness is of paramount importance.

Dipstick and urine culture are the tests of choice for detecting UTI in children. The most cost-effective strategy is to perform urine cultures on all febrile infants in whom UTI is suspected and to begin presumptive treatment on those whose dipstick test are a least moderate (+2) leukocyte esterase or positive nitrite.[6,23] Clearly, the higher the pre-test suspicion of UTI, the more likely the clinician is to believe and treat a positive rapid test result. Therefore, the circumcised male infant with

---

Table 40-4   Rapid Screening Tests for UTI in Children: Sensitivity and Specificity

Microscopy	Sensitivity (%) (range)	Specificity (%) (range)	Reference
≥5 WBC/HPF	67 (55, 88)	79 (77, 84)	Gorelick, et al.[7]
Any bacteria/HPF	81 (16, 99)	83 (11, 100)	AAP[3]
≥5 WBC or bacteria/HPF	99 (97, 100)	65 (67, 74)	Ilyas, et al.[13]
Dipstick			
Any LE	83 (64, 89)	84 (71, 95)	Gorelick, et al.[7]
Any nitrite only	50 (16, 72)	98 (95, 100)	Gorelick, et al.[7]
Any nitrite or LE	88 (71, 100)	93 (76, 98)	Gorelick, et al.[7]
≥Moderate LE or nitrite	73 (62, 81)	99 (98, 99)	Saux, et al.[20]
Both nitrite and LE	72 (14, 83)	96 (95, 100)	Gorelick, et al.[7]
Dipstick + microscopy			
Gram stain, any organism	93 (80, 98)	95 (87, 100)	Gorelick, et al.[7]
Any positive on either LE, nitrite	99 (99, 100)	70 (60, 92)	AAP[3]
≥5 WBC or bacteria/HPF	83 (74, 90)	87 (86, 88)	Saux, et al.[20]
Enhanced urinalysis			
≥10 WBC/mm^3	77 (57, 92)	89 (57, 95)	Gorelick, et al.[7]
≥10 WBC/mm^3 <u>or</u> Gram stain ⊕	94 (83, 99)	84 (82, 86)	Saux, et al.[20]
≥10 WBC/mm^3 <u>and</u> positive Gram stain	75 (61, 86)	99 (99, 100)	Saux, et al.[20]

HPF = high-power field; LE = leukocyte esterase; WBC = white blood cells.

fever and UTI symptoms and a trace leukocyte esterase result would be unlikely to have a UTI. Presumptive treatment should be started in the white female infant, pending the results of the urine culture, if she has 3 days of high fever without a definite cause but has a moderate leukocyte esterase result on dipstick; this patient would be more likely to have a UTI. Any child with a positive nitrite and leukocyte esterase result or a positive Gram stain is likely to have a UTI, and should be started on antibiotic therapy.

An elevated peripheral WBC count, positive C-reactive protein, elevated erythrocyte sedimentation rate, or increased absolute neutrophil counts are non-specific indicators of upper tract infection. A child with fever, clinical signs of UTI, and a positive rapid screen for UTI should be presumed to have pyelonephritis, and must be started on treatment.

TREATMENT OF UTIs IN CHILDREN

Non-pharmacologic treatment enhances elimination of bacteria from the bladder and includes increasing oral fluid intake and the frequency of voiding. Treatment of underlying dysfunctional voiding as well as constipation should be initiated.[1] Cranberry juice alone is not effective in the treatment or prevention of UTIs.

Delay in the treatment of a child with a presumed UTI should be avoided, as it may increase the risk of long-term complications. Treatment is therefore initiated on an empiric basis, and then modified according to the result of the culture when this is available up to 3 days later.

Trimethoprim-sulfamethoxazole (TMP-SMZ) is the most commonly prescribed antibiotic for the treatment of uncomplicated UTI. This has resulted in TMP-SMZ-resistant *E. coli* worldwide. Ampicillin-resistant and ciprofloxacin-resistant *E. coli* strains are also a problem.[6,16] Resistance to one antibiotic increases the likelihood of resistance

to others. Approximately 7% of *E. coli* strains in the US are 'multiple drug resistant' (ampicillin, TMP-SMZ and cephalothin).[16] Observational studies have shown that prescription patterns correlate with the emergence of bacterial resistance, and a reduction in prescription frequency is associated with a reduction in bacterial resistance. There is little resistance of common uropathogens to nitrofurantoin,[1,6,16] because bacteriostatic concentrations of nitrofurantoin in the bladder do not affect the resistance patterns of the intestinal flora.

When the bacterial resistance for a specific antibiotic exceeds 10–20%, it is recommended that an alternative antibiotic is used.[16] However, an antibiotic may still be effective for treating UTI despite resistance *in vitro*. Bacterial resistance is defined by the minimal inhibitory concentration of antibiotic (MIC) that inhibits bacterial growth *in vitro*. Drugs used for the treatment of UTI are often eliminated in the urine in concentrations that are above the MIC. Therefore, the MIC may not appropriately predict the efficacy of eradicating the UTI. Data for local and regional bacterial resistance patterns are generated in large, hospital-based laboratories, where the specimens come from a patient population with high rates of bacterial resistance. These data may therefore not be applicable in a local community. Of note, 60% of adults with resistant *E. coli* causing UTI were cured despite treatment with an antibiotic to which the bacteria were supposedly resistant.[16] However, treatment failures and relapses (defined by infections with an organism with the same resistance pattern 2 weeks or longer after treatment) are significantly more common among these patients compared to patients without bacterial resistance.[16]

Acute Cystitis

Children with acute cystitis are treated with oral antibiotics (Table 40-5). Once the bacterial sensitivities are known, treatment is changed to a narrow-spectrum

Table 40-5 Antibiotic Choices for Empiric Oral Treatment of Cystitis in Children

Drug	Dose	Duration of Treatment
Trimethoprim-sulfamethoxazole[a, b]	8–12 mg TMP/kg/day BID	5 days
Nitrofurantoin[a]	5–7 mg/kg/day QID	5 days
Amoxicillin[b]	25–40 mg/kg/day TID	5–7 days
Sulfisoxasole	120–150 mg/kg/day QID	5–7 days
Amoxicillin-clavulanate	40 mg/kg/day BID	5–7 days
Cefopodoxime[*]	10 mg/kg/day BID	5–7 days
Loracarbef	30 mg/kg/day BID	5 days
Ciprofloxacin[*†]	20–30 mg/kg/day BID	3–5 days

[a]Should not be used in infants aged less than 2 months.
[b]High resistance in *E. coli*.
[*]Very broad-spectrum antibiotics should be avoided if possible.
[†]Not routinely recommended for children aged less than 16–18 years.

antibiotic. The AAP practice guidelines recommend 7 days of antibiotic treatment because prolonged antibiotic therapy is often associated with poor compliance.[3] As this is a risk factor for the development of bacterial resistance, attempts have been made to reduce the length of treatment for uncomplicated cystitis. A 2-day course of TMP-SMZ is safe and efficacious in most women. Two meta-analyses involving 652 children suggested that a 5-day course of antibiotic treatment (according to sensitivities) of *first-time cystitis* is safe and is not associated with increased risk treatment failures or re-infection.[1,16,20] A shorter course of treatment ensures improved compliance and reduces the risk of adverse effects. Patients with recurrent UTIs or a history of recent antibiotic treatment should be treated for a longer period of time (7 days) because of increased risk of treatment failure and recurrence.[17,20] All patients should be instructed to return if symptoms persist, or if there is a relapse (Box 40-2).[1]

Pyelonephritis

Patients with evidence of pyelonephritis should be treated aggressively, and in a timely fashion. Treatment delay increases the risk of renal parenchymal scarring.[14] Neonates, infants aged under 6 months, toxic-appearing children, patients with known urinary tract abnormalities, and those with chronic renal insufficiency should be admitted to hospital for intravenous antibiotic treatment until the fever has defervesced. Patients are usually started on empiric therapy of ampicillin and gentamicin (see Table 40-6 for other drug choices). Once the bacterial sensitivities are known, the antibiotic regimen is adjusted accordingly. The recommended length of treatment is 10–14 days. Neonates should be treated intravenously for the entire duration. Children aged more than 6 months who are not febrile or vomiting can be treated orally. An intravenous loading dose increases the efficiency of this regimen.[10]

Prophylaxis for Recurrent UTI

Low-dose UTI prophylaxis in children with normal urinary tract anatomy increases the risk of infection with

Box 40-2 Patients with Asymptomatic Bacteriuria

- These patients should not be treated.
- Treatment increases the risk of pyelonephritis in these patients.
- Despite not being treated they *do not* have an increased prevalence of renal scarring.

Table 40-6 Antibiotic Choices for Empiric Treatment of Pyelonephritis in Children

Drug	Dose
Ampicillin	100 mg kg/day q. 8–q12 h
Gentamycin	6 mg/kg/day q. 24 h
Tobramycin	5 mg/kg/day q. 8 h
Ceftriaxone[a]	75 mg/kg/day IV or IM q. 12–24 h
Cefotaxime	150 mg/kg/day IV q. 6–8 h
Ceftazidime	150 mg/kg/day IV q. 6–8 h
Ciprofloxacin[†]	20–30 mg/kg/day IV BID
Amoxicillin-clavulanate	40 mg/kg/day PO BID

[a]Should be used in infants aged less than 2 months.
[†]Not routinely recommended for children aged under 16–18 years.

resistant bacteria, without reducing the rate of UTI.[20,24] There are no good prospective randomized trials concerning the use of low-dose antibiotic prophylaxis in children with vesicoureteric reflux (VUR) and recurrent UTI. We recommend that children aged under 5 years with VUR, all patients with grades IV and V reflux, or children with recurrent febrile UTIs should be treated with antibiotic prophylaxis to reduce the lifetime risk of chronic renal scarring (Table 40-7). Prophylaxis should be maintained until the VUR either resolves spontaneously or is treated surgically.

EVALUATION OF THE CHILD WITH UTI

Evaluation of a child should be done after the diagnosis of the first febrile UTI. Several imaging studies are used for this evaluation (Box 40-3 and Figure 40-1). The goal is to identify factors that predispose to recurrent UTI and that increase the risk of renal scarring. Children with recurrent episodes of cystitis also require evaluation.

A small percentage of children are predisposed to UTIs because of underlying anatomical anomalies in the

Table 40-7 Antibacterial Agents Used for UTI Prophylaxis

Drug	Dose
Nitrofurantoin[a]	1–2 mg/kg/day PO QHS
Trimethoprim	1–2 mg/kg/day PO QHS
Trimethoprim-sulfamethoxazole	1–2 mg/kg/day PO QHS TMP
Cefalexin[b]	10 mg/kg/day PO QD

[a]Should not be used in infants aged under 2 months.
[b]Neonates and infants aged under 2 months.

urinary tract. These anomalies are more common in boys (10%) than girls (2%) (Box 40-4).

Renal ultrasound (RUS) evaluates the anatomy of the kidneys and bladder. If there is an abdominal mass in addition to symptoms of pyelonephritis, an urgent RUS must be done to determine if the mass is caused by a urinary tract obstruction. If there is no mass, the ultrasound can be done when the UTI is confirmed. The finding of an area of local swelling in the kidney(s) on RUS suggests acute pyelonephritis.[12] The entire kidney may be enlarged if extensive areas are involved. This swelling may be visualized as a wedge-shaped area of hypoperfusion and/or ischemia by Doppler ultrasonography. RUS is not sensitive enough to make a diagnosis of pyelonephritis. Areas of reduced cortical thickness are found in chronic renal scarring, and the shape of the kidney may be distorted by extensive scarring. The measured kidney length should be compared to known, age-related standard curves. The findings on RUS are an inaccurate predictor of VUR even when the collecting system is dilated; however, hydroureter or hydronephrosis on RUS is suggestive of VUR.[12] A normal RUS in a child with a UTI does not rule out VUR. Although a normal antenatal ultrasound in the third trimester may reduce the yield of abnormal RUS after UTI during infancy,[11] this finding

is not yet generally applicable and we recommend that all infants with UTI should have a RUS as part of their evaluation.

The intravenous pyelogram (IVP) is no longer used for evaluation of the renal anatomy because of an unnecessary high radiation dose and the possibility of contrast-induced allergic reactions.

Acute pyelonephritis can be diagnosed by abdominal computed tomography with contrast. However, we do not recommend its use because it is an expensive alternative to the RUS, requires intravenous contrast, and exposes the patient to unnecessary radiation. Magnetic resonance imaging may be used, but younger patients require sedation, it is expensive, and it does not provide additional information about the urinary tract.

Children with UTI who are aged less than 5 years are evaluated for VUR. There are two ways of doing a voiding cystourethrogram (VCUG): the conventional radiographic technique, and by radionuclide cystography (RNC). The patient's bladder is filled with either a radiopaque contrast medium or a radiolabeled tracer via an in-dwelling catheter. Images of the upper urinary tract are collected during spontaneous voiding after catheter removal. Both of these studies are equally sensitive for the detection of VUR. The conventional VCUG is recommended for the initial evaluation because it better delineates the anatomy of the bladder and ureters. RNC on the other hand does not provide the same anatomical detail, but results in significantly less gonadal radiation and may be used for subsequent evaluations.

[99m]Dimercaptosuccinic acid (DMSA) is a molecule that is taken up by the proximal convoluted tubules after intravenous injection. Because it is stable for 2 to 4 hours, static images of the functioning renal cortex can be obtained. DMSA renal scan or renal cortical scintigraphy has the highest sensitivity (87%) and specificity (100%) for the diagnosis of acute pyelonephritis.[5] In 30–50% of infants who present with fever and laboratory evidence of UTI, the DMSA scan shows no renal

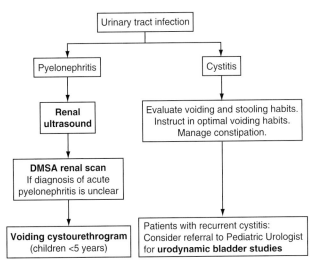

Figure 40-1 Diagnostic algorithm for children with urinary tract infection.

Box 40-5   Risk Factors for Renal Scarring

- Young age (especially <1 year)
- Delayed onset of treatment (>72 hours)
- High-grade vesicoureteral reflux
- Obstruction (anatomic or neurogenic)
- Recurrent episodes of UTI

---

parenchymal involvement.[4,12] Acute parenchymal injury diagnosed by DMSA scan is, in most cases, temporary and regresses over 6–10 months. Only a small proportion of these acute lesions progress to chronic renal scarring. In the absence of VUR, 10% of small renal lesions, involving less than 50% of the kidney, will progress to permanent scar formation. In the presence of VUR this risk increases to approximately 40%. When more than 50% of the kidney is infected, the risk of developing a permanent renal scar approaches 90%.[4]

PROGNOSIS

Several factors are associated with an increased risk of renal scarring (Box 40-5). Chronic renal scarring with large parenchymal scars diagnosed by IVP increases the risk of pre-eclampsia, pre-term delivery, hypertension, and chronic renal insufficiency. The long-term morbidity of small renal scars found by DMSA scans is unknown.

CONCLUSION

Children with recurrent UTI are at risk for renal scarring. The most important tool for preservation of the renal parenchyma is vigilance, with urine analysis and culture added in when the patient presents with fever.

MAJOR POINTS

- A negative rapid screening test for UTI does not eliminate the chance of having a positive urine culture in young infants.
- Fever is often the only sign of UTI in young infants.
- Uncircumcised males and white females with unexplained fever for >2 days are at highest risk for UTI.
- Dysfunctional voiding is the most common cause of recurrent UTIs in a child who presents with the first UTI after completing toilet training.
- Patients with recurrent UTIs are at risk for treatment failures.
- An uncircumcised male infant has a ten-fold increased risk of UTI.

REFERENCES

1. Abrahamsson K, Hansson S, Larsson P, Jodal U. Antibiotic treatment for 5 days is effective in children with acute cystitis. Acta Paediatr 2002;91:55–58.

2. Al-Orifi F, McGillivray D, Tange S, et al. Urine culture from bag specimens in young children: are the risks too high? J Pediatr 2000;137:222–226.

3. AAP, Committee on Quality Improvement, Subcommittee on Urinary Tract Infection: Practice parameter: the diagnosis, treatment, and evaluation of the initial urinary tract infection in febrile infants and young children. Pediatrics 1999;103:843–852.

4. Biggi A, Dardanelli L, Cussino P, et al. Prognostic value of acute DMSA scan in children with first urinary tract infection. Pediatr Nephrol 2001;16:800–804.

5. Goldraich NP, Goldraich IH. Update on dimercaptosuccinic acid renal scanning in children with urinary tract infection. Pediatr Nephrol 1995;9:221–226.

6. Goldraich NP, Manfroi A. Febrile urinary tract infection: *Escherichia coli* susceptibility to oral antibiotics. Pediatr Nephrol 2002;17:173–176.

7. Gorelick MH, Shaw KN. Clinical decision rule to identify young febrile children at risk for UTI. Arch Pediatr Adolesc Med 2000;154:386–390.

8. Gorelick MH, Shaw KN. Screening tests for UTI in children: a meta-analysis. Pediatrics 1999;104:e54.

9. Hoberman A, Han-Pu C, Keller DM, et al. Prevalence of urinary tract infection in febrile infants. J Pediatr 1993;123:17–23.

10. Hoberman A, Wald E, Hickey RW, et al. Oral versus intravenous therapy for urinary tract infections in young febrile children. Pediatrics 1999;104:79–86.

11. Hoberman A, Charron M, Hickey RW, et al. Imaging studies after the first febrile urinary tract infection in young children. N Engl J Med 2003;348:195–202.

12. Ilyas M, Martin ST, Richard GA. Age-related radiological imaging in children with acute pyelonephritis. Pediatr Nephrol 2002;17:30–34.

13. Landau D, Turner ME, Brennan J, et al. The value of urinalysis in differentiating acute pyelonephritis from lower urinary tract infection in febrile infants. Pediatr Infect Dis J 1994;13:777–781.

14. Levtchenko E, Lahy C, Levy J, et al. Treatment of children with acute pyelonephritis: a prospective randomized trial. Pediatr Nephrol 2001;16:878–884.

15. Lohr JA, Portilla MG, Geuder TG, et al. Making a presumptive diagnosis of urinary tract infection by using a urinalysis performed in an on-site laboratory. J Pediatr 1993;122:22–25.

16. Mazzulli T. Resistance trends in urinary tract pathogens and impact on management. J Urol 2002;168:1720–1722.

17. Michael M, Hodson EM, Craig JC, et al. Short compared to standard duration of antibiotic treatment for urinary tract infection: a systematic review of randomized controlled trials. Arch Dis Child 2002;87:118–123.

Boys with Painful Priapism

Ischemia of the corporal bodies may progress to corporal fibrosis if untreated.

Semi-Urgencies

Semi-urgent cases require an appointment within 1–3 days of the problem arising.

Prenatally Diagnosed Hydronephrosis

Postnatal evaluation of prenatally diagnosed hydronephrosis can be started within the first few days of life if the bladder is normal.

Amenorrhea

Females may be uncomfortable because of an imperforate hymen or uterine anomaly that results in poor uterine drainage. Endometriosis and infertility may occur in untreated patients.[73]

Routine Evaluations

Cases considered to be routine will require an appointment within 2 weeks.

Infants with Prenatal Hydronephrosis

Infants with prenatal hydronephrosis without bladder outlet obstruction on the postnatal ultrasound will not require an urgent evaluation provided that:

- there is no bilateral hydronephrosis or thickened bladder wall
- the infant is thriving, with normal serum electrolyte and creatinine concentrations.

Additional tests include an ultrasound, a renal scan to evaluate the relative drainage and percentage of function of the kidneys, and a VCUG to exclude vesicoureteral reflux.

Asymptomatic Hydrocele

In most cases, the hydrocele resolves in the first year. Exceptions are a large hydrocele, or one that is palpable in the inguinal region. An abdominal perineal hydrocele does not spontaneously resolve, and usually enlarges; it should be corrected between 6 and 12 months of age.[57]

Undescended or Absent Testes

Very few undescended testes descend after 3 months of age[7] and orchiopexy is carried out at about 6 months.

Circumcision Complications

Circumcision complications include bleeding, infection, narrowing of the prepucial ring, and urethral meatal stenosis.

> **Clinical Pearl**
>
> Evaluation of circumcision complications can be carried out at the convenience of the family, provided that:
> - there is no active bleeding
> - voiding is normal
> - there is no infection
> - there is no injury to the shaft or glans penis.

Hypospadias

The evaluation of hypospadias is initiated in the newborn period because most parents of a child with a birth defect desire to speak with a specialist as soon as possible.

Varicocele

Varicoceles develop pre-puberty.[63] The varicocele size is determined with an ultrasound examination, and relative testicular volumes are calculated from the three-dimensional measurements on ultrasound.[19] This examination is repeated at intervals of 6 months throughout puberty to assess testicular growth. Surgery is not recommended unless the volume of the left testis provides less than 40% of total testicular volume on two separate ultrasound examinations 6 months apart.

Evaluation for UTI

Completion of the evaluation for UTI is performed after treatment of the initial infection, at the parents' convenience (Chapter 40).

Day or Night Wetting

In the absence of other complicating problems, children with day or night wetting are evaluated routinely. The care of children with nocturnal enuresis is individualized (Chapter 39).

Antenatal Urological Abnormalities

An increasing number of mothers carrying a fetus with hydronephrosis seek prenatal evaluation by the urologist. These visits are scheduled within 1 week unless there are any of the following:
- bilateral hydronephrosis
- oligohydramnios
- significant cystic renal disease in a fetus under 22 weeks.

> **Clinical Pearl**
>
> - Microscopic hematuria in the absence of other symptoms is not an emergency in children

In some cases the decision for discontinuation of a pregnancy may depend on gestational age, therefore a prompt evaluation may be needed.

History

An important first question when taking the history is to ask *'why is the child here?'* The child can often begin to answer these questions, and it is worthwhile early in the interview asking the child a few questions directly. This shows respect for the child, who may be an excellent historian despite their young age. As soon as the child realizes that the interview is directed to him or her, rather than to the parent, he or she will concentrate harder. If future therapy requires behavioral training that involves cooperation from the child, he or she may then be more receptive.

It is important to ask what the patient's and family's goals are. Are they expecting treatment at the facility, or are they after a second opinion to confirm or refute another treatment plan? Do they prefer a reconstructive surgical procedure or the most appropriate non-surgical therapy? Treatment must be tailored to the family's social conditions and to the family's geographic location. Mobile families in the Foreign Service or in the military may require different approaches to surgical problems than families that live near major centers. In some cases, there is more than one approach for a given problem, and the clinician should be prepared to offer choices in order to provide the most appropriate care.

The following sections outline the generalized symptoms in the pediatric patient that the clinician needs to address when preparing a patient's history.

Failure to Thrive (FTT)

FTT describes an individual whose physical growth is below the fifth percentiles for their age. Nephro-urological causes of FTT are chronic UTIs, renal tubular acidosis, diabetes insipidus, and chronic renal insufficiency. The urologist must also be aware of psychosocial or abusive issues that may be contributing to poor growth and development.

Hyperpyrexia

A temperature greater than 41°C is associated with severe infection, hypothalamic disorders, or central nervous system hemorrhage. A urologist must keep in mind other causes of fever, particularly in compromised or at-risk groups.

Abdominal Pain

Abdominal pain usually suggests pyelonephritis, hydronephrosis, or constipation, but may also be due to medical conditions, such as inflammatory bowel disease, serositis, sickle-cell crisis, peritonitis, diabetes, Henoch–Schönlein purpura, and porphyria. It is important to obtain an accurate history of the character of the pain. Details about the character of the pain, time and acuteness of onset, and radiation or migration are important and should, if possible, be obtained from the child. Anorexia, nausea, vomiting, a change in bowel pattern, or icterus may help to distinguish gastrointestinal from genitourinary causes.

Acute Scrotal Pain

An accurate history may prevent an unnecessary surgical exploration. It is particularly important to interview the child as well as the parent. Gradual onset of pain is more consistent with epididymitis, while abrupt pain suggests spermatic cord torsion or torsion of one of the testicular appendices. Associated scrotal wall swelling, erythema, or superior displacement of the testis is suggestive of spermatic cord torsion. An urticarial-purpuric rash, arthralgias, abdominal pain, and hematuria associated with scrotal pain suggest a diagnosis of Henoch–Schönlein purpura.

Perineal or Rectal Pain

The pain of constipation or of bladder spasm may be referred to the penis, testes, scrotum, perineum, or groin.[24]

Voiding Symptoms

Voiding symptoms are discussed elsewhere in this volume: see Chapter 40.

Physical Examination

Vital Signs

Blood pressure and pulse rate are recorded for every new patient, and on all subsequent visits for children with renal anomalies or vesico-ureteral reflux. Reference ranges for blood pressure and pulse rates for boys and girls should be posted in the clinic area where these are measured.[8] Assistants taking the blood pressure should all be aware of the typical variation with age and should notify the team of blood pressure readings greater than the 90th percentile.

Abnormal physical findings suggestive of renal and or urological conditions are discussed in Chapter 3.

Clinical Pearl

- Acute scrotal pain must be presumed to be caused by spermatic cord torsion, regardless of age, until proven otherwise.[85]

Abdomen

Laxity of abdominal muscles with a protuberant abdomen occurs in boys with the prune-belly syndrome, and occasionally in association with other types of bladder outlet obstruction or severe antenatal hydronephrosis. The abdomen must be inspected for ventral hernia, flaring of the rib cage, umbilical leakage, masses, and hernias. The approximate sizes and locations of the kidneys may be determined with deep palpation. An attempt should be made to feel the liver edge and spleen as well as the colon, particularly the descending colon. An estimate should be made of the volume of stool in the descending colon. Separation of the rectus muscles and umbilical hernias are common in the newborn. Unusual masses should be investigated immediately with ultrasonography.

Cystic abdominal masses include: hydronephrosis; multicystic dysplastic kidneys; adrenal hemorrhage; hydrometrocolpos; intestinal duplication; and choledochal ovarian omental or pancreatic cysts. Solid abdominal masses include: neuroblastoma; congenital mesoblastic nephroma; hepatoblastoma; teratoma; and renal venous thrombosis.

The features of renal venous thrombosis are a solid, tender mass in the flank with hematuria, hypertension, and thrombocytopenia. Causes of neonatal onset of renal venous thrombosis are polycythemia, dehydration, maternal diabetes, asphyxia, sepsis, or deficiencies of antithrombin III, protein C or protein S.

Abdominal wall defects may be umbilical (omphalocele) or lateral (gastroschisis). Omphaloceles are associated with Beckwith–Wiedemann syndrome, conjoined twins, trisomy 18, meningomyelocele, and imperforate anus.[13,34,44]

Inguinal Canals

The inguinal canals must be inspected for signs of asymmetry or masses. The examiner's left hand closes the internal inguinal ring to prevent an intracanalicular testis from migrating into the abdomen. The inguinal canal is then palpated for fullness or a mass suggestive of a hernia or spermatic cord hydrocele. The examiner may feel the *silk glove* sign suggestive of a thickened patent processus vaginalis that may be present if a hernia is intermittent. The examiner's right hand is then brought down to the scrotal area, and the testis is then palpated. The testis should be examined with attention to its anatomy, epididymis, and vas deferens.

Clinical Pearl

• As many as two-thirds of neonatal abdominal masses are the result of a renal pathology.[67,70,87]

If the gonadal examination is symmetrical with gonads palpable on each side, or impalpable on both sides, this may suggest a global disorder, such as congenital adrenal hyperplasia or androgen insensitivity. An asymmetrical examination suggests a local problem, such as mixed gonadal dysgenesis or true hermaphroditism.

Undescended Testes

Undescended testes can be palpated if they are in the scrotum or outside the external inguinal ring. Occasionally, a testis in a newborn can be palpated if it is in the inguinal canal, but in many cases, the testis will move in and out of the canal into the abdomen. Retractile testes can be difficult to distinguish from low, undescended testes. Pressure on the femoral artery may help to relax the cremasteric reflex in boys older than 2 years. Placing the child in a squatting or legs-crossed position may relax the reflex and facilitate palpation of the testis.

A testis that feels tethered during manipulation and cannot be manipulated to the base of the scrotum may become an ascending testis. Another examination after 6 to 18 months may help to distinguish a retractile from a tethered testis. An ascending or tethered testis (cryptorchid testis) is more difficult to manipulate into the bottom of the scrotum with increasing age.[14,17,23]

Scrotum

The scrotum in a newborn is relatively large, but may be larger due to the trauma of breech delivery or a hydrocele.

Hydrocele

A hydrocele is distinguished from a hernia by palpation and transillumination, and the absence of a mass in the inguinal canal. A hydrocele that changes in volume suggests a patent processus vaginalis, which increases the risk for inguinal hernia. The processus vaginalis is unlikely to close after birth. Symptomatic hernias should be corrected in the newborn period. In boys with an asymptomatic hernia, outpatient surgery to correct a patent processus vaginalis can be performed between 4 and 6 months of age.

If there are no volume changes within the hydrocele, the processus vaginalis is usually not patent, and the hydrocele involutes by 1 year of age. Persistence of a hydrocele beyond 12 to 18 months, even in the absence of volume changes, is indicative of a patent processus vaginalis.

Clinical Pearl

• A testis is deemed to be descended if it can be manipulated to the base of the scrotum, and remain there after release, for more than a moment.

This requires surgical ligation of the processus vaginalis and incision of the scrotal component of the hydrocele.

Prepuce

Where the foreskin adheres to the glans in the newborn, it should not be separated. The glans should not be inspected if the parents do not want a circumcision. Glandular prepucial adhesions usually separate before 4 years, but may persist for longer periods. The prepuce should not be retracted, but allowed to separate naturally if there is no balanitis or UTI.[39]

Urethral Meatus

The position of the urethral meatus is rarely abnormal in an uncircumcised penis with a circumferential foreskin. A circumcision should not be performed if the ventral foreskin is short, or absent, or if there is ventral or dorsal chordee. The child should be re-examined at a later date, when correction of hypospadias or epispadias can be performed as an outpatient procedure under a general anesthetic.

Hypospadias

The severity of a hypospadia is determined by the position of the urethral meatus, the presence or absence of chordee, and the extent of ventral penile shaft skin coverage. A circumcision should be cancelled if a megameatus is identified. The foreskin may be removed at the time of the urethral repair; however, because normal spongiosum is present on the ventral surface of the penis, repair of the urethra is usually not difficult even after a circumcision.[22]

Penile size

Stretched penile length and girth should be measured. Micropenis in a term baby is less than 19 mm. A karyotype should be performed and the hypothalamic-pituitary-testicular axis should be evaluated in a boy with a micropenis. The penis must be examined in relation to the scrotum for evidence of penile concealment, buried penis, or webbed penis. In these conditions, the size is normal, but it is buried or concealed beneath a prominent pubic fat pad, trapped by a narrow more proximal prepucial ring, or tethered to the scrotum. More penile shaft than indicated is often removed if a newborn clamp circumcision is performed, and this may result in a scar or a secondary trapped penis. Circumcision should be deferred if there is encroachment of the scrotum onto the penile shaft that results in a webbed penis.[11,88]

Varicoceles

Varicoceles are varicosities of the internal spermatic vein. They occur in 10% of adolescent boys but are uncommon under 10 years of age. Varicoceles are almost always on the left and are bilateral in about 10% of cases. Varicoceles are palpable when the boy is standing and drain when supine. A retroperitoneal tumor compressing the vein must be suspected if only the right side is involved or if the varicocele does not decompress when supine.

Testicular size must be determined in a preadolescent or adolescent with a varicocele. Ultrasound examinations can be used to monitor testicular growth. If the testicular volume contribution from the left side normalized to total testicular volume decreases below 40%, surgery may be indicated to correct the varicocele.[26]

Perineal Examination in the Female

Perineal examination in the female is similar to that in a male. Examination of a teenage girl should not be performed in the presence of the father, but can be performed with the mother present as long as the adolescent agrees. A bimanual examination of an adolescent is best performed in the operating room. The girl is placed in a frog-leg position or in a knee-chest position. The clitoris is examined for evidence of hypertrophy that may be suggestive of an intersex condition. The labia majora are gently spread in an inferior direction to permit inspection of the clitoral area and introitus. The vestibule is assessed for discharge.

By gently grasping the labia majora and pulling inferiorly, the perineal folds are better defined and a consistent examination is provided in most cases.[72] An imperforate hymen may cause hydrometrocolpos and a lower abdominal mass. In older girls, a small speculum can be used to evaluate the cervix and interior of the vagina. Palpation of the vaginal walls and cervix and bimanual examination of the uterus completes the examination. A clear vaginal discharge is frequently associated with vaginal voiding and is common in girls who hold urine and subsequently dribble urine into the vagina. Treatment of dysfunctional voiding results in reduced vaginal drainage. Vaginal bleeding in a pre-adolescent may result from a foreign body, such as trapped toilet paper or other foreign bodies that were inserted intentionally or accidentally.

Urethral Prolapse

Urethral prolapse is relatively common, especially in African-American females. The prolapse is through the meatus forming a hemorrhagic, often sensitive, mass that bleeds with palpation or in contact with undergarments. Girls may have difficulty with urination, depending on the size of the prolapse and whether or not it includes the urethral meatus. Urethral prolapse may respond to topical application of estrogen and may be managed expectantly as long as voiding is normal.[72]

Genital Injury

Although genital injuries may be accidental, the possibility of physical or sexual abuse must be considered in all cases of genital trauma in either sex.

Sexual Abuse

'Sexual play' may be defined as viewing or touching of the genitals, buttocks, or chest, by pre-adolescent children separated by not more than four years in age in which there was no force or coercion. 'Sexual abuse' is defined as any activity with a child before the age of legal consent for the purpose of sexual gratification of an adult or a significantly older child. Sexual abuse includes: oral–genital, genital–genital, genital–rectal, hand–genital, hand–rectal, or hand–breast contact; exposure of sexual anatomy; forced viewing of sexual anatomy; showing pornography to a child; and using a child in the production of pornography. Sexual intercourse includes vaginal, oral, or rectal penetration. Penetration is entry into an orifice with or without tissue injury. Younger perpetrators tend to have younger victims but are more likely to have intercourse with older victims. Sex acts perpetrated by young children are learned behaviors and are associated with experience of sexual abuse or exposure to adult sex or pornography. Without detection and intervention, sexual abuse may progress from touching to intercourse.

Sexual abuse is common: 12–38% of adult women are sexually abused by age 18 years. The incidence of sexual abuse of males ranges from 3% to 9%. Approximately one-third of sexual abuse victims are under 6 years of age, one-third are 6–12 years of age, and one-third are 12–18 years of age. Of the total number of reported offenders, 97% are male.[43]

Pedophiles look for positions and opportunities where they have contact with potential victims, and groups of children at particular risk from pedophiles are indicated in Box 41-2.

The abuse of daughters by fathers and stepfathers is the most commonly reported type of incest, although it is thought that brother–sister incest occurs more frequently. Factors that may lead to incest are a father's desire for sexual gratification, a daughter's need for affection and nurturing, an unavailable mother, and a longing to maintain the family unit. Although violence is uncommon in sexual abuse, its incidence increases with the age and size of the victim.

Investigating the possibility of sexual abuse requires supportive, sensitive, and detailed history-taking, preferably by a sexual-abuse team. The key is to be aware of the possibilities when they might exist (Box 41-3) and to invite the sexual-abuse team in early. A pediatric urologist is often asked to evaluate the abdomen and perineum.[43] Examination of the female genitalia with the patient in the frog-leg position for young children or the knee-chest position for older children expedites the examination with minimal touching. Sexual abuse should be considered when the vaginal mucosa is bruised or injected, the vaginal opening is dilated or the hymen is damaged, showing a V-notch or cleft.[86] Despite these guidelines, the diagnosis of sexual abuse is made by the history and not by the physical examination. Suspected abuse must be reported to the police, and the state child-welfare team if the perpetrator is a caregiver or parent.

Perineal Injury

Blunt injury to the perineum may cause a hematoma beneath the perineal skin. Hematomas or contusions do not need treatment. Penetrating injuries of the vaginal area need to be investigated by imaging studies of the urethra and bladder and may require treatment.

Tumors

Benign or malignant tumors of the vaginal area must be considered when vaginal bleeding occurs in young girls. These include capillary hemangioma, rhabdomyosarcoma, neuroblastoma, or carcinoma.

Labia

Labial masses may be associated with hernia or hydrocele of the canal of Nuck.[48] Adhesions of the labia minora are common and are usually asymptomatic. Occasionally, vaginal irritation occurs from pooled urine and, if not separated, the irritation may progress to irregular voiding, which may exacerbate the problem. A short course of estrogen crème applied to the labia may be effective. In many cases, however, separation of the adhesions in the office with local anesthetic crème may be required. A barrier ointment must then be applied within the labia minora to prevent recurrence until the inflammation has resolved.

Box 41-2 Children at Risk from Pedophiles

- Children with mental and physical handicaps
- Children who are unloved and unwanted
- Children who were previously abused
- Children in single-parent families
- Children of drug abusers
- Children with low self-esteem and poor achievement

Box 41-3 Symptoms Suggestive of Sexual Abuse

- Vaginal, penile or rectal pain
- Vaginal, penile or rectal discharge or bleeding
- Chronic dysuria, enuresis, constipation or encopresis
- Sexualized activity with peers, animals, or objects
- Seductive behavior
- Age-inappropriate sexual knowledge and curiosity

Clinical Pearl

A presacral dimple may indicate spina bifida or cord tethering **IF** the dimple is:
- off-center
- more than 25 mm from the anal verge at birth
- deeper than 5 mm.[78]

Labial fusion may be associated with congenital adrenal hyperplasia, gonadal dysgenesis, or a cloaca.[69] A genitosinogram must be performed when the urethra cannot be distinguished from the vaginal orifice.

Imperforate Anus

Meconium is usually passed within 12 hours after birth; 99% of term infants and 95% of premature infants pass meconium within 48 hours of birth. An imperforate anus is not always obvious. An attempt to insert a small finger or rectal tube gently into the anal dimple may be required to confirm the diagnosis. Any child with early and consistent history of constipation must be suspected of having an imperforate anus or a variant thereof.[46]

Lower Back

The dimple or irregularity of skin fold normally present in the sacrococcygeal midline may be mistaken for an actual or potential neurocutaneous sinus.

Tufts of hair over the lumbosacral spine suggest an underlying abnormality, such as spina bifida occulta, sinus tract, or tumor. An ultrasound of the lumbosacral spine must be performed on a newborn if there are sinuses or dimples.[81] The upper and lower extremities and back are examined for asymmetry, length discrepancy, or misalignment of the spine.

OFFICE PROCEDURES IN THE PEDIATRIC UROLOGICAL PATIENT

Urodynamic Suites

The well-equipped urology office will have a urodynamic suite as part of the overall complex. Modern urodynamic systems allow accurate measurements of the intra-luminal bladder pressures before, during, and after bladder contraction. From these measurements, estimates of bladder compliance as well as the bladder outlet resistance may be made. With this information, the pediatric urologist may assess whether the bladder stores at pressures low enough to prevent renal damage and empties well enough to prevent urinary tract infection.

Biofeedback training, designed to help the child to improve bladder emptying, may also be performed in the office. Biofeedback sessions should be performed in a room that is separate from the urodynamic suite because in most cases a different population of patients requires biofeedback training than will undergo urodynamic study.[75,90] Biofeedback, if performed properly, is time consuming, therefore the child must be relaxed for a session to be effective. Biofeedback suites can be equipped with stereo and video, and have low levels of lighting, to help make the child feel more comfortable.

Office Surgical Procedures

Successful outpatient surgery with local anesthetic depends on co-operation from the parents as well as the child. Parents must believe that the convenience of having the procedure in the office outweighs the advantages of a general anesthetic in the main operating room.

Circumcision

Many babies under 4.5 kg (10 lb) may easily undergo an office circumcision through use of an anesthetic crème combined with injected local anesthetic,[37,79] although it is rare to provide office circumcision for older children. Infants older than 3 months are too big to be easily restrained, and the risk of bleeding postoperatively if the skin edges are not sutured is considerable.

A variety of techniques may be used in the clinic for circumcision. Most of these are clamp procedures. An example is the GOMCO clamp, a three-component device which includes a bell that fits over the glans of the penis and separates the glans from the inner preputial skin.[1,32] The clamp is applied, and the foreskin is trimmed away from the clamp. If the clamp is left in place for a considerable amount of time (usually about 10 minutes), there is very little separation of the skin postoperatively. If desired, a small non-stick bandage can be placed beneath a transparent adhesive dressing. The bandage is removed the next day. The boy's parents are instructed to apply petroleum jelly to the incision during the healing period.

Complications following neonatal circumcision include bleeding, wound infection, meatal stenosis, and secondary phimosis resulting from removal of insufficient foreskin or removal of insufficient inner prepucial skin. Potentially serious complications include sepsis, amputation of distal part of the glans, removal of excessive foreskin, and urethrocutaneous fistula.[4,61]

Meatotomy

Meatal stenosis is common following circumcision. It may result from contraction of the meatus following healing of the inflamed, denuded, glans tissue that occurs following retraction of the foreskin, or from damage to the frenular artery at the time of circumcision.[66,82] If the narrowing is pronounced enough to cause deflection of the urinary stream or dysuria, a meatotomy is indicated. This procedure is easily performed in the pediatric urologist's office.

To perform a meatotomy in the office, an anesthetic crème is applied. After 45 minutes, lidocaine with 1% epinephrine is injected using a 26-gauge needle to provide a small wheal at the ventrum of the urethral meatus. The ventral edge of the urethral meatus is clamped, and a small wedge of the scarred tissue is crushed with a straight hemostat and sharply excised. After the procedure, the parents are advised to apply a fine petroleum ointment to the cut edges of the urethral meatus. A small meatal dilator is used twice a day for 4-6 weeks. Postoperatively, these children are seen 2-3 months later to assess the result.

Prepuce

The adhesions that are present between the glans penis and the inner surface of the prepuce in an uncircumcised boy should never be forcefully separated. These filmy prepucial–glanular adhesions rarely result in symptoms and will often re-adhere after they are separated. As the child ages, these adhesions will spontaneously separate.[39] However, following a circumcision, the cut edge of the prepucial surface may occasionally graft to the inflamed glans tissue, forming a prepucial–glanular bridge, which may be incised in the office with application of local anesthetic crème and subsequent injection of local anesthetic. Following injection, the skin bridge is clamped, the clamp is removed, and the skin bridge is sharply incised. In most cases, no suturing is required. This procedure is easy and virtually painless. After the procedure, the parents apply petroleum jelly to the incised edges to prevent them from re-adhering.

VCUG

If a VCUG is required, or if dysuria associated with vaginal pooling of urine contributes to a dysfunctional voiding pattern, labial adhesions can be separated in the office. These membranous adhesions are easy to separate on the midline with a probe or the tip of a curved hemostat. A local anesthetic crème can be applied to the labia to ease the discomfort, which is minimal. After lysis of the adhesions, the child's parent must separate the labia and apply a barrier cream, such as petroleum jelly, at least twice a day for 4-6 weeks while the labial tissue matures. With diligent postoperative care, recurrence is rare.

Summary

The final goal of surgical care of children is to assure as normal an adult life as possible. Children born with complicated problems may require lifelong follow-up by skilled urologists. For boys with prune-belly syndrome or posterior urethral valves, and for children of either sex born with bladder or cloacal exstrophy, pediatric urologists should continue to act as consultants even after he children enter adulthood. As children grow into adults, pediatric teams must develop liaisons with skilled, inter-ested adult teams. In this way, lifetime plans of care may be designed and carried out to assure well-coordinated urological therapy that is capable of addressing the complicated problems unique to this special group of patients.

RADIOLOGICAL EXAMINATION OF THE PEDIATRIC UROLOGY PATIENT

Ultrasound

Ultrasound examination of the kidneys, ureters, and bladder is an extension of the physical examination. Palpable masses within the abdomen can be localized, and even diagnosed, with the aid of ultrasonography performed by a uroradiologist with an interest in pediatrics. The examination should evaluate not only the genitourinary system but also adjacent organs, such as the adrenal, liver, and spleen. The image of the parenchyma of the liver and spleen should be used as a comparison to assess the parenchyma of the right and left kidneys, respectively. The density of the kidney and of the renal medullary pyramids, as well as the wall thickness and configuration of the collecting system, the presence or absence of caliectasis, pelviectasis, or ureterectasis, are all important indicators of renal and ureteral pathophysiology.[38] The lumenal diameter of the ureters, thickness of the bladder wall, and the volume of the bladder (both before and after voiding) should be recorded. If hydronephrosis or ureterectasis is present prior to voiding, the kidneys and ureters should be rescanned after voiding. A skillful ultrasonographer can provide anatomical detail about the insertion of the ureters and the degree of dilation of the ureter, and can identify the jet of urine as it enters the bladder.[47]

Ultrasound is sensitive in detecting solid renal masses, particularly those that measure at least 15 mm in the largest dimension. For smaller renal masses, the ultrasound findings should be considered preliminary and should be confirmed with CT scanning, or magnetic resonance imaging (MRI).[40]

Ultrasonography may also be used to accurately measure post-void residual urine.[15] Increased thickness of the bladder wall may be suggestive of bladder outlet obstruction from posterior urethral valves or urethral atresia. Trabeculation within the bladder, bladder diverticulum, or ureteral duplication or ureterocele are all easily identified with ultrasound.[33] In the absence of comparison studies or appropriate history, ultrasound cannot be used to distinguish obstructive from non-obstructive hydronephrosis. Therefore, a functional study, such as a renal scan, is usually required for diagnosis.

Ultrasound is frequently used to examine the scrotum to assess testicular volume in boys with varicocele.[19] It may also be used to assess blood flow if spermatic cord torsion is suspected, as well as to distinguish between epididymitis and torsion of the appendix testis in cases where tenderness is localized to the upper pole of the testis. It has also been found useful in distinguishing hernia from hydrocele, or identifying abdominoperineal hydroceles.[27,57,80]

Voiding Cystourethrogram

With very few exceptions, children with a proven UTI should undergo VCUG to identify vesicoureteral reflux (VUR), to evaluate the anatomy of the bladder outlet during bladder filling and voiding, and to assess the presence of residual urine following micturition. Additional information regarding trabeculation of the bladder, bladder diverticula, and presence or absence of urachal abnormalities may be identified with a fluoroscopic VCUG.[2,25,31,55,58]

The VCUG begins with a plain film, followed by placement of a feeding tube rather than a Foley catheter. The balloon on a Foley catheter may obscure the anatomy of the bladder neck and trigone, particularly at the beginning of the study. On the plain film, abnormalities of the spine, ribs, and pelvis, and the presence or absence of stones within the kidney, ureter, or bladder, should be noted. The gas pattern and volume of stool is particularly important in infants and in children with dysfunctional voiding in whom constipation may be an important part of the clinical pattern. Gas should normally be present in the rectum on plain film by 24 hours of age. The bladder should be drained, and contrast should be gently infused. In children in whom a ureterocele is suspected, the first few images during filling of the bladder best demonstrate the ureterocele. The bladder is then filled slowly, and the child voids.

Voiding views must be obtained in all cases, this is particularly important if bladder outlet obstruction, such as a posterior urethral valve, is suspected. In children in whom VUR is suspected or in patients with an ectopic ureter, a cyclic VCUG must be performed in which at least two voiding cycles are completed. In some cases, the ectopic ureter that is draining to the bladder neck must empty in order for additional contrast material to reflux. If a second voiding cycle is not performed, one might miss reflux into the ectopic system.[35,68]

It is important to image the bladder neck during voiding in the female as well as the male. The presence of a spinning-top urethra in a school-aged girl may be an important indicator of dysfunctional voiding.[5,49,74] Vaginal voiding should also be noted, which may be seen on the post-void views.

In patients with a genitourinary sinus, the VCUG is modified to image the urethra and vagina simultaneously. In this study, the genitourinary sinus is intubated with a blunt-tipped catheter (which can be made by trimming the cone-shaped end of a feeding tube) placed against the perineal opening. Contrast is injected retrograde to identify the point where the vaginal introitus meets the urethra to form the genitourinary sinus. The genitourinary sinogram will help to differentiate a cervix from a prostatic utricle. If a cloaca is present, the sinogram will provide detail about the position of the rectum, vagina, and urethra, and about the point of confluence and the distance to the perineum.[18,65,76]

Nuclear Cystogram

Nuclear cystogram can be used in follow-up examinations in children with VUR. It can also be used as the first examination to screen for VUR in sisters of children with VUR. The nuclear cystogram may be quantitated by measuring the percentage of the bladder volume refluxing into the ureters during bladder filling. The percentage of bladder filling when the reflux is first identified may also be an indicator of potential resolution of VUR. On subsequent examinations, improvement in VUR may be assumed if a smaller percentage of total bladder volume is refluxing into the ureter or if the reflux occurs at a greater percentage of total bladder filling.[62]

Radionuclide Renal Scan

The radionuclide renal scan is measured in two phases: the cortical imaging phase and tubular imaging phases. Most radionuclide agents will demonstrate renal tubular as well as renal cortical binding. Radionuclide studies are suitable for demonstrating changes in tubular or cortical transit that result from abnormalities of renal perfusion, secretion, and filtration. In most cases, the radionuclide study is inferior to CT scans, MRI, or ultrasound for demonstration of morphologic alterations. When a glomerular filtration excreted agent such as [99m]technetium diethylenetriamine-pentaacetic acid (DTPA) is given, an approximate estimation of glomerular filtration rate (GFR) may be calculated, either *in vivo* by computer-aided scanning or *in vitro* with the collection of one or two blood samples at predetermined time intervals. In addition, it is possible to calculate an 'extraction factor', which estimates the single-kidney GFR during minutes 1 and 2 of the clearance of the radiotracer.[36] The tracer [99m]technetium mercaptoacetyltriglycine (MAG3) is secreted in part by renal tubular function, and may also be used to approximate relative renal plasma flow. If detailed imaging of the renal cortex is required to identify renal scarring, [99m]technetium dimercaptosuccinic acid (DMSA) may be given and the kidneys imaged 3–4 hours after the injection.

Intravenous Pyelogram

Despite the newer imaging techniques that are now available, the intravenous pyelogram (IVP) is useful in selected cases. The plain film of the abdomen should be inspected for calculi, spinal abnormalities, and an abnormal intestinal gas pattern. The nephrogram phase of the IVP identifies mass effects within the kidney and the presence or absence of scarring following pyelonephritis. Subsequent views can sequentially assess the anatomy of the renal cortex, calyces, fornices, renal pelvis, ureters, bladder, and urethra.[77] Subtle anatomic variations in normal anatomy of the renal calyces or of the ureteropelvic junction that may be confusing on ultrasound or CT scan may be clarified with the IVP. Contrast medium may persist in the collecting system for longer than 24 hours.

Spiral CT Scan

In most cases, the spiral CT scan has replaced the IVP as the first line of investigation for children with suspected stone disease. In addition, a CT scan with or without contrast is particularly important as an adjunct in children with suspected focal segmental bacterial pyelonephritis. CT scans are also particularly important in the diagnosis and staging of solid tumors of the chest and abdomen. Contrast-enhanced CT scanning is particularly useful in cases of nephroblastomatosis, where ultrasound shows little displacement of the renal capsule.

Gadolinium Enhanced MRI

MRI has improved the imaging of the pelvic organs in children as in adults.[51,56] Gadolinium enhanced MRI and magnetic resonance angiography (MRA) may provide the best three-dimensional image of the kidneys, ureters, and bladder in children. MRI has also been used to assess ureteral obstruction.[10] Although not routine, MRA is increasingly used frequently in the evaluation and identification of the impalpable testis.[50,92]

Inflammation Seeking Isotopes

Inflammation seeking isotopes ([67]gallium citrate, [111]indium-labeled white blood cells) may be helpful for determining the presence or absence of infection.[91] These techniques may be used to identify and guide therapy for children with focal segmental bacterial pyelonephritis in whom the duration of therapy is uncertain. These are particularly useful in patients with abnormal renal anatomy or in patients with diminished renal function in whom the DMSA scan may be less specific.

REFERENCES

1. Amir M, Raja MH, Niaz WA. Neonatal circumcision with Gomco clamp - a hospital-based retrospective study of 1000 cases. J Pak Med Assoc 2000;50:224-227.

2. Anon. Practice parameter: the diagnosis, treatment, and evaluation of the initial urinary tract infection in febrile infants and young children. American Academy of Pediatrics. Committee on Quality Improvement. Subcommittee on Urinary Tract Infection. Pediatrics 1999;103(4 Pt.1):843-852.

3. Babcook CJ, Goldstein RB, Filly RA. Prenatally detected fetal myelomeningocele: is karyotype analysis warranted? Radiology 1995;194:491-494.

4. Baskin LS, Canning DA, Snyder HM 3rd, Duckett JW Jr. Surgical repair of urethral circumcision injuries. J Urol 1997;158:2269-2271.

5. Batista JE, Caffaratti J, Arano P, et al. The reliability of cystourethrographic signs in the diagnosis of detrusor instability in children. Br J Urol 1998;81:900-904.

6. Bauer SB. The challenge of the expanding role of urodynamic studies in the treatment of children with neurological and functional disabilities [editorial; comment]. J Urol 1998; 160:527-528.

7. Berkowitz GS, Lapinski RH, Dolgin SE, et al. Prevalence and natural history of cryptorchidism. Pediatrics 1993;92:44-49.

8. Bernstein D. History and physical examination. In: Behrman R, Kliegman R, Jenson H, Eds., *Nelson Textbook of Pediatrics*, 16th ed., Philadelphia, PA: WB Saunders Company, 2000;1343-1351.

9. Bokenkamp A, von Kries R, Nowak-Gottl U, et al. Neonatal renal venous thrombosis in Germany between 1992 and 1994: epidemiology, treatment and outcome. Eur J Pediatr 2000;159:44-48.

10. Borthne A, Pierre-Jerome C, Nordshus T, Reister T. MR urography in children: current status and future development. Eur radiol 2000;10:503-511.

11. Casale AJ, Beck SD, Cain MP, et al. Concealed penis in childhood: A spectrum of etiology and treatment. J Urol 1999;162:1165-1168.

12. Chen CJ. The treatment of imperforate anus: experience with 108 patients. J Pediatr Surg 1999;34:1728-1732.

13. Chen CP, Shih SL, Liu FF, et al. Perinatal features of omphalocele-exstrophy-imperforate anus-spinal defects (OEIS complex) associated with large meningomyeloceles and severe limb defects. Am J Perinatol 1997;14:275-279.

14. Clarnette TD, Hutson JM. Is the ascending testis actually 'stationary'? Normal elongation of the spermatic cord is prevented by a fibrous remnant of the processus vaginalis. Pediatr Surg Int 1997;12:155-157.

15. Coombes GM, Millard RJ. The accuracy of portable ultrasound scanning in the measurement of residual urine volume. J Urol 1994;152:2083-2085.

16. Dacher JN, Boillot B, Eurin D, et al. Rational use of CT in acute pyelonephritis: Findings and relationships with reflux. Pediatr Radiol 1993;23:281-285.

17. Davey RB. Undescended testes: Early versus late maldescent. Pediatr Surg Int 1997;12:165-167.

18. De Filippo RE, Shaul DB, Harrison EA, et al. Neurogenic bladder in infants born with anorectal malformations: comparison with spinal and urologic status. J Pediatr Surg 1999;34:825-827, discussion 828.

19. Diamond DA, Paltiel HJ, DiCanzio J, et al. Comparative assessment of pediatric testicular volume: Orchidometer versus ultrasound. J Urol 2000;164:1111-1114.

20. Diven SC, Travis LB. A practical primary care approach to hematuria in children. Pediatr Nephrol 2000;14:65-72.

21. Downs SM. Technical report: Urinary tract infections in febrile infants and young children. The Urinary Tract Subcommittee of the American Academy of Pediatrics Committee on Quality Improvement. Pediatrics 1999; 103:e54.

22. Duckett JW, Keating MA. Technical challenge of the megameatus intact prepuce hypospadias variant: The pyramid procedure. J Urol 1989;141:1407-1409.

23. Eardley I, Saw KC, Whitaker RH. Surgical outcome of orchidopexy. II. Trapped and ascending testes. Br J Urol 1994;73:204-206.

24. Fein J, Donoghue A, Canning DA. Constipation as a cause of scrotal pain in children. Am J Emerg Med 2001;19:290-292.

25. Fernbach SK, Feinstein KA, Schmidt MB. Pediatric voiding cystourethrography: a pictorial guide. Radiographics 2000;20:165-168, discussion 168-171.

26. Fideleff HL, Boquete HR, Suarez MG, et al. Controversies in the evolution of paediatric-adolescent varicocele: Clinical, biochemical and histological studies. Eur J Endocrinol 2000;143:775-781.

27. Finkelstein MS, Rosenberg HK, Snyder HM 3rd, Duckett JW. Ultrasound evaluation of scrotum in pediatrics. Urology 1986;27:1-9.

28. Freedman AL, Johnson MP, Smith CA, et al. Long-term outcome in children after antenatal intervention for obstructive uropathies. Lancet 1999;354:374-377.

29. Gearhart JP. Bladder exstrophy: staged reconstruction. Curr Opin Urol 1999;9:499-506. Review.

30. Glatzl J. Forms of intersexuality in childhood (pathogenesis-clinical aspects-diagnosis-therapy). Wien Klin Wochenschr 1987;99:295-306.

31. Goldman M, Lahat E, Strauss S, et al. Imaging after urinary tract infection in male neonates. Pediatrics 2000;105:1232-1235.

32. Guazzo E. Gomco circumcision. Am Fam Physician 1999;59:2730-2732.

33. Gylys-Morin VM, Minevich E, Tackett LD, et al. Magnetic resonance imaging of the dysplastic renal moiety and ectopic ureter. J Urol 2000;164:2034-2039.

34. Hassink EA, Rieu PN, Hamel BC, et al. Additional congenital defects in anorectal malformations. Eur J Pediatr 1996; 155:477-482.

35. Hellstrom M, Jacobsson B. Diagnosis of vesico-ureteric reflux. Acta Paediatr Suppl 1999;88:3-12.

36. Heyman S, Duckett JW. The extraction factor: an estimate of single kidney function in children during routine radionuclide renography with ^{99m}technetium diethylene-triaminepentaacetic acid. J Urol 1988;140:780-783.

37. Hoebeke P, Depauw P, Van Laecke E, Oosterlinck W. The use of Emla cream as anaesthetic for minor urological surgery in children. Acta Urol Belg 1997;65:25-28.

38. Hulbert WC, Rosenberg HK, Cartwright PC, et al. The predictive value of ultrasonography in evaluation of infants with posterior urethral valves. J Urol 1992;148:122-124.

39. Imamura E. Phimosis of infants and young children in Japan. Acta Paediatr Jpn 1997;39:403-405.

40. Jamis-Dow CA, Choyke PL, Jennings SB, et al. Small (<or= 3-cm) renal masses: detection with CT versus US and pathologic correlation. Radiology 1996;198:785-788.

41. Jeffs RD. Exstrophy and cloacal exstrophy. Urol Clin North Am 1978;5:127-140.

42. Jenkins R. Sexually Transmitted Diseases. In: Behrman R, Kliegman R, Jenson H, Eds. *Nelson Textbook of Pediatrics*, 16th ed., Philadelphia, PA: WB Saunders Company, 2000: 583-586.

43. Johnson C. Sexual Abuse. In: Behrman R, Kliegman R, Jenson H, Eds. *Nelson Textbook of Pediatrics*, 16th ed., Philadelphia, PA: WB Saunders Company, 2000:115-117.

44. Kallen K, Castilla EE, Robert E, et al. OEIS complex-A population study. Am J Med Genet 2000;92:62-68.

45. Kaplan WE. Management of myelomeningocele. Urol Clin North Am 1985;12:93-101.

46. Kim HL, Gow KW, Penner JG, et al. Presentation of low anorectal malformations beyond the neonatal period. Pediatrics 2000;105:e68.

47. Kirby CL, Rosenberg HK. Ultrasound shows masses in pediatric abdomen. Diagn Imaging (San Franc) 1992; 14:168-173.

48. Kizer JR, Bellah RD, Schnaufer L, Canning DA. Meconium hydrocele in a female newborn: an unusual cause of a labial mass. J Urol 1995;153:188-190.

49. Kondo A, Kapoor R, Ohmura M, Saito M. Functional obstruction of the female urethra: relevance to refractory bed wetting and recurrent urinary tract infection. Neurourol Urodyn 1994;13:541-546.

50. Lam WW, Tam PK, Ai VH, et al. Gadolinium-infusion magnetic resonance angiogram: a new, non-invasive, and accurate method of preoperative localization of impalpable undescended testes. J Pediatr Surg 1998;33:123-126.

51. Lang IM, Babyn P, Oliver GD. MR imaging of paediatric uterovaginal anomalies. Pediatr Radiol 1999;29:163-170.

52. Lattimer JK, Hensle TW, MacFarlane MT et al. The exstrophy support team: a new concept in the care of the exstrophy patient. J Urol 1979;121:472-473.

53. Levy DA, Kay R, Elder JS. Neonatal testis tumors: a review of the Prepubertal Testis Tumor Registry. J Urol 1994; 151:715-717.

54. Li FP, Fraumeni JF. Testicular cancers in children: epidemiologic characteristics. J Natl Cancer Inst 1972;48: 1575-1581.

55. Lin DS, Huang SH, Lin CC, et al. Urinary tract infection in febrile infants younger than eight weeks of age. Pediatrics 2000;105:e20.

56. Liu PF, Krestin GP, Huch RA, et al. MRI of the uterus, uterine cervix, and vagina: diagnostic performance of dynamic contrast-enhanced fast multiplanar gradient-echo imaging in comparison with fast spin-echo T2-weighted pulse imaging. Eur Radiol 1998;8:1433-1440.

57. Luks FI, Yazbeck S, Homsy Y, Collin PP. The abdomino-scrotal hydrocele. Eur J Pediatr Surg 1993;3:176-178.

58. McDonald A, Scranton M, Gillespie R, et al. Voiding cysto-urethrograms and urinary tract infections: how long to wait? Pediatrics 2000;105:e50.

59. McGuire EJ, Woodside JR, Borden TA. Upper urinary tract deterioration in patients with myelodysplasia and detrusor hypertonia: A followup study. J Urol 1983;129:823-826.

60. McGuire EJ, Diddel G, Wagner F. Balanced bladder function in spinal cord injury patients. J Urol 1977;118:626-628.

61. Moses S, Bailey RC, Ronald AR. Male circumcision: assessment of health benefits and risks. Sex Transm Infect 1998;74:368-373.

62. Mozley PD, Heyman S, Duckett JW, et al. Direct vesicoureteral scintography: quantifying early outcome predictors in children with primary reflux. J Nucl Med 1994;35:1602-1608.

63. Niedzielski J, Paduch D, Raczynski P. Assessment of adolescent varicocele. Pediatr Surg Int 1997;12:410-413.

64. Noh PH, Cooper CS, Winkler AC, et al. Prognostic factors for long-term renal function in boys with the prune-belly syndrome. J Urol 1999;162:1399-1401.

65. Parrott TS, Woodard JR. Importance of cystourethrography in neonates with imperforate anus. Urology 1979; 13:607-609.

66. Persad R, Sharma S, McTavish J, et al. Clinical presentation and pathophysiology of meatal stenosis following circumcision. Br J Urol 1995;75:91-93.

67. Pinto E, Guignard JP. Renal masses in the neonate. Biol Neonate 1995;68:175-184.

68. Polito C, Moggio G, La Manna A, et al. Cyclic voiding cystourethrography in the diagnosis of occult vesicoureteric reflux. Pediatr Nephrol 2000;14:39-41.

69. Powell DM, Newman KD, Randolph J. A proposed classification of vaginal anomalies and their surgical correction. J Pediatr Surg 1995;30:271-275; discussion 275-276.

70. Raffensperger J, Abousleiman A. Abdominal masses in children under one year of age. Surgery 1968;63:770-775.

71. Ransley PG, Risdon RA. Reflux nephropathy: effects of antibicrobial therapy on the evolution of the early pyelonephritic scar. Kidney Int 1981;20:733-742.

72. Redman JF. Conservative management of urethral prolapse in female children. Urology 1982;19:505-506.

73. Rock JA, Zacur HA, Dlugi AM, et al. Pregnancy success following surgical correction of imperforate hymen and complete transverse vaginal septum. Obstet Gynecol 1982;59:448-451.

74. Saxton HM, Borzyskowski M, Mundy AR, Vivian GC. Spinning top urethra: not a normal variant. Radiology 1988;168:147-150.

75. Schulman SL, Quin CK, Plachter N, Kodman-Jones C. Comprehensive management of dysfunctional voiding. Pediatrics 1999;103:e31.

76. Shaul DB, Harrison EA. Classification of anorectal malformations–initial approach, diagnostic tests, and colostomy. Semin Pediatr Surg 1997;6:187-195.

77. Smellie JM. The intravenous urogram in the detection and evaluation of renal damage following urinary tract infection. Pediatr Nephrol 1995;9:213-219.

78. Soonawala N, Overweg-Plandsoen WC, Brouwer OF. Early clinical signs and symptoms in occult spinal dysraphism: A retrospective case study of 47 patients. Clin Neurol Neurosurg 1999;101:11-14.

79. Taddio A, Ohlsson K, Ohlsson A. Lidocaine-prilocaine cream for analgesia during circumcision in newborn boys. Cochrane Database Syst Rev 2000;93:CD000496.

80. Uehling DT, Richards WH. Abdominoscrotal hydrocele: diagnosis by herniogram and ultrasound. Urology 1992;40:147-148.

81. Unsinn KM, Geley T, Freund MC, Gassner I. US of the spinal cord in newborns: Spectrum of normal findings, variants, congenital anomalies, and acquired diseases. Radiographics 2000;20:923-938.

82. Upadhyay V, Hammodat HM, Pease PW. Post circumcision meatal stenosis: 12 years'experience. NZ Med J 1998; 111:57-58.

83. van der Voort J, Edwards A, Roberts R, Verrier Jones K. The struggle to diagnose UTI in children under two in primary care. Fam Pract 1997;14:44-48.

84. Van Glabeke E, Khairouni A, Larroquet M et al. Spermatic cord torsion in children. *Prog Urol* 1998;8:244-248.

85. Van Glabeke E, Khairouni A, et al. Acute scrotal pain in children: results of 543 surgical explorations. Pediatr Surg Int 1999;15:353-357.

86. Walker R. Evaluation of the Pediatric Urologic Patient. In: Walsh P, Retik A, Vaughan E, Wein A, Eds. *Campbell's Urology*, 7th ed., Philadelphia, PA: WB Saunders Company, 1998;1619-1628.

87. Wedge JJ, Grosfeld JL, Smith JP. Abdominal masses in the newborn: 63 cases. J Urol 1971;106:770-775.

88. Williams CP, Richardson BG, Bukowski TP. Importance of identifying the inconspicuous penis: prevention of circumcision complications. Urology 2000;56:140-142.

89. Wilson DA. Ultrasound screening for abdominal masses in the neonatal period. Am J Dis Child 1982;136:147-151.

90. Yamanishi T, Yasuda K, Murayama N et al. Biofeedback training for detrusor overactivity in children. J Urol 2001;164:1686-1690.

91. Yen TC, Tzen KY, Chen WP, Lin CY. The value of Ga-67 renal SPECT for diagnosing and monitoring complete and incomplete treatment in children with acute pyelonephritis. Clin Nucl Med 1999;24:669-673.

92. Yeung CK, Tam YH, Chan YL, et al. A new management algorithm for impalpable undescended testis with gadolinium enhanced magnetic resonance angiography. J Urol 1999;162:998-1002.

CHAPTER 42

Vesicoureteric Reflux

DOUGLAS A. CANNING, M.D.,

JENNIFER KOLU C.R.N.P., AND

KEVIN E.C. MEYERS, M.B., B.Ch.

INTRODUCTION

The incidence of vesicoureteric reflux (VUR) in the general population is less than 1%.[2] In children with urinary tract infection (UTI), the incidence is as high as 29% to 50%.[11] When reflux coexists with UTI and intrarenal reflux, the kidney is at risk for scarring, and this may lead to end-stage renal disease (ESRD). Progressive scarring following pyelonephritis clearly occurs in children, and is easier to detect in infants and younger children. Therefore, identification of VUR and correct management is important. However, it is important to note that some infants with severe VUR are born with renal dysplasia and have no history of UTI.

DEFINITIONS

VUR exists when there is retrograde flow of urine from the bladder upward toward the kidney. VUR occurs when there is an anatomic or functional abnormality of the usually competent ureterovesical junction. As a result of impairment of the one-way valve mechanism at the ureterovesical junction (UVJ), there is retrograde flow of urine from the bladder into the upper urinary tract (ureters and kidneys). Reflux of infected urine into the upper urinary tract may result in acute pyelonephritis.

EPIDEMIOLOGY AND GENETICS

The indications for testing for VUR are shown in Box 42-1. Infants with prenatal hydronephrosis and VUR usually have high-grade reflux. In contrast to VUR diagnosed following UTI, most children identified with VUR following antenatal hydronephrosis are boys. Up to 50% of children evaluated with a voiding cystourethrogram (VCUG) because of previous UTI have VUR. Toddlers, young children, and girls are more often diagnosed with VUR after UTI than older children and adults. There is a genetic predisposition to VUR. The likelihood that the sibling of a child who has VUR will have reflux demonstrated by VCUG evaluation is 40%. There is a 15% risk in each child of a mother with VUR diagnosed in her childhood. VUR is 10-fold more frequent in white than black children.

PATHOGENESIS

Primary reflux occurs when there is no obvious abnormality of bladder function. VUR can also be caused by high-pressure voiding and is called secondary reflux (Box 42-2).

Box 42-1 Evaluation of VUR

- During the assessment of prenatally diagnosed hydronephrosis
- After an episode of UTI
- After a sibling is diagnosed with VUR

- In boys
  - Posterior urethral valves
  - Prune belly syndrome
- In boys and girls
  - Duplex ureters and trigonal distortion caused by ureteroceles
  - Neurogenic bladder caused by upper motor neuron or lower motor neuron diseases
  - Megaureter
  - Bladder or cloacal exstrophies

The resolution of secondary VUR depends on improvement in the primary anatomical or functional abnormality such as by surgical incision of the urethral valve, or by reconstruction of the trigone following excision of a ureterocele.

The anatomy of the renal papilla is important in preventing or promoting intrarenal VUR.[8] Scarring following bacterial infection occurs most frequently at the polar regions of the kidney where the renal papillae are often confluent, thereby allowing intrarenal reflux (Box 42-3). Scarring does not occur in the absence of infection when voiding pressures are low. Renal scarring – the consequence of recurrent upper UTI – is called reflux nephropathy, and was previously known as chronic pyelonephritis. Reflux nephropathy is an important cause of ESRD.

CLINICAL PRESENTATION

History

Carefully ask about the child's voiding pattern. Dysfunctional voiding is suggested by hesitancy, urgency, or infrequent voiding as well as firm or small stools. High-pressure or dysfunctional voiding must be identified before contemplation of surgery. Even minor

Box 42-3   Factors Predisposing to Renal Scarring

- Younger age
- Delay in treatment
- Recurrent infections
- High-pressure reflux
- Intra-renal reflux
- Recurrent bacterial UTI

abnormalities of bladder function may have an impact on the severity or resolution of reflux. Symptoms of dysfunctional voiding such as urgency, frequency, and diurnal enuresis are frequent in children with VUR. A number of studies have shown that if children with equal grades of reflux and these symptoms are compared to those without symptoms of dysfunctional voiding, the rate at which reflux improves if the abnormal bladder activity is treated appropriately.

If symptoms of dysfunctional voiding are present, care must be taken to improve the coordination of voiding before proceeding with any surgical treatment of reflux, because the failure rate following antireflux surgery in these children is greater.[7] Therefore, we have established a center for the assessment and treatment of voiding dysfunction at The Children's Hospital of Philadelphia. Many children with a history of UTI will have some degree of voiding dysfunction that must be controlled before surgery. Many patients with reflux and recurrent UTI will show a reduction in both the predisposition to infection and the grade of reflux volume with careful treatment of voiding dysfunction.

DIAGNOSIS

VUR is identified directly by voiding cystography. Iodinated contrast is instilled into the bladder for voiding cystourethrography (VCUG), or a radiopharmaceutical such as technetium (NVCUG) is used. Both studies require urethral catheterization and instillation of the agent until the bladder is full and the child voids. Alternatively, indirect radionuclide studies may be diagnostic of high-volume VUR. Reflux is graded on a scale of I to V according to the classification developed by the International Reflux Study Group. Minimal VUR is grade I; grade V is the most severe form of reflux. Grades IV and V are called 'dilating reflux' because of the dilation of the upper renal tracts on the VCUG (Figure 42-1). Neonates with prenatally diagnosed hydronephrosis require postnatal renal ultrasonography and VCUG. Reflux in neonates is often high grade, and is more frequent in boys.

The radiological evaluation for VUR is performed after the diagnoses of a first UTI. Renal ultrasonography is painless, radiation-free, and non-invasive, and is therefore suitable for the initial evaluation of infants and children. Renal ultrasonography is obtained as soon as possible after diagnosis of UTI, especially if the child is toxic and admitted to hospital for intravenous antibiotic therapy. This is important because obstructive abnormalities of the upper urinary tract that may require surgical intervention must be identified.

In boys, VCUG is the initial study because of the anatomic detail provided. Radionuclide studies are used

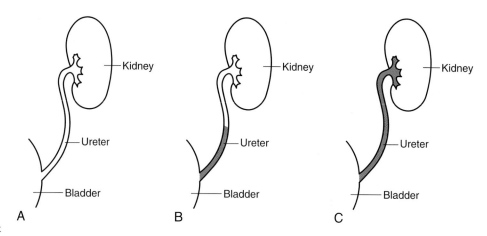

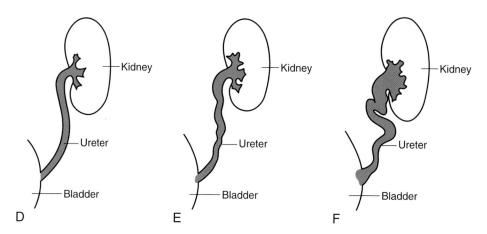

Figure 42-1 Vesicoureteric reflux grades: (A) Normal; (B) Grade I; (C) Grade II; (D) Grade III; (E) Grade IV; and (F) Grade V.

for the follow-up of reflux because anatomical detail is less of a concern, and there is less exposure to radiation.[3]

The renal technetium ^{99m}dimercaptosuccinic acid (DMSA) scan can help to diagnose and manage patients with VUR. DMSA scans permit quantification of the differential function of the kidneys, assessment of cortical defects indicative of scarring, and the visualization of low-uptake areas suggestive of acute pyelonephritis. Evidence of scarring at the time of diagnosis of the first UTI is present in up to 50% of children (Box 42-4).

Box 42-4 Renal 'Scarring' may be due to a Number of Factors

- Prior undetected infections that injured the kidney(s)
- Initial infection damaged the kidney(s)
- Refluxing kidney(s) are intrinsically abnormal at birth in the absence of infection

MANAGEMENT

The management of VUR is divided between medical and surgical therapy. Medical therapy is usually offered initially, while surgery is reserved for patients in whom medical management is unsuccessful (Figure 42-2). Antibiotic prophylaxis is provided whether or not surgery is contemplated. Antibiotics usually are administered continuously at a low dose, and are intended to prevent recurring infections. Children who develop breakthrough UTIs on prophylactic doses of antibiotics require further evaluation.

Medical

Medical management of VUR in the child is based on several observations that have evolved over the past 40 years.[12]

The resolution rate for VUR depends on the initial grade. Approximately 80% of low-grade reflux resolves with medical management, but this may take many years.

VUR GRADE I–II Antibiotic prophylaxis – Endoscopic correction – Open surgery

Age 0–10 y

Unilateral and bilateral

VUR GRADE III–IV Antibiotic prophylaxis – Endoscopic correction – Open surgery

Age 0–5 y

Unilateral and bilateral

Age 6–10 y

Unilateral

VUR GRADE V Antibiotic prophylaxis – Endoscopic correction – Open surgery

Age <1 y

Unilateral and bilateral

VUR GRADE III–IV Endoscopic correction – Open surgery

Age 6–10 y

Bilateral

VUR GRADE V Open surgery

Age 1–10 y

Unilateral and bilateral

Figure 42-2 Treatment algorithm for vesicoureteric reflux (VUR).

Higher grades of reflux resolve much less frequently. Approximately 50% of children have resolution of VUR grades I to III by 3.5 years after diagnosis. Grade IV VUR resolves much less frequently, with resolution in 50% of children projected to 11.5 years. The fact that there is at least an 80% overall resolution rate for low-grade reflux compared with a 20% overall resolution for high-grade reflux helps to decide which children require surgery.[9]

Medical management is generally safe and effective in the absence of high voiding pressures. Medical and surgical management of children with grades III and IV VUR were compared in a multinational prospective study (the International Reflux Study in Children). No advantage of surgical over medical treatment could be found with regard to renal scarring or renal function at the conclusion of the study.[13] Sterile reflux does not cause renal damage in patients who have normal bladder function. The continuous administration of antibiotic prophylaxis is better than intermittent administration of antibiotics for preventing new renal injury in patients managed conservatively. Low-dose continuous antibiotic prophylaxis is safe, although many parents are justifiably concerned about the possibility of adverse effects from long-term antibiotic prophylaxis. The risk of a breakthrough infection and subsequent renal scarring outweigh any potential deleterious antibiotic adverse effects. However, the use of prophylaxis for low-grade VUR in children with normal voiding is currently being challenged by trials that are examining this question.

The standard of care at this time continues to be continuous low-dose antibiotic prophylaxis for all children with UTI who have any grade of VUR.

The following factors are taken into consideration when considering the appropriate follow-up of a child on antibiotic prophylaxis for VUR: (i) low-grade reflux tends to resolve whereas high-grade VUR tends to persist; (ii) unilateral VUR rather tends to resolve more often than bilateral VUR; and (iii) reflux tends to resolve more often with normal bladder function (Box 42-5).

Surgical

After a diagnosis of VUR, all children are placed on antibiotic prophylaxis and carefully followed. The more aggressive surgical approach is recommended:
- when care-givers are considered unreliable with regard to follow-up visits or administration of prophylactic antibiotics;
- for all patients with breakthrough UTI despite antibiotic prophylaxis.

Endoscopic treatment of VUR by subureteral injection (STING) is a less invasive technique for correcting one of the most common pediatric urologic problems. The technique is straightforward, and is usually performed as an outpatient procedure. It does require general anesthesia, but repeat injections may be required, particularly in patients with high-grade reflux. Endoscopic injection therapy has not yet become the procedure of choice for most

---

Box 42-5   Follow-up of a Child on Antibiotic Prophylaxis for VUR

- Serial imaging studies are used to follow the progress of the reflux; this is achieved by annual radionuclide cystography
- Upper urinary tract imaging by renal ultrasonography or by DMSA renal scanning is performed at less frequent intervals
- Younger children require serial imaging to follow renal growth and to detect any evidence of evolving renal scars
- A renal scar from a UTI may take months, or even years, to evolve
- The presence of a renal scar in an otherwise healthy child is of questionable significance
- The most sensitive technique for detecting renal scars is the DMSA renal scan
- It is unnecessary to obtain routine urine cultures in an asymptomatic child
- Urine culture is indicated whenever there is an unaccounted febrile illnesses

---

patients with VUR despite the ease of treatment, obviation of an open incision, and minimal hospital stay. This is because two problems exist: (i) until recently there has been no single implant substance that can provide the safety and durability; and (ii) it is less successful for high-grade reflux.

Recently the substance Deflux® (Q-Med Scandinavia) has become available and FDA approved. This substance is extremely promising and may well increase the indications for correction of low-grade reflux.

A year after the first study follow-up, nuclear cystography is carried out to measure aspects of bladder function:
- The bladder volume when the bladder is filled to capacity.
- The bladder volume at which reflux is first noted.
- The volume of urine refluxing into either ureter.

Improved resolution rates are found in patients in whom reflux occurs only after the bladder is more than 60% full, or if the volume of urine refluxing into either ureter is 2.6% of the bladder volume at capacity.[6] If the child continues to have high-volume reflux early in bladder filling, then surgical correction is considered. If high-volume reflux persists at the second study and the patient is not a dysfunctional voider, then again surgical correction is considered. Although medical management in the absence of infection is safe, this may not be the most effective way to manage the patient with high-volume VUR. Even if symptoms of dysfunctional voiding do not exist in the patient with high-volume VUR, a prolonged period of medical management may be necessary before resolution can be expected. Surgical correction of VUR, if it becomes necessary later on, may be emotionally more

difficult for an older child. Many families elect to proceed with surgery when faced with the prospect of numerous radiological studies and years of antibiotic prophylaxis without a guarantee of spontaneous resolution of VUR. The option for surgical correction is more attractive with the relatively less invasive technique of STING.

Secondary Reflux

The management of secondary reflux is directed toward the anatomical pathology. The reflux often improves as the bladder pressures return towards normal. Anti-reflux surgery should be performed only after careful evaluation in patients with posterior urethral valves, neuropathic bladder, or severe dysfunctional voiding. In these patients a vesicostomy is usually a better option than anti-reflux surgery. In many cases, high-volume VUR effectively improves capacity in the valve bladder, and should be allowed to remain as long as the patient does not have an upper UTI.

PROGNOSIS AND OUTCOMES

Children with VUR are followed for at least 1 year, regardless of their reflux grade. In many of these children the grade of reflux decreases with control of UTI improvement in voiding. Infants with high grades of reflux benefit from a period of monitoring because reflux improves most dramatically within the first year.[10] At the same time, the infant bladder increases in volume most rapidly during the first 18 months.[14] Infants with severe VUR void with high pressures, and this may become less evident with age. Anti-reflux surgery is safer and more effective when the severity of reflux decreases and bladder volume increases.

Almost all patients undergo ultrasonography as the initial study to assess the shape of the kidney and the presence of scarring. The potential for renal failure is estimated using the echotexture of the renal parenchyma relative to the liver or spleen, and the presence or absence of corticomedullary junctions correlate with future renal function.[5] A renal scan is obtained to assess preoperative function and drainage if there is significant scarring, if the volume of renal parenchyma is small, or if the echo texture of the kidney is increased, or if the corticomedullary junctions are obscure. The kidney and ureter can be removed if the function is poor (<10%). In rare cases there is a secondary ureteropelvic junction (UPJ) obstruction. If there is a UPJ obstruction as well as VUR, this should be corrected prior to, or at the time of anti-reflux surgery if the obstruction appears to be primary. On the other hand, if the UPJ obstruction is secondary to high-grade VUR it must be carefully monitored after anti-reflux surgery.[4] The bladder volume must be adequate to allow for low-pressure storage following voiding whether attempting endoscopic or open repair of VUR. If the bladder empties poorly or is poorly compliant, then recurrent infections, progressive upper tract dilation or renal scarring may result. Attempts to correct reflux by any means usually fail if bladder capacity is reduced.

MAJOR POINTS

- Vesicoureteric reflux is as much a medical as a urological problem.
- Primary reflux may improve with maturation.
- Secondary reflux usually does not improve with maturation.
- The symptoms and signs of UTI are non-specific in neonates and infants.
- A UTI must be suspected in all infants and toddlers with persistent fever, lethargy, stomach upset, or vomiting.
- The diagnosis of UTI is best made on a urine specimen obtained by urethral catheterization.[1]
- There is no need to wait for 6 weeks after UTI to perform a VCUG.
- The VCUG can be performed safely as soon as the urine is sterile.
- Antibiotic prophylaxis is the cornerstone of management for children with VUR.
- Newly diagnosed patients with VUR should initially be given daily antibiotic prophylaxis.
- Low-grade reflux tends to resolve, whereas high-grade VUR tends to persist.
- Unilateral VUR rather tends to resolve more often than bilateral VUR.
- Reflux tends to resolve more often with normal bladder function.
- Sterile reflux does not cause renal scars but persistent reflux of infected urine may cause renal scarring.
- Patients *fail* medical management because of persistent reflux lasting into adolescence, breakthrough UTI, or failure to adhere to maintenance prophylactic regimens.
- Bladder training is imperative to promote the resolution of VUR.
- Surgery is the initial treatment to prevent kidney damage for higher risk groups: older children, higher grades of reflux, breakthrough UTIs.
- Endoscopic correction is a less invasive approach for patients on antibiotics who continue to have reflux.
- A second injection is attempted if the first does not cure the reflux; however, open surgery is the next step if two injections fail.

REFERENCES

1. AAP, Committee on Quality Improvement, Subcommittee on Urinary Infection. Practice parameter: the diagnosis, treatment, and evaluation of the initial urinary tract infection in febrile infants and young children. Pediatrics 1999;103:843-852.
2. Bailey R. Vesicoureteric reflux and reflux nephropathy. In: Schrier R, Gottschalk C (eds), *Diseases of the Kidney.* Little, Brown, Boston, 1988, pp. 747-783.
3. D'Errico G. The role of nuclear medicine in evaluation of vesicoureteral reflux and/or reflux nephropathy. Rays 2002; 27:149-154.
4. Hollowell JG, Altman HG, Snyder HM, Duckett JW. Coexisting ureteropelvic junction obstruction and vesicoureteral reflux: diagnostic and therapeutic implications. J Urol 1989;142:490-493.
5. Hulbert WC, Rosenberg HK, Cartwright PC, et al. The predictive value of ultrasonography in evaluation of infants with posterior urethral valves. J Urol 1992;148:122-124.
6. Mozley PD, Heyman S, Duckett JW, et al. Direct vesicoureteral scintigraphy: quantifying early outcome predictors in children with primary reflux. J Nucl Med 1994:35: 1602-1608.
7. Noe HN. The role of dysfunctional voiding in failure or complication of ureteral reimplantation for primary reflux. J Urol 1985;134:1172-1175.
8. Ransley P, Risdon R, Godley M. High pressure sterile vesicoureteral reflux and renal scarring: an experimental study in the pig and minipig. Contrib Nephrol 1984;39:320-343.
9. Schwab W, Wu H, Selman H, et al. Spontaneous resolution of vesicoureteral reflux: a 15 year perspective. J Urol 2003; 168:3.
10. Skoog SJ, Belman AB, Majd M. A nonsurgical approach to the management of primary vesicoureteral reflux. J Urol 1987;138:941-946.
11. Walker R, Duckett J, Bartone F, McLinn P, Richard G. Screening schoolchildren for urologic disease. Birth Defects 1977;13:399-407.
12. Walker R. Vesicoureteral reflux. In: Gillenwater J, Grayhack J, Howard S, Duckett J (eds), *Adult and Pediatric Urology,* 2nd edn. Year Book, Chicago, 1992, pp. 1889-1920.
13. Weiss R, Duckett J, Spitzer A. Results of a randomised clinical trial of medical versus surgical management of infants and children with grades III and IV primary vesicoureteral reflux (United States). J Urol 1992;148:1667-1673.
14. Zerin JM, Chen E, Ritchey ML, Bloom DA. Bladder capacity as measured at voiding cystourethrography in children: relationship to toilet training and frequency of micturition. Radiology 1993;187:803-806.

CHAPTER 43

Pathogenesis, Clinical Features, and Management of Intersexuality

THOMAS F. KOLON, M.D.

Introduction

Female Pseudohermaphroditism (FPH)

Congenital Adrenal Hyperplasia (CAH)

CYP21 (21 α-Hydroxylase) Deficiency

CYP11B1 (11 β-Hydroxylase) Deficiency

Gonadal Dysgenesis

Complete Gonadal Dysgenesis (CGD)

XY Gonadal Dysgenesis (XY Sex Reversal or Swyer Syndrome)

46XX Pure Gonadal Dysgenesis

45X Gonadal Dysgenesis (Turner Syndrome)

Partial Gonadal Dysgenesis (PGD)

Male Pseudohermaphroditism (MPH)

Leydig Cell Aplasia/Hypoplasia

Testosterone Biosynthesis Enzyme Defects

StAR Deficiency

3 β-Hydroxysteroid Dehydrogenase Deficiency (3 β-HSD)

CYP17 Abnormality

17 β-Hydroxysteroid Dehydrogenase Deficiency

5 α-Reductase Deficiency

Androgen Insensitivity Syndrome (AIS)

Persistent Müllerian Duct Syndrome (Hernia Uteri Inguinali)

Dysgenetic Male Pseudohermaphroditism (46XY Gonadal Dysgenesis)

SRY Mutations

DAX–1 Mutations

ATR-X Syndrome

Denys–Drash Syndrome (DDS)

WAGR Syndrome

Campomelic Dysplasia

Vanishing Testes Syndrome

True Hermaphroditism

Sex Chromosome Anomalies

46XX Sex-Reversed Males

History and Physical Examination of Intersexuality

Laboratory Studies

Treatment Options and Indications

Female Pseudohermaphroditism

Congenital Adrenal Hypoplasia

Gonadal Dysgenesis

True Hermaphroditism

Male Pseudohermaphroditism

5 α-Reductase Deficiency

Persistent Müllerian Duct Syndrome

Dysgenetic Male Pseudohermaphroditism (46XY Gonadal Dysgenesis)

Male CAH

Androgen Insensitivity Syndrome

INTRODUCTION

The first sections of this chapter provide a basic science template for the etiology of intersex. However, it may be worthwhile to read the history, physical examination, and evaluation descriptions first, and then begin again at the start of the chapter to keep this subject in perspective.

Human sexual determination occurs in an organized, sequential manner (Box 43-1). Sexual differentiation is regulated by more than 50 different genes on both the sex chromosomes and autosomes. These genes encode

---

Box 43-1 Human Sexual Determination

- Chromosomal sex is established at fertilization and directs the undifferentiated gonads to develop into testes or ovaries.
- Phenotypic sex results from the differentiation of internal ducts and external genitalia under the influence of hormones and transcription factors
- Intersexuality is the result of discordance among the processes of chromosomal, gonadal, or phenotypic sex determination

transcription factors, gonadal steroid and peptide hormones, and tissue receptors. The sex determination genetic cascade involves the *SRY* gene (sex-determining region on Y) as the testis-determining factor. Other upstream (*SF-1*, *WT-1*) and downstream (*DAX-1*, *AMH*, *HOXA10*) genes are also involved. The female phenotype represents the default pathway in sexual development. Failure of testis determination results in the development of the female phenotype. Genetic alterations resulting in partial testicular development cause a spectrum of abnormal masculinization. The timing of hormonal exposure is also critical to appropriate development.

FEMALE PSEUDOHERMAPHRODITISM (FPH)

FPH is the most common intersex disorder (Figure 43-1). The ovaries and Müllerian derivatives are normal, and the sexual ambiguity is limited to virilization of the external genitalia. A female fetus is masculinized only if exposed to androgens. The degree of masculinization is determined by the stage of differentiation at the time of exposure (Figure 43-2). Masculinization also can occur secondary to exogenous maternal steroids.[1]

Congenital Adrenal Hyperplasia (CAH)

CAH accounts for most of the patients with FPH. Inactivating or loss of function mutations in five genes involved in steroid biosynthesis can cause CAH: *CYP21*, *CYP11B1*, *CYP17*, *HSD3B2*, and *StAR* (Figure 43-3 and Table 43-1). All of these biochemical defects are characterized by impaired cortisol secretion, but only *CYP21* and *CYP11B1* are predominantly masculinizing disorders. The female fetus is masculinized due to overproduction of adrenal androgens and precursors. Affected males have no genital abnormalities.

HSD3B2, *CYP17*, and *StAR* deficiencies block cortisol synthesis and gonadal steroid production. These affected males have varying degrees of male pseudohermaphroditism (MPH) while females have normal external genitalia. Inheritance is autosomal recessive.[4,19]

CYP21 (21 α-Hydroxylase) Deficiency

The *CYP21* gene is located within the major HLA locus on chromosome 6p21.3. HLA types are co-dominantly inherited, and can be used as a marker to distinguish homozygous, heterozygous, and unaffected individuals. Two *CYP21* genes are located on chromosome 6 between HLA-B and HLA-DR. Recombination between *CYP21B* and the homologous but inactive *CYP21A* account for approximately 95% of 21 α-hydroxylase deficiency mutations.[19] In the classic salt-losing 21 α-hydroxylase deficiency, gene deletions or conversions severely reduce

the enzyme's activity.[19] Patients with simple virilizing 21 α-hydroxylase deficiency have a conversion mutation (Ile→Asn) causing severely decreased enzyme activity, but sufficient aldosterone production to prevent salt wasting. Non-classical CAH conversion mutations have 20–50% of normal activity. Since some mutations cause more than one phenotype, other genes that code for extra-adrenal 21 α-hydroxylase activity may be involved.

The identification of a fetus with a *CYP21* deficiency by HLA typing of amniotic fluid cells in mothers with a previously affected offspring has led to mixed results of experimental prenatal treatment of CAH.[18,22]

CYP11B1 (11 β-Hydroxylase) Deficiency

Cytochrome P450 is a terminal oxidase on the inner mitochondrial membrane. Two enzymes, CYP11B1 and CYP11B2, are encoded by two tandem and homologous genes at 8q21-22. *CYP11B1* encodes *11 β-hydroxylase* that converts 11-deoxycorticosterone to corticosterone and 11-deoxycortisol to cortisol. This gene's protein is expressed in the adrenal zona fasciculata, and is primarily under the influence of corticotropin. *CYP11B2* encodes for aldosterone synthetase that converts deoxycorticosterone (DOC) to corticosterone and 18-hydroxycorticosterone to aldosterone. It is expressed in the zona glomerulosa, and is under the influence of angiotensin II and potassium. Cortisol deficiency results in increased secretion of 11-deoxycortisol, DOC, corticosterone, and androgen by the adrenal gland. Hypertension, in two-thirds of patients, may be a consequence of excess DOC-induced salt and water retention. Excess androgen secretion *in utero* masculinizes the external genitalia of the female fetus. After birth, untreated males and females progressively virilize and have rapid somatic growth and skeletal maturation.

There are 20 known mutations of the *CYP11B1* gene. Although *CYP11B1* and *CYP11B2* are extremely homologous, both genes are functional. Therefore in contrast to 21 α-hydroxylase deficiency, gene conversions are not the cause of impaired enzyme activity. Alterations with less enzyme activity usually result in more severe phenotypes, but heterogeneity can occur. Mutations in the *CYP11B2* gene impair the conversion of DOC to aldosterone, causing hyponatremia, hyperkalemia, and failure to thrive, but do not affect virilization. This disorder can be detected prenatally. and the masculinization of the fetus can be decreased by in-utero dexamethasone treatment.

GONADAL DYSGENESIS

Gonadal dysgenesis disorders comprise a spectrum of anomalies ranging from complete absence of gonadal development to delayed gonadal failure. Complete (pure)

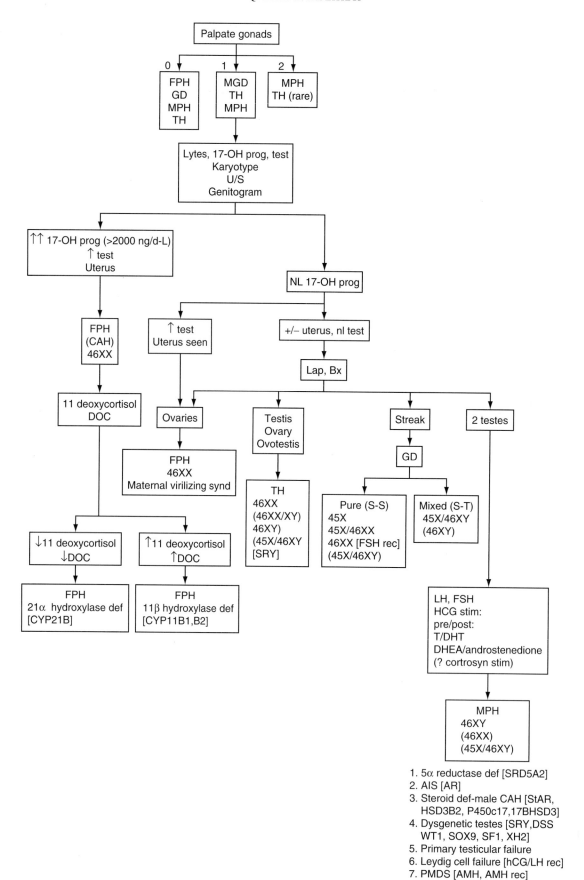

Figure 43-1   The decision pathway of evaluation for intersex.

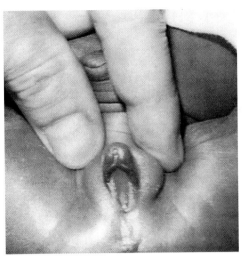

Figure 43-2 A 46XX patient with moderate masculinization due to congenital adrenal hyperplasia.

gonadal dysgenesis includes failed gonadal development in genetic males and females due to abnormalities of sex or autosomal chromosomes. Partial gonadal dysgenesis refers to disorders with partial testicular formation at some point in development including mixed gonadal dysgenesis, dysgenetic MPH, and some forms of testicular regression.

Complete Gonadal Dysgenesis (CGD)

The bipotential gonad differentiates into an ovary if testicular formation fails. However, if an X chromosome

is present, the gonad develops into an ovary but then degenerates into a streak gonad with ovarian-like stroma and few or no germ cells.

XY Gonadal Dysgenesis (XY Sex Reversal or Swyer Syndrome)

This occurs secondary to the absence of testes, despite a Y chromosome. It is a heterogeneous condition that can result from deletions of the short arm of the Y chromosome. *SRY* gene mutations, alterations in autosomal genes, or duplications of the DSS locus on the X chromosome.[6,16] Inheritance is X-linked recessive or male-limited autosomal dominant. The other genetic alterations that may cause this type of gonadal dysgenesis are *WT-1, DAX-1, SOX-9, 10qdel*, and *9pdel*.

46XX Pure Gonadal Dysgenesis

This is characterized by normal stature, normal external and internal female genitalia, sexual infantilism, and bilateral streak gonads. It is a heterogeneous condition occurring sporadically or, when familial, as an autosomal recessive trait. A locus maps to chromosome 2p with a homozygous missense mutation for the follicular stimulating hormone (FSH) receptor gene.

45X Gonadal Dysgenesis (Turner Syndrome)

A 45X constitution may be caused by non-disjunction or chromosome loss during gametogenesis in either

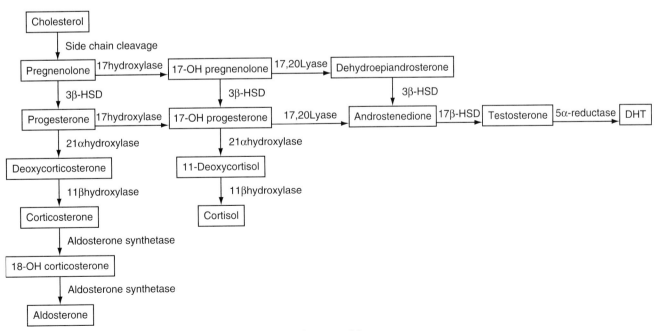

Figure 43-3 The intersex steroid biosynthetic pathways, with responsible enzymes.

Table 43-1 Genetic Characteristics of Intersex Disorders

Syndrome	Karyotype	Genital Phenotype	Gene	Locus
21-Hydroxylase deficiency	XX	Virilized	CYP21B	6p21.3
11-Hydroxylase deficiency	XX	Virilized	CYP11 (B1,B2)	8q21-22
3 β-HSD deficiency	XX XY	Ambiguous	HSD3B2	1p13.1
17 α-Hydroxylase or 17,20 Lyase deficiency	XX XY	Ambiguous	CYP17	10q24-25
17 β-HSD deficiency	XY	Ambiguous	17BHSD3	9q22
Lipoid adrenal hyperplasia	XX XY	Female Ovarian failure (XX)	StAR	8p11.2
Leydig cell failure	XY	Ambiguous	hCG/LH receptor	2p21
Androgen insensitivity	XY	Ambiguous (Female – AIS 7)	AR	Xq11-12
5 α-reductase deficiency	XY	Ambiguous, pubertal virilization	SRD5A2	2p23
Persistent Müllerian duct	XY	Male	AMH AMH II receptor	19q13.3 12q13
Gonadal dysgenesis:				
Complete	XX 45X, 45X/46XX XY	Female Sexual infantilism	FSH receptor X monosomy SRY DSS (DAX-1) SOX9 WT-1	2p16-21 Paternal X loss Yp53.3 Xp 21-22 17q24.3-25.1 11p13
Mixed	45X/46XY XY	Ambiguous	Unknown	Unknown
Dysgenetic MPH	XY 45X/46XY	Ambiguous	SRY DSS (DAX-1) XH-2 WT-1 SOX9 SF-1	Yp53.3 Xp 21-22 Xq13.3 11p13 17q24.3-25.1 9q33
True hermaphrodite	XX XX/XY XY	Ambiguous	SRY Testis cascade Downstream genes	Yp53.3 Unknown
Klinefelter's syndrome	47XXY 46XY/47XXY	Variable androgen Deficiency	XY	Sex chromosome Non-disjunction
Male sex reversal	XX	Ambiguous to normal	SRY	Y translocation to X

parent resulting in a sperm or ovum without a sex chromosome. 45X/46XX mosaicism may be present in up to 75% of Turner syndrome patients. Since approximately 99% of 45X fetuses spontaneously abort, it is theorized that mosaicism may increase survival in Turner syndrome. Familial studies of X-linked traits indicate that loss of the paternally derived X chromosome is more common (77%). Maternal imprinting, however, does not appear to affect fetal survival in 45X^m individuals.[5] Turner stigmata can be seen in patients with deletions involving the X or Y chromosomes. It is theorized that homologous genes that are not X-inactivated are present, and normally prevent the Turner phenotype. Other rare forms of X chromosome anomalies including mosaicism, trisomies, deletions, rings, or isochromosomes occur. These individuals usually have somatic stigmata that are less severe than classic 45X patients.

Partial Gonadal Dysgenesis (PGD)

PGD is a result of impaired testicular determination in the presence of SRY, resulting in partial gonadal dysgenesis. The phenotypes vary including bilateral testicular dysgenesis (dysgenetic MPH), a testis and a streak gonad (mixed gonadal dysgenesis; MGD), and absence of one or both testes (testicular regression). The majority of MGD patients have a 45X/46XY karyotype, but 46XY is also seen. In contrast to patients presenting with genital ambiguity and mosaicism, 95% of prenatally detected 45X/46XY mosaics have a normal male phenotype.[24] This contradiction may be related to separate cell lines in the streak gonad and the testis. Mutations in the pseudoautosomal region of the Y chromosome upstream of the SRY gene have been identified in partial gonadal dysgenesis.[17] Many of the previously discussed mutations associated with CGD (*WT-1, DAX-1, 10qdel*) have also been reported in PGD, although the etiology of gonadal dysgenesis remains unknown in most cases.

MALE PSEUDOHERMAPHRODITISM (MPH)

MPH is a heterogeneous disorder in which testicles are present but the internal ducts and/or the external genitalia are incompletely virilized. The phenotype ranges from completely female external genitalia to mild male ambiguity, such as hypospadias or cryptorchidism. Causes of MPH are listed in Box 43-2.

Leydig Cell Aplasia/Hypoplasia

This autosomal recessive condition has a variable phenotype.[1] In its complete form, patients are 46XY, but are cryptorchid and phenotypically female. Wolffian structures are present due to the secretion of anti-Müllerian hormone (AMH) by intact Sertoli cells. The underlying abnormality is a failure of Leydig cell differentiation secondary to an abnormal luteinizing hormone (LH) receptor (LHR).[13] LH is elevated, testosterone is markedly decreased, and FSH levels are unaffected. There is no testosterone surge on human chorionic gonadotropin (hCG) stimulation. This disorder highlights the importance of LHR for Leydig cell growth and differentiation. The human LH/CG receptor (*hLHCGR*)

gene is mapped to chromosome 2p16-21. The variable phenotype is determined by the effect that the mutation has on the biological activity of the *hLHCGR*. Mutations in the receptor may affect either the extracellular binding domain or its signal transduction activity. More severe phenotypic abnormalities occur in patients with hLHCG receptors that are not expressed on the cell surface or fail to transduce the signal for hormone binding. Leydig cell hypoplasia is a genetically heterogeneous condition that may occur in the presence of an intact LH receptor gene.[25]

Testosterone Biosynthesis Enzyme Defects

Defects in four steps of the steroid biosynthetic pathway from cholesterol to testosterone may produce genital ambiguity in the male (see Table 43-1).

StAR Deficiency
Congenital lipoid adrenal hyperplasia is a rare, autosomal recessive disorder caused by mutations in the *StAR* (steroidogenic acute regulatory) gene.[14] Mutation of the *StAR* gene on chromosome 8p11.2 severely disrupts the synthesis of all adrenal and gonadal steroids.

3 β-Hydroxysteroid Dehydrogenase Deficiency (3 β-HSD)

This results in impaired adrenal aldosterone and cortisol synthesis, as well as gonadal testosterone and estradiol formation. Male infants have variable degrees of MPH. Females commonly have clitoromegaly and mild masculinization. The masculinization is a result of conversion of the Δ5 precursors to testosterone via placental and peripheral tissue fetal 3 β-HSD. There may be salt wasting. 3 β-HSD2 is the isoenzyme responsible for this syndrome.[21] Treatment with glucocorticoids is similar to that of 21-hydroxylase deficiency, and mineralocorticoids are added to treat the salt-wasting forms. Sex steroid replacement may be necessary at puberty.

CYP17 Abnormality
The *CYP17* gene is located on chromosome 10q24.3 Combined 17 α-hydroxylase and 17,20 lyase deficiency causes deficient production of cortisol and sex hormones.[26] Genetic females have sexual infantilism due to a lack of ovarian estrogen synthesis at puberty. Genetic males have a spectrum ranging from a normal female phenotype to an ambiguous hypospadiac male. Overproduction of 11-deoxycorticosterone (DOC) and corticosterone leads to hypertension, hypokalemic alkalosis, and carbohydrate intolerance.

Genetic males with isolated 17,20 lyase deficiency also have variable degrees of incomplete masculinization.[8] However, they do not suffer from the associated

---

Box 43-2 Causes of Male Pseudohermaphroditism

- Leydig cell aplasia/hypoplasia due to hCG/LH receptor defect causes testicular unresponsiveness to hCG and LH
- Enzyme defects in testosterone biosynthesis. Some are common to CAH (StAR, HSD3B2, CYP17, 17-β HSD3)
- Androgen insensitivity syndrome caused by defects in androgen-dependent target tissues
- Defect in the enzymatic conversion of testosterone to DHT caused by 5 α-reductase deficiency
- Persistent Müllerian duct syndrome caused by defects in the synthesis, secretion, or response to anti-Müllerian hormone (AMH) or Müllerian inhibiting substance (MIS)
- Testicular dysgenesis caused by aberrations in testicular gonadogenesis
- Vanishing testes caused by primary testicular failure
- Maternal ingestion of progesterone/estrogen or environmental toxins

abnormalities in cortisol secretion and hypertension that occurs in patients with combined 17 α-hydroxylase/17,20 lyase deficiencies. They need to be monitored for hypertension, because 17 α-hydroxylase activity diminishes with age. Studies reveal an accumulation of C21 precursors combined with depressed C19 steroid levels. This disorder highlights the importance of 17,20 lyase in sexual maturation. Adrenarche, which occurs between ages of 8 and 10 years, involves the selective activation of 17,20 lyase leading to a dramatic increase in adrenal dehydroepiandrosterone (DHEA) synthesis without affecting cortisol/ACTH secretion or 17 α-hydroxylase activity. 17,20 Lyase activity of human p450c17 is approximately 30-fold greater with Δ5 substrates than with Δ4 substrates. Therefore, virtually all of the androstenedione is derived from DHEA by the action of 3 β-hydroxysteroid dehydrogenase, and virtually all human sex steroid production is from DHEA. Only insignificant quantities of androstenedione are synthesized from 17-OH progesterone. Thus, these patients require only surgical repair of the external genitalia and sex steroid replacement at the time of puberty.

17 β-Hydroxysteroid Dehydrogenase Deficiency

There are five known isoenzymes of 17 β-HSD.[7] Type 3 17 β-HSD (9q22) catalyzes the reduction of androstenedione to testosterone, and is expressed only in the testis. Different isoenzymes catalyze the isoreduction of estrone to estradiol and androstenedione to testosterone. These patients have elevated plasma androstenedione (up to 10 times as high) levels, low plasma testosterone (increased androstenedione:testosterone ratio after hCG stimulation in prepubertal patients), elevated LH, and normal to high FSH levels. In these patients, more than 90% of plasma testosterone is produced from the extragonadal conversion of androstenedione to testosterone, compared to <1% in normal males. Plasma dihydrotestosterone (DHT) may be normal in some patients, suggesting conversion from androstenedione.

The inheritance is autosomal recessive, and there is no evidence that the phenotypic expression of those affected with 17 β-HSD3 deficiency correlates with a particular 17 β-HSD3 gene mutation. Patients with 17 β-hydroxysteroid dehydrogenase deficiency are usually 46XY males with ambiguous or female external genitalia and normal internal Wolffian structures, including inguinal testes and a blind vaginal pouch. This occurs because there is little or no peripheral conversion of androstenedione to testosterone and DHT during early gestation by the other 17 β-HSD isoenzymes. Additionally, increased aromatization of androstenedione to estrogen by the placenta may leave little substrate available for conversion to testosterone and DHT. These children are often raised as girls, but may virilize at puberty and adopt a male gender role, similar to that

seen in 5αRD-2 deficiency.[11] At puberty, the expression of other 17 β-HSD isoenzymes in the peripheral tissues partially compensates for testicular 17 β-HSD3 deficiency; however, the phenotype is variable. Some patients develop gynecomastia at puberty, depending on their testosterone:estradiol ratio.

5 α-Reductase Deficiency

5 α-Reductase deficiency (5αRD) is an autosomal recessive condition with variable phenotype.[10] It was initially called 'pseudovaginal perineoscrotal hypospadias' because of the striking genital ambiguity/female external phenotype. Two 5 α-reductase isoenzymes share 50% homology. The *5αRD-1* gene (5p15) is extragonadal and is mostly expressed in the liver. The mutated gonadal *5αRD-2* gene (2p23) causes male pseudohermaphroditism.

Androgen Insensitivity Syndrome (AIS)

The broad phenotypic spectrum in these 46XY patients varies from normal female external genitalia (AIS7 or testicular feminization) to normal males with infertility (AIS1) (Figure 43-4). This X-linked disorder affects 1 in 20,000 live male births. The androgen receptor (*AR*) gene is located in the pericentromeric region of the long arm of chromosome X at Xq11-12, and contains eight exons.[3,15] The 3′ region of exon 4 and exons 5 through 8 encode the steroid-binding domain that confers ligand specificity. Binding of DHT or testosterone to this receptor ligand-binding domain results in activation of the receptor. The majorities of *AR* gene mutations affect the steroid-binding domain, and this results in receptors that are unable to bind androgens or that bind androgens but exhibit qualitative abnormalities.

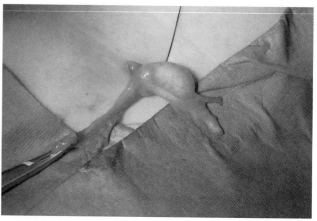

Figure 43-4 Abdominal testis identified at time of inguinal hernia repair in a 46XY patient with complete androgen insensitivity syndrome.

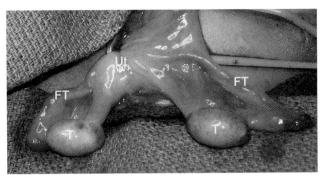

Figure 43-5 Retained Müllerian structures in a 46XY patient with unilateral cryptorchidism and persistent Müllerian duct syndrome. FT = Fallopian tube; T = testis, Ut = uterus.

Persistent Müllerian Duct Syndrome [PMDS] (Hernia Uteri Inguinali)

This is a rare autosomal recessive disorder that arises from a lack of AMH (or Müllerian inhibiting substance; MIS) action on the Müllerian ducts, resulting in the presence of Müllerian structures in a normally virilized XY male (Figure 43-5). PMDS is due to either a mutation in the *AMH* gene or from a defect in the AMH type II receptor.[9] The *AMH* gene is located on chromosome 19p13.3.

Dysgenetic Male Pseudohermaphroditism (46XY Gonadal Dysgenesis)

Patients with dysgenetic gonads have ambiguous development of the internal genital ducts, the urogenital sinus, and the external genitalia (Figure 43-6). Mutations or deletions of any of the genes involved in testis determination cascade can cause dysgenetic MPH.

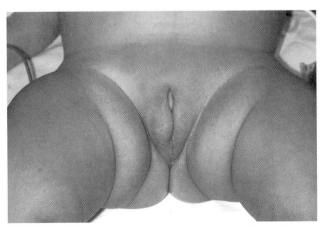

Figure 43-6 A 46XY patient with severe hypospadias and unilateral cryptorchidism due to dysgenetic male pseudohermaphroditism.

SRY Mutations

SRY is a single-exon gene located on the short arm of the Y chromosome near the pseudoautosomal region. Histological analysis of dysgenetic gonads of XY males revealed that those with normal *SRY* had some element of rete testis and tubular function, while those with *SRY* mutations had completely undifferentiated gonads similar to those of 45XO individuals. *SRY* may have a direct role in testicular formation in addition to its indirect role in initiating the male differentiation cascade.

DAX-1 Mutations

Duplication of the DSS (Dosage-Sensitive Sex reversal) locus is associated with dysgenetic MPH and other anomalies.[12,25] It maps to the Xp21 region that contains the *DAX-1* gene (DSS-AHC critical region on the X chromosome, gene 1). Mutations in *DAX-1* can cause X-linked congenital adrenal hypoplasia and hypogonadotropic hypogonadism.

ATR-X Syndrome

This is characterized by 46XY dysgenetic MPH, mental retardation, and α-thalassemia. Mutations in the *XH2* gene at Xq13.3 have been described in this syndrome. Other chromosomal deletions have been reported (10q26-qter and 9p24-pter).

Denys–Drash Syndrome (DDS)

Male patients with DDS have ambiguous genitalia with streak or dysgenetic gonads, progressive nephropathy, and Wilms' tumor. These patients have heterozygous mutations of the Wilms' tumor suppressor gene (*WT-1*) on 11p13, and are usually missense mutations mostly in exon 9. Most *WT-1* mutations in DDS occur *de novo*, and act as dominant-negative mutations.

WAGR Syndrome

The Wilms' tumor, aniridia, genitourinary abnormalities, mental retardation (WAGR) syndrome is also associated with *WT-1* alterations (heterozygous deletions). The genitourinary abnormalities anomalies in the WAGR syndrome are usually less severe than in Denys–Drash syndrome.

Campomelic Dysplasia

The *SOX9* gene is associated with campomelic dysplasia, an often-lethal skeletal malformation, and dysgenetic MPH. The sex reversal locus maps to 17q24.3-25.1.

Affected 46XY males have phenotypic variability from normal males to normal females, depending on the function of the gonads. The SOX9 protein is expressed in the developing gonad, rete testis, and seminiferous tubules as well as skeletal tissue. The *SOX9* gene has 71% homology to the *SRY* gene.

Vanishing Testes Syndrome

Vanishing testes syndrome (congenital anorchia) describes the spectrum of anomalies resulting from cessation of testicular function. Loss of testes prior to 8 weeks' gestation results in 46XY patients with female external and internal genitalia with agonadism or streak gonads. Loss at 8–10 weeks causes ambiguous genitalia and variable ductal development. Loss of testis function after the critical male differentiation period (12–14 weeks) results in a normal male phenotype externally and internally, but anorchia. There are sporadic and familial forms of unilateral and bilateral anorchia, including discordant and concordant monozygotic twins.

TRUE HERMAPHRODITISM

True hermaphroditism (TH) requires the presence of both ovarian and testicular tissue in the individual. This uncommon condition may be classified into three groups:

1. Lateral: testis and ovary (usually left).
2. Bilateral: ovotestis and ovotestis.
3. Unilateral (most common): ovotestis and testis or ovary.

The genital development is ambiguous with hypospadias, cryptorchidism, and incomplete fusion of labioscrotal folds. Genital duct differentiation generally follows that of the ipsilateral gonad.

TH can result from sex chromosome mosaicism, chimerism, or Y chromosomal translocation.[23] The most common karyotype is 46XX, followed by 46XX/46XY chimerism, mosaicism, and 46XY. Most 46XX TH are SRY-negative, and the genes responsible have not yet been identified. A mutated downstream gene in the sex determination cascade likely allows for testicular determination.

While sex chromosome mosaicism arises from mitotic or meiotic errors, 46XX/46XY chimerism is usually a result of double fertilization (an X sperm and a Y sperm) or, less commonly, the fusion of two normally fertilized ova. Chimeric patients have two distinct cell populations. The least common form of TH, 46XY, may result from a cryptic 46XX cell line or gonadal mosaicism with a mutated sex determination gene.[2]

SEX CHROMOSOME ANOMALIES

46XX Sex-Reversed Males

One in 20,000 phenotypic males has a 46XX karyotype. Categories of 46XX sex reversal include classic XX male individuals with apparently normal phenotypes, nonclassic XX males with some degree of sexual ambiguity, and XX true hermaphrodite. Some 80–90% of 46XX males result from an anomalous Y to X translocation involving the *SRY* gene during meiosis. The amount of DNA material involved in the exchange varies but, in general, the greater the amount of Y-DNA present, the more virilized the phenotype. However, 8–20% of XX males have no detectable Y sequences, including SRY. Most of these patients have ambiguous genitalia, but there are reports of classic XX males without the *SRY* gene.

HISTORY AND PHYSICAL EXAMINATION OF INTERSEXUALITY

The history must include the gestational age, ingestion of hormones used in assisted reproductive techniques, or oral contraceptives during pregnancy. Obtain a family history of consanguinity, urologic abnormalities, neonatal deaths, precocious puberty, and infertility. Determine if the mother has signs of virilization or cushingoid appearance. Obtain information regarding antenatal ultrasound studies, and discordance between fetal karyotype genitalia (see Figure 43-6).

Look for dysmorphic features of Turner syndrome such as a short broad neck, puffy hands and feet, and widely spaced nipples. The baby should be examined in a warm room while supine in the frog-leg position with both legs free. Note the width and stretched length measurements of an abnormal phallus. Describe the position of the urethral meatus and the amount of chordee (ventral curvature) and note the number of orifices: three in normal girls (urethra, vagina and anus), and two in boys (urethra, anus). A rectal examination is performed to palpate a uterus. With warmed hands, one should begin the inguinal examination at the anterior superior iliac crest and sweep the groin from lateral to medial with a non-dominant hand. Once a gonad is palpated, grasp it with the dominant hand and continue to sweep toward the scrotum with the other hand in an attempt to bring the gonad to the scrotum. Soap or lubricant on the fingertips can aid this examination. It is important to check size, location, and texture of both palpable gonads. An undescended testis may be found in the inguinal canal, the superficial inguinal pouch, at the upper scrotum or rarely in the femoral, perineal, or contralateral scrotal regions. One should also note the

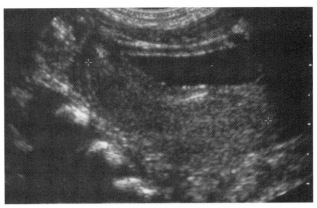

Figure 43-7   Ultrasound investigation in newborn, showing large uterus filled with debris (between cursors) behind the bladder.

development and pigmentation of the labioscrotal folds and any other congenital anomalies of other body systems. It is important to determine whether or not the gonad is palpable (Box 43-3). Unless associated with a patent processus vaginalis, ovaries and streak gonads do not descend, while testes and rarely an ovotestis may be palpable. In 46XY boys, hypospadias and cryptorchidism without an underlying intersex cause are a diagnosis of exclusion only after a full evaluation.

LABORATORY STUDIES

The following must be obtained in all patients:
- Serum electrolyte concentrations, and levels of 17-OH-progesterone, testosterone, LH, and FSH (Box 43-4)
- An immediate karyotype
  - An ultrasound can detect gonads in the inguinal region, but is only 50% accurate for an intra-abdominal testes

- A computed tomography scan and a magnetic resonance imaging scan may help to delineate the anatomy and identify a uterus (Figures 43-7 and 43-8)
- A genitogram evaluates a urogenital sinus and the entry of the urethra in the vagina. A cervical impression can be identified on the vaginogram
- An open or laparoscopic exploration with bilateral deep longitudinal gonadal biopsies for histological evaluation of infants in whom TH, MGD, or MPH is considered

During the first 60 to 90 days of life there is a normal gonadotropic surge with a resultant increase in the testosterone level. Therefore, during this period one can forego the hCG stimulation for androgen evaluation.

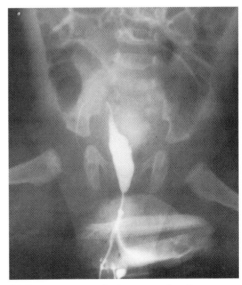

Figure 43-8   Contrast study demonstrating the uterus and right Fallopian tube in a 46XY patient.

TREATMENT OPTIONS AND INDICATIONS

Female Pseudohermaphroditism

Congenital Adrenal Hypoplasia

First, correct dehydration and salt loss with electrolytes (excluding potassium) and fluid, and with mineralocorticoid replacement.[4] Glucocorticoid replacement is added upon confirmation of the diagnosis. Infants that are going to be raised as girls usually undergo clitoral reduction and vulvovaginoplasty in early infancy, but the timing of surgery is controversial and all aspects must be considered prior to making a decision. Many surgeons advocate early surgery for technical and psychological reasons and understand that vaginal revision may be needed after puberty. The three main aims of surgery are to reduce the size of the enlarged masculinized clitoris, to reconstruct the female labia, and to increase the opening and possibly length of the vagina. Surgical technique attempts to optimize the external appearance and functional size while maintaining adequate sensation. Clitorectomy to remove the entire clitoris and clitoral recession without reduction are no longer performed. Reduction clitoroplasty is the operation of choice for most infants with clitoromegaly. A vulvoplasty is carried out by extending the incision for the clitoroplasty on either side of the midline strip of tissue down to the level of the vaginal orifice. Redundant labial scrotal skin is brought down as preputial flaps to form the labia minora.

The position of the vagina should be accurately determined preoperatively by the genitogram. There are four main types of vaginal repair: a simple 'cut-back' of the perineum; a 'flap' vaginoplasty; a 'pull-through' vaginoplasty; or a more extensive rotation of skin flaps or segmental bowel interposition.

Gonadal Dysgenesis

A streak gonad does not descend, but may be palpable as a small remnant of tissue in an inguinal hernia sac. If the testis is in the inguinal position, it can be removed using an incision in the groin, as for a traditional orchiopexy or hernia repair. If the gonad is in the abdomen – as is usually the case with the gonadal dysgenesis – then the treatment options include open abdominal exploration and removal of the gonads, or preferably a laparoscopic gonadectomy. When the anatomy is purely female, such as in Turner syndrome (Box 43-5) or Swyer syndrome (Box 43-6), no treatment may be necessary. These girls have sexual infantilism at puberty marked by absence of secondary sexual development. Since gonadoblastoma does not occur in the absence of Y chromosome material, removal of the

---

Box 43-5 Features of 45X Gonadal Dysgenesis (Turner Syndrome)

- The cardinal features include webbed neck, shield chest, short stature, cardiac anomalies (coarctation of the aorta), and sexual infantilism
- Bilateral streak gonads are the rule, but primary follicles are found in the genital ridges of some 45X individuals correlating with the rare occurrence of menarche
- Conceptions are documented despite only 45X cell lines

---

streak gonads is not required. Growth hormone is usually recommended early in childhood, and estrogen therapy is begun after puberty to optimize the height. Most are infertile, although there are reports of rare cases of spontaneous pregnancy.

Noonan syndrome patients have Turner-like features, including short stature, webbed neck, and right-heart disease.[20] They have a normal sex chromosome constitution, often with cryptorchidism of hypoplastic testes. Puberty is delayed and there may be androgen deficiency. However, fertility may occur in the absence of cryptorchidism. Most cases are sporadic, but there may be autosomal dominant inheritance.

True Hermaphroditism

Generally, a female sex has been assigned to most patients due to the presence of a vagina, uterus, and ovarian tissue. Less commonly, male sex assignment is more appropriate if the patient has a 46XY karyotype with adequate penile development and no uterus. The decision of sex of rearing should always be deferred until the child has had an adequate evaluation of his genitourinary system. Usually, the internal organs need to be visualized and the gonads biopsied. If raised as

---

Box 43-6 Swyer Syndrome (Gonadal Dysgenesis, XY Female)

- Point mutations or deletions of the *SRY* gene
- In some cases there are changes in the X chromosome
- Look like normal females at birth and appear to be normal females
- Do not develop secondary sexual characteristics at puberty, have amenorrhea, and have streak gonads

a female, the child should have dysgenetic testicular tissue removed due to the risk of malignancy. A vaginoplasty can be performed early or deferred until puberty. If the child is raised as a boy, any degree of hypospadias or cryptorchidism must be repaired in infancy. Testosterone supplementation may be needed if the amount of testicular tissue is inadequate to begin or continue puberty. A persistent Müllerian duct, such as a uterus and Fallopian tubes, usually has not fully regressed and connects to the urethra near the bladder at the verumontanum. If the decision is made to rear the child as a boy, the structures are generally removed – taking care not to injure the vas deferens, which usually runs alongside the uterus. Extensive dissection behind the bladder neck and up to the area where the Müllerian structures insert into the urethra is usually contraindicated in order to avoid damage to the sphincter mechanism and risk incontinence. Both open and laparoscopic excision has been reported. Arguments for removal of the Müllerian structures include the possibility of cyclic hematuria post puberty, or the formation of stones or chronic urinary tract infections if continuity with the urethra is maintained and stasis occurs in a dilated Müllerian remnant. Arguments against removal maintain that complications from the structures are uncommon and their removal risks injury to the vas deferens, the bladder neck, and the urethral sphincter.

Male Pseudohermaphroditism

Decreased masculinization (hypospadias with cryptorchidism or more ambiguous development) is seen in most patients with male pseudohermaphroditism.

5 α-Reductase Deficiency

These patients often have a clitoris-like phallus, severely bifid scrotum, and perineoscrotal hypospadias. Some patients have less severe genital ambiguity. Other findings are normal Wolffian structures, cryptorchidism, and a rudimentary prostate. In untreated patients with 5 α-reductase deficiency, significant virilization occurs at puberty as testosterone levels increase into the adult male range, while DHT levels remain disproportionately low. The treatment of this enzyme deficiency is unclear when it is diagnosed in infancy. Male gender assignment has been recommended because the natural history of this deficiency is virilization at puberty with subsequent change to male gender. However, this decision requires surgical hypospadias repair and orchiopexy with male hormonal replacement.

At puberty, the signs of virilization are increased muscle mass, deepening of voice, substantial growth of phallus, rogation, and hyperpigmentation of the scrotum, and normal libido. They do not have gynecomastia

or male pattern balding, facial hair is decreased, and their prostate remains infantile. Although these patients are usually oligo- or azoospermic, fertility can occur via intrauterine insemination. These patients are often raised as girls but adopt a male gender role at puberty. Therefore, they should be reared as males, if possible. DHT cream is applied to the genitals to induce growth of the phallus and facilitate hypospadias repair. DHT cream may also increase facial and body hair growth in adulthood. Early correction of cryptorchidism may theoretically preserve fertility. Psychiatric counseling and parental reassurance that their child will have a normal male puberty is also critical.

Persistent Müllerian Duct Syndrome

The diagnosis is often made at surgery for cryptorchidism or inguinal hernia repair. Patients with type I PMDS will have low or undetectable levels of serum AMH, whereas those with type II PMDS secondary to a defective AMH receptor will have high normal or elevated serum AMH levels. Treatment consists of orchidopexy. Leaving the uterus and Fallopian tubes *in situ* may be optimal, to avoid injury to the vas deferens. The retained Müllerian structures are not at risk for malignant degeneration.

Dysgenetic Male Pseudohermaphroditism (46XY Gonadal Dysgenesis)

Patients with dysgenetic testes rarely have fully masculinized external genitalia. The surgical issues depend on the degree of virilization in each individual case. This will also influence the decision process of sex assignment. If a 46XY infant with testicular dysgenesis is going to be raised as a male, he will need a hypospadias repair, orchiopexy, or possibly orchiectomy. Müllerian ducts have usually not fully regressed, and they may be fully or partially removed at the time of other repairs in order to facilitate orchiopexies. As previously discussed, retained female structures have the potential for urinary tract infections, stones or even cyclic hematuria at puberty. Dysgenetic testes may appear normal grossly, but microscopically they are disorganized and poorly formed; thus, a biopsy of the gonad is recommended in most children undergoing intersex evaluation. Currently, the recommendation is to remove an undescended dysgenetic testis because of the risk of malignancy. In 45X/46XY patients, if the biopsy is normal and the testis is scrotal or can be placed in the scrotum, it should not be removed, but a risk of malignancy correlates with the extent of testicular decent. Tumors have also been reported in scrotal dysgenetic testes. A scrotal testis needs to be followed very closely for this reason. The possibility for a male gender exists in these patients, who would need a hypospadias repair and yet would

Box 43-7 Diagnosis of Complete Androgen Insensitivity Syndrome

- Usually diagnosed at puberty when there is amenorrhea
- Occasionally discovered at the time of inguinal hernia repair
- May be diagnosed when a prenatal karyotype does not match the external phenotype of the neonate

require removal of severely dysgenetic testis and replacement hormones.

Male CAH

Affected boys with errors in testosterone production are undermasculinized, with varied degrees of hypospadias, cryptorchidism, bifid scrotum, or a blind vaginal pouch. For the patient reared as a boy, testosterone therapy may be indicated to augment penile size and to aid in the hypospadias repair. The natural history in some of these patients when untreated is virilization at puberty with a gender role change from female to male. Therefore, many recommend a male gender assignment diagnosis. Some enzyme deficiencies require glucocorticoid and mineralocorticoid replacement, and all of these patients need testosterone replacement at puberty for masculinization. Gonadectomy is required in 46XY patients raised as girls in order to address the risk of tumor formation. Traditionally, a child with complete AIS would be raised as a girl (Box 43-7).

Androgen Insensitivity Syndrome

If the child is to be raised as a female, then an orchiectomy is required. The testes are at risk for cancer development post-puberty, with an incidence of 5–10%. Seminoma is the most frequent tumor. The risks are greater in older patients and in those with complete AIS. In patients with partial AIS, orchiectomy is recommended as soon as the diagnosis is made in order to avoid further virilization in patients who will be raised as females. Male gender assignment is usually successful in patients with a predominantly male phenotype. However, predicting the adequacy of masculinization in adulthood may not be possible. Some children do respond well to high-dose androgen therapy, but its durability is not yet clear.

The best time to perform the orchiectomy is controversial. Traditionally, in an infant with complete AIS, the testes are left in place until after puberty to take advantage

of the hormonal function, and in this way, natural female pubertal changes can occur by testosterone conversion to estrogen. After puberty is completed, the testes would be removed and replacement estrogen begun. Risks with this approach are as follows: no cancers have been reported in prepubertal children, but carcinoma in-situ may occur. If the testes happen to be in the inguinal region, they can easily be injured. One also needs to explain to a mature post-pubertal patient of the need to remove the testes. Delaying the surgery also increases the risks of testis cancer if the patient is lost to follow-up care. If orchiectomy is performed early, replacement hormones are required for pubertal changes (Box 43-8).

Up to 30% of dysgenetic testes may develop a tumor that is usually a benign gonadoblastoma. However, although this tumor does not spread, it can develop into a malignant dysgerminoma. Patients with a 45X/45XY mosaic karyotype also have an increased risk of carcinoma in-situ. Ultrasound is then performed yearly until the age of 20, when a repeat biopsy is performed.

The patient whose hypospadias was repaired as a child should continue to be followed-up to identify and correct any long-term complications of the surgery. It is also important to document adequate control of voiding and the force of urinary stream. There appear to be no issues regarding fertility from a urethral point of view rather than that previously described for cryptorchidism.

Girls who have undergone a feminizing genitoplasty require long-term follow-up for issues of menstruation, intercourse, and sensation. With a proper assignment of sex of rearing and a continued management with continuity of care, intersex individuals should be able to lead well-adjusted lives and ultimately obtain sexual satisfaction.

Box 43-8 On-Going Treatment

- Boys must be evaluated 1 year after orchiopexy for testes size, location, and viability
- Starting at puberty, boys must be shown how to perform monthly testicular self-examinations
- Parents should be made aware of the issues regarding cancer and infertility
- The risks for malignant testicular tumor development in cryptorchidism are 22-fold that in the general population
- Orchiopexy does not protect against testis cancer development but allows easier palpation for subsequent physical examinations
- Some surgeons recommend ultrasound examination and biopsy of a testis at puberty

MAJOR POINTS

- Intersex is one of the most complex subjects in medicine.
- There are numerous emotional, psychological, social, endocrine, genetic and surgical problems.
- The important issue with any intersex evaluation is not to get bogged down by the vast range of possibilities in the differential diagnosis.
- Work slowly through the pathway based on the physical examination and laboratory findings.
- Many possible diagnoses will be removed from contention by this approach.
- The most common cause of genital ambiguity is deficiency of CYP21 (cytochrome $P450_{c21}$).
- Some centers include screening for 17-hydroxy-progesterone levels at 3–5 days of life with screening for inborn metabolic diseases.
- 1 in 14,500 infants are homozygous for the classic (simple [25%] or salt-wasting [75%]) forms of CYP21 deficiency.[18,22]
- 1 in 60 infants is a heterozygote.[18,22]
- A distinction must be made whether or not the gonad is palpable for purposes of differential diagnosis and treatment.
- Much current research is aimed at understanding the influence of androgens on fetal and newborn brain and its relationship to gender identity.
- Diagnosis and management is individualized.
- Starting immediately after birth, there must be a team approach including the neonatologist, nurses, social workers, pediatric urologist, endocrinologist, geneticist, and parents.
- It is important to individualize treatment whenever feasible.
- Issues that parents must discuss with the pediatric urologist, endocrinologist, geneticist, and psychiatrist are testosterone imprinting *in utero*, need for hormones pre- and post-puberty, degree of masculinization, function of the testis, and the extent of surgery.
- Comprehensive discussions among all the involved physicians, nurses and social workers *and* the parents must take into account parental anxieties, as well as their social, cultural and religious views in order to facilitate appropriate gender assignment.
- Treatment of the child with intersex should not end with the first postoperative visit.

REFERENCES

1. Berthezene F, Forest MG, Grimaud JA, Claustrat B, Mornex R Leydig cell agenesis: a cause of male pseudohermaphroditism. N Engl J Med 1976;295:969–972.

2. Braun A, Kammerer S, Cleve H, et al. True hermaphroditism in a 46XY individual caused by a postzygotic somatic point mutation in the male gonadal sex-determining locus (SRY): molecular genetics and histological findings in a sporadic case. Am J Hum Genet 1993;52:578–585.

3. Chamberlain NL, Driver DE, Miesfeld RL. The length and location of CAG trinucleotide repeats in the androgen receptor N-terminal domain affect transactivation function. Nucleic Acids Res 1994;22:3181–3186.

4. Scriver CR, Sly WS, Valle D. The metabolic and molecular basis of inherited disease. In: Donohue P, Migeon CJ (eds), *Congenital Adrenal Hyperplasia,* 7th edn. McGraw-Hill, New York, 1995, pp. 2929–2966.

5. Epstein CJ. Mechanisms leading to the phenotype of Turner syndrome. In: Rosenfield RG, Grumbach MM (eds), *Turner Syndrome.* Marcel Dekker, New York, 1990.

6. Ferguson-Smith MA. SRY and primary sex reversal syndromes. In: Scriver CR, Sly WS, et al. (eds), *The Metabolic and Molecular Basis of Inherited Disease.* McGraw-Hill, New York, 1995.

7. Geissler WM, Davis DL, Wu I, et al. Male pseudohermaphroditism caused by mutations of testicular 17β-hydroxysteroid dehydrogenase 3. Nature Genet 1994;7:34–39.

8. Geller DH, Auchus RJ, Mendonca BB, Miller WL. The genetic and functional basis of isolated 17,20-lyase deficiency. Nature Genet 1997;17:201–205.

9. Imbeaud S, Belville C, Messika-Zeitoun L, et al. A 27 base-pair deletion of the anti-mullerian type II receptor gene is the most common cause of the persistent müllerian duct syndrome. Hum Mol Genet 1996;5:1269–1277.

10. Imperato-McGinley J, Peterson RE, Gautier T, Sturla E. Male pseudohermaphroditism secondary to 5 alpha-reductase deficiency – a model for the role of androgens in both the development of the male phenotype and the evolution of a male gender identity. J Steroid Biochem 1979; 11(1B):637–645.

11. Imperato-McGinley J, Peterson RE, Stoller R, Goodwin WE. Male pseudohermaphroditism secondary to 17 β-hydroxysteroid dehydrogenase deficiency: gender role change with puberty. J Clin Endocrinol Metab 1979;49:391–395.

12. Kolon TF, Ferrer FA, McKenna PH. Clinical and molecular analysis of XX sex reversed patients. J Urol 1998;160: 1169–1172.

13. Latronico AC, Anasti J, Arnhold IJ, et al. Brief report: testicular and ovarian resistance to luteinizing hormone caused by inactivating mutations of the luteinizing hormone-receptor gene. N Engl J Med 1996;334:507–512.

14. Lin D, Sugawara T, Strauss JF 3rd, Clark BJ, et al. Role of steroidogenic acute regulatory protein in adrenal and gonadal steroidogenesis. Science 1995;267:1828–1831.

15. MacLean HE, Zajac JD. Defects of androgen receptor function: from sex reversal to motor neurone disease. Mol Cell Endocrinol 1995;112:133–141.

16. McElreavey KD, Vilain E, Abbas N, et al. XY sex reversal associated with a deletion 5′ to the SRY 'HMG box' in the testis-determining region. Proc Natl Acad Sci USA 1992;89: 11016–11020.

17. McElreavey K, Vilain E, Barbaux S, et al. Loss of sequences 3' to the testis-determining gene, SRY. Proc Natl Acad Sci USA 1996;93:8590-8594.

18. Miller WL. Genetics, diagnosis, and management of 21-hydroxylase deficiency. J Clin Endocrinol Metab 1994;78: 241-246.

19. New MI. Genetic disorders of steroid hormone synthesis and metabolism. Baillières Clin Endocrinol Metab 1995; 9:525-554.

20. Noonan JA. Noonan syndrome: an update and review for the primary pediatrician. Clin Pediatr 1994;33:548-555.

21. Simard J, Rheaume E, Sanchez R, et al. Molecular basis of congenital adrenal hyperplasia due to 3 beta-hydroxy-steroid dehydrogenase deficiency. Mol Endocrinol 1993; 7:716-728.

22. Speiser PW. Prenatal treatment of congenital adrenal hyperplasia. J Urol 1999;162:534-536.

23. Spurdle AB, Ramsay M. XX true hermaphroditism in southern African blacks: exclusion of SRY sequences and uniparental disomy of the X chromosome. Am J Med Genet 1995;55:53-56.

24. Sugarman ID, Malone PS. Mixed gonadal dysgenesis and cell line differentiation: case presentation and literature review. Clin Genet 1994;46:313-315.

25. Swain A, Narvaez V, Burgoyne P, Camerino G, Lovell-Badge R. DAX1 antagonizes SRY action in mammalian sex determination. Nature 1998;391:761-767.

26. Yanase T. 17α-Hydroxylase/17,20-lyase defects. J Steroid Biochem Mol Biol 1995;53:153-157.

Calculi

DAWN S. MILLINER, M.D.

INTRODUCTION

The diagnosis of urinary tract calculi is being made with increasing frequency in pediatric patients. Population-based studies from earlier decades reported urolithiasis at a much lower prevalence rate in children and adolescents than is true in middle-aged adults.[16] However, recent appreciation that presenting symptoms may be different in children, combined with improved radiographic techniques used more liberally than in the past, have enhanced the recognition of urinary tract stones in young patients. The frequency of occurrence has been influenced by factors predisposing premature infants to nephrocalcinosis and urinary tract stones, as well as by advances in medical care that have resulted in the improved survival of increasing numbers of patients with medical conditions, such as cystic fibrosis, that are associated with urolithiasis. In addition, there is an increasing incidence of urolithiasis overall in industrialized countries in recent decades.[16] The perception that urinary tract calculi are uncommon in children and adolescents is changing.

DIAGNOSIS

Symptoms

Symptoms of renal colic and gross hematuria, pathognomonic of urolithiasis in adults, are seen less reliably in children. Flank or abdominal pain or hematuria accounted for presenting features in 94% of adolescents, 72% of school-age children, and just 56% of those from birth to 5 years of age with urinary tract stones (Figure 44-1). In younger children with pain, typical renal colic was the exception. Most reported or were observed to have non-specific, generalized abdominal pain. Indeed, among children aged up to 5 years the diagnosis of urolithiasis was made following a urinary tract infection, or as an incidental radiographic finding during the evaluation of other problems in 44% of the patients.[14]

Imaging of Urinary Tract Stones

Imaging studies for the confirmation of urolithiasis should be performed whenever the diagnosis is under consideration. In North American series, 60–78% of urinary tract calculi are in the kidney at the time of diagnosis.[6,14] Of calculi found in the ureters, bladder, or urethra, the majority have originated in the kidneys. The bladder appears to be the site of stone formation in less than 10% of North American children, though in other areas of the world bladder calculi more commonly occur.[6] They are often referred to as 'endemic bladder stones,' and appear related to dietary factors in developing countries.[16] Calculi that form in the bladder in North American children are nearly always associated with bladder malformations or prior surgery such as augmentation cystoplasty, and are characterized by infection.

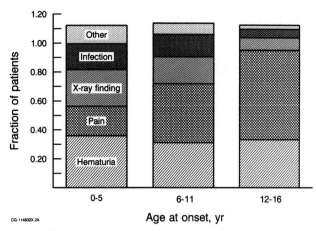

Figure 44-1 Presenting symptoms by age in children with urolithiasis. Reprinted with permission from Milliner DS, Murphy ME. Mayo Clin Proc 1993;68:241-248.

The composition of stones reported in several pediatric series is calcium oxalate in 40-60%, calcium phosphate in 15-25%, mixed (usually calcium oxalate and calcium phosphate) in 10-25%, magnesium ammonium phosphate (struvite) in 15-30%, cystine in 6-10%, and uric acid in 2-10%.[14,22,26] Their appearance on radiographs varies from densely radiopaque (calcium oxalate and calcium phosphate stones) to intermediate (struvite and cystine stones) to radiolucent (uric acid and xanthine) (Table 44-1).

Plain abdominal radiographs readily demonstrate radiopaque stones in the kidney, along the course of the ureter, or in the bladder (Figure 44-2). Stones of intermediate density, such as cystine or struvite stones (Figure 44-3), may be difficult to see if small. Radiolucent stones, such as those comprised of uric acid, are not visible. In order to visualize radiolucent stones by standard radiography, administration of intravenous contrast is needed, following which they can be seen as filling defects in the renal pelvis, ureter, or bladder. Ultrasonography of the kidneys and urinary tract is reliable for detection of stones in the kidneys, but less so for stones in the ureter or bladder. Ultrasonography provides valuable additional information regarding the presence or absence of hydronephrosis and can detect many structural malformations of the urinary tract that may predispose to stone formation (Figure 44-4). Accordingly, it is an excellent screening tool. Non-contrast computed tomography (CT) scanning is sensitive in the detection of even very small stones and ureteral stones, provides visualization of stones of intermediate density and of most stones that are radiolucent by conventional techniques, and detects hydronephrosis when present (Figure 44-5).

The importance of initial non-contrast images is illustrated by Figure 44-6, in which a stone clearly evident on tomography is obscured by contrast in a patient with a ureteropelvic junction (UPJ) obstruction. When obstruction of the urinary tract is suggested by symptoms, but is not confirmed on ultrasound or non-contrast studies, or when renal colic is suggested by symptoms but a responsible stone is not identified, repeat imaging following administration of a contrast agent should be considered. Confirmation of partial or complete obstruction by a urinary tract stone, as well as detailed anatomic information regarding the structure of the urinary tract, is provided by intravenous pyelography or by CT urography. In many centers, CT with or without urography has replaced the intravenous pyelogram (IVP) for the evaluation of pain or other symptoms consistent with urolithiasis. Depending on the technique used, helical CT has the potential to result in higher radiation exposure than other imaging modalities. However, when performed with attention to the radiation dose, the radiation exposure can be minimized. Individualization of imaging is of importance to obtain the necessary diagnostic information with a minimum of radiation exposure.

MANAGEMENT OF UROLITHIASIS

Stones causing obstruction, acute renal colic, stones with a high potential for acute obstruction (e.g., a large stone in the renal pelvis), and infected stones may

---

Table 44-1   Stone Composition and Radiographic Appearance

		Imaging Modality		
Stone Composition*	**%**	**Radiography**	**Ultrasound**	**CT**
Calcium oxalate	50	Densely opaque	↑ Echogenicity with shadowing	High density
Calcium phosphate	20	Densely opaque	↑ Echogenicity with shadowing	High density
Struvite	15	Intermediate density	↑ Echogenicity with shadowing	Medium density
Cystine	8	Intermediate density	↑ Echogenicity with shadowing	Medium density
Uric acid	5	Radiolucent	↑ Echogenicity with shadowing	Low density
Other	2-3	Variable**	↑ Echogenicity with shadowing**	Variable**

*Mixed composition, most often Ca oxalate and Ca phosphate, is found in 10-25% of stones.

**Indinavir stones and matrix stones (which are rare) are radiolucent on radiographs. They are of low density on CT, and are difficult to distinguish from surrounding soft tissue by both CT and ultrasound.

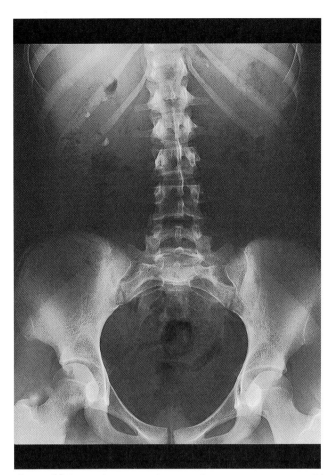

Figure 44-2   Radiopaque calcium oxalate stones in a 13-year-old girl with primary hyperoxaluria, type I. Three stones are seen in the right kidney, and one in the left kidney.

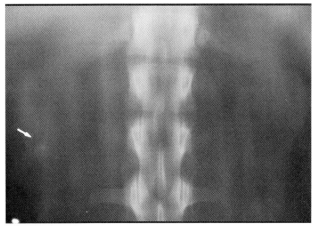

Figure 44-3   Cystine stones of moderate size (arrow) visualized on nephrotomography in a 15-year-old with cystinuria. With standard radiography, cystine stones are much less dense than calcium-containing stones.

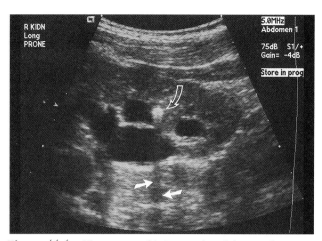

Figure 44-4   Ultrasonographic image of a calcium oxalate stone (open arrow) in the right kidney of a 4-year-old boy with idiopathic hypercalciuria and congenital ureteropelvic junction obstruction. Characteristic acoustic shadowing (solid arrows) is seen below the stone, which is sufficiently dense to block the sound waves. The stone is not obstructing urine flow.

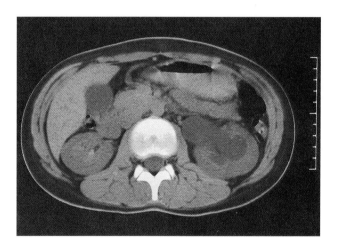

A

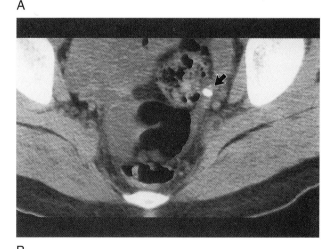

B

Figure 44-5   (A) Hydronephrosis of the left kidney of a 15-year-old girl seen on non-contrast computed tomography. (B) A large dense stone is obstructing the ureter at the level of the pelvis (solid arrow).

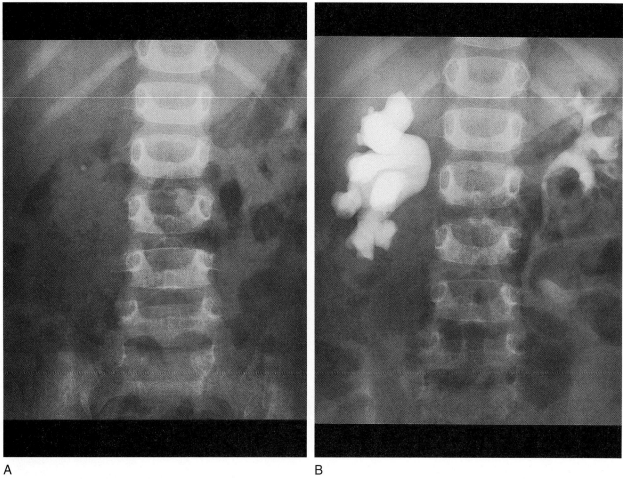

A   B

Figure 44-6 (A) A calcium oxalate stone in the pelvis of the right kidney readily seen on renal tomography is obscured by contrast (B) in the hydronephrotic right renal pelvis on the intravenous pyelogram in a 3-year-old boy.

require surgical intervention and should be evaluated jointly with a urologist. Renal colic due to stones that are progressing down the ureter, and are of a size that may spontaneously pass, can be managed initially with hydration, analgesics, and watchful waiting.[21] If complete obstruction develops, or the stone does not pass within a few days, surgical intervention is likely to be needed. The range of effective surgical interventions continues to increase, and now even very young patients can often undergo extracorporeal shock wave therapy (ESWL), ureteroscopic lithotripsy or removal, or percutaneous ultrasonic lithotripsy procedures.[2,6,14] Open lithotomy is rarely required. Due to the potential for high-energy shock waves to permanently damage renal tissue, there has been concern regarding the possible long-term adverse effects of ESWL on the developing kidney. One study suggested impaired growth of kidneys in children following ESWL. However, most information with second- or later-generation lithotriptors does not suggest clinically significant renal parenchymal scarring, impaired growth, permanent renal function abnormalities, nor hypertension in children following ESWL treatment.[2] Information to

date is still limited, however, particularly in children under the age of 6 years at the time of treatment.

Small stones within the papillary tips or in the collecting system that are not causing obstruction and are not infected often remain asymptomatic for years and can be managed medically. The goal of most medical management is to prevent the formation of new stones, and the growth of existing stones. Only a few stones, such as those comprised of uric acid, can be reduced in size or dissolved with medication. For effective medical management, common approaches valuable for all stone-formers are used in conjunction with interventions specific to the individual patient's stone profile.

For all forms of urolithiasis, increased oral fluid intake to maintain a daily urine volume of greater than 750 ml in infants, 1000 ml in children aged under 5 years, 1500 ml up to the age of 10 years, and more than 2000 ml in preadolescence and adolescence is most helpful to minimize stone formation. The avoidance of dietary excesses of calcium, oxalate, and sodium is also important. However, strict reduction, particularly with regard to dietary calcium intake, may be problematic with respect to nutritional adequacy and normal growth. Reduction to the appropriate recommended daily allowance (RDA) for age for calcium, and not lower, is suggested, even in children with known hypercalciuria.[26] Indeed, recent epidemiologic studies in adults suggest that a reduction in dietary calcium is associated with an *increased* likelihood of urolithiasis, perhaps due to greater absorption of dietary oxalate when less calcium is present in the intestinal tract. Dietary sodium limitation is of particular importance in patients with hypercalciuria and those with cystinuria.[1,9] Diets very high in protein are disadvantageous in stone-formers. A high dietary protein intake results in an increased urinary excretion of uric acid, calcium, and oxalate, and a reduced excretion of citrate and pH – all of which favor calcium oxalate urolithiasis.[16] Ketogenic diets, used for the management of seizure disorders, also predispose to urolithiasis. Hypercalciuria, reduced urine citrate, and reduced oral fluid intake characteristic of such diets result in urinary tract stone formation in 3–10% of children receiving this form of therapy. In children on such diets who form stones, the benefit of the diet must be balanced against the risk of further urolithiasis.

Treatment directed to address specific causes of stone formation in individual patients is based upon an evaluation of each patient for metabolic factors, obstruction, and infection (Table 44-2). In patients with no identifiable risk factors or modest abnormalities such as mild hypercalciuria as an isolated finding, increased oral fluid intake combined with prudent diet recommendations is sufficient as initial therapy. The patient should then be monitored over time for additional stone formation. If further stone formation is documented despite these measures, medication treatment may be indicated. Patients with significant metabolic findings most often require medication management of stone disease from the outset.

CAUSES OF STONE FORMATION

Among children and adolescents with urolithiasis, approximately 75% have identifiable predisposing causes for stone formation. From a compilation of studies that included 492 North American pediatric patients with urolithiasis,[14,22,26] metabolic causes accounted for 40%, urinary tract abnormalities 25%, and infection-related stones 10% (Table 44-3). In some pediatric studies, especially from Europe, a higher proportion of patients have infection cited as the cause of urolithiasis.[5] In most series, infants and young children more frequently have infection-related stones than do older children or adolescents. No contributing cause for stone formation (idiopathic) was able to be identified in 25% of patients. Adolescents account for the majority of those with idiopathic stone disease. It is common to find more than one predisposing factor in a given patient (Figure 44-7).[14]

Table 44-2 Treatment of Urolithiasis

Type of Stone Disease	Treatment
All stone-formers	High fluid intake Avoid dietary excess of calcium, sodium
Hypercalciuria	Limit dietary sodium Thiazides Citrate
Hyperoxaluria	Limit diet oxalate (idiopathic, enteric hyperoxaluria) Neutral phosphate Citrate Pyridoxine (primary hyperoxaluria)
Cystinuria	Limit dietary sodium Urine alkalinization Mercaptopropionylglycine D-penicillamine Captopril
Hyperuricosuria	Limit diet protein to RDA Urine alkalinization Allopurinol
Hypocitric aciduria	Citrate
Xanthinuria	Urine alkalinization Allopurinol
Infected stones	Antibiotic Removal of stone material from urinary tract
Stones due to stasis/ obstruction	Alleviate obstruction Avoid infection

Infection and urinary tract abnormalities frequently coexist, and are also frequently observed in conjunction with metabolic factors (see Figure 44-4). Infection by bacteria that produce urease (species of *Proteus, Klebsiella, Staphylococcus, Pseudomonas, Ureaplasma,* some anaerobes, and others) results in an increased urinary pH and increased urinary magnesium ammonium phosphate concentrations – conditions which favor the formation of struvite stones. Genitourinary tract abnormalities favor stone formation by stasis or obstruction. However, the incidence of urolithiasis among children

Table 44-3 Causes of Urolithiasis in Children

Primary Cause	Patients (%)
Metabolic	40
Stasis/obstruction	25
Infection	10
Idiopathic	25

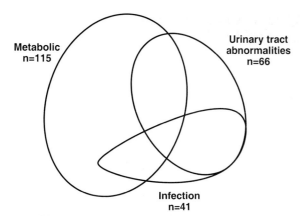

Figure 44-7   Metabolic factors (n=115), structural abnormalities (n=66), and infection of the urinary tract (n=41) identified in 221 pediatric and adolescent patients with urolithiasis.[14] As illustrated by the diagram, many of the patients had more than one predisposing factor. Concordance between urinary tract abnormalities and infection was particularly high. A few patients demonstrated all three types of predisposing factor.

with infected, obstructed, or structurally anomalous urinary tracts is low. Stone formation, when it does occur, is often influenced by coexisting metabolic abnormalities. Thus, infected, obstructed, or structurally anomalous urinary tracts do not obviate the need for careful metabolic assessment in all young patients who form stones.

A complete assessment of stone-forming factors is indicated in all children and adolescents with urolithiasis due to the high likelihood of identifying causes for stone formation, the early onset, and the potential for many future years of stone-forming tendency. Because of the overlap among predisposing metabolic abnormalities, infection, and structural contributors, the assessment should always include a metabolic evaluation.

High urinary concentrations of calcium, oxalate, uric acid, or cystine resulting from either increased renal excretion or low urine volume result in supersaturation of the urine for the respective crystal systems, thus favoring crystal and stone formation. In addition to the promoting effects of high solute concentrations, a role for naturally occurring urine inhibitors of crystal and stone formation is recognized.[22,25] Some authors have suggested that higher concentrations of inhibitors in the urine of children than in adults may explain, in part, their lower incidence of stone disease.[17] Citrate, magnesium, and pyrophosphate are the best defined of the naturally occurring inhibitors. A number of urinary macromolecules including glycosaminoglycans, osteopontin, and urinary prothrombin fragment 1 also appear to play a role in inhibition of stone formation, but as yet these are not well studied in children and adolescents.[23] Identification of the specific predisposing metabolic

factors in each patient is of importance in developing the most effective therapeutic regimen.

Patient Evaluation

Recommendations for the initial evaluation of children or adolescents with urolithiasis are shown in Box 44-1.[22,26] Medical, family, and diet histories are included. An estimate of daily fluid intake is an important aspect of the dietary history, as is an estimate of the daily intake of salt, calcium, and oxalate. Inquiry should be made regarding use of over-the-counter food supplements, vitamins, minerals, or herbal preparations, as well as prescription medications. Serum levels of calcium, phosphorus, uric acid, bicarbonate, sodium, potassium, creatinine, alkaline phosphatase, and albumin should be measured. Whenever stone material is available following spontaneous stone passage or surgical intervention, its composition should be determined. Urine analysis with determination of pH, osmolality or specific gravity, and the presence or absence of crystals, and a urine culture are needed. Urine concentrations and, whenever possible, excretion rates of solutes should be measured. Urine should be analyzed for calcium, oxalate, citrate, uric acid, sodium, cystine, creatinine, and total volume. In infants or young children or older children with developmental delay, random urine specimens with solute to creatinine ratio can be useful. However, caution is advised since normal values for such ratios often vary by age, prandial state, and diurnal status. Whenever a child is able to cooperate, a timed 24-hour urine collection will provide more complete information, including assessment of daily urine volume. Completeness of the collection is assessed by the creatinine excretion rate in mg/kg per 24 hours. A metabolic evaluation should be performed while the patient is on his or her usual diet, usual fluid intake, and normal activity. The studies should not be performed shortly after ESWL or a stone removal procedure, and should not be conducted when

---

Box 44-1   Evaluation of the Patient with Urolithiasis

- Medical and family history
- Diet history
- Radiographic appearance of urinary tract and stones
- Stone analysis
- Urine analysis and culture
- Serum potassium, bicarbonate, calcium, phosphorus, alkaline phosphatase, uric acid, creatinine
- Urine volume, pH, calcium, oxalate, citrate, phosphorus, uric acid, sodium, cystine, and creatinine

Table 44-4 Urine Chemistry Normal Values in Children*

	Random	Timed	Comments
Calcium	<0.21 mg/mg creatinine	<4 mg/kg/day	Higher in infants
Oxalate	<0.15 mmol/mmol creatinine	<0.45 mmol/1.73 m²/day	Oxalate/creatinine ratios are higher in infants and young children and decrease progressively through early adolescence
Citrate	>300 mg/g creatinine	>300 mg/g creatinine	Higher in infants and younger children. Normal values not well defined in childhood
Uric acid	3.3 mg/dl GFR⁺, in term infants; <0.53 mg/dl GFR in children aged over 3 years	<815 mg/1.73 m²/day	Age-dependent. Higher in infants
Cystine	<75 mg/g creatinine	<60 mg/1.73m²/day	Detects homozygotes and some heterozygotes

*Values provided are for children aged over 2 years, except where specified.
⁺Uric acid exereted/GFR.

the child is receiving intravenous fluids. If abnormalities are found, specific additional metabolic studies may be indicated.

Normal values for urine analytes in children above 2 years of age are shown in Table 44-4. Infants have higher analyte to creatinine ratios and higher excretion rates.[26,27] Uric acid excretion rates vary with age during childhood.[27] Uric acid excretion can also be expressed as mg/dl GFR and determined on either a random or timed urine specimen. When expressed as mg/dl GFR, the normal range does not change from 3 years of age through adolescence.[27] Urine oxalate/creatinine normal values vary considerably by age,[26] but excretion rates, when determined as mg/1.73 m² per day, remain the same from 2 years of age through adolescence.

Metabolic Factors Predisposing to Stone Formation

The metabolic causes of urolithiasis are listed in Box 44-2.

Solute Excess

Hypercalciuria

Hypercalciuria is the most common metabolic factor predisposing to stone formation, and is found in 30–50% of children with urolithiasis.[22] Defined as >4 mg/kg per day of urinary calcium or as a urinary calcium/creatinine ratio >0.21 (higher in infancy), hypercalciuria occurs in 3–4 % of healthy children,[19] and can predispose to hematuria, dysuria, urinary urgency, and perhaps urinary tract infections[3] as well as to urolithiasis. Causes of hypercalciuria are shown in Box 44-3. Most hypercalciuria is idiopathic, and identified as an isolated finding. It may occur sporadically or it may be inherited. Inherited forms have been well described, and may account for up to 40% of patients with idiopathic hypercalciuria, with most data

suggesting an autosomal dominant pattern.[8] The gene(s) responsible remains to be identified. Among children with idiopathic hypercalciuria, two subtypes have been described, one related to an enhanced gastrointestinal absorption of calcium (absorptive hypercalciuria) and the other related to reduced renal tubular reabsorption of calcium from the glomerular filtrate (renal leak hypercalciuria).[14, 27] The former subtype is characterized by a normal urine calcium/creatinine ratio in the fasting state

---

Box 44-2 Metabolic Causes of Urolithiasis

Solute excess
- Hypercalciuria
  Isolated finding (idiopathic)
  Secondary
  Renal tubular transport disorders
- Hyperoxaluria
  Idiopathic
  Enteric diseases
  Primary hyperoxaluria, genetic
- Cystinuria
- Hyperuricosuria
  Idiopathic
  Secondary to diet or medication
  Tumor lysis
  Myeloproliferative disorders
  Inborn errors of metabolism
  Lesch–Nyhan syndrome
  Partial hypoxanthine phosphoribosyl transferase deficiency

Inhibitor deficiency
- Hypocitric aciduria
  Metabolic acidosis
  Hypokalemia
  Renal tubular acidosis

Box 44-3   Causes of Hypercalciuria

- Idiopathic
  - Sporadic
  - Inherited
- Secondary
  - Dietary calcium, sodium excess
  - Corticosteroids
  - Furosemide
  - Vitamin D excess
  - Phosphate depletion
  - Immobilization
  - Primary hyperparathyroidism
  - Hypercalcemia
  - Metabolic acidosis
- Renal tubular transport disorders
  - Renal tubular acidosis
  - Dent's disease

with hypercalciuria following an oral calcium intake. Renal leak hypercalciuria is present in the fasting as well as the postprandial state. Oral calcium loading tests have been advocated to distinguish between the types, but these tests often do not allow clear separation. This is in part due to the confounding role of sodium in urine calcium excretion, and the recognition that some children identified as idiopathic hypercalciuria have sodium-dependent hypercalciuria related to a high dietary sodium intake. Other physiologic mechanisms have been postulated as responsible for idiopathic hypercalciuria, including a renal tubular phosphate leak, increased 1,25-dihydroxyvitamin D synthesis, increased renal prostaglandin E_2 production, and enhanced bone resorption.[27]

Among children with idiopathic hypercalciuria who do not have urolithiasis, the likelihood of developing calculi was 13% in one 3-year follow-up study of 30 patients, and 4% in a 4- to 11-year follow-up study of 33 children.[1,27] The risk of urolithiasis appears to increase with age. In addition to urinary tract symptoms, idiopathic hypercalciuria may be associated with reduced bone mass. For children with hypercalciuria who develop urolithiasis or other symptoms, treatment with thiazides and avoidance of excess dietary salt is usually effective in reducing renal excretion of calcium.

Secondary forms of hypercalciuria (see Box 44-3) are also common,[22] and occur most often in response to dietary salt excess, to chronic use of corticosteroids, and to the administration of loop diuretics such as furosemide. Prolonged immobilization in children or adolescents or excess intake of calcium or vitamin D as well as high concentrations of circulating parathyroid hormone all predispose to hypercalciuria. Any cause of hypercalcemia is likely to result in secondary hypercalciuria.

Metabolic acidosis results in mobilization of calcium from bone, followed by excretion in the urine. In distal renal tubular acidosis (RTA), the deficiency in acid secretion leads to metabolic acidosis, which in turn results in hypercalciuria. Once the metabolic acidosis is fully corrected with exogenous administration of base, the hypercalciuria resolves.

Rare, inherited forms of hypercalciuria include X-linked disorders related to mutations of the CLCN5 chloride channel.[24] Mutations of this channel have now been demonstrated in four conditions, previously described as separate clinical entities: X-linked nephrolithiasis with renal failure, Dent's disease, X-linked recessive hypophosphatemic rickets, and low molecular-weight proteinuria with hypercalciuria and nephrocalcinosis. All are now included under the term Dent's disease. These conditions have in common hypercalciuria, nephrolithiasis, nephrocalcinosis, renal tubule dysfunction characterized by low molecular-weight proteinuria and impaired absorption of phosphorus, and progressive renal insufficiency.[24] Affected males demonstrate proteinuria of renal tubular origin with particular elevation of retinol binding protein, and often develop nephrocalcinosis and/or urinary tract stones during childhood. Thiazides are effective in reducing the hypercalciuria in Dent's disease. Carrier females also occasionally develop clinical findings. Other rare, inherited disorders are associated with hypercalciuria, including mutations of the calcium-sensing receptor leading to hypocalcemia and hypercalciuria, and familial hypomagnesemia-hypercalciuria.[25]

Hyperoxaluria

Hyperoxaluria is observed in 2 to 20% of children and adolescents with urolithiasis.[14,22] Mild idiopathic hyperoxaluria may be seen, and elevations of urinary oxalate and calcium are frequently observed together in patients with idiopathic urolithiasis. A large dietary excess of oxalate may contribute to hyperoxaluria, though under normal circumstances less than 10% of dietary oxalate is absorbed and the majority of oxalate in the urine is derived from body metabolism. Diets low in calcium predispose to hyperoxaluria due to reduced binding of oxalate to calcium in the intestinal lumen, leaving oxalate free to be absorbed.[16] Certain anaerobic bacteria are capable of metabolizing oxalate, populate the intestinal tract of healthy individuals, and may play a role in the disposition of oxalate in the intestinal tract. Definition of the role of such bacteria awaits further study. Abnormalities of the intestinal tract that result in malabsorption of fat typically result in enhanced absorption of oxalate, referred to as 'enteric hyperoxaluria'.[22] In these conditions, the binding of calcium by fatty acids leaves less calcium in the intestinal lumen to combine with oxalate, such that oxalate is absorbed more avidly. In addition, bile salts cause injury to the colonic epithelium, thereby promoting enhanced oxalate absorption. The degree of hyperoxaluria caused by enteric dysfunction can vary from mild to severe and is influenced by dietary content of both oxalate and calcium.

The primary hyperoxalurias are associated with moderate to marked elevation of urine oxalate excretion due to inborn errors of metabolism.[15] These autosomal recessive disorders are due to deficiency of hepatic alanine: glyoxylate aminotransferase (type I) or glyoxylate reductase/hydroxypyruvate reductase (type II). Both of these enzymes are important in the metabolic disposition of glyoxylate, a precursor of oxalate found in hepatic cells. When there is a deficiency of the activity of either of these enzymes, oxalate is formed in large amounts and must be eliminated by renal excretion. Due to the degree of the resulting hyperoxaluria and the presence of the abnormality from birth, primary hyperoxaluria is characterized by particularly aggressive stone formation. Over time, due to repeated stone episodes which can be complicated by obstruction and infection, nephrocalcinosis, and other effects of oxalate on the renal tubular cells and interstitium, renal failure often results.[4] The primary hyperoxalurias are the most severe of all forms of urolithiasis. They are rare, with type I accounting for a large majority of those reported to date.[4] Approximately one-half of patients with type I primary hyperoxaluria respond to pharmacologic doses of pyridoxine (vitamin B_6), with reductions in the amount of oxalate produced. In the remaining patients with type I disease and those with type II disease, pyridoxine appears to have no effect. Other treatment approaches include the administration of neutral phosphate or citrate, which inhibit calcium oxalate crystallization and stone formation in the urine.[15] At present the inborn error of metabolism can only be corrected by liver transplantation in type I disease, and combined liver/kidney transplantation is often performed in type I patients with renal failure.

Cystinuria

Cystinuria accounts for 2–8% of stones in children and adolescents. An inherited defect in the renal tubular reabsorptive transport of cystine and the dibasic amino acids (ornithine, arginine, and lysine) accounts for the high concentrations of cystine in the urine of patients with this disorder.[13] Stones composed of cystine form due to cystine concentrations that exceed solubility at usual urine volumes. The increased urinary concentrations of the other dibasic amino acids and the accompanying intestinal dibasic amino acid transport defects appear to be without clinical consequence. Cystine solubility is enhanced at an alkaline urine pH, such that alkalinization of the urine is an important component of treatment.[9] However, even at an optimal urine pH of 7, cystine solubility in the urine is limited to approximately 1250 μmol (300 mg) per liter of urine. Cystine excretion

increases with urine sodium excretion, such that low-salt diets are beneficial. For patients whose stone formation cannot be adequately controlled with these measures and high oral fluid intake, the use of mercaptopropionyl glycine (Thiola) or D-penicillamine can be beneficial.[9] The use of captopril has been advocated, but results with this agent have been inconsistent.[9]

The prevalence of cystinuria in the general population in the United States and Europe is estimated at 1 in 7000. Three clinical subtypes have been described, based on the level of urinary cystine in obligate heterozygotes. Type I accounts for approximately 70% of patients with clinically evident cystinuria, and is completely recessive. Patients with type I/I show a mean cystine excretion rate of 4500 μmol/g creatinine,[7] with 50% or more developing stones within the first decade of life.[7] Mutations of the *SLC3A1* gene on chromosome 2p encoding the rBAT protein which is important in dibasic amino acid transport have been shown to be responsible. Types II and III were identified by elevated cystine excretion in obligate heterozygotes, and are caused by mutations of the *SLC7A9* gene on chromosome 19.[13] Heterozygotes with type II/N have cystine excretion from 400 to 2400 μmol/g creatinine, and may form stones. Those with III/N have lower cystine excretion and typically do not develop urolithiasis. Patients with types II/II and III/III have cystine excretion rates similar to those for I/I. Compound heterozygotes are common. Type I/III patients appear to excrete less cystine, and are unlikely to form stones within the first decade of life.[7] Other compound heterozygotes have not been as well studied. Due to immaturity of renal tubule function during infancy, the incomplete recessive nature of types II and III, and the complexity of compound heterozygosity, it is difficult to establish definitively the diagnosis of cystinuria prior to 1 year of age.

Hyperuricosuria

Hyperuricosuria is found in 2–10% of children with urolithiasis. Mild idiopathic hyperuricosuria may be a cause of hematuria,[27] and is often found in conjunction with hypercalciuria.[14,27] A defect in renal tubular transport of uric acid, either due to reduced proximal tubular reabsorption or to increased secretion has been implicated. Idiopathic renal hyperuricosuria is often familial and asymptomatic. Secondary hyperuricosuria may result from diets high in protein, or to ketogenic diets and from medications including probenecid, salicylates, and citrate as well as pancreatic extract therapy in patients with cystic fibrosis.[27] It can be seen in association with diabetes and the syndrome of inappropriate secretion of antidiuretic hormone.

Although uric acid crystals in the urine may contribute to urolithiasis by forming a nidus for calcium oxalate crystallization, uric acid stones are uncommon in childhood. Uric acid stones, when they occur in children, are generally due to marked overproduction of uric acid as occurs in tumor lysis syndrome, myeloproliferative disorders, or rare inborn errors of metabolism such as complete (Lesch–Nyhan syndrome) or partial deficiencies of hypoxanthine phosphoribosyl transferase (HPRT) enzyme activity.

Other Solute-Related Causes
Urinary tract stone disease in childhood or adolescence may result from urinary solute excess due to other rare inborn errors of metabolism including dihydroxyadeninuria, xanthinuria, orotic aciduria, and alkaptonuria.

Inhibitor Deficiencies
Deficiency of urinary inhibitors may also predispose to urolithiasis.[14,22,25] Citrate is a naturally occurring inhibitor of calcium oxalate and calcium phosphate crystallization, and has been found in some series to be reduced in the urine of children with calcium stones when compared with healthy children. The administration of potassium citrate has been shown to be of benefit in idiopathic stone-formers. Deficiency of urinary citrate occurs predictably as a result of hypokalemia, systemic or intracellular acidosis. However, in most such situations, the hypocitric aciduria is transient. In RTA, hypocitric aciduria persists until the metabolic acidosis is corrected. Interpretation of urinary citrate concentrations is complicated by the limited number of published studies of urinary citrate in normal children of various ages, and the fact that citrate is influenced by prandial state, dietary composition, and age. Pyrophosphate and magnesium in the urine are also known to act as inhibitors of calcium oxalate and calcium phosphate crystal formation. Deficiencies of pyrophosphate or magnesium have not been described as a primary cause of urolithiasis, although both neutral phosphates (which leads to increased urinary pyrophosphate concentrations) and magnesium have been used therapeutically to reduce stone formation.

A variety of urinary macromolecules appear to inhibit calcium oxalate crystal formation. Those studied include glycosaminoglycans, osteopontin, nephrocalcin, and urinary prothrombin fragment 1, among others.[23] Relatively lower concentrations of some of these inhibitors have been observed in children who form stones when compared with healthy children.[23] However, there is controversy regarding the role of urinary macromolecules in clinical disorders of stone formation.[23]

Clinical Conditions Associated with Urolithiasis
Lithogenic factors are associated with certain clinical conditions (Box 44-4). Premature infants are at risk of nephrocalcinosis and nephrolithiasis (Figure 44-8). In three prospective studies, renal calcifications occurred

Box 44-4 Clinical Conditions Associated with Urolithiasis

- Prematurity
- Inflammatory bowel disease
- Cystic fibrosis
- Glycogen storage disease
- Medullary sponge kidney
- Autosomal dominant polycystic kidney disease
- Distal RTA

in 64%, 16%, and 27% respectively of infants born at less than 1500 g or less than 32 weeks' gestation.[16,20] The likelihood of renal calcification appears greater in smaller infants, in those receiving furosemide or post-natal corticosteroids, with a longer duration of mechanical ventilation and parenteral nutrition, of white race, and with a family history of urolithiasis.[10,11] Metabolic disturbances including hypercalciuria, hypophosphatemia and hypercalcemia (both of which can induce hypercalciuria), and hyperoxaluria related to parenteral nutrition have been implicated.[11,16,20] Abnormalities of urine composition related to renal tubule immaturity may also play a role. Nephrocalcinosis resolves in approximately half of the patients, and new stone formation appears to cease with renal maturity. However, longer term studies performed at 4 to 12 years of age in very low birth weight children who had a history of renal calcifications demonstrated reduced ammonium excretion in response to furosemide, hypercalciuria, and hypocitric aciduria when compared with a control group of children born at term.[18] At the time of study, 18% of the children still had renal cortical

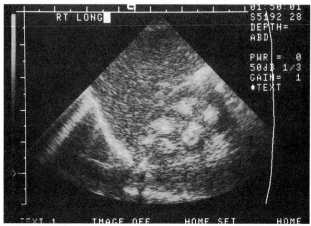

Figure 44-8 Ultrasonography showing dense renal medullary pyramids characteristic of nephrocalcinosis in a premature infant.

hyperechogenicity and 9% had urolithiasis. Whether the persistent abnormalities are the long-term result of renal tubular immaturity at birth, secondary to renal damage from nephrocalcinosis, or due to other factors remains to be established.

Inflammatory bowel disease and other diseases of the gastrointestinal tract associated with malabsorption can cause hypocitric aciduria and hypomagnesuria due to loss of bicarbonate and magnesium in the stool, hyperoxaluria from enhanced enteric oxalate absorption, hyperuricosuria due to increased cell turnover, and low urine volume because of diarrhea. These factors result in both reduced inhibitor activity and high solute concentrations in the urine. Urolithiasis and nephrocalcinosis occur with greater frequency in patients with cystic fibrosis when compared with healthy children and have been attributed to hyperoxaluria, hypocitric aciduria, and to increased urine uric acid related to large doses of pancreatic enzyme replacement. Hypercalciuria is also sometimes found in this patient group. Renal tubular damage related to antibiotic treatment has been implicated by some authors as a contributing cause.

Distal RTA results in hypocitric aciduria, hypercalciuria, and high urine pH. Multiple calcifications comprised of calcium phosphate and/or calcium oxalate in the region of the papillary tips of the kidneys are typical and are seen with both incomplete and complete forms of distal RTA. Hereditary forms of distal RTA are well described, some associated with deafness or osteopetrosis. Mutations in the red cell anion exchanger (Band 3, AE1) gene have been confirmed in several reported families. Secondary distal RTA such as occurs in Wilson's disease and Sjögren's syndrome has also been associated with urolithiasis. Hypercalciuria and hypocitric aciduria (which worsen with age) and distal RTA have been implicated in the nephrolithiasis associated with type 1a glycogen storage disease. Although proximal renal tubular acidosis is associated with hypercalciuria, urine citrate concentrations are usually normal and may protect against stone formation. Urolithiasis is not typically associated with proximal RTA, nor with type IV RTA.

Medullary sponge kidney is frequently associated with recurrent calcium urolithiasis. Hypercalciuria, hypocitric aciduria, incomplete RTA, and increased urine pH have been variably observed in such patients. Patients with autosomal dominant polycystic kidney disease have an increased likelihood of stone formation. Hypocitric aciduria, hypercalciuria, and hyperuricosuria are observed in this clinical setting. Thin basement membrane nephropathy is associated with hypercalciuria, hyperuricosuria, and resulting nephrolithiasis. Urolithiasis and nephrocalcinosis have also been observed in association with cystinosis.

Pharmacologic Agents Causing Urolithasis

Pharmacologic use of a variety of medications can result in urolithiasis (Box 44-5). Calculi may result from excretion of the medication or a metabolite into the urine at concentrations that exceed solubility, or they may occur due to secondary metabolic effects. The protease inhibitor indinavir, which is used widely in the treatment of human immunodeficiency virus (HIV), precipitates in the urine as crystals and stones. It is the parent drug that is poorly soluble in the urine at a pH of greater than 5 and forms radiolucent stones. The indinavir crystals or small stones may also act as a nidus for calcium oxalate or calcium phosphate, and can be associated with stones of mixed composition that may be radiopaque. Urinary tract stones have been observed in 2 to 28% of patients treated with this agent, and are frequently associated with ureteral obstruction and colic. There are a number of such reports in children. Due to the radiolucent nature of indinavir stones, they are not visible on non-contrast renal tomography, and their similarity to the density of soft tissue makes them difficult to see on CT scanning. Ultrasonography, intravenous pyelography, or CT urography may be needed to demonstrate indinavir stones and associated ureteral obstruction. Dissolution of stone material may be observed with discontinuation of indinavir, increased fluid intake, and urine acidification. Other medications that can precipitate to form urinary tract stones are ceftriaxone, sulfonamides, triamterene, guaifenesin, phenazopyridine, and acyclovir. Urinary tract stones are rarely observed with these agents.

Carbonic anhydrase inhibitors, which are administered for the management of epilepsy and glaucoma (among other uses), result in alkaline urine, reduced urine citrate, and hypercalciuria. Agents of this class – including zonisamide, topiramate, and dorzolamide – have been

Box 44-5 Pharmacologic Agents Associated with Urolithiasis

- Urinary excretion of agent with low solubility
  - Indinavir
  - Sulfonamides
  - Ceftriaxone
  - Triamterene
  - Guaifenesin
  - Pancreatic enzymes
- Metabolic effects
  - Furosemide
  - Corticosteroids
  - Carbonic anhydrase inhibitors
  - Vitamin D

reported to be associated with calcium phosphate and calcium oxalate urolithiasis in children. Corticosteroids, calcium supplements, vitamin D and its analogues are associated with hypercalciuria, and can predispose to stone formation. Aminophylline results in hypercalciuria, alkaline urine, and phosphaturia countered, in part, by its diuretic effects.

Infection as a Lithogenic Factor

Urease that is produced by certain strains of bacteria leads to hydrolysis of urea, with resulting production of ammonium and bicarbonate ions in the urine. In the presence of the increased pH, dissociation of phosphate occurs; with supersaturation of the urine for magnesium ammonium phosphate (struvite) and subsequent precipitation of stone material.[22] A variety of bacterial species produce urease, including *Proteus, Staphylococcus, Klebsiella, Providentia, Pseudomonas, Ureaplasma urealyticum*, and some anaerobes. A particular calculous encrustation of the pelvis of the kidney has been observed with *Corynebacterium urealyticum* infection, another urea-splitting organism. This encrusted pyelitis is typically observed in immune-suppressed patients (e.g., after renal transplantation), and may be associated with significant compromise of kidney function.

Although infection with urease-producing organisms can produce de-novo urolithiasis, most often the infection exacerbates underlying metabolic factors. With careful evaluation, 30–60% of patients with struvite or other infection stones can be also be demonstrated to have metabolic factors predisposing to stone formation.[14] Stasis due to urinary tract abnormalities also predisposes to infection.

Chronic bacteriuria can be a troublesome cause of stones. Struvite may deposit rapidly, and often forms staghorn calculi. It is difficult to eradicate infection as the bacteria reside in the interstices of the stone where antibiotic does not penetrate well. Bacteriuria quickly recurs when antibiotics are discontinued. Less than half of patients with infected staghorn calculi are rendered stone free by ESWL, and retained stone fragments are a nidus for early recurrence. Combined procedures, which may include percutaneous ultrasonic lithotripsy, are often needed. Any manipulation of infected stone material, but ESWL in particular, may distribute bacteria into the urinary tract and precipitate pyelonephritis. The use of parenteral antibiotic is advisable immediately prior to and following ESWL of stones known or suspected to be infected.

Structural Abnormalities of the Urinary Tract

Structural abnormalities of the urinary tract, whether congenital or acquired, are often associated with stasis of urine. Stasis predisposes to stone formation and to infection by compromising the normal continuous flow of urine in the upper tracts and the regular and complete emptying of urine from the bladder. Urolithiasis has been associated with a wide range of structural abnormalities including calyceal diverticulae, medullary sponge kidney, ureteropelvic junction obstruction, horseshoe kidney, ureteroceles, primary megaureters, posterior urethral valves, and the bladder extrophy-epispadius complex. Enterocystoplasty and urinary diversion employing intestinal mucosa are particularly prone to local formation of stones, with 30–50% of patients with enterocystoplasty reported to form bladder stones.[12] The difficulty in eradicating bacteria from the enteral mucosa, stasis, an alkaline urine pH due to infection or to exchange of chloride for bicarbonate across the mucosa, and the presence of mucous in the bladder all favor stone formation.[12] Foreign bodies such as sutures or staples or indwelling stents also can act as a nidus for stone formation.

However, with the exception of enterocystoplasty, the overall incidence of stones in children with structurally anomalous, obstructed, or infected urinary tracts is low, on the order of 1–5%.[14] This suggests that while stasis and infection promote stone formation, children who form stones may also have underlying metabolic abnormalities. Hypercalciuria, hyperoxaluria, or hypocitric aciduria have been identified in 60–80% of patients with structural abnormalities of the urinary tract and urolithiasis, and in 30–60% of those with infected stones in whom a metabolic evaluation was performed. For example, patients with myelodysplasia often have impaired bladder emptying, recurrent urinary tract infections, and hypercalciuria from relative immobility. Partial obstruction can result in deficient renal acidification with accompanying hypocitric aciduria. Accordingly, complete metabolic evaluation is just as important in children with structural abnormalities of the urinary tract or infection related stones as it is in those without.

LONG-TERM MANAGEMENT OF UROLITHIASIS

Treatment should be directed to the patient's individual predisposing factors (see Table 44-2). Evaluation of metabolic stone-forming activity over time, as determined by growth in the size of existing stones or the formation of new stones, is an important aspect of management. Periodic renal imaging is needed, the frequency of which will depend upon the type and number of stones and the severity of the abnormalities detected. In most circumstances, and in the absence of symptoms or infection, once yearly or every other year imaging is sufficient. Patients with significant metabolic problems such as primary hyperoxaluria, cystinuria, marked hypercalciuria, and those with infected stones (which can develop and grow quickly) may require more frequent evaluations. Ultrasonography has the advantage of visualization of radiolucent as well as radiopaque stones, detection of hydronephrosis, and the absence of radiation exposure and is preferred for most routine follow-up assessments. However, lack of sensitivity for detection of small stones, difficulty in comparing size of individual stones over time, lower sensitivity for visualization of ureteral stones, and the possibility of obstruction in the absence of hydronephrosis will at times dictate other imaging modalities. During follow-up, acute symptoms should prompt re-evaluation, including imaging studies.

Urolithiasis in children and adolescents, like that in adults, frequently recurs. Recurrence rates of 20-40% have been reported with variable follow-up periods. In one study of 221 children followed for a mean of 59 months (median 36 months), 67% demonstrated two or more stones during initial evaluation and follow-up.[14] Because of the usual persistence of underlying metabolic

abnormalities and known risk of recurrence, long-term follow-up with periodic reassessments of the activity of stone formation are indicated. If new stone formation occurs despite treatment, a more intensive management program should be implemented. Additional studies can be helpful in identification of therapies most likely to be effective. Such studies include determination of crystalluria by phase-contrast microscopy, supersaturation of the urine, and measurement of urinary inhibitor activity. Response to treatment is typically excellent in children of all ages.

MAJOR POINTS

- Urolithiasis occurs in children and adolescents of all ages, and should be included in the differential diagnosis of hematuria, flank or abdominal pain, and urinary tract infection. In children aged less than 5 years, non-specific abdominal symptoms are more common than pain with features of renal colic.
- The majority of urinary tract stones in children and adolescents are formed in the kidneys and are composed of calcium oxalate.
- Stones causing obstruction or acute renal colic, stones with a high potential for obstruction, and infected stones may require surgical intervention and should be evaluated jointly with a urologist. Other stones can be managed medically.
- Metabolic abnormalities, infection, and urinary stasis or obstruction predispose to formation of urinary tract calculi. One or more of these factors are found in the majority of children with urolithiasis.
- Metabolic evaluation and evaluation for stasis/obstruction and infection is indicated in every child or adolescent with urolithiasis.
- Hypercalciuria is the most common metabolic abnormality found in stone-formers.
- A number of clinical conditions including prematurity, inflammatory bowel disease, and primary and secondary RTA are associated with urolithiasis.
- High oral fluid intake and moderation in dietary calcium and sodium (to the RDA for age) are of benefit to nearly all stone-formers. These measures should be used along with treatment directed to the specific predisposing factors of each patient.
- Long-term follow-up and management are indicated due to the risk of stone recurrence.

REFERENCES

1. Alon US, Berenbom A. Idiopathic hypercalciuria of childhood: 4- to 11-year outcome. Pediatr Nephrol 2000; 14:1011-1015.
2. Brinkman OA, Griehl A, Kuwertz-Broking E, et al. Extracorporeal shock wave lithotripsy in children. Eur Urol 2001;39:591-597.
3. Cervera A, Corral MJ, Gómez Campdera FJ, et al. Idiopathic hypercalciuria in children. Acta Paediatr Scand 1987; 76:271-278.
4. Cochat P, Deloraine A, Rotily M, et al. Epidemiology of primary hyperoxaluria type I. Nephrol Dial Transplant 1995;10:3-7.
5. Diamond DA. Clinical patterns of paediatric urolithiasis. Br J Urol 1991;68:195-198.
6. Gearhart JP, Herzberg GZ, Jeffs RD, Childhood urolithiasis: experiences and advances. Pediatrics 1991;87:445-450.
7. Goodyer P, Saadi I, Ong P, et al. Cystinuria subtype and the risk of nephrolithiasis. Kidney Int 1998;54:56-61.
8. Harangi F, Mehes K. Family investigations in idiopathic hypercalciuria. Eur J Pediatr 1993;152:64-68.
9. Joly D, Rieu P, Mejean A, et al. Treatment of cystinuria. Pediatr Nephrol 1999;13:945-950.
10. Karlowicz MG, Katz ME, Adelman RD, et al. Nephrocalcinosis in very low birth weight neonates: Family history of kidney stones and ethnicity as independent risk factors. J Pediatr 1993;122:635-638.
11. Katz ME, Karlowicz MG, Adelman RD, et al. Nephrocalcinosis in very low birth weight neonates: sonographic patterns, histologic characteristics, and clinical risk factors. J Ultrasound Med 1994;13:777-782.
12. Khoury AE, Salomon M, Doche R, et al. Stone formation after augmentation cystoplasty: the role of intestinal mucus. J Urol 1997;158:1133-1137.
13. Langen H, von Kietzell D, Byrd D, et al. Renal polyamine excretion, tubular amino acid reabsorption and molecular genetics in cystinuria. Pediatr Nephrol 2000;14:376-384.
14. Milliner DS, Murphy ME. Urolithiasis in pediatric patients. Mayo Clin Proc 1993;68:241-248.
15. Milliner DS, Eickholt JT, Bergstralh E, et al. Primary hyperoxaluria: results of long-term treatment with orthophosphate and pyridoxine. N Engl J Med 1994;331:1553-1558.

16. Milliner DS. Epidemiology of calcium oxalate urolithiasis in man. In: Kahn S (ed.), *Calcium Oxalate in Biological Systems.* CRC Press, Boca Raton, 1995, pp. 169–188.

17. Miyake O, Yoshimura K, Yoshioka T, et al. High urinary excretion level of citrate and magnesium in children: potential etiology for the reduced incidence of pediatric urolithiasis. Urol Res 1998;26:209–213.

18. Monge M, Garcia-Nieto VM, Domenech E, et al. Study of renal metabolic disturbances related to renal lithiasis at school age in very low birth weight children. Nephron 1998;79:269–273.

19. Moore ES. Hypercalciuria in children. Contrib Nephrol 1981;27:20–32.

20. Narendra A, White MP, Rolton HA, et al. Nephrocalcinosis in preterm babies. Arch Dis Child Fetal Neonatal 2001;85:F207–F213.

21. Pietrow PK, Pope JC, Adams MC, et al. Clinical outcome of pediatric stone disease. J Urol 2002;167:670–673.

22. Polinsky MS, Kaiser BA, Baluarte HJ. Urolithiasis in childhood. Pediatr Clin North Am 1987;34:683–710.

23. Ryall RL. Glycosaminoglycans, proteins, and stone formation: adult themes and child's play. Pediatr Nephrol 1996;10:656–666.

24. Scheinman SJ. X-linked hypercalciuric nephrolithiasis: clinical syndromes and chloride channel mutations. Kidney Int 1998;53:3–17.

25. Scheinman SJ. Nephrolithiasis. Semin Nephrol 1999;19: 381–388.

26. Stapleton FB. Clinical approach to children with urolithiasis. Semin Nephrol 1996;16:389–397.

27. Stapleton FB. Hematuria associated with hypercalciuria and hyperuricosuria: A practical approach. Pediatr Nephrol 1994;8:756–761.

Index

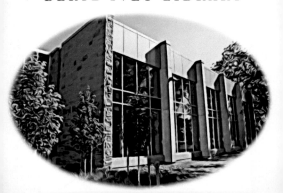

UNIVERSITY COLLEGE

Brescia

BERYL IVEY LIBRARY

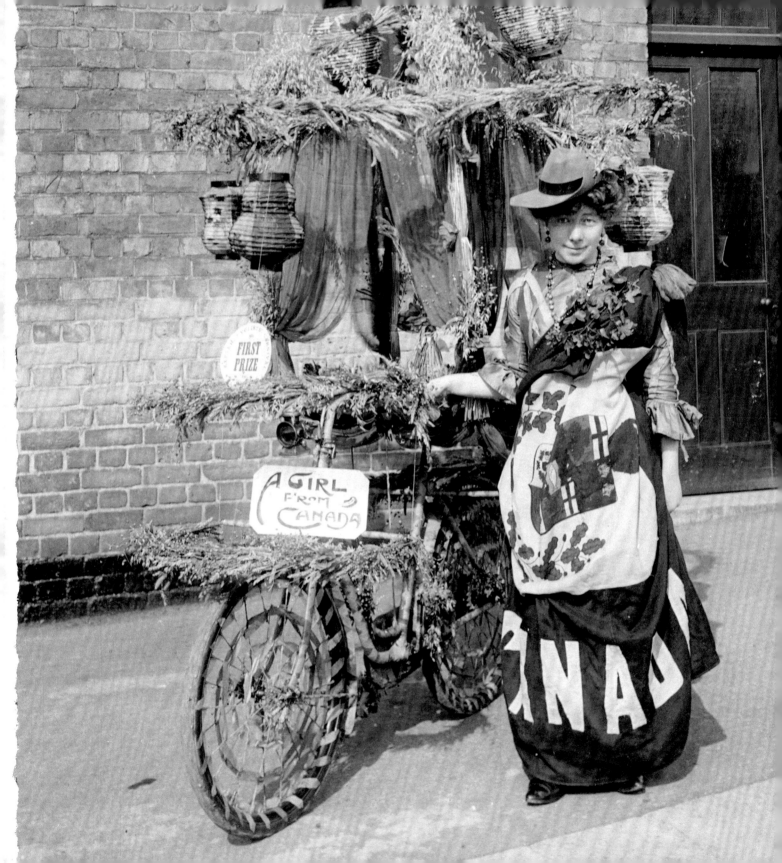

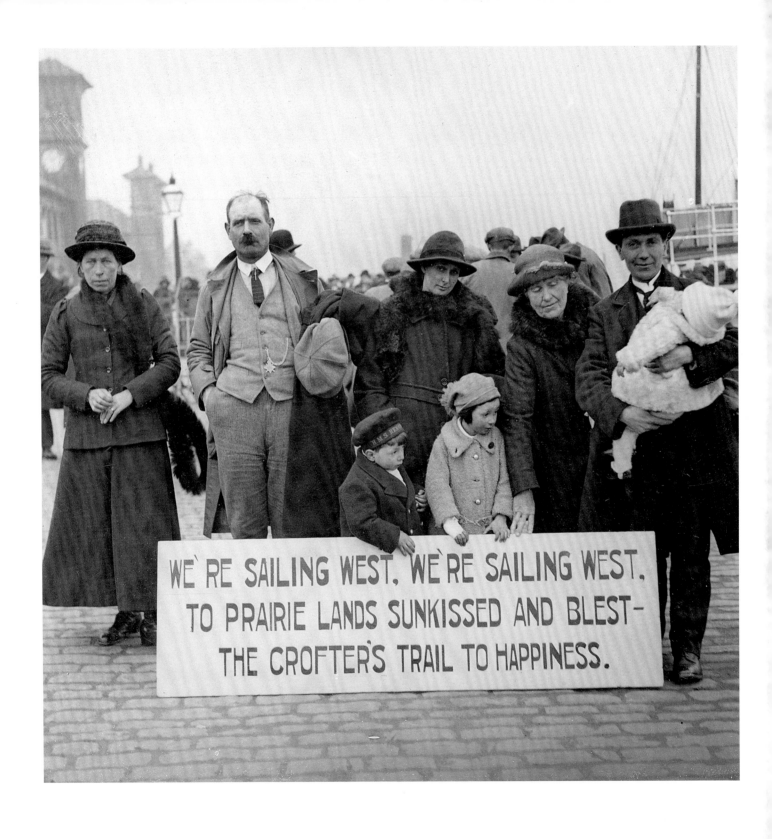

WE'RE SAILING WEST, WE'RE SAILING WEST, TO PRAIRIE LANDS SUNKISSED AND BLEST— THE CROFTER'S TRAIL TO HAPPINESS.

DANIEL FRANCIS

SELLING CANADA

Three propaganda campaigns
that shaped the nation

Stanton Atkins & Dosil Publishers / *Vancouver*

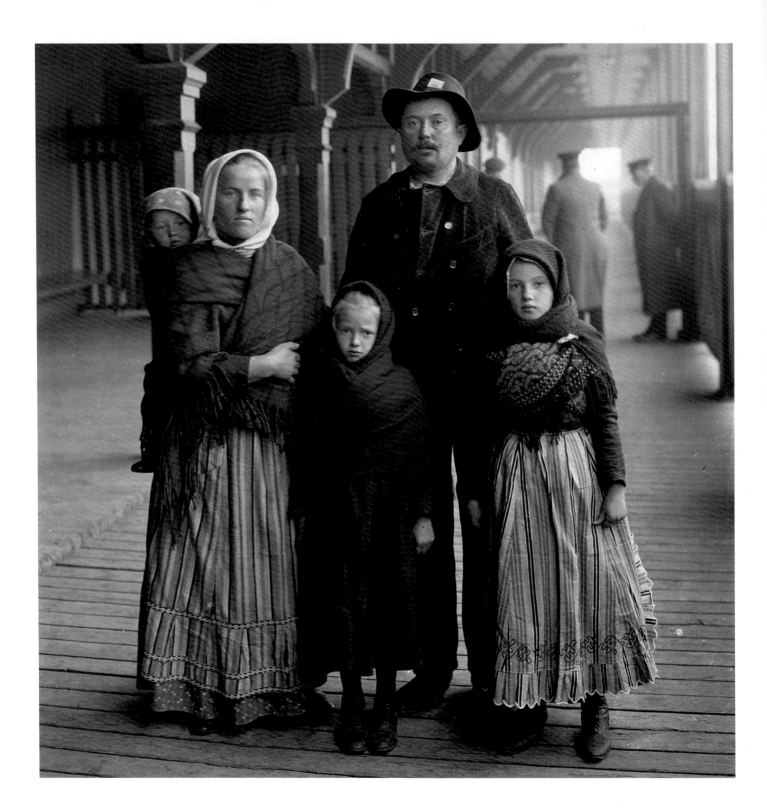

CONTENTS

JAMES OLIVER CURWOOD

Back to God's Country

Thirteen stirring tales of love and adventure set in the wilderness of the north country

PROMOTING GOD'S COUNTRY

Not far from the rugged and storm-whipped north shore of Lake Superior,
and south of the Kaministiqua, yet not as far south as the Rainy River
waterway, there lay a paradise lost in the heart of a wilderness world.
   – JAMES OLIVER CURWOOD, *The Country Beyond*, 1922

WHEN HE WAS A YOUNG BOY GROWING UP IN OWOSSO, MICHIGAN, JAMES OLIVER
Curwood took every opportunity he could to sneak away from school to trap
rabbits in the woods. An impulsive youth, eager to win the admiration of the
other youngsters, he once brought a pistol to class to impress his friends and
on another occasion attacked his teacher with his fists. "Under my white skin I
was almost an Indian," he later said of his childhood self, meaning that he was
happiest running wild on his own.

   When he wasn't off playing in the woods or getting into trouble at school,
Curwood spent time training himself to be a writer. "Before I was fifteen years
old," he recalled, "I had written more than a hundred stories ranging in length
from five hundred to twenty thousand words." He mailed them off to magazines
around the country and the rejection slips he collected only seemed to make
him more determined. On one occasion he copied a poem by Lord Byron out of
a British magazine and sold it as his own for fifty cents. When the truth came
out the editor who accepted it was too embarrassed at not having recognized the
fraud to complain. Finally, in 1898, when he was nineteen years old, Curwood
sold his first story for five dollars to a magazine in Cincinnati and the career of
one of North America's most successful popular writers was launched.

   Curwood studied at the University of Michigan but his literary ambitions
trumped his academic ones and he quit school to take a job at a Detroit newspaper. At the same time he continued to grind out magazine articles and then
began publishing books. It was in Detroit that the young writer met M.V. Mac-
Inness, a representative of the Canadian Immigration Department. The pre-
World War I immigration boom was on in Canada and the department's agents
were stationed all over the United States encouraging likely settlers to pick up

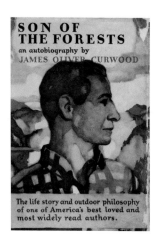

SON OF
THE FORESTS
an autobiography by
JAMES OLIVER CURWOOD

The life story and outdoor philosophy
of one of America's best loved and
most widely read authors.

James Oliver Curwood's autobiography, *Son of the Forests* (Grosset & Dunlap, 1930), tells the story of his years working as a "wilderness freelance" for the Canadian government. Curwood's many books established the image of Canada as a northern wilderness, "God's Country."

and move to "The Last, Best West," the Canadian prairie. Through his contact with MacInness, Curwood received an offer he could not refuse. The Canadian government would pay him $1,800 a year, about three times the income of an average working family, plus expenses, to travel around northern and western Canada gathering eyewitness material, which he would then incorporate into articles and stories that would publicize the benefits of western settlement. For a decade Curwood spent a part of each year in western Canada working, as he put it, "as a prairie and wilderness freelance for the Canadian government." He took what he saw of what was then a raw frontier and transformed it into wholesome melodrama for the reading public, producing more than thirty books. Titles included *The Honour of the Big Snows, Nomads of the North, The Courage of Marge O'Doone* and *The Valley of the Silent Men*. (He once said that his ambition was to produce stories "of brave men and beautiful women who dared much, loved greatly, and died bravely.") Curwood coined the term "God's Country" to describe the wilds of Canada, and for most of his readers the term became synonymous with Canada itself. Where was it exactly? Not very helpfully, Curwood once called it "the land where the lean wolves run," and the publicity for one of the Hollywood adaptations of his stories said it was "away in the timber lands of the North where the purity of women is placed above all else." Clearly God's Country was a fantasy, a land of the imagination that Curwood's government paymasters were happy to have people believe exemplified Canada.

In 1915 the Canadian team of Ernest Shipman and his young wife Nell made one of Curwood's stories into a silent film. *God's Country and the Woman* was set in Canada but filmed on location in the mountains of California and it made a star out of Nell, who also produced and directed. From then on she was

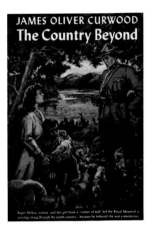

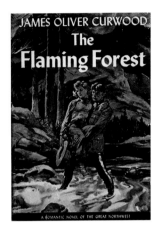

known as "the girl from God's Country" – which she actually was; she was born in Victoria, moving to Seattle as a teenager. In 1918 Curwood struck a deal with the Shipmans, who acquired rights to his stories in return for Nell agreeing to appear exclusively in films based on them. The first, and as it turned out only, result of this partnership was *Back to God's Country,* filmed in Calgary and at Lesser Slave Lake. Notorious for including the first nude scene in Canadian cinema – hardly the sort of wholesome entertainment, one would have thought, that the Canadian government was looking for – the movie was a hit with audiences. But it turned out that there was temptation in God's Country. Nell ran off with the film's production manager and the Shipman marriage foundered. Curwood was collateral damage in this domestic skirmish; the Shipmans' breakup brought an end to their business deal.

But it was not the end of the writer's romance with Hollywood. Curwood formed his own production company, which made two films, *Nomads of the North* (1920) starring Lon Chaney, and *The Golden Snare* (1921) with Wallace Beery. Several more movies made by other producers were inspired by his stories, one as recently as 1989 when French director Jean-Jacques Annaud made *The Bear,* a wildlife adventure based on the 1916 novel, *The Grizzly King.* (On this occasion the mountainous Dolomite region of northern Italy stood in for the wilds of British Columbia.) Curwood himself used his considerable earnings to build a replica French château, Curwood Castle, on the banks of the Shiawassee River in his hometown of Owosso where he lived when he was not away on fishing or hunting trips. Ironically for someone so identified with the great outdoors and its fierce wildlife, Curwood died in 1927, age forty-nine, of complications from a spider bite. His castle is now a museum.

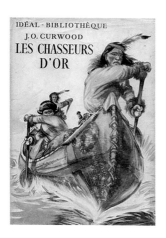

Les Chasseurs D'Or was a French-language translation of one of Curwood's earliest novels, *The Gold Hunters*, published in 1909.

THE CANADIAN GOVERNMENT GOT REASONABLE VALUE FOR ITS INVESTMENT IN James Curwood's literary talents. Hundreds of thousands of readers devoured his stories and just as many saw silent versions of them at the cinema. Curwood's northern romances may have been a little over the top when it came to portraying Canada as a northern wilderness full of desperadoes and other predatory animals. Still, no publicity was bad publicity, and a country striving to create a name for itself needed all the help it could get. Curwood's wilderness potboilers portrayed a place where opportunities for outdoor adventure were plentiful, the scenery was stunning, and square-jawed Mounties always got their man. In other words, Canada was exotic (but safe), adventureful (but well governed) and wild (but beautiful and accessible); just the sort of country that might appeal to a British or American tourist looking for somewhere exciting to visit or an immigrant looking for a new place to call home.

James Curwood may have been the only professional writer the Canadian government put on retainer, but he was not the only propagandist to work at selling Canada to outsiders or to promote a particular vision of Canada to her own citizens. Far from it.

In the 1890s Ottawa employed a small army of functionaries, some on staff, others on contract, whose job it was to extol the virtues of the Dominion to any potential immigrant who would listen. Canada needed settlers and was not very particular about where they came from. Agents travelled across the United States and Europe spreading the good word about Canada and offering incentives to anyone wishing to relocate there. With the completion of the transcontinental railway in 1885, the prairie West became in easy reach of anyone wishing to make a new start. Both the government and the railway company carried on an intensive, and sometimes misleading, advertising campaign to attract settlers. During World War I the job of promoting Canada turned inward as the government recognized that the military effort required the unswerving support of everyone on the home front. Once the initial wave of enthusiasm for the war had ebbed, it began to dawn on Canadians that they were in for a long struggle against a determined foe. In response, the government launched a second major propaganda campaign, this one aimed at stiffening the resolve of the public to see the conflict through. And from the late 1800s to the present, tourism promoters have been waging a third advertising campaign, one aimed at visitors to Canada. This campaign began with the construction of the railways and the creation of the first national parks, and continued with the "branding" of Canada as a wilderness paradise that was both exotic and civilized.

In each campaign, whether the audience consisted of immigrants, Canadian citizens or tourists, the government and its allies unleashed the relatively new techniques of advertising and propaganda to shape the country's public image in order to "sell Canada."

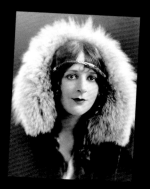

Back to God's Country was Curwood's first foray into filmmaking. The 1919 drama featured silent-film star Nell Shipman (above), who was born Helen Foster-Barham in Victoria, BC, in 1892. *Back to God's Country* gave Curwood's version of Canada the full Hollywood treatment.

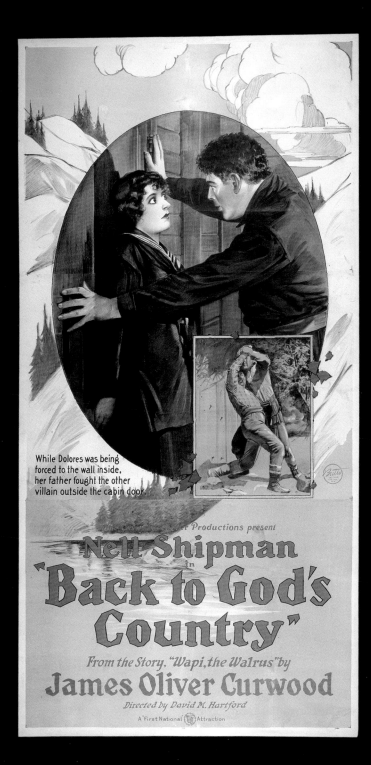

While Dolores was being forced to the wall inside, her father fought the other villain outside the cabin door.

...t Productions present

Nell Shipman
in
"Back to God's Country"

From the Story, "Wapi, the Walrus" by
James Oliver Curwood

Directed by David M. Hartford

A First National Attraction

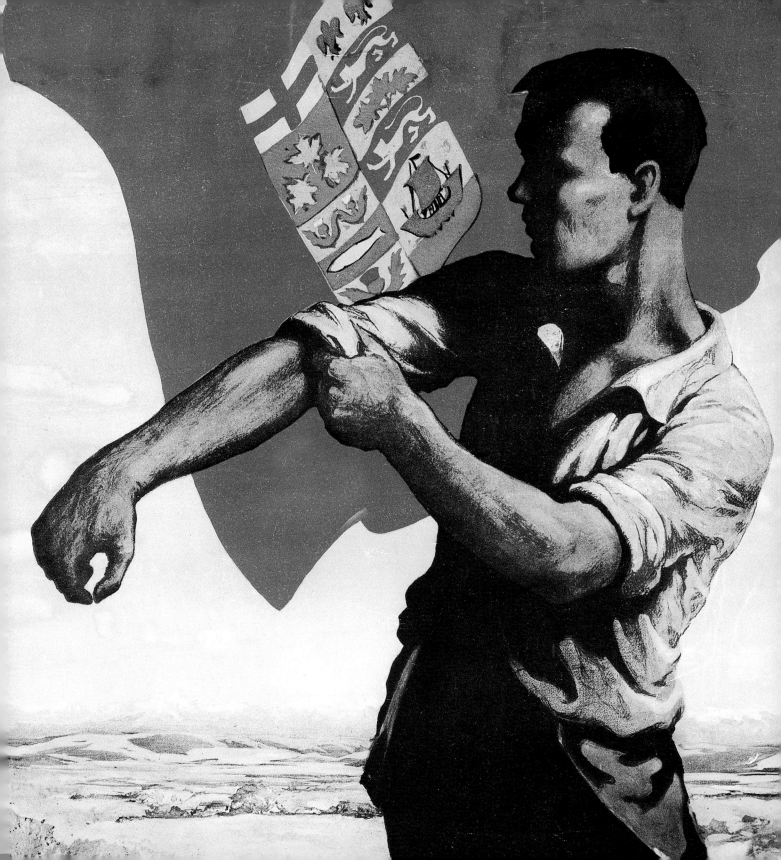

A PROMISED LAND:
Selling Canada to Immigrants

CHAPTER ONE

*Oh, it is all very fine, when I was at home, reading about this
sort of thing; but I confess the reality sometimes appals me.*
  – British immigrant to the Canadian West, 1890

AT THE TURN OF THE TWENTIETH CENTURY, Canada put out the welcome mat and opened its door to the world. "I don't care what language a man speaks, or what religion he professes," the government minister responsible for immigration, Clifford Sifton, declared in the House of Commons in 1899. "If he is honest and law-abiding, if he will go on that land and make a living for himself and his family, he is a desirable settler."

Newcomers responded to Sifton's invitation enthusiastically. In 1896, when the Laurier government of which he was a member took office, 16,835 immigrants came to Canada. By 1901 that number had more than tripled, to 55,747, and in another five years it had almost quadrupled again.

This flood of immigrants was not unique to Canada. It was part of an unprecedented international flow of people from Europe and, to a lesser extent, Asia, into North and South America. Tens of millions of people left their homes in search of new opportunities across the ocean. Eager to divert this human stream toward its own North-West, so recently opened to settlement, the Canadian government launched an aggressive advertising campaign aimed at potential immigrants. The product for sale was nothing less than Canada itself.

CANADA HAD ACQUIRED THE NORTH-WEST (basically, the land west and north of Ontario all the way to the Rockies) through negotiation and force of arms. In 1869 the government in Ottawa, then just two years old, struck a deal with the Hudson's Bay Company (HBC) and the British government to take ownership of Rupert's Land, the company's vast fur-trade territory in the interior. Prime Minister John A. Macdonald chose not to absorb the region into Canada as a province or provinces, but instead to administer it as the North-West Territories. When the Metis residents of the Red River Colony objected to what they experienced as high-handed colonial rule and set up their own government under their leader, Louis Riel,

OPPOSITE This image from a Canadian Pacific Railway poster conveys the central theme of the immigration campaign: that western Canada was a fertile paradise for newcomers who were not afraid to roll up their sleeves and get to work.

Land in the North-West was a commodity the government used to reward friends and public servants. This certificate, dated February 24, 1880, grants a quarter section (64 hectares) to Sub-Constable William Johnson, a member of the North West Mounted Police. The prospect of receiving land from a grateful government in return for service encouraged many young men to join the force.

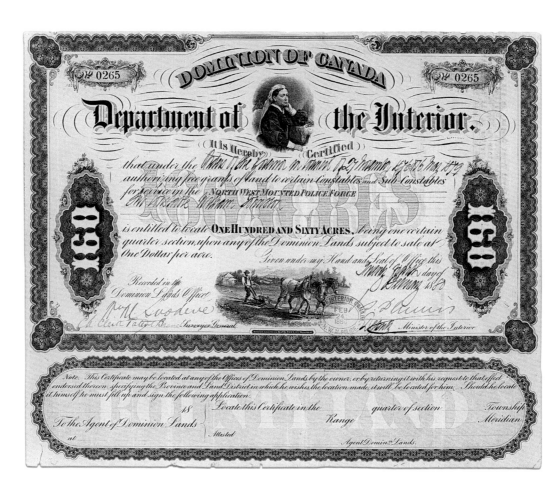

Prime Minister John A. Macdonald was determined to make the North-West part of Canada, and his response to the Red River uprising showed that he was willing to use force to do so. In addition to sending troops to oppose Riel and his followers, Macdonald also initiated policies that prepared the way for a peaceful influx of settlers. In 1895, four years after his death, the citizens of his hometown, Kingston, unveiled a statue in his memory in City Park. This souvenir commemorates the event.

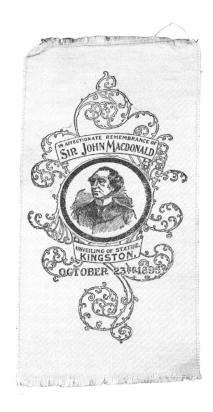

Macdonald sent in troops to assert Canadian authority. Riel, a wanted man, bolted for the United States, but many of his demands were realized with the creation of the Province of Manitoba in July 1870. The new "postage-stamp" province, a rectangle roughly 160 kilometres square surrounding the confluence of the Assiniboine and Red Rivers, was only a fraction of its present size. The rest of the North-West remained territories controlled from Ottawa.

With the matter of Canadian ownership settled, the challenge was to populate the new land with settlers. Macdonald was not an enthusiastic colonizer but he recognized that if Canada did not act, the Americans might. "I would be quite willing, personally, to leave that whole country a wilderness for the next half century," he remarked, "but I fear if Englishmen do not go there, Yankees will." Macdonald instructed the lieutenant-governor of Manitoba to suggest the best policies "for the removal of any obstructions that might be presented to the flow of population into the fertile lands that lie between Manitoba and the Rocky Mountains." His government negotiated with a private company, the Canadian Pacific, to build a transcontinental railway (completed in 1885). It initiated a survey of the territory and in 1872 opened the land to settlers by way of the Dominion Lands Act. This legislation allowed any male at least twenty-one years old to obtain a quarter section of land (64 hectares), known as a homestead, for a ten-dollar fee so long as he lived on the land, made improvements, started cultivating it and became a British subject. After 1882 women who were the head of a family were welcome to apply for land as well. Homesteaders might also place a pre-emption on an adjoining quarter section for which they had three years to meet the same requirements, or they could buy land belonging to one of the railways. Macdonald also created a police force, the North West Mounted Police, to impose Canadian law, and negotiated a series of treaties with the First Nations in order to extinguish their rights to the land. All of this was done to clear the way for settlement.

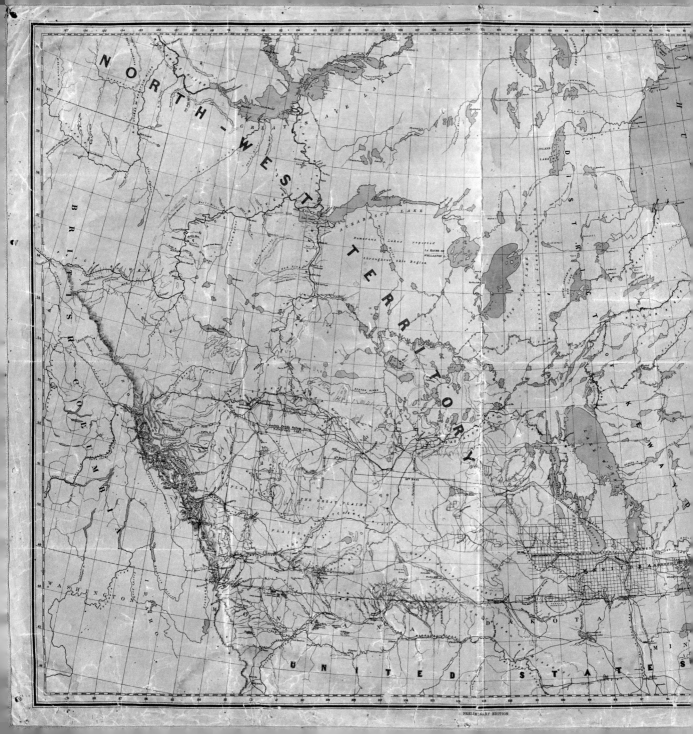

NORTH-WEST TERRITORY

BRITISH COLUMBIA

WASHINGTON

IDAHO

MONTANA

DAKOTA

UNITED STATES

PRELIMINARY EDITION.

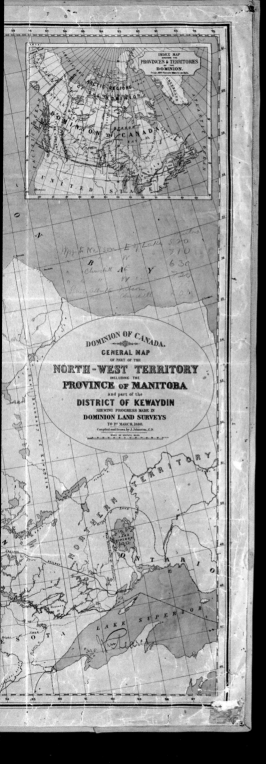

DOMINION OF CANADA.
GENERAL MAP
OF PART OF THE
NORTH-WEST TERRITORY
INCLUDING THE
PROVINCE OF MANITOBA
and part of the
DISTRICT OF KEWAYDIN
SHEWING PROGRESS MADE IN
DOMINION LAND SURVEYS
TO 1ST MARCH, 1880.
Compiled and Drawn by J. Johnston, C.D.

LEFT Before settlement by outsiders began, teams of surveyors from the Dominion Lands Branch arrived in the North-West to lay out the checkerboard grid system that would divide the territory into homestead lots. The survey began in 1873, following passage of the Dominion Lands Act, and continued for several years. This map shows the progress that had been made up to March 1, 1880. Note that while the "postage-stamp" province of Manitoba is rendered completely, much of the rest of the North-West remains to be surveyed. Metis residents were suspicious of the surveyors and afraid that their property rights were being ignored. These anxieties fed the unrest that later culminated in the North-West Rebellion of 1885.

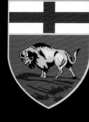

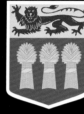

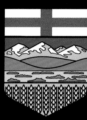

ABOVE Unlike European heraldic devices, which frequently feature mythical beasts, the coats of arms for Canada's western provinces feature real animals and hint at the promise of a magnificent and fertile land. Manitoba's shield (1) includes a bison, while wheat sheaves figure prominently on Saskatchewan's shield (2) and the Rocky Mountains predominate on Alberta's shield (3).

William Francis Butler was thirty-two years old when he came to Canada with the Red River military expedition in 1870. This force was sent to Manitoba in the wake of an uprising of Metis who feared their land would be taken from them. Butler was commissioned to report on conditions in the territories west of Manitoba, and that summer he completed a 6,000-kilometre trip to the Rocky Mountains and back. His report, published in England in 1872 as *The Great Lone Land*, is a celebrated Canadian travel narrative. Later Butler served in several imperial military campaigns in Africa. He died in 1910.

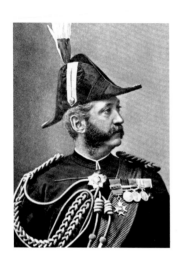

As well as practical policies for settlement, there had to be a revolution in the way the outside world imagined the North-West. For decades, the powerful Hudson's Bay Company had been telling whoever would listen that its Rupert's Land territory was a frozen wasteland inhabitable only by Indians and hardy fur traders. In 1812 the British noble Thomas Douglas, Earl Selkirk, had attempted to establish a farm settlement at the confluence of the Red and Assiniboine rivers but in the end this struggling colony, afflicted by locusts, floods and the hostility of the local Metis, seemed only to prove that Rupert's Land was hostile to settlers. Certainly the HBC did not want anyone getting the idea that its jealously guarded empire might be suitable for agriculture. "I do not think that any part of the Hudson's Bay Company's territories is well adapted for settlement," the company's governor, Sir George Simpson, told a British parliamentary committee in 1857. At the same time, the widely held perception of the interior plains was that they were a desert, incapable of supporting farming. This image was fortified by the British adventurer William Francis Butler, who rode across the prairies on horseback in 1870. Butler titled the book that he wrote about his experiences *The Great Lone Land*, a memorable phrase that neatly summed up the prevailing view of the North-West. "There is no other portion of the globe in which travel is possible where loneliness can be said to live so thoroughly," he informed his readers. Butler described a vacant region that seemed to exist outside of time, outside of history. "This ocean has no point – time has been naught to it; and men have come and gone, leaving behind them no track, no vestige, of their presence... One saw here the world as it had taken shape and form from the hands of the Creator."

Butler's presentation of the North-West as a primordial wilderness was already losing credibility even as his book was published. The process of reimagining the region had started earlier in the nineteenth century as explorers, scientists and railway surveyors ventured into the North-West and discovered that it was not the

IN THE SUMMER OF 1881 THE Marquis of Lorne, Canada's governor general, made a tour of the North-West, accompanied by four journalists from England. The party travelled by rail as far as Portage la Prairie, Manitoba, on the Canadian Pacific line, which was still under construction. From there they struck out overland by wagon to Calgary. It was an impressive cavalcade, including not only Lorne, his staff, various government officials and the foreign journalists, but a troop of North West Mounted Police as well. In all, seventy-seven men, twenty-seven wagons and ninety-six horses made their way across the rutted trail toward the foothills.

The purpose of Lorne's "royal tour" was to publicize western Canada, especially in Britain. "I have great hope that this journey may be of some use in advertising the new territories," he wrote. Not only did the government want to illustrate the agricultural potential of the area, it also wanted to show that peace and security prevailed, unlike in the United States where Indian wars were raging. Lorne was the son-in-law of Queen Victoria. How better to impress the British public than to show a member of the royal family swanning around the Canadian

West in perfect safety? A speech he gave in Winnipeg on his return trip eastward predicting a great future for the western plains was produced as a pamphlet and distributed widely in Europe.

One of the journalists who accompanied Lorne was Sydney Prior Hall, a reporter-artist with the London *Graphic*. Hall's dispatches were typical in their positive attitude toward emigration. The North-West "comprises the best and most desirable lands now open for free settlement in any quarter of the globe," he told his readers. Hall made one hundred sketches of the expedition for the *Graphic*. One recorded a

meeting at Blackfoot Crossing in southern Alberta with Chief Crowfoot, the venerated Blackfoot leader. The Blackfoot, who had signed a treaty with Ottawa in 1877, were suffering terribly from the disappearance of the buffalo and the failure of the government to fulfill its promises to provide food rations. In Hall's sketch, Crowfoot can be seen gesturing with a tin cup, indicating the poverty of his people and making a plea for assistance. While the government tried to sell the West as a land of opportunity to outsiders, it was neglecting the welfare of the original inhabitants for whom settlement posed many challenges.

THE GOVERNOR GENERAL JOINS THE PUBLICITY TRAIL

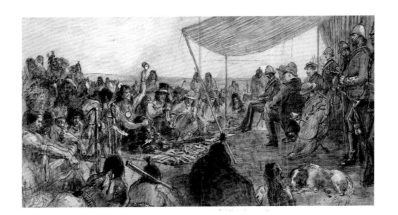

A pencil sketch by Sydney Prior Hall of Chief Crowfoot and a party of Blackfoot meeting with the Marquis of Lorne at Blackfoot Crossing on September 10, 1881.

The sketch was the basis for a larger pastel, which in turn was the basis for a finished oil painting commissioned for the marquis.

In overpopulated Britain, government posters regularly advertised settlement opportunities in Canada, Australia, South Africa and other parts of the Empire. This poster promotes Canada as a destination that is much easier to reach than any of the other colonies.

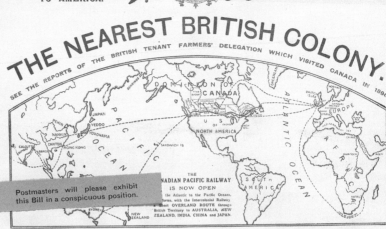

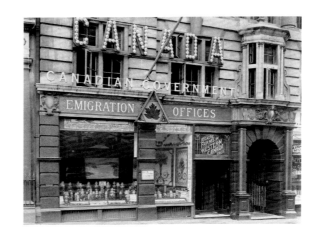

arid wasteland that Governor Simpson liked to pretend. During the 1850s two government expeditions visited, one sponsored by the United Canadas (today's Ontario and Quebec) and the other by the British. Both reported back that the region held significant economic potential. By the time the Canadian government acquired Rupert's Land from the HBC in 1869, the image of western Canada was changing from desert to oasis. It was to help this process along, and to counter the stereotype of a western wilderness inimical to farm settlement, that the Canadian government launched its ambitious and wide-ranging propaganda campaign to rebrand the region as a settlement frontier and to redirect the flow of immigrants away from the US, Australia and South America toward the Canadian West.

UNDER THE BRITISH NORTH AMERICA ACT, immigration was a responsibility shared by Ottawa with the provinces. At a meeting in 1868, the year after Confederation,

provincial and federal representatives agreed that the national government would take a leading role in immigration promotion. To this end Canada opened one immigration office in London and another on the European mainland, and as the years passed offices opened in other cities when the need was identified. At the same time, provinces were free to have their own agents working in the field. This joint activity led to competition between provinces and at a subsequent federal-provincial meeting delegates agreed to a set of guidelines that once again asserted Ottawa's primacy in the area. Between Confederation and 1892 the federal Department of Agriculture held responsibility for immigration, which then shifted to the Department of the Interior until 1917, when immigration became its own department in the federal bureaucracy.

In the early days, immigration promotion took the form of simple pamphlets extolling the benefits of western settlement. One of the authors of these early

tracts was Thomas Spence, "the father of western immigration pamphlets." An immigrant from Scotland himself, he had arrived with his family in the Red River Settlement in 1866 and became a vocal advocate of the North-West's union with Canada. Following the creation of Manitoba, he was appointed clerk of the Legislative Council and in that position he published his first pamphlet. Forty-six pages long, it bore the quaintly cumbersome title, *Manitoba and the North-West of the Dominion, Its Resources and Advantages to the Emigrant and Capitalist,* and trumpeted the advantages of the Canadian prairie over the western United States. "The North-West," enthused Spence, "the future destiny of which will be a great and glorious one, possesses all the true elements of future greatness and prosperity." A harsh climate? Don't believe it, wrote Spence. The weather was as mild as England, with less snow than fell in the settled parts of eastern America. It was "a climate of unrivalled salubrity," and "one of the healthiest in the world." The land

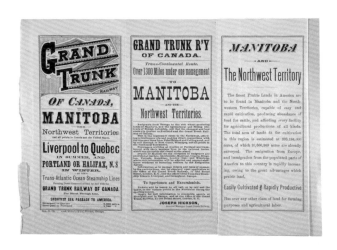

This pamphlet produced in 1880 represents the early days of immigration promotion, when publications were bland in design and presentation. It promises that "the finest Prairie Lands in America are to be found in Manitoba and the North-western Territories." Millions of acres of "easily cultivated and rapidly productive" land are available, the pamphlet says, "affording every facility for agricultural productions of all kinds." As time passed, promotional literature became easier on the eye and ever more boastful in its language.

was fertile, and best of all there was lots of it available to the energetic pioneer willing to be in the vanguard of settlement. *Manitoba and the North-West* was one of six pamphlets that Spence wrote, all of them mixing useful information for the "emigrant" with exaggerated claims for the good life, setting the pattern for the many hundreds of similar pamphlets that would follow.

The overheated prose of these thin publications had to make up for their blandness of design and production. Printed on flimsy paper, featuring no photographs or illustrations of any kind, they were the best that the print technology of the period could produce. Nonetheless, they were distributed in the hundreds of thousands across Canada and throughout western Europe. Historian Douglas Owram notes that the names of Thomas Spence and Acton Burrows, another pamphleteer, "were probably more widely known in Europe than were those of Charles G.D. Roberts and Charles Mair." A single pamphlet might have 300,000 copies in print;

one early government publication, *Information for Intending Emigrants*, had a print run of one million.

Early government promotional efforts focused on Britain and in 1872 an immigration office opened in London. From there, William Dixon, the senior immigration agent, managed the work of sub-agents in several other cities. The offices distributed information about Canada, making sure that it was prominently displayed in railway stations and post offices around the British Isles. Agents also went into the field, delivering lectures in the small rural communities where they were most likely to find the type of agriculturalist Canada was looking for. Many of these lectures were reprinted in local papers and ended up as pamphlets. Agents were admonished to be truthful and accurate in their presentations but inevitably a certain amount of exaggeration crept in as they tried to convince prospective immigrants of the charms of Canada. "Enthusiasm rather than fraud typified the writings on the North-West,"

BELOW In an attempt to reach farming communities outside the large urban centres, an assortment of horse-drawn publicity wagons travelled the countryside of the United Kingdom in the early twentieth century. This small wagon toured Wales.

RIGHT This large, heavily laden wagon carried examples of agricultural produce of all kinds around the Scottish countryside. The containers would have held seed samples of different grains and vegetables.

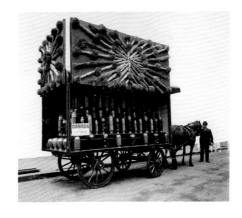

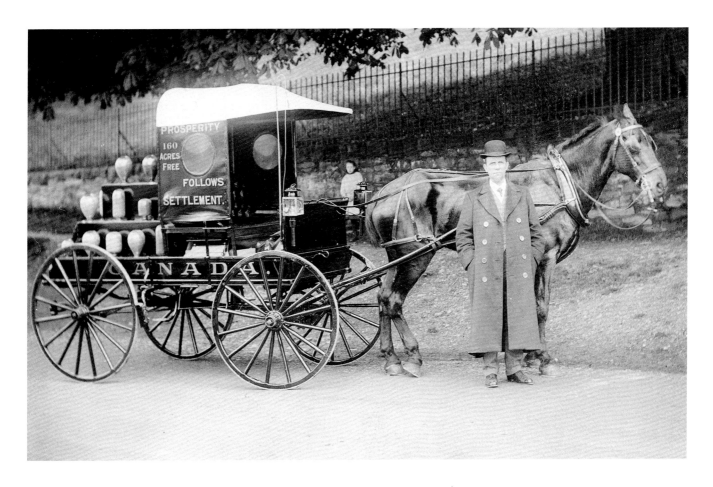

The Allan line of trans-atlantic steamships, based in Montreal, rose to dominate shipping between Canada and Great Britain, especially with the help of lucrative government mail contracts. The Allan vessels also carried immigrants to Canada, paid for by government subsidy. This poster illustrates the advances in print technology that allowed for the use of colour and appealing images.

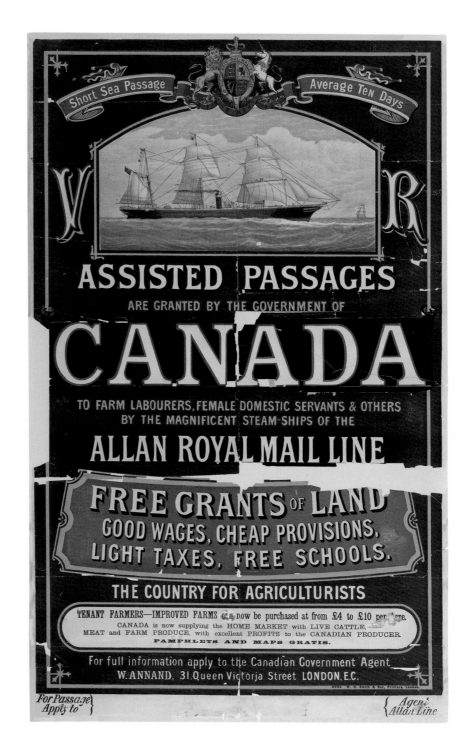

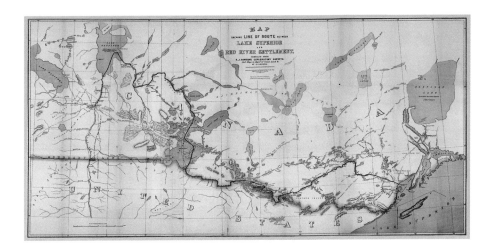

is how Douglas Owram generously puts it.

Initially the sales campaign was unsuccessful. Despite the best efforts of the government agents, Canada did not enjoy a high profile abroad. Some settlers migrated west from Ontario into Manitoba, making it an English-Canadian province and earning it the nickname "Ontario West." With most of their province's good farmland occupied, expansionists in Ontario hoped that the North-West would turn out to be an agricultural hinterland for central Canada, a situation that naturally alarmed the local French-speaking Metis population and contributed to the tensions that erupted as a second episode of violent unrest in 1885. Meanwhile, a few thousand people came from Europe. Mennonites from Russia, lured by government promises of religious freedom and exemption from military service, began settling on the prairie south of Winnipeg in 1874, then spread westward into Saskatchewan. A group of Icelanders created a colony on the shores of Lake Winnipeg at Gimli in the mid-1870s, while parties of Mormons migrated north from the United States into southern Alberta beginning in 1887. But as historian Gerald Friesen points out, each of these groups came to Canada as a result of special-case negotiations with the government, not the blandishments of the early immigration promoters.

In fact, the advertising campaign had little impact. The 1881 census showed that the prairies had only 66,000 settlers; during the next couple of years more people left the area than arrived. The Canadian West was still remote and hard to reach. Prior to the completion of the transcontinental railway in 1885, travellers came by boat to the head of Lake Superior, then embarked on the Dawson road to Manitoba, a combination wagon trail and steamboat service that one person who experienced it described as "the worst piece of business that I ever saw anywhere." International grain prices were low and even if a newcomer wished to get into farming, the western US and other destinations such as Australia and

This map traces the so-called Dawson road, the all-Canadian land and water route to Manitoba pioneered by the surveyor and engineer Simon James Dawson. From 1868 to 1885 it was the main route to the interior. Travellers took at least a month to make the trip and it was more of an impediment to immigration than an asset. After 1885 immigrants used the newly completed Canadian Pacific Railway to reach the North-West.

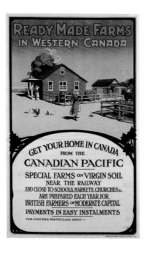

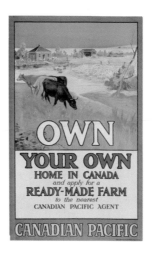

Well into the 1920s the Canadian Pacific Railway was selling land it had received in the 1880s in return for building the transcontinental rail line. Settlers buying CPR land could also purchase ready built houses and barns from the company in a wide range of sizes and prices.

South America still had plenty of available land. In fact, until the first decade of the twentieth century, more people migrated from Canada to the US than entered Canada as immigrants.

———

THE CANADIAN GOVERNMENT WAS NOT the only agency promoting the North-West to immigrants. It was joined in the propaganda effort by the Canadian Pacific Railway, the largest private landowner in the country. As part of the agreement to construct its transcontinental rail line, the CPR had received ten million hectares of land between Ontario and the Rocky Mountains. Naturally it was eager not only to sell some of it, but to see the territory settled so that the company might profit from the traffic, both freight and passenger, that would result. "The efforts of the CPR in the matter of settling Manitoba and the North-West has been as great, and probably more methodical, than the government's," claimed a writer in the *Manitoba Daily Free Press* in 1889.

Even before the track was complete, the CPR had published its first promotional brochure, *The Great Prairie Provinces of Manitoba and the Northwest Territories* (1881). The following year it launched its own sales campaign in London, orchestrated by Alexander Begg, a former journalist and the company's general emigration agent. Begg lectured and wrote brochures extolling the benefits of western settlement. These were produced in several languages and distributed throughout the British Isles and in northern Europe. Begg, and his successor Archer Baker, also undertook a variety of other publicity efforts that prefigured similar initiatives that the Canadian government would later undertake. For instance, Begg advertised "homes for all" in hundreds of publications in Britain and on the continent. He dispatched touts into the countryside to talk up Canada as a destination for emigrants, and supported them with formal lecturers equipped with maps, posters, charts and lantern-slide projectors – cumbersome contrap-

BELOW A display for potential immigrants sponsored by the CPR in the English market town of Devizes, Wiltshire, in 1894. A sign reads "150 Acres of Land as Free Gift to Every Settler." Like the government, the CPR was eager to attract new settlers to its extensive land holdings in the Canadian West.

RIGHT A CPR exhibition railcar visits a rural area somewhere in eastern Canada or the northern US with the intention of inspiring farmers there to resettle out West.

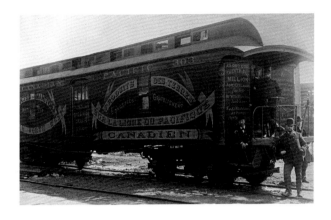

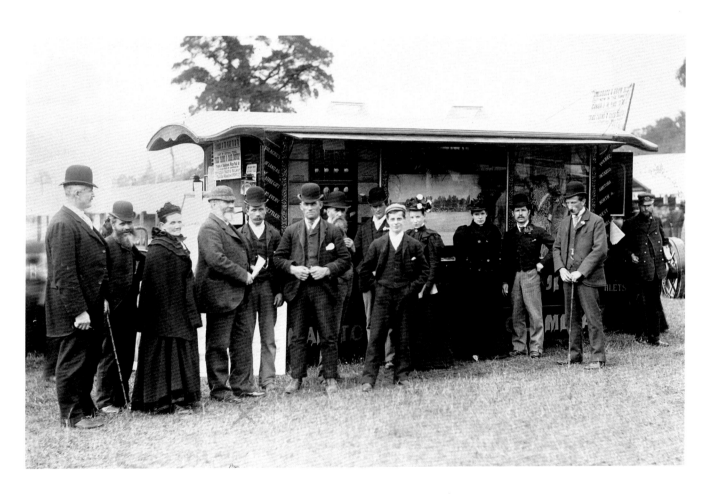

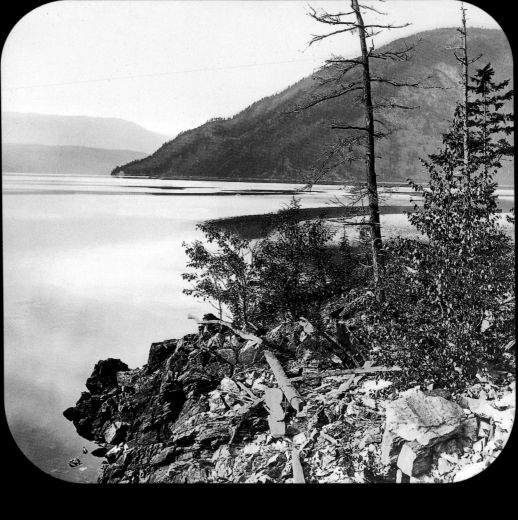

A tinted photograph of Shuswap Lake on the CPR line near Sicamous in central British Columbia in 1889. The photograph was taken by William McFarlane Notman of the Montreal-based photographic firm William Notman and Son. W.F. was the son of the company's founder and took over the business when his father died. The CPR hired the Notmans to produce images of western Canada for promotional material designed to attract immigrants and tourists. On this particular trip, W.F. was accompanied by his younger brother Charles. When W.F. died in 1913, Charles took over management of the operation and it was he who finally sold the company in 1935, ending an illustrious history that began in 1856 when William Notman, a young Scottish immigrant, opened a portrait studio in a room in his brick house on Bleury Street in Montreal.

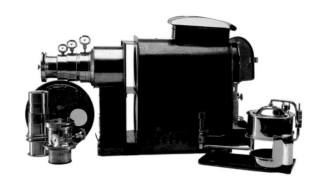

The magic lantern was the forerunner of the modern slide projector. Lecturers used it widely at the end of the nineteenth century. Light from a lamp – first oil, then electric – was projected through a glass plate with a photograph printed on it, casting an enlarged image onto a screen.

tions also known as magic lanterns that projected photographs printed on glass plates onto a screen.

The CPR also sent the first horse-drawn exhibition van into the countryside, much like a travelling circus, to educate British farmers about the Canadian West. "The system followed is to be present at the various towns on market days, wherever possible," explained Baker. "Handbills are sent on a few days in advance to ministers, and for display in hotels and public houses, announcing the day on which the Van will arrive. On arriving at a town or village a place on the market (if there be one) is obtained. If there is no market the most prominent position available is secured. The Van is opened out and publications are distributed to applicants." The van, emblazoned with slogans, contained samples of all kinds of Canadian produce, from wheat to nuts, intended to impress visitors with the fertility of the country. "In 1893," writes geographer Ronald Rees, the van attracted "1.75 million viewers in 593 different places."

Similar exhibition railcars travelled to eastern Canada and into the United States.

One of the more successful immigration initiatives undertaken by the CPR during this period was the wooing of Count Paul Esterhazy, Hungarian nobleman and emigration agent. In 1885 the railway sponsored a visit to the North-West by Esterhazy, who then organized the relocation of groups of Hungarians, who had earlier settled in Pennsylvania, to the Minnedosa area of Manitoba and to Saskatchewan's Qu'Appelle Valley. The railway offered free train travel and helped the newcomers get settled. The success of these Hungarian colonies was a stimulus to later immigration by other eastern European groups.

To provide images of the North-West for its publicity efforts, the CPR hired photographers and sent them out to take pictures of the country. In 1884 the company engaged the well-known Montreal photographic firm, William Notman and Son. William McFarlane Notman, eldest son of the firm's founder, made eight

trips to the West, travelling in his own specially outfitted railcar, Photographic Car No. 1, containing a darkroom, kitchen, sitting room and staterooms. The CPR projected Notman's photographs as lantern slides, used them in promotional material and sold them separately as postcards, prints and viewbooks. They were the first encounter many prospective immigrants had with the country they were thinking of making home.

In Canada itself, the CPR publicity machine was driven by George Ham, another former journalist, hired by company president William Van Horne in 1891 to be chief passenger agent at the Montreal headquarters. For the next couple of decades Ham was the railway's propagandist-in-chief, leading tours of journalists, speaking on the CPR's behalf, showing up wherever he was needed to burnish the company's reputation with travellers and immigrants. He was an outsized figure: tall, shambling, dressed in baggy suits, with a walrus moustache and an affable manner. A witty, expansive speaker, Ham was

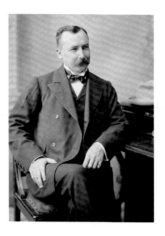

As minister of the interior in the federal Liberal government from 1896 to 1905, Clifford Sifton (shown here in 1900) was the driving force behind attempts to sell western Canada to prospective settlers.

dubbed the Mark Twain of Canada and made friends for the railway wherever he went, a glass of liquor never far from his elbow and the pockets of his rumpled suit always overflowing with cigars.

Unlike government land, which was basically free to homesteaders, CPR land was available for $2.50 per acre. Buyers were required to bring most of it under cultivation within four years; for each acre producing a crop within that period they received a rebate of $1.25. But despite the aggressive publicity effort, CPR land sales sputtered, basically for the same reasons that the government was finding it difficult to attract settlers to the North-West: isolation, lack of transportation, better opportunities elsewhere. In an attempt to quicken the pace, the CPR sold 2.2 million acres to a British syndicate, the Canada North-West Land Company. The Land Company was one of several colonization firms that acquired vast tracts of western land at a reduced rate with the intention of selling to colonists. But the company was unable to market its land either and went

bankrupt in 1893, most of the remaining land reverting to the CPR.

———

FINALLY, IN THE 1890S, THE SITUATION began to improve for Canada. Grain prices rose, the cost of shipping it across the oceans fell, the American frontier closed and new techniques for dry-land farming emerged along with new grain varieties; all these factors combined to make the North-West a better bet for immigrants. At the same time, population increases in European countries continued to encourage people to look elsewhere for economic opportunities. Rural poverty, urban unemployment, land hunger, political and religious repression: all had a role in convincing emigrants to take a chance on the New World. If Canada played its cards right, it could take advantage of this perfect storm of circumstances favouring the North-West as a destination for immigrants.

With the election of the Liberal government of Wilfrid Laurier in 1896, the set-

tlement of the West became a national priority as never before. Laurier named Clifford Sifton, a thirty-five-year-old Manitoba lawyer, minister of the interior and put him in charge of filling the West with people. Pierre Berton called Sifton "a man of impressive strengths and glaring flaws." The strengths included tireless energy, strict self-discipline, dynamic intelligence, a genius for organization and a talent for being out of the room when the oil of patronage was greasing the wheel of politics. It was no wonder he became one of the most powerful and effective ministers in the Laurier cabinet. The flaws were no less impressive and included an aloof manner, a tendency to flaunt his substantial wealth, a towering ambition, an odour of corruption that trailed behind him for most of his career, an antipathy toward French Canadians, and an arrogance that won him few friends but many enemies. In other words, he came by his nickname, "the young Napoleon," honestly.

When Sifton took charge of the Department of the Interior he famously described

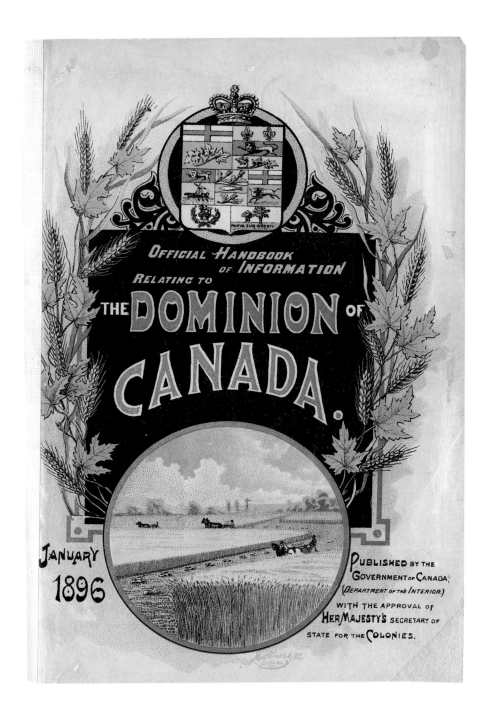

The Department of the Interior published several "Official Handbooks" for immigrants during the mid-1890s. The harvest scene on the cover set the pattern for promoting the Canadian West for the next thirty years: farmers harvesting a bountiful crop of golden grain beneath a sunny sky. Because some colonial governments were publishing misleading information, Canadian government publications such as this one had to be approved by the British secretary of state for the colonies before it could be circulated in Britain.

CANADIAN PACIFIC

THE BEST WAY TO

YOUR OWN FARM IN CANADA

FREE PASSAGES FOR CHILDREN

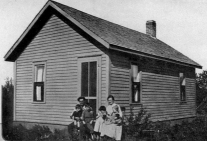

LOANS FOR THE PURCHASE OF FARMS

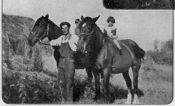

BRITISH SETTLERS ON THEIR CANADIAN FARMS.

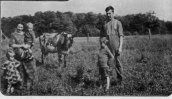

SPECIAL FARES TO CANADA

From British Ports to the following Canadian Pacific Centres

Halifax, Nova Scotia	-	£3 : 0 : 0	Saskatoon, Saskatchewan	- £6 : 0 : 0
Saint John, New Brunswick		3 : 0 : 0	Regina, Saskatchewan	- 6 : 0 : 0
Quebec	- - - -	3 : 0 : 0	Moose Jaw, Saskatchewan	- 6 : 0 : 0
Montreal	- - - -	4 : 0 : 0	Edmonton, Alberta	- - 6 10 : 0
Toronto, Ontario	- -	4 10 : 0	Calgary, Alberta	- - 6 10 : 0
Winnipeg, Manitoba	-	5 10 : 0	Vancouver, British Columbia	9 : 0 : 0

For further Particulars APPLY WITHIN

THOMAS & SONS, LTD., Printers, 26, QUEEN STREET, LONDON, E.C. 4

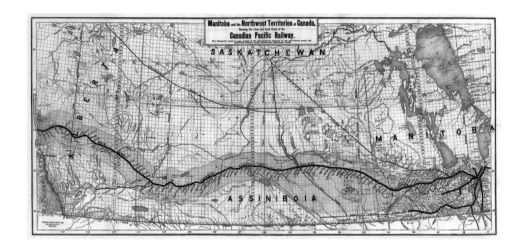

This map shows the Canadian Pacific main line from the Red River to the Rockies. The company received ten million hectares of land in return for building the railway, much of it in the green shaded area close to the track.

it as "a department of delay, a department of circumlocution." Given a mandate by Laurier to change things, he was determined to do so in a hurry.

In the nine years he held the portfolio Sifton more than quadrupled the departmental budget. First off he fired the two most senior bureaucrats and replaced them with his friend James Smart, the mayor of Brandon. Then he purged another twenty-three senior members of the department, replacing them with his own Liberal Party loyalists, and hired a small army of agents to represent Canada south of the border and in Europe. (The civil service was still relatively young and it was accepted practice for the minister to arbitrarily hire and fire employees; the most important qualifications for a job were political affiliation and personal connections.) Sifton pressured private landholders who were withholding their large blocks of land from settlement for speculative purposes – particularly the railways, and even more particularly the CPR – to open their holdings. "The whole

fertile belt was looked upon as railway reserves," he told the House of Commons, and it was preventing homesteaders having access to the best land. He also promoted irrigation projects and streamlined land granting procedures, all with the aim of making the North-West more attractive to immigrants. "The first thing to do was to settle the empty West with producing farmers," he pronounced; "this was also the second, third, fourth and fifth thing to do." As John W. Dafoe, Sifton's first biographer, wrote: "The regulations of the Department and its organization were all directed towards putting the individual John Doe on 160 acres of land, keeping him there, making his conditions of life tolerable, supplying him with railway facilities; and then multiplying the performance a countless number of times."

Along with doing what he could to remove all obstructions that stood in the way of settlement, Sifton launched a vast publicity campaign to trumpet the benefits of Canada to the world. So long as he was minister, the Department of

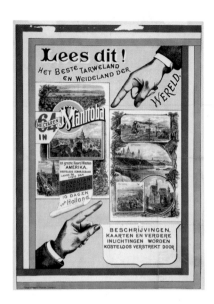

In order to attract European settlers to the West, Canadian Pacific advertised in many languages. This Dutch-language poster, circa 1890, is offering free land and free rail transportation to reach it.

the Interior might more accurately be described as the ministry of propaganda. "In my judgement," Sifton told the House of Commons in 1899, "the immigration work has to be carried on in the same manner as the sale of any commodity; just as soon as you stop advertising... the movement is going to stop." The government published millions of posters and pamphlets in as many as twelve languages portraying Canada as a land of milk and honey. In 1902–1903 the immigration division spent over $200,000 on promotional literature in Great Britain alone. By 1905 the budget for Sifton's entire publicity campaign reached $4 million.

———

THE GOVERNMENT DID NOT VALUE EVERY immigrant equally. First and foremost the propaganda campaign targeted the British Isles. The immigration office in London produced a steady stream of promotional literature. Journalist Ralph Stock described being buttonholed by one of Canada's insistent sales represent-

atives. "Unctuous gentlemen met you in the street with six page pamphlets," he wrote, "imploring you to come to such and such an address and hear of the fortunes in store for the man of initiative who would take the plunge and emigrate to Canada." These proselytizers were known as "Canadian crackers" and were primed with an encyclopedic store of information, and misinformation, about Canada. Promotional materials, some no more than a single page folded on itself, were distributed widely through post offices, reading rooms, clubs and hotels. On at least one occasion the government distributed a pamphlet to every farmer in Great Britain. Writer Edward McCourt later called this propaganda "the richest, purplest fiction ever written about the Canadian West."

By the new century, much of the literature had become quite sophisticated. Many employed photographs showing the best side of Canadian life taken by photographers Horatio Topley and John Woodruff, employees of the Topley Studio

"The Last Best West" was the most common slogan used to advertise the Canadian Prairies. It referred to the fact that land in the American West was becoming scarce and expensive, and that Canada offered a better, cheaper alternative destination.

SOME OF THE MOST ICONIC PHOTO-graphs of the immigration period feature immigrants and their families on the dock at Quebec City shortly after their arrival. Clutching babies and a few personal belongings, the newcomers stare straight ahead at the camera, their stoic expressions disguising the anxiety they must have felt as they embarked on their new life on a new continent.

Most of these images were taken by photographers from the Topley Studio, Ottawa's leading photographic firm at the turn of the century. William Topley (1845–1930) got his start in photography as an apprentice in the renowned Montreal studio of William Notman. (His brothers Horatio and John George also came to work at the Notman studio.) When he was just twenty-two years old, in 1868, William Topley began managing the new studio that Notman had opened on Wellington Street in Ottawa, building it into the premier photographic studio in the national capital. In 1875 he launched his own business in a Sparks Street studio. By the end of the decade the Topley Studio was the official photographer to the governor general. His brothers joined him in Ottawa, where Horatio later joined the Department of the Interior as a staff photographer and John George eventually opened his own business. The Topley Studio went into decline after the war and closed in 1923.

The immigrant photographs, mostly taken in 1910 and 1911, were commissioned by the immigration branch of the Department of the Interior. They were copied, printed in various publications and distributed to agents who used them as lantern slides in their lectures. They were meant to encourage other potential immigrants to follow in the footsteps of their compatriots.

THE TOPLEY STUDIO

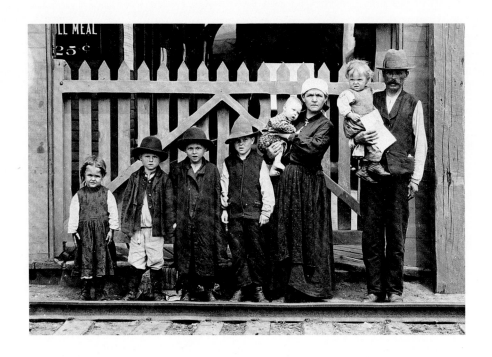

A family of Galicians (Ukrainians) photographed by the Topley Studio at the immigration sheds at Quebec City in 1910.

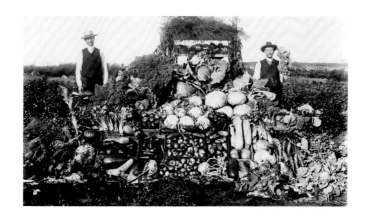

in Ottawa. Woodruff and Topley, who eventually became a full-time employee of the interior department, were dispatched on cross-Canada tours to take photographs that were then used in the immigration pamphlets. The photographs were also used in the lantern slides employed by lecturers to enliven their talks.

No age group was safe from Canada's army of propagandists. During the 1890s Sir Charles Tupper, Canada's high commissioner in London, managed to initiate an essay contest in British schools, offering five pounds sterling for the best essay about Canada and its resources. This idea was picked up by James Smart, who donated wall maps and atlases of Canada to every school in Britain and a specially prepared textbook, *Canada: A Descriptive Textbook*, to every British schoolchild. Students were expected to use these resources to write essays for the competition. The winning entries won bronze medallions engraved with the Canadian coat of arms.

Books and pamphlets were supplemented by posters. The earliest posters, rudimentary in design, contained simple text messages. Then, as printing technology improved, they became elaborate, multicolour combinations of words and images intended to capture the imagination of the viewer. Featuring breezy slogans such as "The Last Best West" and "The Richest Land on Earth," they evoked images of a fertile promised land overflowing with abundance, populated by happy, prosperous farmers. These posters hung in town halls, railway stations, post offices, mechanics' institute and hotels – wherever there was public wall space available. Ralph Stock reported that London was "plastered from end to end with flaring posters, representing fields of yellow grain and herds of fat stock tended by cowboys picturesquely attired in costumes that have never been heard of outside the covers of a penny dreadful."

Of course, residents of London were not the intended target for this blizzard of propaganda. Canada did not want urban dwellers, it wanted farmers. And so the message had to be taken to the country.

Horatio Topley took this photograph of a pair of farmers posing with a staged arrangement of fruits and vegetables intended to illustrate the fecundity of the Canadian West.

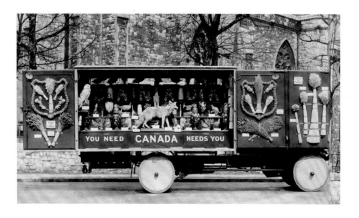

A post-war motorized exhibition van fitted out with an array of agricultural products to impress Britons with the possibilities of the Canadian West. To add a touch of the exotic, the van also contains some stuffed examples of wildlife, including a fox and an owl. The slogan centring on the word "Canada" (to be read as "You need Canada" and "Canada needs you") is reminiscent of wartime posters declaring "Your country needs you."

The government dispatched lecturers to carry the message to rural communities. Equipped with maps, charts, photographs and exhibits, these salesmen swamped the British countryside with information about Canada. A ubiquitous sight on the back roads during this period was the Canadian Advertising Wagon, painted bright red and filled with examples of produce to impress the British farmer with the fertility of the North-West. After the turn of the century this horse-drawn vehicle was supplemented with a motorized exhibition van. "It is safe to say," reported Canada's immigration agent in 1907, "there is not a highway, nor a village, nor an important by-way of any consequence...[to which the wagons have] not penetrated with literature, exhibits of Canadian grains and grasses, and drawing the attention of the agricultural people to the claims of Canada." One particularly bizarre exhibit was a huge buffalo that appeared at the Royal Agricultural Show in 1913. The animal, which had died at the Banff zoo, had been stuffed and sent

to Europe as an example of Canada's exoticism and natural abundance. It was displayed alongside pyramids of Quebec cheeses and bowls of prairie grain.

———

AFTER GREAT BRITAIN, THE SECOND MOST important target for the propaganda campaign was the United States. When Sifton came into office, there were six immigration agents selling Canada south of the border; within three years there were three hundred. Americans were considered to be very desirable settlers. "They are a strong, vigorous people," Sifton remarked, "capable, very alert, and progressive in their ideas." Sifton's successor as minister, Frank Oliver, concurred. "They are people of intelligence, of energy, of enterprise, of the highest aspirations," he enthused. "They speak the same language, they worship in the same churches, they have the same political ideals, although they have enjoyed different political institutions." For the most part Americans were experienced farmers who arrived

BELOW Immigration to western Canada was promoted at trade shows and farm exhibitions across the American West and Midwest. This Canadian government exhibit at the Oklahoma State Fair in 1913 was intended to interest fair-goers with a rural background. Attempts at targeting specific audiences with a specific message were new to advertising when Canada started its immigration campaign.

RIGHT A "mammoth cheese" made at the Dominion Experimental Dairy Station in Perth, Ontario, on display at the World's Columbian Exposition in Chicago in 1893. The cheese was 1.8 metres tall and 8.5 metres around, and weighed almost 10,000 kilograms. It took roughly 90,000 litres of milk to produce. The purpose was to promote Canadian cheese, the dairy industry, and Canadian agriculture generally.

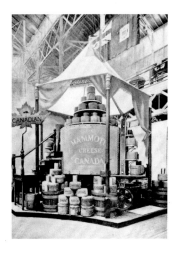

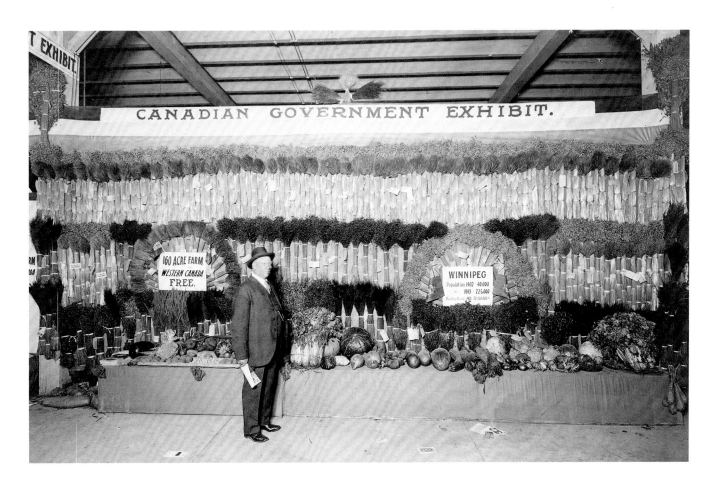

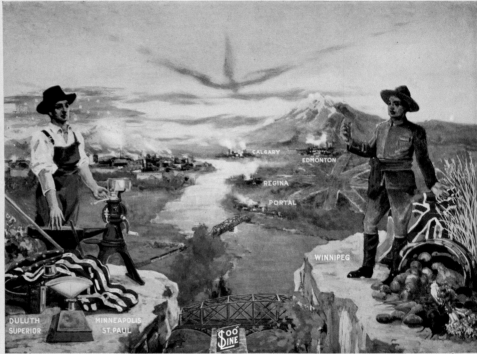

A 1911 poster advertises cheap rail fares for American farm labourers wanting to travel west to help with the harvest. Immigration promoters hoped that many of them would like what they saw and become permanent settlers. The welcoming Canadian figure on the right is wearing what appears to be a North West Mounted Police uniform and points to the familiar overflowing basket of farm produce.

"Welcome stranger" is the American-style caption on this calendar illustration meant to appeal to the British public's fascination with the American West. The friendly man on horseback in a field of golden wheat waves howdy to a new settler family arriving in "the most fertile country in the world."

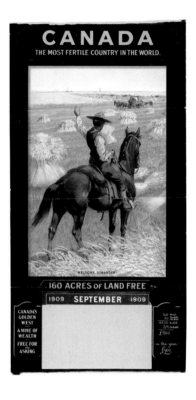

with a nest egg of capital they had already accumulated. They spoke English, and they appreciated the availability of cheap land and the absence of Indian wars and the frontier mayhem that characterized the American wild west. ("Is it well to carry a revolver?" asked one pamphlet in its question-and-answer section. The answer? "It is most unusual and almost unnecessary to do so under ordinary circumstances.") Whereas earlier the US had been a rival in the competition to attract newcomers, for Sifton it became a source of immigrants, including Canadians who had moved south and now desired to return home and Europeans who might be disillusioned with their initial homestead experience on the American plains.

Sifton put his friend William J. White, editor of the *Brandon Sun* newspaper, in charge of the US campaign. White oversaw a far-flung empire of twenty-one immigration offices, plus twenty-seven travelling agents and hundreds of subagents contracted to receive three dollars for every man, two dollars for every woman and a dollar for every child they convinced to come to Canada. In their offices the agents interviewed prospective immigrants, answered queries and dispensed literature. As did their counterparts in Great Britain, they also took to the road, giving lectures, planting information in schools and libraries, holding street-corner meetings, erecting displays at county and state fairs, and placing advertisements in local newspapers. Nothing was considered as effective as a chance to meet farmers face-to-face in their own communities. A cross between a secretary and a travelling salesman, an agent was also a facilitator who eased the way for farmers once they decided to move north. Sometimes agents even accompanied their recruits to their destinations. Most importantly they provided each migrant with a Settlers' Certificate that guaranteed cheap rail travel from the Canadian border to the new homestead. Since an agent's pay depended, at least in part, on how many settlers he sent north, the competition for recruits was intense.

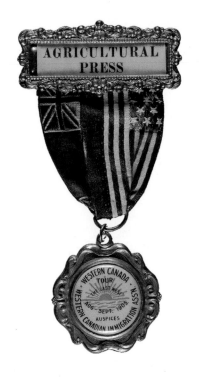

This bronze medallion was presented to American agricultural journalists who toured western Canada from August to September 1905 at the invitation of the Western Canadian Immigration Association, a group of private land agents. A great many tours were organized by Canadian government officials, who wined and dined American writers, newspaper editors and agricultural scientists in anticipation of positive write-ups when they returned home.

In such an atmosphere, agents naturally felt pressure to oversell the benefits of moving to Canada.

Foreign journalists, both American and European, were invited to tour the North-West so that they would write flattering articles when they returned home. "Train-loads of compliant editors, lubricated by good whiskey and warmed by the best CPR cuisine, raced across the prairies at government expense," writes Pierre Berton, "stopping at wheat fields and handsome farms (carefully selected) or for banquets at the major cities." As we have seen, one of these writers was the American popular novelist James Oliver Curwood.

All this activity south of the border bore impressive results. The flow of migrants out of Canada to the US was reversed as the number of people moving north from the US more than quadrupled between 1900 and 1905, from about ten thousand a year to forty-five thousand. Between 1896 and World War I, nearly six hundred thousand Americans moved north to Alberta and Saskatchewan alone.

ALONG WITH THE TRADITIONAL SOURCES of Great Britain and the United States, Canada welcomed newcomers from continental Europe. Here the situation was more complicated. Germany would not allow foreign governments to advertise for settlers, while Scandinavians had already shown a marked preference for the American West. Sifton decided to focus on Austria-Hungary, where he believed suitable homesteaders abounded. But immigration agents could not work as freely there as in Great Britain and the US. For instance, the Canadian government routinely paid agents for steamship companies a bonus for every immigrant they signed up for passage to Canada. But this practice of paying agents skirted the law in some European countries, which did not like to see foreign governments openly soliciting people to emigrate. As a result, Sifton made a secret deal in 1899 with the North Atlantic Trading Company (NATC), based in Amsterdam, to promote Canada in continental Europe and Scandinavia on the government's behalf.

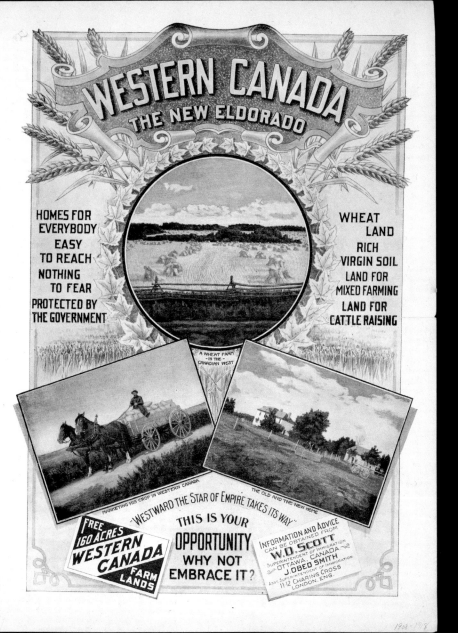

This poster presents western Canada as "the New Eldorado" and uses the message at the bottom – "Westward the Star of Empire Takes Its Way" – to portray settlement of the Canadian West in the light of an imperial destiny. The poster also promises that settlers have "nothing to fear" and will be "protected by the government," perhaps a response to anxiety about the American wild west, or perhaps a subtle way to reassure prospective settlers that Canada's Aboriginal people, who rarely got a mention in immigration material, were peaceful.

Cards like these, advertising "160 Acres of Free Land" in various languages, were distributed across Europe by agents of the shadowy North Atlantic Trading Company.

On the back a map shows possible sea routes to Canada. The NATC was active from 1899 until 1906 when accusations of impropriety led to its demise.

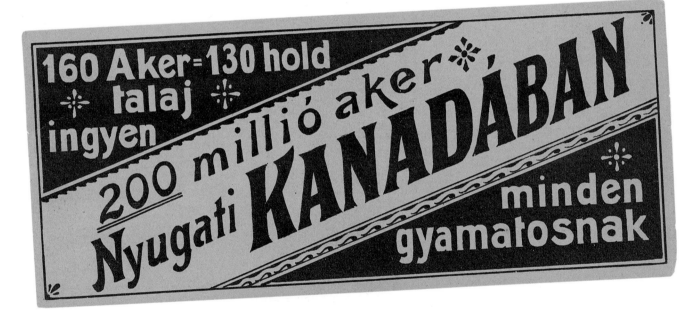

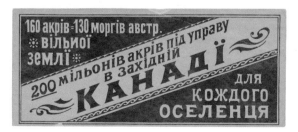

The government published descriptive handbooks for potential immigrants in many languages, including this one for Scandinavians in 1899.

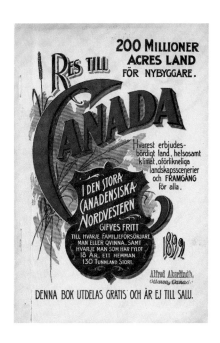

The NATC has a murky history. It was set up by a former organizer for the Liberal Party with a long record of political dirty tricks, W.R.T. Preston, who had been rewarded for his loyalty to the party with the job of Canada's immigration inspector in London. With the connivance of Sifton's deputy, James Smart, the company acquired a monopoly over immigration promotion on the continent and worked behind a veil of secrecy. For each agricultural settler (man, woman and child older than twelve) that it delivered to Canada, the NATC received a five-dollar bonus. The company also received an annual fee for promotional literature. Preston claimed the company was distributing pamphlets in several languages, advertising in newspapers and sending agents to rural areas in central and eastern Europe to scare up potential immigrants, but whether or not the company did these things no one actually knew. He said the North Atlantic Trading Company was responsible for delivering thousands of new settlers to Canada, but was he merely taking credit, and money, for migrants who would have made the move anyway? Again, there was no accountability whatsoever so no one knew.

When the arrangement with the NATC became public in 1905 it caused a scandal in Parliament. There was so much secrecy surrounding the company that the Opposition naturally suspected it was up to no good. Conservative Member of Parliament George Foster called the NATC "a headless, houseless, homeless monstrosity" that was stealing from Canadian taxpayers under the pretext of performing a service that it did not fulfill. In 1906 the new minister of the interior, Frank Oliver, ended the arrangement with the company. Pierre Berton describes the NATC as "very largely a boondoggle" created by Preston to line his own pockets. Historian D.J. Hall, Sifton's biographer, is more charitable, concluding that the company did effective work. A more recent study by historian Jaroslav Petryshyn sides with Berton. Petryshyn concludes that the NATC was a scam and that

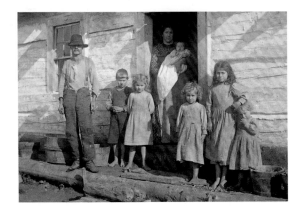

Preston and Smart "used their positions for personal gain at the public expense."

What the episode reveals is that immigration promotion at times was nearly indistinguishable from what later generations would call human trafficking. The enthusiasm for selling Canada abroad at times provided a pretext for some very dubious characters to profit personally from the ambitions of many humble European farmers to make new lives for themselves in the North-West. While men like Preston became wealthy and agents received payment for sending immigrants to Canada, immigrants themselves did not receive any form of payment for resettlement. Free land and the benefits of a liberal democracy were considered by the government to be payment enough.

_____

EVERY ELEMENT OF THE PROPAGANDA campaign that was deployed to woo immigrants conveyed the same message: Canada, and more particularly the Canadian North-West, was a land of unlimited opportunity where success was almost guaranteed if a settler was willing to work hard for it. One popular pamphlet had a cover showing a one-room log cabin, labelled "1st Year," compared to an illustration of a prosperous farm, labelled "5th Year." The message was clear: western Canada meant success, prosperity, progress. This same optimistic sense of possibility was expressed in the work of the Manitoba poet and novelist, Robert Stead (1880–1959), who wrote about homesteading in his poem "The Plough":

> *You came. Straightway the silent plain*
> *Grew mellow with the glow of golden*
> *grain;*
> *The axes in the solitary wood*
> *Rang out where stately oak and maple*
> *stood;*
> *The land became alive with busy din,*
> *And as the many settled, more came in;*
> *The Earth gave up her hoard, and in a*
> *stream*
> *The gold poured forth behind your*
> *busy beam!*

In the words of one poster, western Canada was "the new Eldorado." In this version of the Canadian West, newcomers shed all the prejudices and restraints of the Old World and breathed the air of freedom. "In God's great blue all things are possible, and all things are fair," enthused the writer Emily Murphy, a transplanted Ontarian. Settlers who had already experienced its benefits were considered to be the best spokespeople for immigration. Many pamphlets featured first-hand accounts by settlers who had come to Canada and prospered. "We consider Western Canada the best country in the world for the poor man," attested two American homesteaders. "Any man with a good team and money enough to buy provisions and seed for six months can become rich there in five years," agreed a trio of German immigrants.

Especially in the early years, the literature worked hard to dispel negative notions about the Canadian climate. Words like "snow" and "cold" were not in the pamphleteer's vocabulary; indeed,

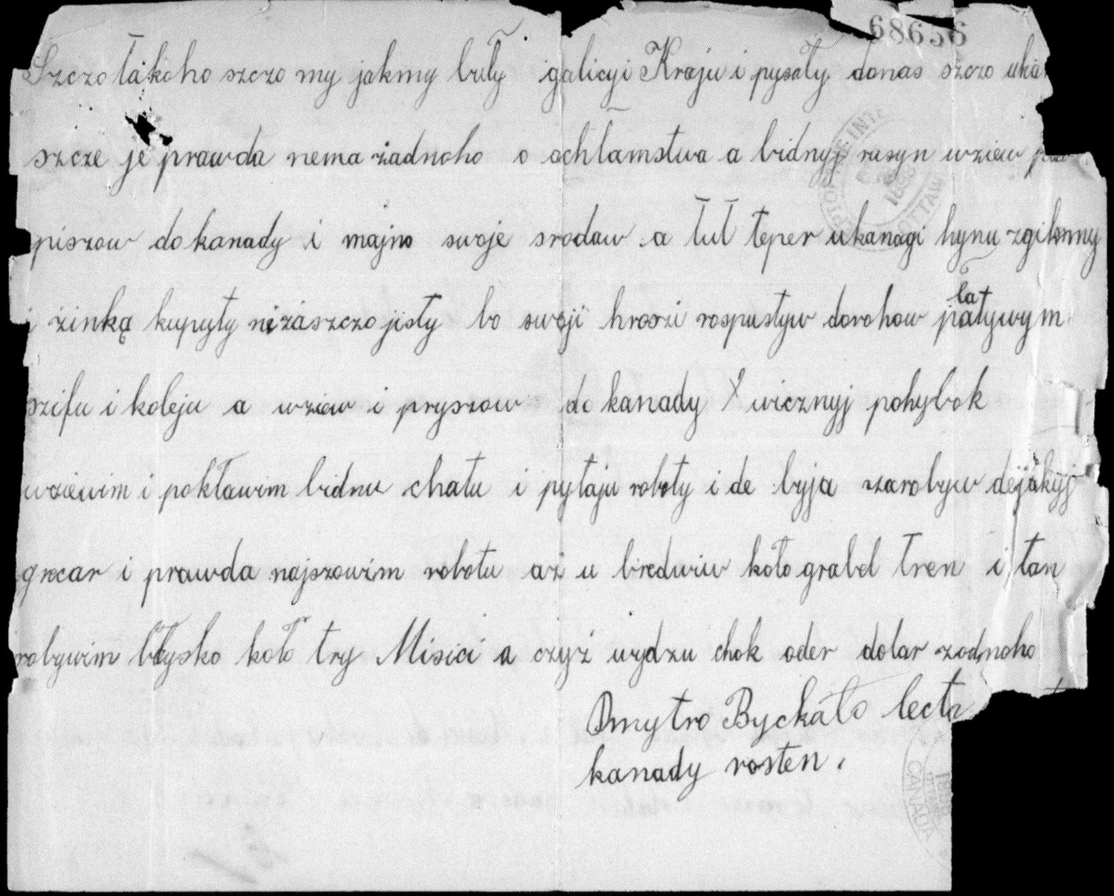

[handwritten letter in Ukrainian cursive, signed]

Dmytro Byckalo
kanady rosten.

The reality of life in western Canada frequently belied what immigrants had been led to expect by the glowing accounts in the propaganda. This letter to a government agent from Dmytro Byckalo, a Ukrainian who immigrated to Saskatchewan with his family in the 1890s, shows how one family was disappointed. The translation reads: "We heard in Galicia that we can find in Canada truth and I sold my property and I went to Canada. I die now in Canada with my wife and children. I have nothing to eat because I spent all my money on journey from Galicia to Canada. I put a small house on my farm and went to work. I found work. I worked nearly three months but I didn't get one cent for my work. After while I worked one month and five days I earned $4 but I got only $1 from Mr. Ens in Rosthern. I earned second month $24 and near Moose Jaw $3.25 but for all my work I got only $1. I have to starve because I cannot write English or speak and I have here nobody to ask in that case. I could buy a cow for that money that I made. Now I have some more trouble. I sent my daughter in service for $3 per month to one German, but I didn't get one cent. I don't know what I can do. Now I write to you and ask you to help me because that is my only hope. We Ruthenian people let you know about our trouble, we can't get our wages for our work. I write you only the truth. I don't understand Canadian law. I know only that I worked whole summer for nothing."

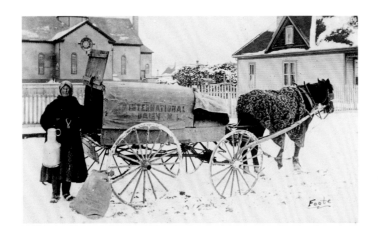

A Ukrainian woman delivering milk in Manitoba, circa 1900. Many immigrant women took work outside the home when they could to help make ends meet for the family.

Sifton himself banned them from government publications. Instead the climate of the North-West was "bracing" and "salubrious." *The Atlas of Western Canada*, produced by the Department of the Interior in 1901, describes it as "very agreeable." "Spring commences about the first of April. Some seasons, however, seeding is begun early in March, the snow having entirely disappeared. But spring scarcely puts in an appearance before it is followed by summer, and it is almost impossible to describe the delights of that pleasant season, with its long days and cool nights." Far from being a negative, a northern climate was presented as an asset, the incubator of a new, more energetic, industrious race of people. It "gives quality to the blood, strength to the muscles, power to the brain," wrote Thomas Spence in one of his pamphlets. "Indolence is characteristic of people living in the tropics, and energy of those in temperate zones." When snow was mentioned it was dismissed as unimportant, even beneficial. "Less snow falls on the prairies than in

the East," claimed a department pamphlet from 1906, "and on account of the dryness of the air, it brushes off one's coat like dust...The snow protects the autumn-sown wheat from the frost, aids the lumberman in drawing his timber from the forest, and also the farmer in hauling his produce to market, and so contributes alike to business and pleasure."

The result of such a pleasing climate was not just a healthy population but a tremendous productivity of the soil that seemed to make success as a farmer a mere matter of dropping a few seeds on the ground. A 1903 pamphlet, *Evolution of the Prairie by the Plow,* described the rise of "tall, red, hump-shouldered elevators, where settlements have clustered into villages," and "the fenceless, unbroken expanse" of "nothing but wheat, wheat, wheat." Posters showed western homesteads spilling over with fresh produce, rippling fields of grain, and contented farm families. Pamphlets portrayed nothing but success stories. "Altogether the whole district is very encouraging and

LEFT British emigrants could take advantage of subsidized fares to different parts of the Empire aboard passenger liners operated by various shipping companies, including the White Star and Red Star lines. This poster, with its image of a farmer in stetson hat and riding boots leading a glamorous life on the western Canadian frontier, was designed to encourage farmers and farm labourers to take advantage of these special fares. As always, the harvest shown is plentiful and the weather is perfect.

RIGHT The happy, healthy woman depicted in this poster is definitely "the right type" of English immigrant worker. On the wall beside the kitchen window hangs a picture of the White Star liner that brought her to Canada. Another farm on the horizon suggests there are neighbours nearby and that social isolation is not the problem so many immigrant families actually found it to be.

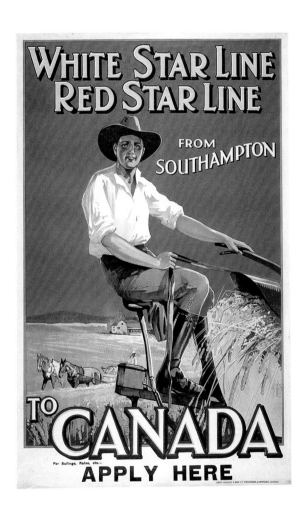

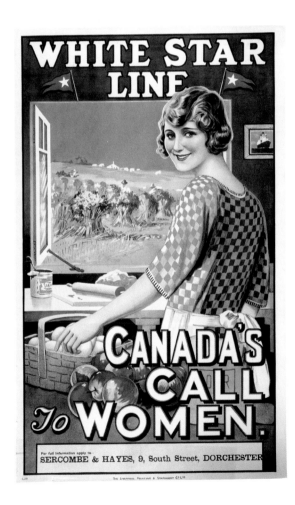

IN ITS EFFORTS TO POPULATE CAN-
ada, the government sometimes
targeted a particular occupational
group. This was the case in the
late 1800s when both farmers and
members of the growing urban
middle class needed help with
housework and child rearing. At
that time household service was
the single largest wage-earning
occupation in the country. There
were not nearly enough Canadian
women willing to fill these positions, and so young immigrant
women, usually single, were imported to make up the difference.
In the decade before the outbreak
of World War I, close to 80 percent of these women (90,028)

came from Great Britain, where
women were considered to have
the proper morals and upbring-
ing to adapt easily to Canadian
society. About 40 percent found
work in Ontario while an equal
number were destined for the
Prairies and British Columbia.

The government recruited
female domestics by offering
immigration agents five dollars
for every individual they sent to
Canada. Pamphlets were distributed throughout Great Britain targeting young women directly; in
1910, for example, immigration
agents in Britain handed out one
hundred thousand copies of *Canada Wants Domestic Servants*, one

of the department's more popular
pamphlets. These pamphlets
assured prospective immigrants
that life in Canada was far better
than in Britain, with a healthy
climate, higher wages and a more
democratic work environment.
Some of the young women agreed
to work without wages for as
much as a year to pay for the cost
of their passage; in practice, they
were indentured servants.

There were also private organizations and societies devoted
to resettling women abroad. The
largest were the British Women's
Immigration Association and the
Salvation Army, both of which
recruited women and supervised

their relocation to Canada. The
women travelled in groups in
the care of a chaperone and were
often assisted by local charities
and welcome homes on their
arrival. Once they arrived the
women sometimes found that
circumstances were not what
they were promised. Household
servants were a status symbol
for middle-class families, and
a necessity in an age before the
introduction of most labour-
saving domestic devices such as
washing machines and vacuum
cleaners. But that did not mean
servants were always well treated
by their employers. The work
was difficult, occupying long
hours of every day with arduous
physical demands. Most of the
women lived in their employer's
house under the watchful eye
of a mistress who monitored
their behaviour closely to ensure
respectability. They would have
had little opportunity in the
small amount of free time they
had to make friends or develop a
life outside the home. Their low
wages meant they had almost no
money to spend on themselves
and their social status meant they
had to endure the condescension
of their "betters." Poor, isolated,
lonely, denied a chance at normal
sexual relations, unfamiliar with
the local society: it is not hard
to imagine that many domestic
servants regretted their decision
to come to Canada.

CANADA WANTS DOMESTIC SERVANTS

There were many open-
ings for domestic ser-
vants on farms in the
western provinces. A
bright future awaited
British domestics out
West, as one pamphlet
suggested, especially if
they were looking for a
husband: "Canada has
an ever growing excess
of males over females of
no less a number than
150,000... as a matter of
fact, a very large percentage enter the matrimon-
ial state shortly after
their arrival, [and] in turn
become themselves mis-
tresses requiring help in
their household duties."

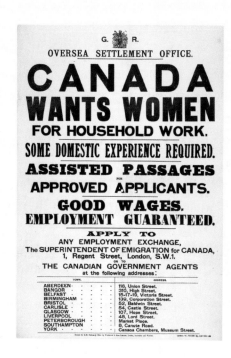

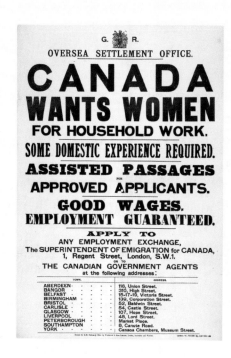G. R.
OVERSEA SETTLEMENT OFFICE.
CANADA WANTS WOMEN
FOR HOUSEHOLD WORK.
SOME DOMESTIC EXPERIENCE REQUIRED.
ASSISTED PASSAGES
FOR
APPROVED APPLICANTS.
GOOD WAGES.
EMPLOYMENT GUARANTEED.
APPLY TO
ANY EMPLOYMENT EXCHANGE,
The SUPERINTENDENT OF EMIGRATION for CANADA,
1, Regent Street, London, S.W.1.
OR TO
THE CANADIAN GOVERNMENT AGENTS
at the following addresses:

TOWN.		ADDRESS.
ABERDEEN	· · ·	116, Union Street.
BANGOR	· · ·	316, High Street.
BELFAST	· · ·	15-17-19, Victoria Street.
BIRMINGHAM	· · ·	139, Corporation Street.
BRISTOL	· · ·	52, Baldwin Street.
CARLISLE	· · ·	54, Castle Street.
GLASGOW	· · ·	107, Hope Street.
LIVERPOOL	· · ·	48, Lord Street.
PETERBOROUGH	· · ·	Market Place.
SOUTHAMPTON	· · ·	8, Canute Road.
YORK	· · ·	Canaaa Chambers, Museum Street.

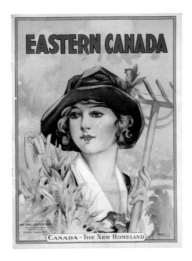

hopeful to us," reported a delegation of visitors whose impressions ostensibly were recorded in a typical promotional publication. "It is a nice prairie, covered with beautiful grass, and dotted here and there with little poplar forests which gives the whole a very romantic appearance. The settlers whom we visited look forward to a very happy and contented future."

GIVEN THAT THE GOVERNMENT'S PRIORITY was to populate the prairie West, farmers were Sifton's preferred class of immigrant. "Experience shows that workingmen from the cities and towns are the most helpless people in the world when they are placed upon the prairie and left to shift for themselves," he once wrote and he wanted little to do with them. Of course urban workers and middle-class professionals were by no means banned from coming, but neither were they encouraged as the agricultural class was. "We do not want anything but agricultural labourers and farmers," Sifton bluntly told a col-

league. This attitude was reflected in the promotional literature. "Clerks, shop assistants and persons desiring situations, are advised not to emigrate," warned an 1899 pamphlet, *Western Canada*. For this reason Sifton wanted nothing done to encourage Jewish or Italian immigration, judging both groups to be uninterested in and unsuited to agriculture. The majority of newcomers from overseas did not head out west at all but in fact remained in central Canada, where they found jobs in the factories and offices of the major cities or in the work camps of the hinterland. Nonetheless, the government propaganda machine was aimed almost exclusively at selling the North-West.

ONE CHARACTERIZATION USED BY THE government to populate the North-West promoted Canada as a place where religious freedom was respected. By and large this was done through negotiations with particular groups. Many religious leaders in Europe believed that the Canadian

West offered their followers a better life, not only materially but also because it promised to be free of the religious persecution some sects experienced at home. Groups such as the Mennonites, Hutterites and Doukhobors all joined the flood of immigration into Canada.

The Doukhobors were especially noteworthy because after their arrival they became the focus of an anti-immigrant backlash. Members of this Russian religious sect were persecuted in their homeland for their unorthodox beliefs and their pacifism. Thanks in part to the intervention of the great Russian novelist Leo Tolstoy, the world learned of the Doukhobors' plight. Sympathetic friends, among them a Toronto university professor named James Mavor, intervened on their behalf and found an ally in Clifford Sifton, who believed the Russian refugees were exactly the type of agricultural immigrant the Canadian West needed. In 1899 the first seventy-five hundred Doukhobors arrived in what became Saskatchewan and established three

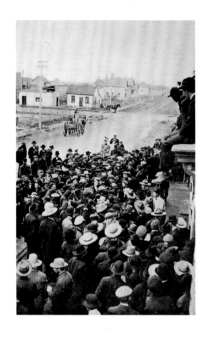

Initially the government allowed the Doukhobors who came to Canada beginning in 1899 to live in communal villages. But government policy changed with the resignation of Clifford Sifton, and Doukhobor families were required to become naturalized and to occupy individual homesteads. In 1907 some decided to leave the territory and their land became available, sparking a frantic land rush in Yorkton, where other land-hungry settlers gathered to try to acquire the abandoned lots.

communal settlements. Under a special agreement with the government, they were allowed to own their land, buildings and equipment collectively and received guarantees of exemption from military service. It looked like a win-win situation.

But public opinion began to turn against the newcomers, especially after a zealous splinter group known as the Freedomites staged a nude march to renounce worldliness in 1903. Sifton continued to stand up for the Doukhobors. When the political opposition tried to stir up animosity toward them, Sifton declared: "The cry against the Doukhobors and Galicians [Ukrainians] is the most absolutely ignorant and absurd thing that I have ever known in my life. There is simply no question in regard to the advantages of these people. The policy of exciting racial prejudice is the most contemptible possible policy." But Sifton's successor, Frank Oliver, was less sympathetic. He cancelled some of the Doukhobors' privileges and required that they swear allegiance to the British Crown. When they would not apply for homesteads in the conventional manner, he stripped the colonies of much of their land. In response, about five thousand Doukhobors began migrating to southeastern British Columbia in 1908 to establish new communities on land their leader Peter Verigin had purchased there. The rest stayed on the prairie where they adapted to the individual homestead system.

It was not only religious sects that immigrated to Canada in groups. In 1902 a fifty-five-year-old Anglican cleric from Ontario named Isaac Barr began circulating a plan in London to install a group of British homesteaders on the Canadian prairie. "Let us take possession of Canada," he wrote. "Let our cry be 'Canada for the British.'" After confirming the cooperation of the Canadian government, Barr rounded up a party of nineteen hundred would-be immigrants and embarked for Canada aboard a transatlantic steamship on March 31, 1903. The group was a mixed bag of office clerks, tradespeople, unskilled workers, city professionals and farmers.

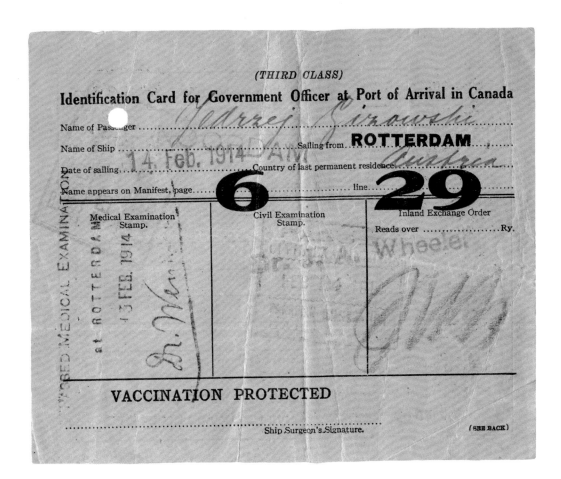

An identification card issued to a new immigrant from Austria arriving in Canada in February 1914. Stamps verify that the newcomer has passed a medical examination and been interviewed by an immigration officer. The back of the card states, in twelve languages, that the document must be kept for three years and shown to government officials on demand.

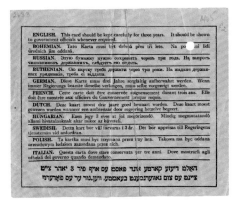

BELOW The Barr Colonists were a group of British immigrants who came to Saskatchewan in 1903, led by Anglican cleric Isaac Barr. At Saskatoon they left the train to continue their journey by wagon.

RIGHT Like most homesteaders, the Barr colonists took jobs locally until they could get their own farms established. These men are laying ties on the Canadian Northern Railway line between Saskatoon and Lloydminster.

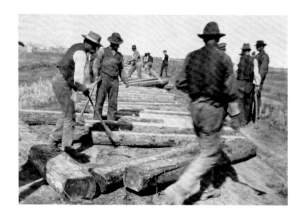

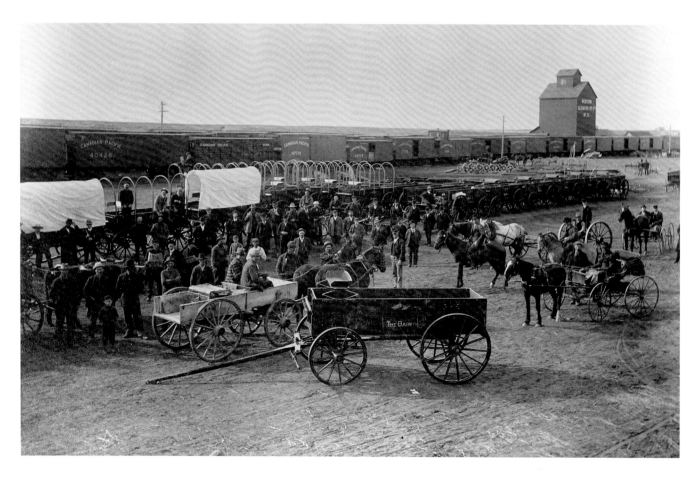

"The Wonderful Canadian Arch in Whitehall," as the London *Sphere* called it, was erected on the ceremonial route from Buckingham Palace to Westminster Abbey for the coronation of King Edward VII in August 1902. Clifford Sifton's staff seized the moment to combine imperial sentiment with a magnificent advertising opportunity. Photographs of the arch appeared in newspapers throughout Britain. Messages on both sides of the arch were lit with electric lights so they were visible day and night. "Canada. Britain's Granary. God Bless Our King and Queen" appeared on the side facing Buckingham Palace, while the message on the other side, visible in this photograph, read "Canada. Free Homes for Millions. God Bless the Royal Family." The arch, which stood 17 metres high and 18 metres wide, was decorated with wheat sheaves and capped by an open lantern with a roof in the shape of a crown.

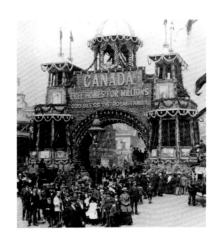

But they had all read the promotional literature and what they shared was the dream of owning their own piece of the Canadian West.

Joining the group was a second Anglican cleric, forty-two-year-old George Lloyd, who had visited Canada and believed in its potential as a settlement frontier for Britons. As the colonists made their way toward the land that had been reserved for them in Saskatchewan, the steady, reliable Lloyd began to win their confidence as the incompetent Barr lost it. The journey was a miserable one. The ship and the railcars used were overcrowded. In Saskatoon the travellers were housed in army surplus tents. Supplies were costly and the trail to the colony, negotiated on wagons drawn by oxen, was rough and dangerous. Some of the newcomers turned back. The rest, disgruntled with Barr's leadership, feeling that he had misled them about conditions in the North-West, voted to depose him in favour of Lloyd and an elected committee. Finally, early in May, they arrived at the reserve and began staking their homesteads. Despite the hardships of the early years the colonists made a success of the settlement and the town, named Lloydminster, that grew up to service it. In 1905, when the provinces of Alberta and Saskatchewan were created, the border between them passed right through the middle of the community.

———

DESPITE FALTERING STARTS, THE PUBLICITY campaigns mounted by the government and the CPR eventually succeeded in sparking a population explosion in western Canada. In 1896, Laurier's first year in office, 16,835 immigrants came to Canada; in the year of his election defeat, 1911, that number had jumped to 331,288, and in the year before the Great War broke out the number of immigrants topped 400,000. (Compare that to the approximately 235,000 immigrants Canada welcomed in 2007.) In the first two decades of the century, Canada's population increased by 64 percent. Out West the

...lantic steamships to bring immigrants from Europe to North America, as this poster promises, in "only four days" on the open sea. In 1915 the company organized its steamer operation as Canadian Pacific Overseas Services, later Canadian Pacific Steamship Ltd.

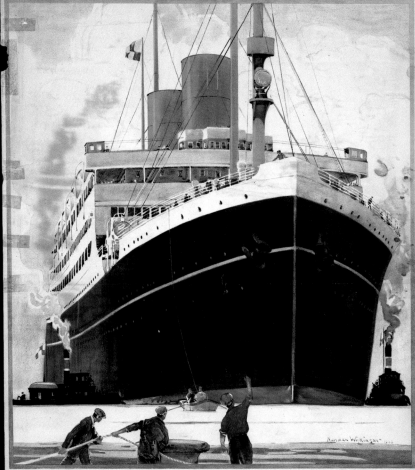

CANADIAN PACIFIC

TO CANADA & U.S.A

ONLY FOUR DAYS OPEN SEA

Apply:-

Canada West was a magazine published annually by the federal government from 1904 to 1930 as part of the campaign to attract immigrants. Covers like the ones shown here presented an idealized – some would say misleading – image of life on a prairie homestead. The magazine provided thirty to forty pages of practical information for would-be settlers, including colour maps of each of the four western provinces.

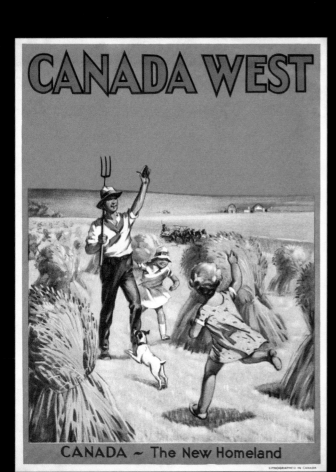

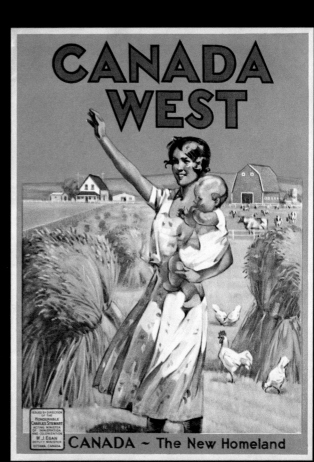

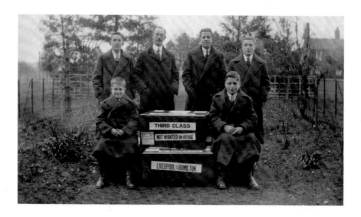

Young English immigrant boys prepare to leave for Canada with their trunks stamped "Liverpool to Hamilton." Canada received more than 100,000 juvenile immigrants between 1869 and the 1930s. The idea was to rescue youngsters who were orphans or the victims of poverty and give them a chance at a new life overseas.

increase was even more dramatic. In 1901 the territory that would become Saskatchewan held fewer than 100,000 people; by 1911 that number was almost 500,000, a fivefold increase. Alberta was the same story, growing from 73,000 inhabitants to almost 375,000, more than a fourfold increase. Manitoba had a larger population to begin with, but still came close to doubling in size during the same period. In a speech he gave in 1902, Clifford Sifton told his Toronto audience he knew that "you have for a good many years looked upon [the West] as a land of large promise but somewhat slow and poor performance." All that had changed, he assured them. "Where we counted our incoming settlers by hundreds we now count them by thousands, and the whole situation has undergone an alteration that is little short of phenomenal."

The success of the campaign was revealed not just in the raw statistic indicating growth, but also in the personal testimony of immigrants. "When I went to school," recalled one young English-

man, "on my way home every day I stopped to look at a big coloured poster of a wheat field in stook. On it was printed '160 acres land free.' I made up my mind, 'That's what I want,' and I got all the pamphlets on it and read all about it." With money saved by working in a hotel, this young immigrant made his way to Winnipeg where he found work on a farm and after two years was homesteading in Saskatchewan, proof positive that, as promised, Canada was the land of opportunity.

As the architect of the Liberal government's immigration campaign, Clifford Sifton was not around to enjoy its success for very long. In February 1905, newly elected to his Brandon seat in the recent federal election, Sifton suddenly resigned from Wilfrid Laurier's cabinet. He said it was because he could not support the government's school policies in the two new provinces of Alberta and Saskatchewan, and perhaps it was, though it may also have been a pretext for a semi-retirement he had been contemplating for some time, or a way of dodging a scandal

connected to rumours of an affair with a married woman. Regardless, Sifton was gone and responsibility for the great campaign to sell Canada to immigrants was turned over to his ministerial successor, Frank Oliver.

Oliver, an Edmonton newspaper editor, did not share Sifton's enthusiasm for "the stalwart peasant in a sheepskin coat." He believed that certain "races" were incompatible with Canadian society, would never fit in here, and should be discouraged. The races he had in mind were most particularly the eastern Europeans who had been so important to Sifton's policies. With Oliver's appointment, the "open door" was closed. Immigration became much more controlled. As Oliver said, his policy was "restrictive, exclusive, and selective." Changes to the Immigration Act in 1906 increased the number of categories of prohibited immigrants and allowed for easier deportation of individuals who were deemed "undesirable." Four years later, in 1910, another even more restrictive Immigration Act gave the

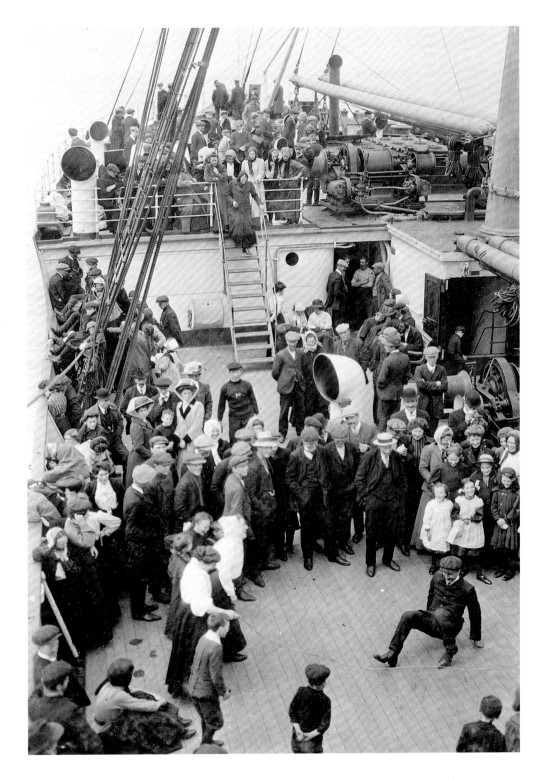

Immigrants passing the time aboard the SS *Empress of Britain*, one of the Canadian Pacific passenger liners, during a transatlantic crossing in 1911. Immigrants generally travelled third class and did not mingle with other passengers.

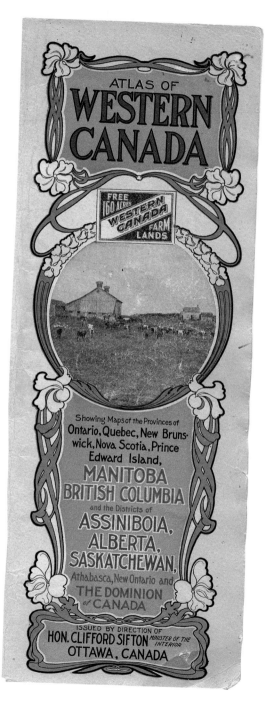

The federal government gave copies of this *Atlas of Western Canada* to every school in Britain for use as a reference for youngsters writing essays about Canada. Immigration officials expected that parents would also take a look and perhaps think about emigrating.

government authority to prohibit "immigrants belonging to any race deemed unsuited to the climate or requirements of Canada." At the same time, Oliver stepped up efforts to recruit newcomers from Great Britain, where he increased the bonus paid to booking agents, opened several new immigration offices and appointed many new government agents. The campaign to sell Canada was not over, but it shifted its focus back to more traditional sources of immigrants; that is to say, it targeted mainly Britons and Americans, who were believed to correspond to the kind of society the government was hoping to create in western Canada.

Clifford Sifton was not allowed a peaceful retirement. He was dogged by a series of scandals dating back to his time in the cabinet. Basically, the Opposition alleged that he had used his position as minister of the interior to line the pockets of his political cronies by granting them access to valuable timber, grazing and First Nations lands. Still, no matter how questionable his tactics, Sifton wasn't charged with

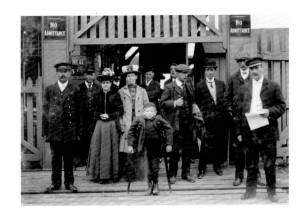

wrongdoing and he went down in history as the great promoter of Canadian immigration and the Canadian West. As Pierre Berton concludes, "Sifton is remembered as the man who brought people and prosperity to the West, not as the minister who presided over a corrupt department."

———

OF COURSE, THE PROMOTIONAL LITERATURE tended to exaggerate the sunny side of settlement, literally and figuratively, and ignore or minimize the dark side. "The ones that are not a pack of lies are a pack of rubbish," one disgruntled homesteader wrote about the government pamphlets that had played a role in luring him to the West. "So many books, pamphlets, etc. (mostly untrue) have been written about the charms and beautiful climate of the North-West of Canada and none about the hardships that have to be endured...I think it high time someone should let the public know the true state of affairs in that region of the world." Inevitably, the reality of homesteading in the Canadian

West did not live up to the promises made by the immigration boosters and these stanzas from two popular songs circulating before World War I express some of the disappointment newcomers felt:

> *We've reached the land where we*
>   *were told*
> *Was chocolate soil and full of gold*
> *And naught was known of storm*
>   *nor cold,*
> *Alberta Land, Alberta Land*
>   (from "Alberta Land")

> *Saskatchewan the land of snow*
> *Where winds are always on the blow*
> *Where people sit with frozen toes*
> *And why we stay here no one knows*
>   (from "Saskatchewan")

Life on a western homestead was much harsher than most newcomers anticipated. Sod houses, back-breaking labour, drought, hail and severe winter cold: these were a part of life in the North-West that official propaganda did not mention. One farm

"Undesirable" immigrants wishing to enter Canada were sent back to their departure points at the expense of the steamship company that brought them. Those barred from entering included people suffering from a range of mental and physical conditions, and prostitutes and their pimps.

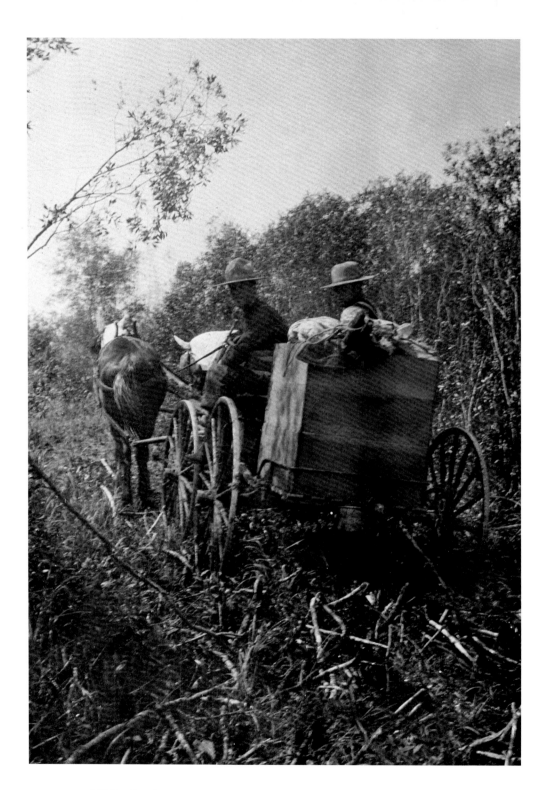

Optimistic settlers penetrated every corner of the Canadian West, including north of Edmonton beyond the Athabasca River and into the Peace River Country where these travellers are shown heading for their homestead in 1910.

One of the most difficult aspects of life for new immigrants on a prairie homestead was the isolation. Lack of company drove some settlers to abandon their farms, but it also led many to come together for work parties and social events.

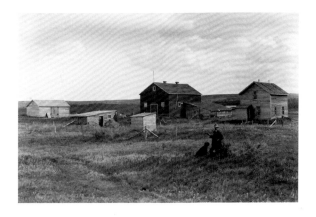

wife from Yorkshire in England who had read the pamphlets describing "the beauties of Canada, showing pictures of cattle knee deep in prairie grass" discovered instead, on her arrival at Estevan, Saskatchewan, banks of snow higher than she had seen before, sub-zero temperatures and everyone walking around "muffled up to the eyes in furs...Certainly the pamphlets we read on Canada did not describe that side of the country to us." Edward Roper, a British writer and artist who toured the West in 1889, asked one new homesteader to say what he felt about Canada. "Now I am here," the fellow answered, "and look around me and see what it is, really what a great piece of land I own, and think that here, and out of it, I've got to make my fortune, I begin to fancy I've done wrong in coming. Then the loneliness, the utter want of congenial society, the roughness, the immense distances, and the prospect of the dreadful winter. Oh, it is all very fine, when I was at home, reading about this sort of thing; but I confess the reality sometimes appals me."

The rigours of life on a homestead are reflected in some astonishing statistics. It has been estimated that 40 percent of homestead applicants failed; that is, they did not meet the requirements to obtain ownership of the land. In Saskatchewan that figure climbed above 50 percent. Historians have concluded that as many as two-thirds of the American incomers to the West did not remain but instead, not liking what they found, returned south of the border. Europeans had crossed an ocean to come to Canada and did not have the same opportunity to return home easily. Instead they had to make do with the situation as they found it.

The propaganda left the impression that all land in the West was of equal quality, but it wasn't. The selection of the right quarter section was crucial to success. There had to be ready supplies of wood and water, access to transportation, good soil, of course, and preferably a community nearby. Climate and landscape aside, there were many practical difficulties. Many newcomers arrived with little or no

capital with which to establish a home and begin farming. Seduced by promises of "free" land, they neglected to consider how they were going to pay for the necessaries. They learned soon enough that they had to hire themselves out as labour to established farmers, or find seasonal jobs in the western mines and railway construction camps. Social isolation was a serious problem. The sectional survey system had the effect of isolating homesteaders on their farms many kilometres from their nearest neighbours. The lack of a social life was felt harshly by the newcomers, especially the women, and was a significant reason why so many left the land.

"I used to get so hungry I would eat grass," recalled one Saskatchewan homesteader. Another, Johanne Frederiksen, her husband Ditlev and five children, emigrated from Denmark in 1911. Her letters home to relatives describe the hardships of life in the Canadian West and the culture shock experienced by the newcomers. "It is said that life is a struggle and if we did not know it before, urban department store. To serve these distant customers, the T. Eaton Company in Toronto opened a mail-order catalogue business. Eaton's offered its first catalogue in 1884 (this one dates from 1887–1888) and by 1896 it was shipping more than 200,000 parcels per year to mail order customers. In 1905 the company opened a Winnipeg store with its own catalogue operation serving western Canada.

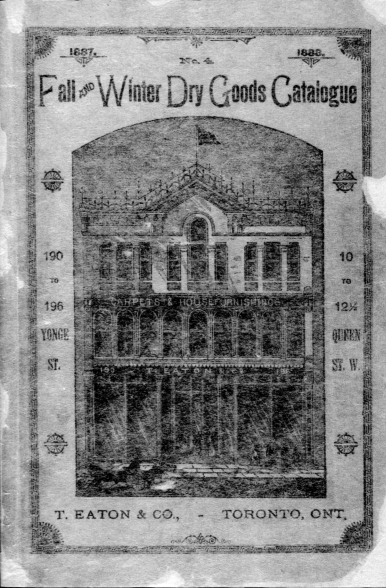

LEFT The Robert Simpson Company opened a department store in downtown Toronto in 1894 and for many years it was the main competition for Eaton's.

RIGHT The Montreal retailer Samuel Carsley was the pioneer of the mail-order catalogue in Canada, issuing his first catalogue in 1882, two years before Eaton's. This one dates from 1902 and celebrates the coronation of King Edward VII that summer.

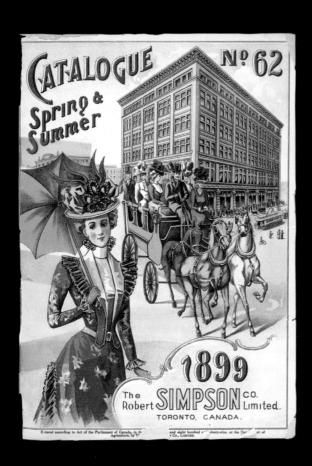

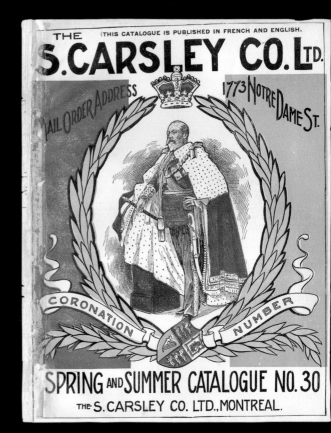

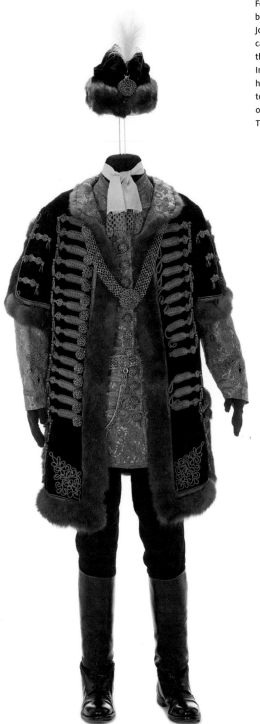

Following World War I two brothers from Hungary, Josef and Endre Csavossy, came to Alberta where they purchased a ranch. In Hungary the brothers had belonged to the aristocracy and enjoyed lives of wealth and privilege. They brought with them a train car load of personal items to remind them of their old way of life, including this fine suit of clothes for wearing at court. The Csavossy brothers made a success of their ranch but they always maintained links to eastern Europe. They brought four families with them to work on the ranch; eventually, each family acquired its own land and remained in Alberta.

we surely notice it here," Johanne wrote in one letter. "Not as before a struggle against wild animals and man, but against nature's fury, the unyielding soil, the harsh climate, it is a struggle for existence, a struggle against the loss of culture's benefits: church, school parish, community." Welsh newcomer Evan Davies echoed this sense of alienation from an unfamiliar landscape. "There was something so impersonal about this prairie," he wrote, "something that shattered any hope of feeling attached to it, or ever building a home on it." These were the testimonials that never made it into the publicity material that lured so many immigrants to the North-West. It is not so much that the government lied to the newcomers as that it only told the truths that were convenient.

———

SOME CRITICS, AT THE TIME AND LATER, have argued that the propagandists were their own worst enemies, luring to Canada people who were completely unsuited to

L'Ouest canadien offered prospects of a new life in western Canada to a special group of American residents: expatriate French Canadians. Quebec-based *missionaires colonisateurs* employed by the immigration branch distributed the pamphlet in the US. *L'Ouest canadien* contained favourable reports from French-Canadian farmers living in the western US who had toured Manitoba and the North-West as guests of the Canadian government. Despite these efforts, neither Canadian nor American French speakers were attracted to the Canadian West in large numbers. By 1901 only 23,000 French-speaking settlers lived in the region.

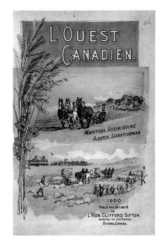

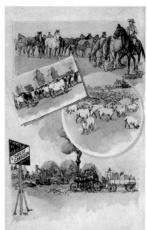

pioneering. They expected "all those beautiful, poetic and aristocratic privileges promised them by the honey-tongued immigrant agent and the reliable settler's guide," writes one contemporary critic, Professor Adam Shortt of Queen's University. Instead, many of them encountered, and were overwhelmed by, the realities of frontier life. A feeling of betrayal entered western political culture. Some historians have argued that behind many of the economic grievances of western farmers – opposition to the tariff policy and antagonism to the grain companies, the banks and the railways – was a basic resentment of a government that had enticed them to settle an inhospitable region with false promises and left them without the necessary supports they needed to survive.

The Liberal publicity campaign was also misleading to the degree that it presented Canada as a place that was open to everyone. For one thing, Clifford Sifton wanted farmers and he had firm ideas about who made the best farmers: northern and eastern Europeans, Britons and Americans, not Italians or Jews or Blacks or Asians. He thought of southern Europeans and Jews as essentially urban dwellers, unsuited to a life on the land. If the government did not stop them from immigrating, it did not actively encourage them. They were not the target of the propaganda campaign. Neither did Sifton encourage francophones from Quebec to come to the North-West. He preferred a unilingual West that did not replicate the often combative relations between French and English in eastern Canada. And of course the original inhabitants, the First Nations, played no role at all in the government's vision of a new North-West. For them, shunted away on their reserves, encouraged to become farmers but denied the land, training and supplies that would have made the transition possible, the influx of outsiders must have seemed less like settlement and more like conquest.

Two immigrant groups, Blacks and Asians, stand out as the recipients of special treatment at the hands of the

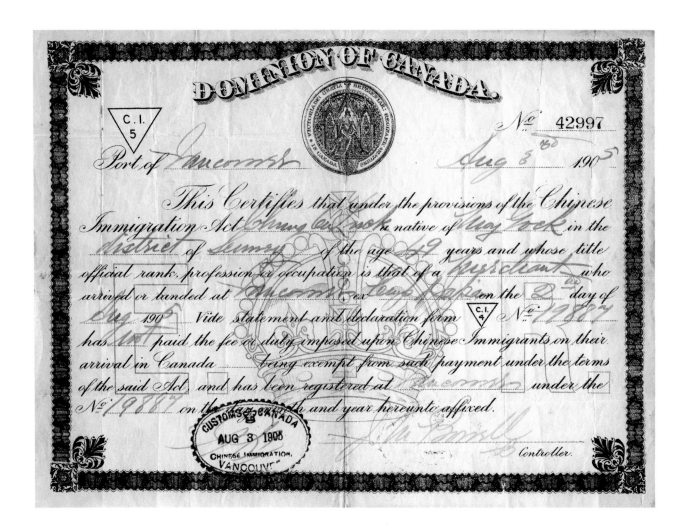

Unlike Americans, Britons and many continental Europeans, Asians were not welcome as immigrants to Canada. In 1885 the federal government introduced its notorious head tax, requiring a $50 payment for every Chinese immigrant. (The tax eventually rose to $500.) There were exceptions, however, as this certificate shows. Dated August 3, 1905, it exempts the holder from paying the head tax. In this case the individual, whose name is hard to read but may be Chung Gu Luok, was a merchant. Five categories of Chinese were exempted from paying the tax: merchants, students, diplomats, tourists and "men of science." Three of these groups would have been exempted because they were not really immigrants at all but merely visitors. Merchants and men of science were presumably exempted because they brought with them knowledge or material assets that made them valuable to Canadian society.

The only group actually banned from entry to Canada were African Americans and then only for a brief two-month period. Despite the cool reception given to Black people, some did move from the US to the Canadian West, especially after Oklahoma became a state in 1908 and began implementing racial segregation and denying Blacks fundamental rights. The majority of Blacks settled in Alberta, where this photograph was taken and where about a thousand Blacks were living by 1911, usually in their own communities.

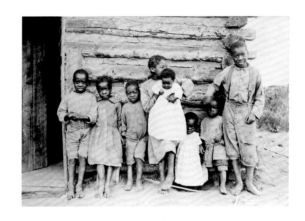

government. A small number of Black settlers from Oklahoma began arriving in Saskatchewan in 1905 as part of the tide of American migration. As their number increased, so did concerns in Canada about their "suitability" as pioneers in what most people expected would be, and should be, a "white man's country." Immigration officials agreed, pulling all advertisements from newspapers in Black communities in the United States. In August 1911 the federal government passed an order-in-council declaring that the "Negro race" was "unsuitable to the climate and requirements of Canada." The order was rescinded two months later and was never used, but it stands as the only example of the government actually banning a particular racial or ethnic group from Canada, as opposed to simply discouraging them with discriminatory regulations. In 1912 William Scott, the superintendent of immigration, made explicit the government's antagonism to African-American immigration. "It is to be hoped that climatic conditions will prove unsatisfactory to those new settlers," he wrote, "and that the fertile lands of the West will be left to be cultivated by the white race only."

As for Asian immigrants, whether from China, Japan or India, they also met a wall of discriminatory legislation. The Canadian Pacific Railway imported thousands of labourers from China to build the transcontinental line, especially the section through British Columbia. With the job finished, many of these men settled in Canada, again particularly in British Columbia but also on the Prairies. Anti-Asian sentiment ran high. Asian immigrants – Chinese but also Japanese and South Asians – were despised and resented. White Canadians believed they were culturally unassimilable as well as being a detriment to the economy because they accepted low-paying jobs. In 1885 the federal government responded to the anti-Asian sentiment by passing its infamous head tax, a $50 charge (later raised by increments to $500) imposed on every Chinese immigrant entering Canada.

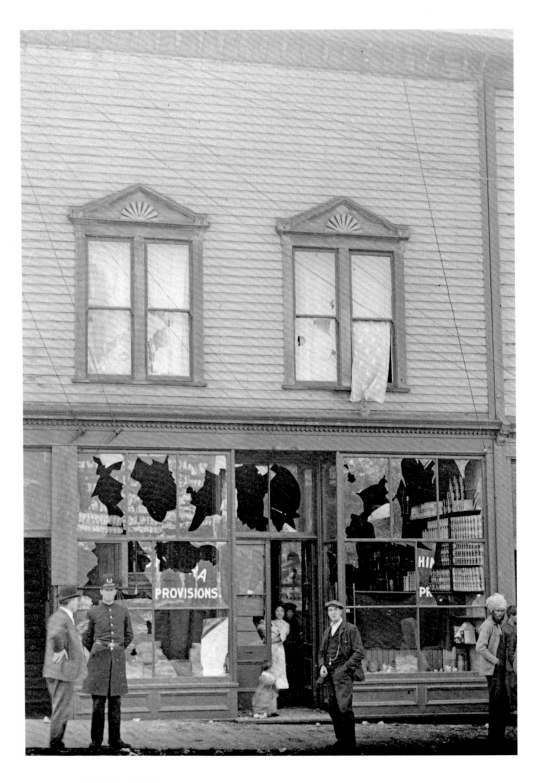

Anti-Asian feeling peaked in Vancouver in September 1907 when a rally organized by the Asiatic Exclusion League erupted into violence. Rioters roamed the streets of Chinatown and the nearby Japanese neighbourhood, threatening residents and damaging homes and businesses. Of the two dozen people arrested, five were found guilty and sent to jail.

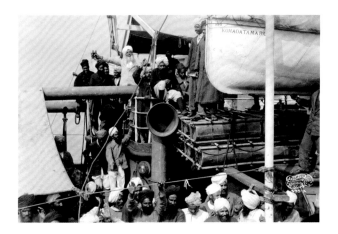

Sikh passengers wait aboard the *Komagata Maru* in Vancouver harbour, June 1914. After a standoff lasting almost two months, the arrivals were turned away and forced to return to India. In 2008 the federal government officially apologized for the incident.

Chinese and Japanese newcomers were denied certain jobs, confined to certain neighbourhoods and not allowed to vote or hold public office. In Vancouver, anti-Asian sentiment boiled over in September 1907 when a mob ran riot through the streets of the Chinese and Japanese quarters, breaking store windows and smashing property. This incident led to the federal government negotiating new restrictions on immigration from Japan.

By the spring of 1914 the focus of anti-Asian sentiment had settled on immigration from India. One of the ways Ottawa conspired to restrict the number of newcomers from Asia involved the "continuous passage regulation." This meant that any immigrant arriving in Canada had to have made a continuous voyage from his or her home port. Since there was no direct shipping connection between India and Canada, the effect was to stop South Asian immigration. On May 23, 1914, a steamship named the *Komagata Maru* arrived in Vancouver harbour carrying 376 passengers, mainly Sikhs from the Punjab desiring to enter British Columbia. They were refused admittance and a standoff began that lasted almost two months. After lengthy hearings and negotiations the Canadian naval vessel HMCS *Rainbow* ushered the *Komagata Maru* out of the harbour and it returned with its passengers to India. For this group of Sikhs, and most other Asian immigrants, the celebrated open door was not just closed – it was slammed shut.

FOR ALL THAT IT WAS MISLEADING AND racially biased, the campaign to sell Canada, especially western Canada, to immigrants was successful. By 1911 more than 80 percent of the inhabitants of the Prairie provinces had been born outside Canada. While it was hailed as a key to national development, this influx of newcomers at the same time provoked anxiety about what kind of society Canada was becoming. "Foreigners in large numbers are in our midst," wrote the Ontario-born Methodist minister and founder of Canadian socialism, J.S. Woodsworth, in his 1909 book *Strangers Within Our Gates*. "More are coming. How are we to make them into good Canadian citizens?" It was a frequently asked question: How do we Canadianize newcomers, many of whom speak foreign languages, worship at different churches and practise different customs?

By and large, British and American immigrants were exempt from this concern. They were seen to share the Anglo-Saxon values that dominated mainstream Canadian society. But for the others, the true "foreigners," what was to be done? Many observers feared that they were "mongrelizing" Canada, diluting its true, British character. Ethnic diversity and multiculturalism were concepts for the future. Most opinion leaders, in English-speaking Canada at least, preferred a bicultural Canada and a unicultural western Canada. In the words of one Member of Parliament, Canada had become "the dumping ground for the refuse of every country in the world." Others were more circumspect

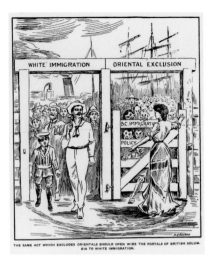

THE SAME ACT WHICH EXCLUDES ORIENTALS SHOULD OPEN WIDE THE PORTALS OF BRITISH COLUMBIA TO WHITE IMMIGRATION.

in their language but basically said the same thing. For instance, Frank Oliver, speaking in the House of Commons, suggested that many immigrants were "of such class and character as will deteriorate rather than elevate the condition of our people and our country." It was a paradox of the publicity campaign: at the same time the government was abroad so aggressively selling Canada as a promised land for immigrants, Canadians at home were making so many of them feel inferior and unwelcome.

Concerns about the cultural implications of immigration led to the imposition of restrictions on the inflow of immigrants from non-preferred sources; in other words, the closing of the open door. But the more pressing issue related to the proper assimilation of newcomers who were already in the country. By 1911, for instance, 15 percent of the population of the Prairies were recent arrivals from central and eastern Europe. These people were at the centre of the debate about how to ensure that immigrants were

inoculated with mainstream Protestant, Anglo-Saxon values. First of all, the newcomers had to learn to speak English. "If our people are to become one people, we must have one language," declared Woodsworth (conveniently ignoring the existence of Quebec). Beyond that, Canadians looked to the schools and the churches to do the necessary work of assimilating the newcomers who, it was felt, had to learn the ideals and values of mainstream Canadian society. Minority groups such as the Doukhobors and Mennonites watched in dismay as the tolerance of diversity that had characterized Clifford Sifton's approach gave way to a more rigorous emphasis on cultural conformity. The openness that had attracted so many immigrants to the country was giving way to a very narrow interpretation of what constituted the Canadian nationality.

With the outbreak of World War I in 1914, the debate about "Canadianization" was suddenly interrupted. The forging of a nationality had to be postponed while

attention turned to the more pressing emergency in Europe. Initially, the conventional wisdom was that the war would be over in a hurry. But as it settled into a long, drawn-out struggle, the government found it needed to formulate another propaganda campaign, aimed this time not at foreigners but at the hearts and minds of Canadians themselves. Techniques developed in the earlier publicity campaign were turned to promoting the war effort, often with the same paradoxical results.

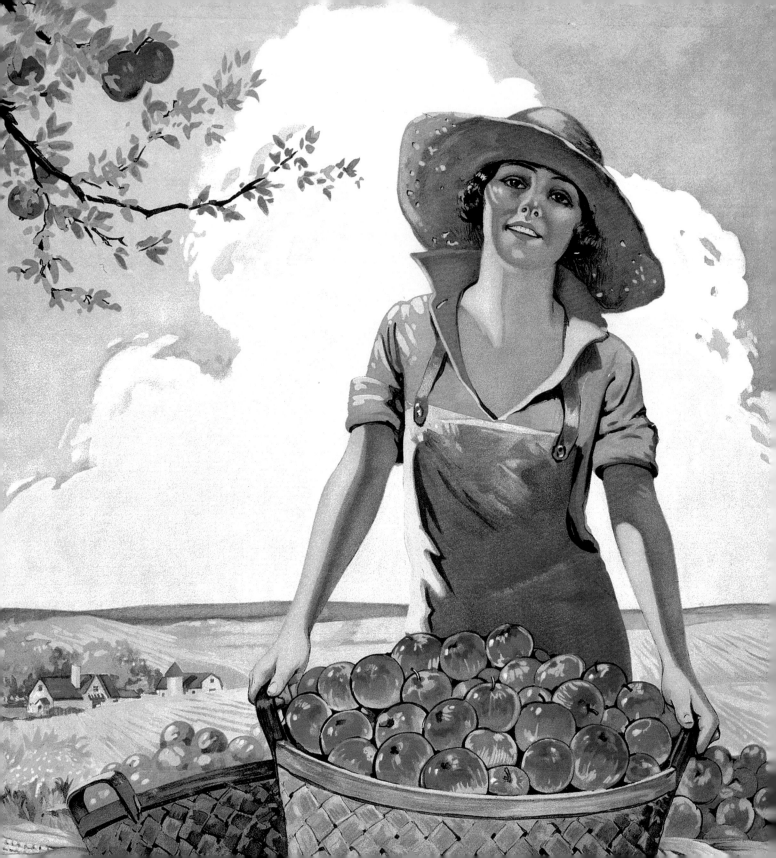

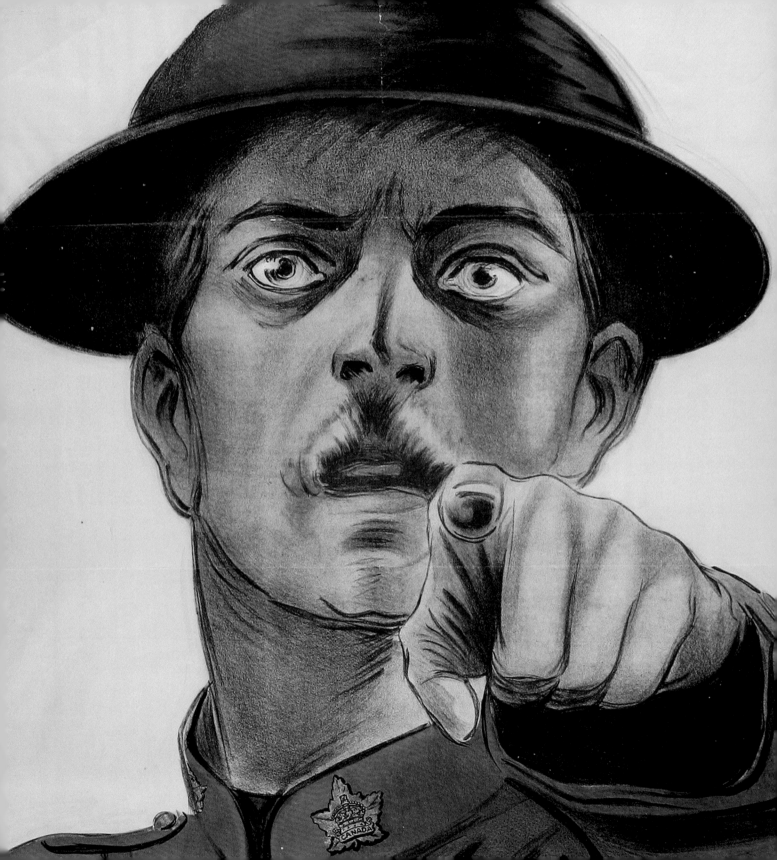

YOUR COUNTRY NEEDS YOU:
Selling the Great War to Canadians

CHAPTER TWO

*I have seen sights in the bloodstained trenches of Flanders that
I will never forget. If the people at home could see the real horrors
of the battle-field they would be worried to death.*
   – Canadian infantryman

IN THE RETROSPECTIVE GLOW OF NOSTALGIA the summer of 1914 is remembered as a blissful time of innocence and peace. The weather in the last weeks before World War I began was sunny and warm. While the well-to-do vacationed at the lake or seashore, the working class enjoyed time at park and playground. Charles Gordon was typical. The prominent Presbyterian clergyman and popular novelist (under the pen name Ralph Connor) was camping with his family at Lake of the Woods near Kenora, Ontario. "It was glorious weather," he later recalled. "With our canoes and boats, with our swimming and tennis, with our campfires and singsongs our life was full of rest and happy peace. It was a good world. On Thursday, July 30th, our boat returning with supplies from the little town brought back a newspaper with red headlines splashed on its front page. Austria had declared war on Serbia." Even the prime minister, Robert Borden, was enjoying a brief holiday. He was swimming and golfing in the sunshine at Port Carling in the Muskoka Lakes district of Ontario

when he was called back to Ottawa on July 31 by the developing crisis in Europe. A time of blue-sky innocence abruptly interrupted by unspeakable horror: that is how we remember the onset of the Great War.

And even then, the horror of what was to come was delayed by a naive euphoria, a festive sense that a fabulous storybook adventure was getting under way. When Canada joined the fight on August 4, young men hurried to enlist, worried that "it would all be over by Christmas" and they would have missed it. "The country went mad!" recalled Bert Remington, a telephone company employee in Montreal who joined the rush to the recruiting office. "People were singing on the streets and roads. Everybody wanted to be a hero, everybody wanted to go to war." In Toronto, the downtown streets were filled with a cheering throng. "It was the voice of Toronto," reported the *Telegram* newspaper, "carried away with patriotic enthusiasm at the thought that Britain, longing for peace, had determined to give the bully

OPPOSITE A detail from a World War I poster asking Canadians to buy Victory Bonds in support of the war effort. The pointing soldier is based on a celebrated 1914 image of Lord Kitchener, the British war minister, exhorting young Britons to join the army.

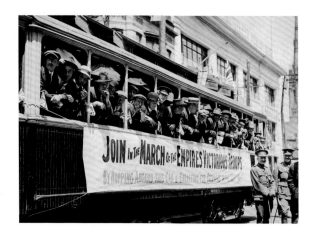

A streetcar in downtown Toronto loaded with eager recruits. The outbreak of war was greeted with enthusiasm by most Canadians, who naively believed that it would be a great adventure.

of Europe a trouncing." Within the first five weeks of war, 32,665 volunteers signed up. British-born Canadians, of which there were many, rallied to the defence of their homeland. Teenagers lied about their ages to get in on the excitement. Wives eagerly gave permission for their men to fight, as required by the law. Looking back, one of the saddest things about the Great War in all its slaughter is the enthusiastic clamour with which it started.

At the outbreak of war, Canada was overwhelmingly a "British" country. The torrent of immigration from the European continent that characterized the pre-war period did not alter this fundamental fact. The Dominion was linked constitutionally, economically and culturally to Great Britain. When war broke out, Canadians naturally responded as if they themselves were threatened. "All are agreed," Prime Minister Borden told the House of Commons on August 19, 1914, "we stand shoulder to shoulder with Britain and the other British dominions in this quarrel." The Leader of the Opposition, Wilfrid Laurier,

agreed. "When Britain is at war," he announced, "Canada is at war also." Even Quebec nationalist leader Henri Bourassa argued in favour of joining the conflict. It was Canada's "national duty," he wrote in the newspaper Le Devoir, "to contribute... to the triumph and above all the endurance of the combined efforts of France and England."

At first there was no need to "sell the war." It sold itself. Canadians overwhelmingly supported it and expected it to be effortless. They saw it as a crusade for freedom and civilization against the barbarity of "the Hun." (This widely used epithet referred to the warlike Asiatic people who invaded Europe in the fourth and fifth centuries; their most famous leader was Attila.) Secondarily, many men saw the military as a sensible alternative to low-paying jobs, or no jobs at all, at home. The Winnipeg labour activist Roger Bray spoke for many when he explained why he joined up: "I had no job and a large family." In city and village from coast to coast crowds lined the

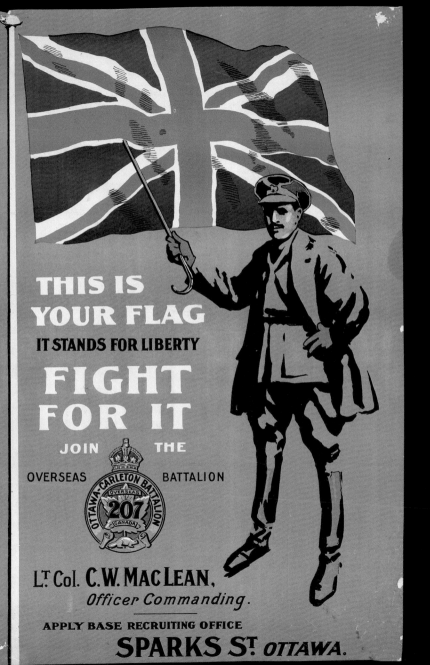

A recruiting poster for the 207th (Ottawa-Carleton) Overseas Battalion. The 207th was formed in 1916 and arrived in England in June 1917. The officers and men were then dispersed to other infantry units fighting at the front. The flag that recruits were urged to fight for was, of course, the British Union Jack since Canada had no official flag of its own.

A recruiting poster for the 148th Overseas Battalion, formed in Montreal in late 1915. The battalion was based at McGill University and drew heavily from the city's anglophone community. After the battalion arrived in England in September 1916 its men were absorbed into other infantry units. More than three thousand McGill students and alumni enlisted in the war; 383 died. The black eagle was a familiar symbol of the German enemy.

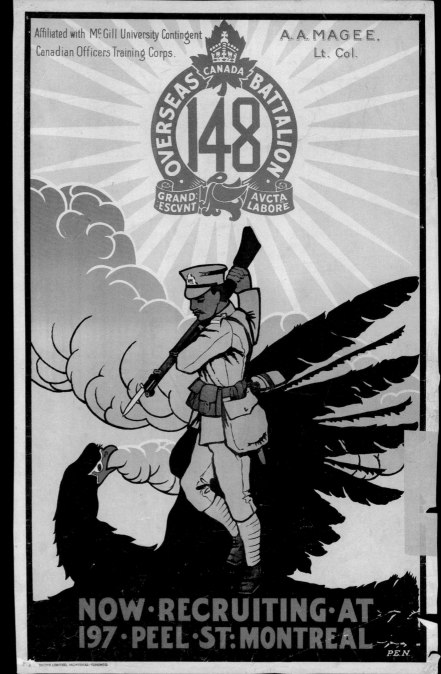

LEFT The 245th Grenadier Guards was an infantry battalion recruited in Montreal in 1916. The battalion sailed to England the following year and was broken up for reinforcements. The commanding officer, Charles Colquhoun Ballantyne, was a prominent manufacturer appointed by Prime Minister Borden to cabinet in October 1917 as minister of public works and then minister of marine and fisheries.

RIGHT A recruiting poster highlights the actions of Canadian soldiers at the battles of St. Julien and Festubert. St. Julien was part of the Second Battle of Ypres in April–May 1915, when Canadian and British troops were exposed to the enemy use of poison gas for the first time. Festubert took place later in May. It resulted in minimal gains at the cost of 661 Canadian dead. Recruiters relied on heroic words and images from both battles to maintain patriotic enthusiasm at home.

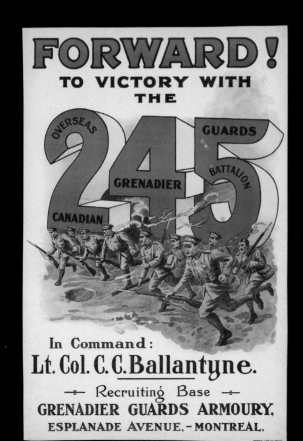

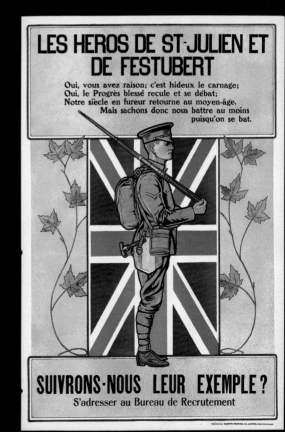

BELOW The 109th Regiment uses a streetcar to do some mobile recruiting in the streets of Toronto, drawing several curious youngsters along with a crowd of eligible-looking men. It was the winter of 1915–1916 when recruits were getting harder to find but the government was promising more and more men for the front.

RIGHT J.W. Geddes, a recruiting officer, seeks volunteers in front of city hall in downtown Toronto during the summer of 1916. By this time Prime Minister Borden had promised to provide half a million Canadian soldiers for the fight. Mayor Tommy Church leans casually against the vehicle beside the Presbyterian chaplain J.D. Morrow.

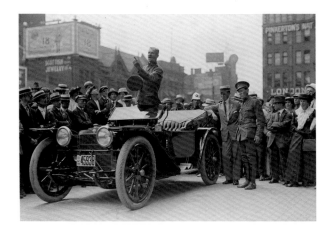

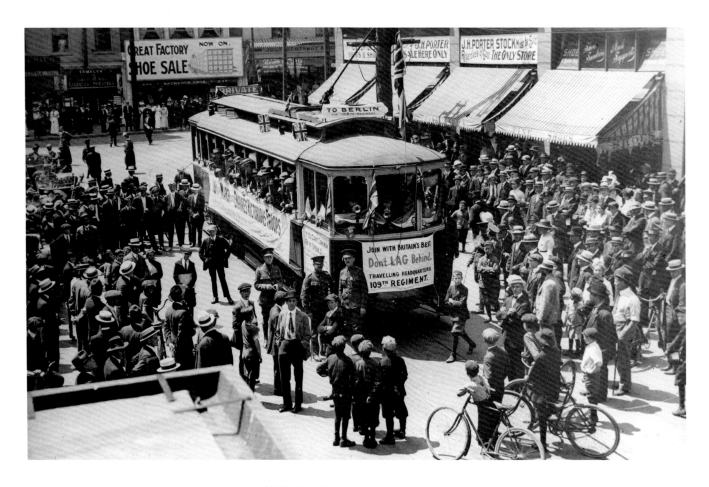

BELOW RIGHT This primitive-looking hood was an early gas mask, known as a P.H. helmet. Masks like this one were uncomfortable, left soldiers gasping for breath, irritated the skin and permitted limited visibility. They were soon replaced by more effective equipment.

RIGHT These wounded Canadian soldiers are on their way from the front to England for medical treatment. Canadians were appalled when they began to learn of the terrible suffering their soldiers were enduring. Propagandists had to carefully manage information from the front lines to convince the public that the sacrifice was worthwhile.

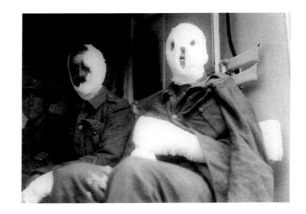

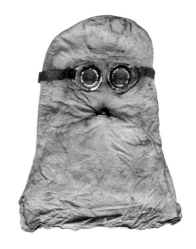

streets to cheer enthusiastically as eager recruits led by brass bands paraded to the trains and ships that carried them off to the assembly point at Valcartier, Quebec, and then to Europe. "They had this terrific propaganda," said New Brunswicker Jack Burton, who at thirteen was not old enough to enlist when war broke out, "and there were recruiting officers at every corner. They'd practically grab you by the back of the neck and take you in and put a uniform on you. You know, banners waving and bands playing! It was just like a fever." There was a sense of urgency; Lloyd's of London was giving even money odds that the war would be over by year's end.

This initial blaze of enthusiasm lasted through the first winter of war. But then the bad news began arriving from overseas, and with it the realization that the enemy was not going to be as easily overwhelmed as had been imagined. Canadians came to recognize that the war was going to be a struggle requiring unprecedented suffering and sacrifice. It was to justify that suffering and to encourage that sacrifice

that Canada's second great propaganda campaign was launched.

————

THE FIRST CONTINGENT OF THE EXPEDITIONary force reached England in October 1914 to begin training on Salisbury Plain. The following March the First Canadian Division was deemed battle-ready and made its way into the trenches of the Western Front where already hundreds of thousands of French, German and British soldiers had been killed or maimed. In mid-April the Canadians advanced to defend the town of Ypres in Belgium, where the Germans unleashed a deadly gas attack, "the first lethal chlorine gas attack in the history of warfare." When French and Algerian soldiers, with no gas masks and no experience of chemical warfare, fell back, the Canadians came forward to plug the gap in the lines. After a week of furious combat, the German advance was halted, at a cost of 6,036 dead and wounded Canadians. For the first time, family and friends at home

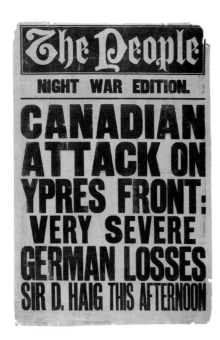

The People

NIGHT WAR EDITION.

CANADIAN ATTACK ON YPRES FRONT: VERY SEVERE GERMAN LOSSES SIR D. HAIG THIS AFTERNOON

As news spread about the terrible losses at Ypres in the spring of 1915 it began to dawn on the Canadian public that the war would not be the easy victory they had anticipated.

read the appalling list of casualties in the newspapers.

Ypres was followed, in early May, by a German submarine attack on the British passenger liner *Lusitania* off the Irish coast in which 1,195 people died, including almost one hundred children. Soon after that, details from the Bryce Report began circulating in the newspapers. The British government had appointed Viscount Bryce and his Committee on Alleged German Outrages to look into war crimes that allegedly occurred during the German invasion of Belgium. "Murder, lust and pillage prevailed over many parts of Belgium on a scale unparalleled in any war between civilised nations during the last three centuries," declared Bryce. With its sensational accounts of enemy atrocities, the report had a huge impact on public opinion in Allied countries, including Canada. Even someone as dispassionate as the writer Nellie McClung, a noted pacifist, began to see the enemy as evil incarnate. "It was the *Lusitania* that brought me to see the whole truth," she wrote.

"Then I saw that we were waging war on the very Prince of Darkness... I knew that no man could die better than in defending civilization from this ghastly thing which threatened her!" Interestingly it was also the *Lusitania* that made former US president Theodore Roosevelt change his mind about the war. Roosevelt had supported armed neutrality for the Americans, but with the *Lusitania* sinking he became the most prominent advocate of US intervention.

As horror mounted on horror, it became clear that the war was not going to be a short-lived escapade after all. It was going to be brutal and drawn-out and a determined enemy was going to do everything it could to win. Civilization itself seemed to be hanging in the balance. In Canada, public opinion was all but unanimous in support of the war effort. But in a prolonged conflict this support could not be relied upon to sustain itself without encouragement, which is why the propaganda campaign became so important.

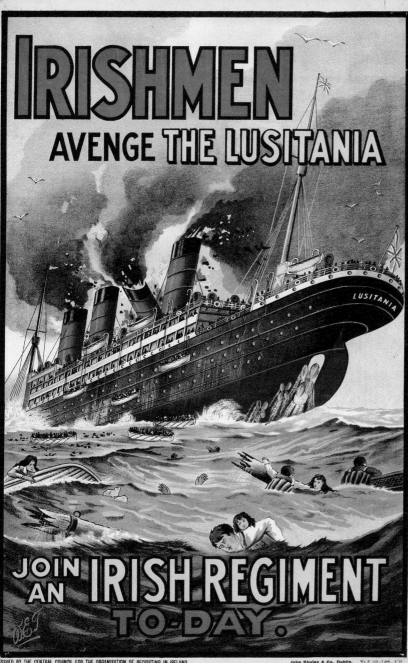

The sinking of the *Lusitania* off the Irish coast in early May 1915 was used to rouse public passions and stimulate recruiting throughout the British Empire. Depictions of the many innocent lives lost – see the women and child featured in this poster – were used to inspire contributions to the war effort.

BELOW At Toronto's Union Station the 180th Battalion leaves for war. The photographer, William James, came to Canada from his native England in 1906 at the age of forty and became Toronto's first press photographer, documenting daily life in the city for a variety of publications. During the war he concentrated on scenes from the home front like this one.

RIGHT Immediately after war was declared, existing units recalled their members from across the country. On August 9, 1914, this telegram reached Robert Kane from his commanding officer, asking him if he intended to volunteer for active service and telling him to report to Kingston, Ontario. Kane did serve. He died of a gunshot wound to the chest on December 12, 1915, and is buried near Ypres, Belgium.

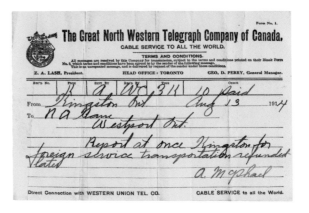

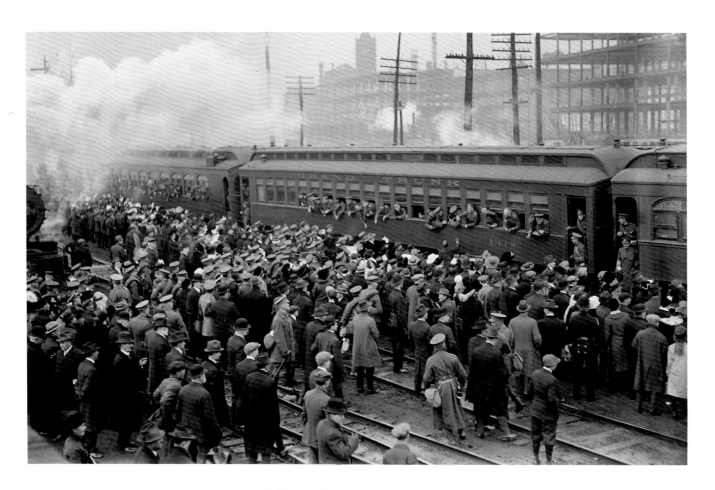

Soldiers outside the recruiting office of the 155th Battalion in Stirling, Ontario. The battalion began recruiting in late 1915 and left for England a year later. The sign on the balcony reads: "Who would be a conscript – No man – Your King and Country need you – Join now."

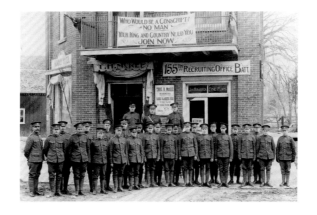

THE FIRST OBJECTIVE OF THE CAMPAIGN was to convince young Canadians to volunteer for the fight. At the outbreak of war Canada had promised to contribute twenty-five thousand men, but as the conflict unfolded the Canadian Division, later renamed the Canadian Corps, required more and more recruits. By the beginning of 1916 Prime Minister Borden had increased the Canadian commitment to half a million men (the population of Canada at the time being less than eight million). The front lines were chewing up soldiers at a rate that no one had anticipated. In April 1917, for example, during five days of fighting at Vimy, the Corps sustained 10,602 casualties. Later that same year, at Passchendaele, the cost to Canada was even higher, over fifteen thousand dead and wounded. Many thousands of new recruits were needed every month to make up for the losses, and as the war dragged on the pool of available volunteers grew smaller and smaller.

The recruitment effort was not centrally organized. It depended instead on a nationwide spirit of enthusiastic volunteerism. "There has not been, there will not be, compulsion or conscription," Borden promised in December 1914. Wealthy industrialists funded their own regiments and a wide variety of institutions and organizations lent their support to a grassroots campaign to raise an army. Clergymen gave sermons extolling the virtue of armed service and counselled their young male parishioners to enlist. Armchair soldiers thundered the same message from the columns of the daily newspapers. Universities introduced military training programs. Teachers pressured their students to volunteer. In Ontario, a group of business and professional leaders established the Speakers' Patriotic League as a central agency to provide orators to rouse public sentiment in favour of the war. Recruiting Leagues popped up in communities across the country. Aimed specifically at signing up recruits, the groups later worked to mobilize public opinion in favour of conscription.

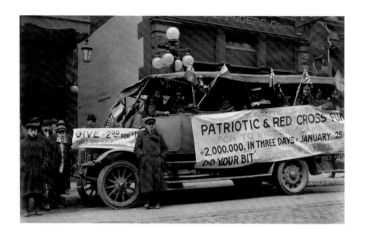

A transport van loaded with soldiers tours downtown Toronto collecting money for the Canadian Patriotic Fund and the Red Cross. To a large extent, the war was paid for by the donations of everyday Canadians.

Another leading group involved in the informal support-the-war movement was the Canadian Patriotic Fund, initiated by the wealthy Montreal manufacturer and politician Herbert Ames to provide financial support for dependants of men who had volunteered to fight. The fund was intended to reassure potential recruits that if they enlisted, their families would be cared for. After all, a soldier was only receiving $1.10 a day, about half the average wage for a production worker back home. The amount paid out to a wife or dependent mother varied over time but it began at $30 per month and by 1916 the fund was supporting fifty-five thousand families. By the middle of the war the federal government had stepped in to provide pensions for widows and dependents of the war dead, the first planks in the public social welfare system that would develop during the subsequent decades.

As the war continued, donations flowed into the Canadian Patriotic Fund from wealthy philanthropists, the business community, local governments, service clubs, women's organizations, youth groups, labour unions and thousands of individual Canadians. Contributors to the fund, which enjoyed the patronage of the governor general, the Duke of Connaught, who threw his considerable prestige behind the fundraising efforts, received a button they could display proudly on their lapels. As well, the fund mobilized thousands of volunteers to comfort soldiers' families with advice and moral support.

While soldiers and their families were praised and supported, able-bodied males who had not signed up were made to feel like either cowards or traitors. The unofficial anthem of the recruiting movement was a new song, "Why Aren't You in Khaki?" It was a confident individual who could withstand the pressure of family, the accusing looks from strangers who had loved ones at the front, or the guilt of not serving while others did. Robert Swan, a young Nova Scotian, recalled that "young girls were going along and they would meet what looked

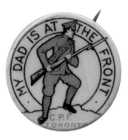
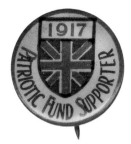
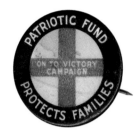
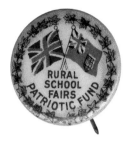

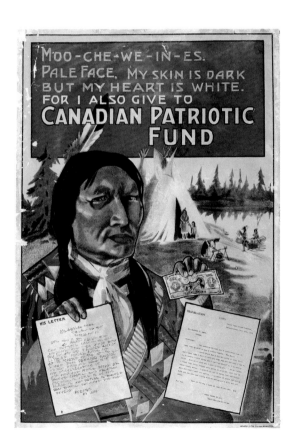

MOO-CHE-WE-IN-ES. PALE FACE, MY SKIN IS DARK BUT MY HEART IS WHITE. FOR I ALSO GIVE TO CANADIAN PATRIOTIC FUND

LEFT The condescending depiction of an Aboriginal Canadian ("my heart is white") used in this 1916 poster was meant to inspire contributions to the Canadian Patriotic Fund. The poster features a Cree man holding a letter of support written in Cree syllabics with an English translation on the right. An estimated four thousand Aboriginal men volunteered to fight overseas.

ABOVE A series of buttons handed out by the Canadian Patriotic Fund, which provided financial aid to the families of soldiers. On the left, a button distributed to youngsters whose fathers were overseas proudly proclaims "My Dad Is at the Front." On the right, a button awarded during a rural schools fundraising drive displays the British Union Jack and the Canadian Red Ensign, Canada's flag until 1965. The two buttons in the middle were given to anyone who made a contribution to the fund.

This poster for a battalion of the Queen's Own Rifles encouraged members of the public to reveal the identities of able-bodied men who they thought should be in the army. The power of public opinion was mobilized to make young men ashamed to remain on civvy street.

As the war continued, wounded soldiers became a common sight on the streets of Canadian cities. These three wounded veterans pose in Toronto beside some graffiti scrawled on a wall warning "slackers" that conscription was around the corner.

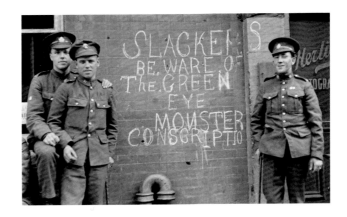

like a pretty good able-bodied man and they'd pin something white on them – called them a coward in other words, because they weren't in the army." Another witness, this time in Toronto, watched a group of women patrol the streets with feather dusters doused with talcum powder. "They used to shower the powder over any person that they thought was a slacker." And if shame was not incentive enough, it was not unheard of for gangs of soldiers to strong-arm reluctant "volunteers" into the local recruiting office. The military even organized "Give Us His Name" campaigns to encourage members of the public to hand over the names of anyone they knew who might be eligible for service and had not yet enlisted. "In the cities of the West," reported Manitoba's chief justice, T.G. Mathers, "the man who is not in uniform is made to feel that he is a sort of social outcast. No man who joins the ranks today does so voluntarily. He does so because he can no longer resist the pressure of public opinion."

Of course, when raw recruits marched off to fight, some enthusiastically, some reluctantly, the families they left behind felt the departure with pride mixed with sorrow and apprehension. Nellie McClung captured the horrible catch-22 faced by loved ones when she wrote in her diary:

Dec. 4, 1915: This morning we said goodbye to our dear son Jack at the CNR station where new snow lay fresh and white on the roofs and on the streets, white, and soft, and pure as a young heart. When we came home I felt strangely tired and old though I am only 42. But I know that my youth has departed from me. It has gone with Jack, our beloved, our first born, the pride of our hearts. Strange fate surely for a boy who never has had a gun in his hands, whose ways are gentle, and full of peace... What have I done to you, in letting you go into this inferno of war? And how could I hold you back without breaking your heart?

McClung alienated many of her pacifist friends in the suffrage movement when she came out publicly in favour of the war effort as a necessary evil.

⸻

IF RECRUITMENT WAS ONE OBJECTIVE OF the propaganda campaign, the encouragement of a spirit of sacrifice and patriotism in the population at large was another. Canadian society was totally mobilized for war. Employees got time off from their jobs to go and fight. In school, students learned about the war effort and engaged in patriotic lessons. Ontario teachers were even provided with special textbooks and instructed to include the subject as part of the history curriculum. Families raised their own vegetables in Victory Gardens intended to relieve the demand for food domestically and make more food available for the troops. Industry retooled to produce war material instead of consumer goods, which were considered frivolous in an emergency. Children gathered scrap metal for munitions; their mothers knitted socks, scarves and other "comforts"

BELOW A helmet and face guard worn by early tank crews. The armoured goggles and chain-mail mouth shield were supposed to protect the face from small arms fire and from metal fragments flying around the interior of the vehicle.

RIGHT The motorized tank was an innovation of the war, used for the first time in combat in 1916. Many hoped this armour-plated vehicle would break the dead-lock of trench warfare. For the public the tank was a great curiosity, as can be seen by the crowds getting their first sight of one in downtown Toronto.

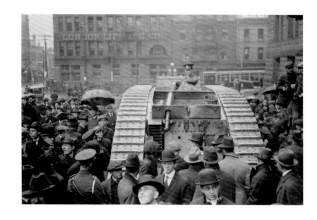

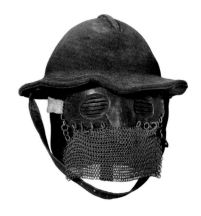

for the men at the front. The country even put up with prohibition so that grains previously used in the production of alcohol could be diverted to feed the soldiers. So much effort and personal inconvenience could only be sustained by constant reminders that the cause was noble, the sacrifice worth it.

At the most basic level, the government needed money to prosecute the war. By 1917 it was costing Canadians almost a million dollars a day. That year Thomas White, the finance minister, reluctantly imposed the nation's first income tax, promising it would only last for the duration of the conflict. Rates were set so low, however, that few people made enough income to pay the tax and other funding sources had to be found. The more effective option was to borrow the money from the Canadian people by selling them bonds. There were five different bond offerings between 1915 and 1919 and the proceeds from them far exceeded expectations. The first Victory Bond drive collected $100 million, twice the anticipated amount and many times more than any previous bond issue in Canadian history. The 1918 campaign raised more than $600 million in just three weeks.

Bond drives were accompanied by aggressive publicity campaigns orchestrated by the Victory Loan Dominion Publicity Committee. Dramatic posters went up across the country emphasizing the need for funds to prosecute the war. Advertisements appeared in newspapers and giant rallies stirred up public enthusiasm. In Toronto a tank joined a parade through the streets; for most people in the city it was the first time they had seen the great lumbering weapon that would have such an impact on modern warfare. But of all the public events that were held to support the bond drives, few drew as many curious spectators as a gathering in the streets of downtown Vancouver on October 31, 1918, just days before the end of the war. It was billed as a Victory Bond event but most of the people were there to watch "The Human Fly," Harry Gardiner,

BELOW Knitted socks were among the "comforts" made for soldiers serving overseas. Here a load of socks intended to warm the feet of men in the trenches is photographed outside the offices of the *News-Telegram* in Calgary. On the home front, everyone pitched in to show their support for the war effort.

RIGHT The children of Brantford, Ontario presented tin chocolate boxes like this one to soldiers and sailors in 1914.

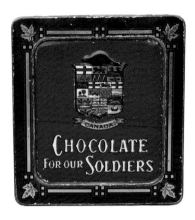

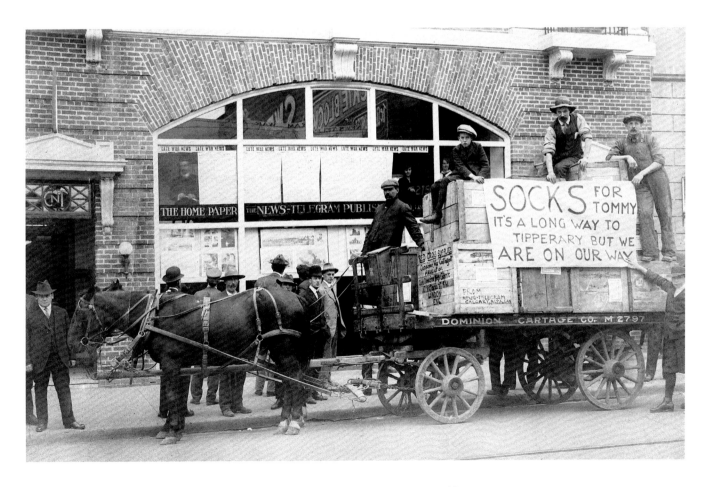

SHORTLY AFTER THE OUTBREAK OF war, eighty-two artists contributed canvases to a large exhibition of paintings and sculptures mounted to raise money to support the families of military personnel. The Canadian artists' exhibition kicked off in Toronto in December 1914, then travelled to Winnipeg, Halifax, Saint John, Quebec City, Montreal, Ottawa and Hamilton. It raised $10,514 for the Patriotic Fund and impressed on the public that artists were as capable as anyone else of contributing to the war effort.

As the war continued, artists were also encouraged to describe what was going on at the front. Two paintings produced by war artists Richard Jack and Frederick Varley reveal a changing perception of the conflict. "The Second Battle of Ypres, 22 April to 25 May, 1915" by Jack, a British painter, was the first canvas commissioned by the Canadian War Memorials Fund established by Max Aitken to memorialize in art Canada's contribution to the war effort. Jack was not at the battle – he painted the canvas in his London studio – but viewers at the time believed he had captured the gallant bravery of the Canadian soldiers. Modern critics have been less kind. Art historian Maria Tippett wrote: "In order to glorify the Canadian troops, Jack employed every hackneyed nineteenth-century battle art convention." This romantic view of war stands in contrast to Varley's "For What?"– a much more sombre, even despairing, expression of the pointlessness of war. "You'll never know dear anything of what it means," Varley wrote to his wife. "I'm going to paint a picture of it, but heavens, it can't say a thousandth part of a story."

ARTISTS SUPPORT AND DESCRIBE THE WAR

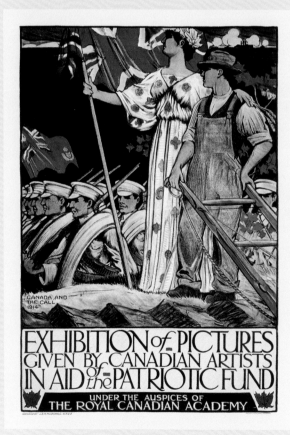

This poster advertises the exhibition of Canadian art that toured the country in 1914–1915 in support of the Patriotic Fund.

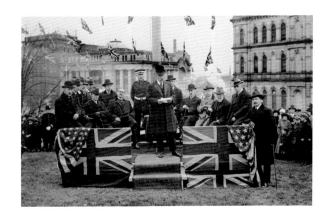

as he scaled the outside of the city's tallest building, the seventeen-storey World Tower. It was the largest crowd Vancouver had ever seen. At precisely noon Gardiner emerged from the front door of the building, dressed in a white canvas suit so as to be visible from a distance to the naked eye, and began his ascent. There was a fire truck parked in the street with its ladder extended about three storeys into the air and a young woman named Lottie Fletcher clambered to the top and unfurled a banner encouraging everyone to buy Victory Bonds. Then attention reverted to the tiny white speck as Gardiner continued his assault on the tower. Finally, after an hour and a half, he scrambled up the copper dome to the summit. "Then," wrote a reporter in the *Vancouver Sun*, "crowned by the brilliant sunlight, he waved once again to the crowd, now scarcely able to see him, and vanished into the interior of the building."

Buying a bond was considered a way that Canadians at home could show solidarity with the brave boys fighting overseas. Money raised would be spent on weaponry that could make the difference between life and death, victory and defeat. When a community purchased enough bonds, it was awarded a Victory Loan honour flag that could be flown proudly in the civic square. In total, Victory Bond drives raised over $2 billion, including $680 million by the post-war 1919 campaign that focused on support for returned soldiers.

———————

POSTERS WERE ONE OF THE MOST EFFECTIVE media for manipulating public opinion, whether to raise money by the sale of Victory Bonds, to promote enlistment or to demonize the enemy. Mass media outlets were in their infancy. Newspapers flourished – by 1891, 80 percent of Canadians were literate – but there was no radio, no television. In their stead, posters served as an accepted and familiar public art form and source of information. People were used to seeing posters in store windows, post offices, factories, town

Robert Borden addresses a crowd gathered on Parliament Hill in Ottawa during a 1917 campaign for Victory Bonds – a new and hugely successful way of financing the heavy costs of war. No pre-war bond issue had ever raised more than $5 million, yet the first Victory Bond drive brought in $100 million and subsequent drives even more.

RIGHT Each Victory Bond drive was accompanied by a new marketing campaign and a new set of posters. In this one, a soldier doffs his coat to prepare for the fight and urges Canadians to "finish the job."

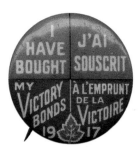

ABOVE Buy a bond, get a button. This bilingual button was evidence that its wearer had bought a 1917 Victory Bond and was supporting the soldiers overseas.

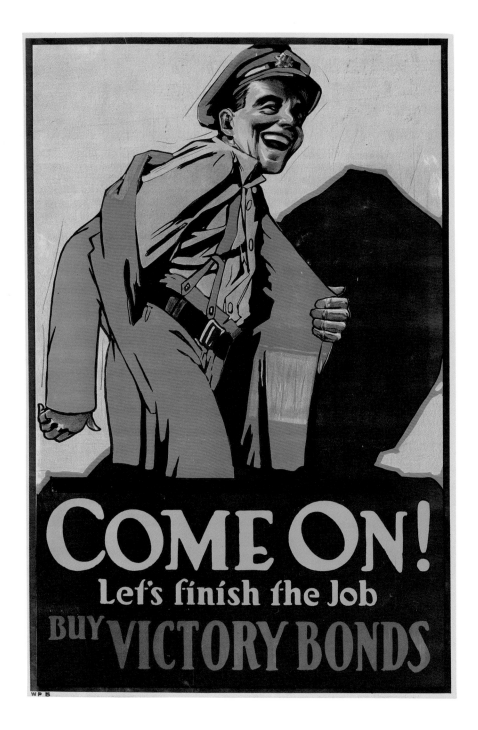

Images taken by war photographers sometimes ended up in publicity campaigns at home. An unknown photographer snapped this picture of Canadian troops (right) returning from the front at Vimy Ridge in 1917. The image was transformed into a poster (below) used to sell Victory Bonds. Note that the road ahead is paved with bonds and the men are smiling and celebrating, an uplifting image of war that seemed to indicate victory was just around the corner.

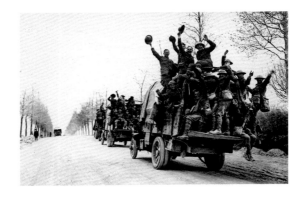

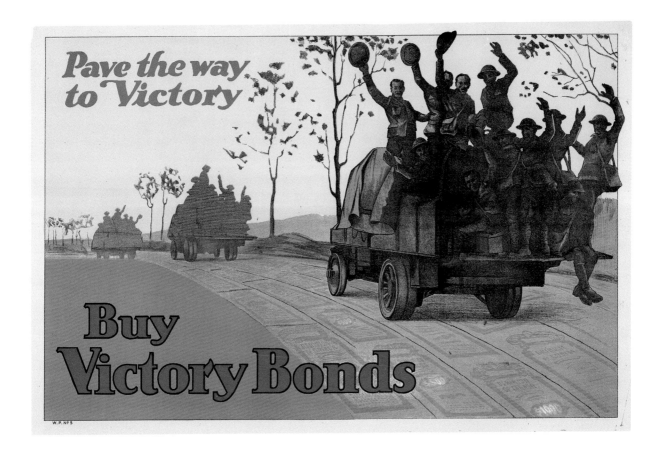

Khaki University (initially Khaki College) was a Canadian educational institution set up and managed by the general staff of the Canadian Army in Britain from 1917 to 1919 during World War I and again from 1945 to 1946 in World War II. Some 50,000 soldiers took courses in the Khaki University system from 1917 to 1919. Most took primary, elementary, or high school courses, but several hundred were accepted into universities such as Oxford, London, and Edinburgh. Henry Marshall Tory, the president of the University of Alberta, organized the program; his name is signed at the bottom of this certificate.

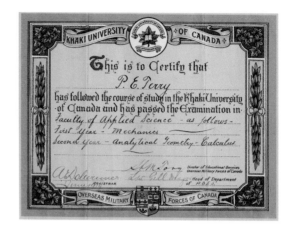

halls, theatres, banks, wherever there was space available and something worth advertising. They were reasonably cheap to produce in large quantities and, if designed effectively, delivered a direct, emotionally charged message. Initially the federal government did not produce posters itself but left it to local businesses, civic groups or regiments to produce their own. Then, in 1916, the War Poster Service was established to coordinate the production and distribution of posters in both official languages. Most of these posters were lithographs produced by large printing companies in Toronto, Montreal and Hamilton.

The best posters featured a single dominant image and a simple slogan so that the message could be absorbed quickly and felt forcefully. For the most part, the horrors of the front lines were avoided, although sometimes atrocities were featured, as in the Victory Loan poster that depicted the sinking of the hospital ship *Llandovery Castle*. The positive images most popular with illustrators were the Union Jack, then considered to be Canada's national flag, the maple leaf and a single heroic figure – often a nurse or a soldier. One hero featured in a poster produced in Quebec was the iconic Dollard des Ormeaux, who held off an Iroquois assault on the young colony of New France in 1660. The poster evoked the spirit of bravery and sacrifice supposedly embodied by Dollard and his small party of French traders and First Nations allies. The negative images used to represent the enemy included the spiked helmet, the German eagle and a grotesque caricature of "the Hun."

Simple slogans emphasized the threat to Canadian values ("Kultur vs. Humanity") or made appeals to manly pride ("Your Chums Are Fighting, Why Aren't You?" or "Daddy, What Did You Do In the War?"). One recurring image was the "Pointing Soldier" with some variation of the message, "Your Country Needs You." This image was based on a magazine cover designed by the commercial illustrator Alfred Leete in Britain in 1914 showing Lord Kitchener, the war minister, pointing out at the viewer with his index finger and asking for recruits. A parliamentary committee responsible for recruiting adapted the cover for use as a poster. In the United States, "Uncle Sam Wants You" was modeled on the Leete illustration, which was also popular in Canadian versions.

POSTERS AND OTHER FORMS OF PROPAganda were intended to convey positive messages about the war to the public. At the same time, the government imposed a strict censorship on negative information that it felt might jeopardize the military effort or weaken public resolve. In *The First Casualty*, his classic study of the war correspondent, Phillip Knightley claims that "more deliberate lies were told [during World War I] than in any other period of history, and the whole apparatus of the state went into action to suppress the truth." Knightley was writing about Britain, but Canadian authorities eagerly

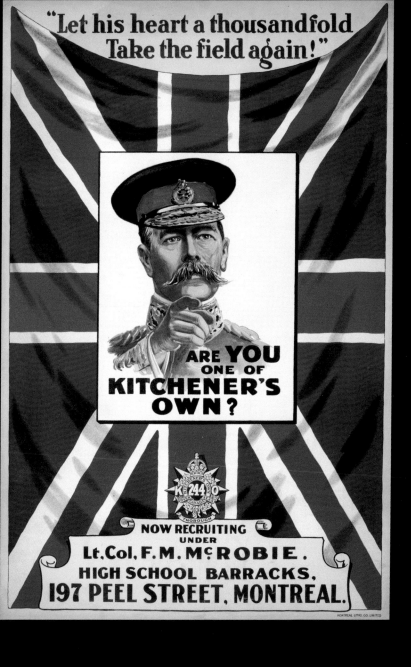

A recruiting poster for the 244th (Kitchener's Own) Battalion, based in Montreal. The image of Lord Kitchener, the British war minister, was used widely in war propaganda. He died travelling to Russia in June 1916, when the cruiser he was on struck a mine and sank.

one for a francophone audience suggests that the privileged fat cats who continued to live in luxury were in fact supporting the enemy by wasting food and other precious resources. The message was that all Canadians, rich and poor alike, should make sacrifices. One of the grievances felt by many working people was that the rich were not being asked to bear their fair share of the costs of war.

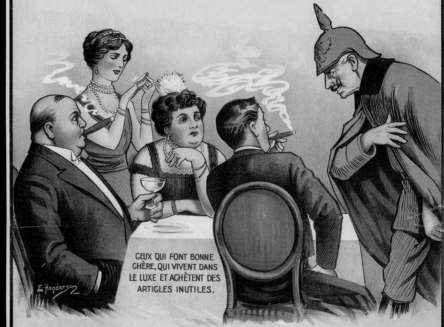

ETES-VOUS UN AMI DU KAISER?

CEUX QUI FONT BONNE CHÈRE, QUI VIVENT DANS LE LUXE ET ACHÈTENT DES ARTICLES INUTILES.

E. Henderson

(LES EXTRAVAGANTS)
"Oui! Guerre ou pas de Guerre, Nous vivons comme d'habitude."
(LE KAISER)
"Merci, mes Amis, car vous êtes vraiment mes Amis"

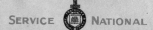

SERVICE NATIONAL

urged to eat less wheat, meat and sugar so these foodstuffs could be sent overseas to keep the army fed.

ages had become a reality on the home front. The government created the Canadian Food Board to monitor food sales and encourage consumers to use substitutes for high-demand foodstuffs. The

series of posters urging the public to save food and warning them that it was unpatriotic to hoard.

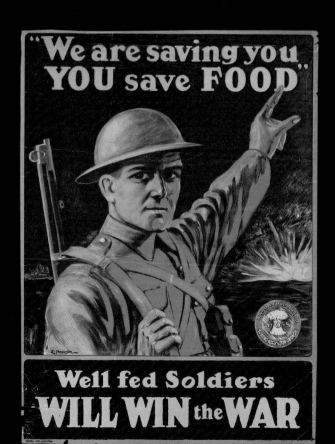

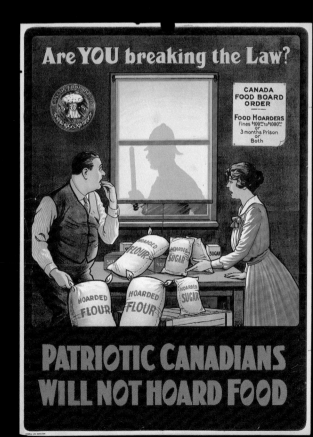

ON JUNE 27, 1918, A GERMAN U-boat torpedoed the unarmed hospital ship HMHS *Llandovery Castle* off southern Ireland, killing 234 people, including 88 medical staff, 14 Canadian nurses among them. The ship was returning to England from Halifax and no patients were aboard.

When some of the survivors tried to escape in lifeboats, the submarine surfaced and strafed them with machine-gun fire. Only twenty-four people in one lifeboat survived. Naturally the attack outraged the Canadian public.

This poster shows how dramatized images from the war were used to arouse public indignation against the enemy. Here a Canadian soldier cradles the dead body of a nurse while defiantly shaking his fist at the German war machine. Canadians were urged to buy Victory Bonds to support the war effort that would put an end to this kind of barbarity.

News of the incident reached the front lines as well and when Canadian soldiers took part in the Battle of Amiens in early August they dubbed their operation *Llandovery Castle* and saw it as a revenge mission. They got their revenge. On the first day of the battle the Allies delivered a devastating blow that turned out to be the beginning of the end for the enemy. General Erich Ludendorff, the German commander on the Western Front, famously called it "the black day of the German army in the history of the war."

Following the war the captain of the submarine and two of his officers were charged with war crimes. The captain disappeared; his two lieutenants were convicted but later escaped custody.

SINKING OF THE *LLANDOVERY CASTLE*

As the war progressed, the poster campaign began to demonize Germans as conscienceless killers of innocent women and children. The ironic use of the German word for culture in "Kultur vs. Humanity" was meant to show that the sinking of an unarmed hospital ship had placed Germany outside the community of civilized nations.

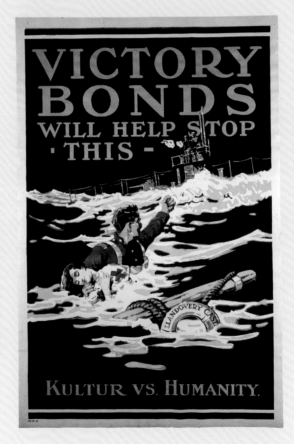

Sheet music for the American anti-war song "I Didn't Raise My Boy to Be a Soldier." The Americans did not join the war until April 1917 and isolationist sentiment remained strong there. The chorus of the song makes this clear: "I didn't raise my son to be a soldier, I brought him up to be my pride and joy, Who dares to put a musket on his shoulder, To shoot some other mother's darling boy? Let nations arbitrate their future troubles, It's time to lay the sword and gun away, There'd be no war today, If mothers all would say, I didn't raise my boy to be a soldier." In Canada, a small segment of the population supported pacifism.

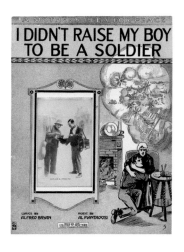

joined the campaign of subterfuge. Censorship was considered to be crucial for maintaining public morale. "I have seen sights in the bloodstained trenches of Flanders that I will never forget," wrote an infantryman from the front. "If the people at home could see the real horrors of the battle-field they would be worried to death." Government leaders agreed. They feared that if Canad-ians knew the truth about the carnage, their determination to see the war through might crack.

News from the battle lines was severely limited. Letters home from soldiers were censored routinely. There were no "embedded" journalists covering the Great War; indeed, Lord Kitchener threatened to arrest any correspondent discovered in the field. Initially the Allied press relied on communiqués from the army. A single correspondent, approved by the Allied high command, filed most of the highly generalized, highly patriotic dispatches that Canadians read in their daily papers. At the same time the British government had established a War

Propaganda Bureau, headed by Charles Masterman, a former literary journalist and member of the Liberal cabinet. Masterman used his contacts with the literary community to ask many leading writers, including Arnold Bennett, James Barrie, John Galsworthy, Arthur Conan Doyle and H.G. Wells, to produce pamphlets and books in support of the war effort. By the spring of 1915 the absolute ban on field correspondents was relaxed to the extent that small numbers of selected writers were allowed to visit the front under carefully controlled circumstances, but even these dispatches were censored. Often when newspaper reporters were allowed brief visits to France they were not allowed within many kilometres of the fighting.

Canada's own first war correspondent was Max Aitken, later Lord Beaverbrook, a financier from New Brunswick who had moved to England before the war. Aitken, who won election to the British parliament and embarked on a successful career as a newspaper owner, was the

Canadian government's man in London. At first he was named to the rather nebulous position of Canada's "eyewitness" to the war. Then he was made director of the Canadian War Records Office, a clearing house for documents recording Canada's contribution to the war – a self-described "official reporter of what was good to report." In March 1915, Aitken began writing press articles for Canadian consumption, gathering information during lightning visits to the front in his Rolls-Royce. His account of the Battle of Ypres in April 1915, published on front pages across the country, made it seem like Canadian soldiers had won a great victory all by themselves. "As long as brave deeds retain the power to fire the blood of Anglo-Saxons," he wrote, "the stand made by the Canadians in those desperate days will be told by fathers to their sons." Early in 1916 Aitken published his version of the battle in *Canada in Flanders,* a book called "supremely patriotic, sanitized and uncritical" by one historian. Aitken and his staff then

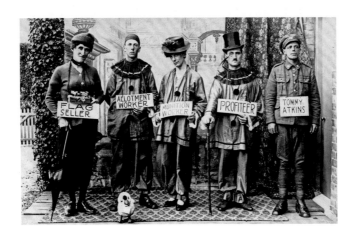

The Woodpeckers were an entertainment troupe composed of members of the 126th Company of the Canadian Forestry Corps. They are pictured here at Downham Hall in Suffolk, England. As the war proceeded, almost every division had its own entertainers helping to maintain good morale.

followed up on the runaway success of the Flanders book with two more volumes that brought comfort and inspiration to tens of thousands of Canadians. The office also produced three volumes of *Canada in Khaki,* collections of stories and eyewitness accounts from soldiers, all carefully selected for their upbeat tone and patriotic content.

Aitken's accounts of stirring bravery and Canadian pluck set the standard for much of the early press coverage of the fighting. Even when Canadian newspapers began sending their own correspondents to the front, articles adhered to the patriotic, uplifting tone established by Aitken, rather than reporting grimly on the slaughter and mayhem. As historian Tim Cook has pointed out, Aitken's London-based publicity machine also succeeded in promoting an image of the Canadian soldier as a steadfast, fearless warrior, already prepared for battle by the hard life on the Canadian frontier. This "hardy breed of men, the stalwart children of nature" were, so the propa-

ganda from the Canadian War Records Office had it, peculiarly suited to war.

———

CANADIAN NEWSPAPERS WOULD HAVE had difficulty printing accurate accounts of the war even if they had wanted to. Under the War Measures Act, passed by Parliament shortly after the outbreak of the war, the government gave itself unprecedented emergency powers, including the powers of censorship and suppression of all material that might be considered detrimental to the war effort. In June 1915 Ernest Chambers was appointed Chief Press Censor, a position that gave him almost unlimited authority to control what Canadians read and heard about the war. Chambers, a former newspaper reporter and a long-time member of the militia, attacked his new job with relish. He and his group of editors and translators applied themselves to suppressing any information that was not wholly supportive and benign in its view of the conflict. They kept a particularly watch-

SIR ROBERT BORDEN'S NATIONAL SERVICE CAMPAIGN

CANADIAN DAILY RECORD

ISSUED BY CANADIAN WAR RECORDS OFFICE TO UNITS OF THE CANADIAN EXPEDITIONARY FORCE.

No. 1.   TUESDAY, JANUARY 16, 1917.   GRATIS.

HOW CANADIANS STAND THE STRAIN OF WAR AT THE FRONT.

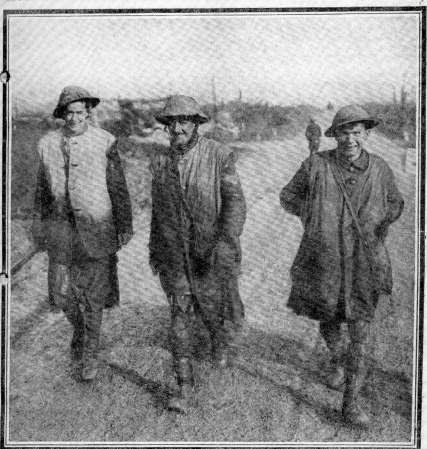

A Trio of Happy Canadian Soldiers—torn and warworn and bespattered with the mud of the trenches, but brisk and jovial as ever.
(Canadian Official Photograph.)

The *Canadian Daily Record* was a semi-official service newspaper published by the Canadian War Records Office and issued to Canadian Expeditionary Force units. It contained information from Canadian newspapers on events at home and frequent depictions of Canadian soldiers as captured by the official photographers. The newspaper was relentlessly cheerful and rarely depicted the horrors of war.

NOTHING is to be written on this side except the date and signature of the sender. Sentences not required may be erased. If anything else is added the post card will be destroyed.

[Postage must be prepaid on any letter or post card addressed to the sender of this card.]

I am quite well.

~~I have been admitted into hospital~~

{ ~~sick~~ } ~~and am going on well.~~
{ ~~wounded~~ } ~~and hope to be discharged soon.~~

~~I am being sent down to the base.~~

{ letter dated _____
~~I have received your~~ { telegram „ _____
{ parcel „ _____

Letter follows at first opportunity.

~~I have received no letter from you~~
{ ~~lately~~
{ ~~for a long time.~~

Signature } *Best*
only }

Date *Sept. 2nd 1917*

Wt. W34977293   29246.   6000m.   9716.   C. & Co., Grange Mills, S.W.

Mail was important to soldiers serving in the trenches. Letters from home were distributed daily and provided solace and support, though this could not always be said about the letters sent by soldiers in return. As this 1917 card from the front lines shows, mail from soldiers was heavily censored by their officers and told those at home very little about what was happening.

ful eye on foreign-language publications and newspapers published by labour groups and radical political parties. This surveillance culminated in 1918 with government regulations banning a long list of left-wing organizations, everything from the mainstream Social Democratic Party to groups that were avowedly anarchist and revolutionary. But censorship extended well beyond fringe, anti-war publications. In 1916, for example, Chambers stopped fourteen mainstream American newspapers belonging to the Hearst chain from crossing the border because they contained articles critical of the United Kingdom.

Chambers' remit included not just print sources – newspapers, magazines and books – but photographs, newsreels and movies as well. Photographs that showed the carnage of war were banned because they might dishearten the public. In one extreme example, Chambers banned several British temperance pamphlets because of the supposedly negative view they presented of drunk-

During the war a total of 21,453 men and women served in the Canadian Army Medical Corps as doctors, nurses and stretcher-bearers. This canvas field surgery kit held all the instruments needed for general surgery at the front. With it the surgeon could extract bullets and shell fragments and sew up wounds.

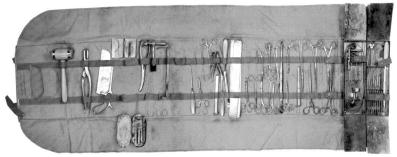

enness in Great Britain and the impact this might have on morale in Canada. On another occasion a film from Great Britain had to be edited for viewing in Canada because Chambers believed the sight of wounded soldiers would cause women in theatres to become hysterical. The Chief Censor's powers were almost total; he was permitted to request telephone operators to listen in on calls, telegraphers to provide copies of all their messages and postal workers to open all suspicious letters or parcels. He basically controlled everything Canadians listened to, saw, read and talked about, right down to the songs they sang and the pictures they looked at.

Still, the information blackout was not complete. Authorities did not wish to demoralize people at home but there was also propaganda value in allowing Canadians a glimpse of the horrors of war in order to stiffen their resolve to fight on. Casualty figures appearing in the local press made it obvious that young soldiers were dying in large numbers. In October 1916 filmgoers in Toronto got a chance to see actual footage from the front lines of Allied soldiers fighting, and dying, in battle. The film screened at a downtown theatre continuously all day every day for more than a week. Then two more theatres began showing the film in order to accommodate the demand. More than one hundred thousand Torontonians were introduced to life, and death, in the trenches.

———————

WHILE IT WAS PRESENTED BY THE GOVernment as a moral crusade that united Canadians in support of their fighting men and women, the Great War became in many ways a divisive force, revealing and intensifying deep fractures in Canadian society. English speakers doubted the commitment of French speakers. Imperialists who thought the war was a defence of the British Empire disagreed with nationalists who thought it was about Canada's independent role in the world. As the cost of living rose and wages failed to keep pace, working people wondered if their employers were making an equal sacrifice. When Charles Gordon returned home in early 1917 from France, where he had been serving as a front-lines chaplain to the 79th Cameron Highlanders, he was deeply discouraged by the public mood that he encountered. "What had come over the Canadian people?" he wondered. "I remembered how my heart had been filled with a new hope for a new national unity that would wipe out forever from true Canadian hearts all the racial and religious jealousy and hate that had darkened the future of our Canadian life. Now all was back again, and in a more disgraceful and dangerous form. Small wonder that recruiting of men had grown slack."

Prior to the war Canada welcomed hundreds of thousands of immigrants from Europe. Many of these newcomers came from countries that suddenly, in August 1914, became the enemy. People from Germany, Austria-Hungary, Turkey and Bulgaria, some of them residents of long standing, were transformed into

IN THE SPRING OF 1916, MAX Aitken, director of the Canadian War Records Office in London and chief publicist for the war in Canada, convinced British military authorities to allow him to dispatch photographers to the front to "shoot the war." The photographs that resulted – about seven thousand in total – provided a dramatic record of Canadian soldiers in combat. "Before we can realize the patience, the exhaustion and the courage of the modern fighting man," wrote Aitken, the public needs "to see our men climbing out of the trenches."

Not all the photographs were as accurate as they seemed to be, however. A famous series of images depicting Canadians going "over the top" were actually cooked up behind the lines. What they showed was real enough and gave some sense of wartime experience to the public back home, but in the end the photographs were works of sanitized propaganda, showing Canadian troops in the best possible light. Aitken organized them into books and mounted travelling exhibitions that toured the United Kingdom and Canada. In July 1917, for example, a huge photograph (6.7 metres by 3.3 metres) showing Canadians in action at Vimy Ridge went on display at a gallery in London as part of the Official Canadian War Photographs Exhibition.

SHOOTING THE WAR

Exhibitions of war photography were one way the public at home got some understanding of what life was like for soldiers in the trenches.

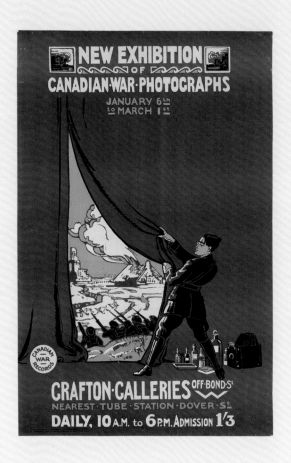

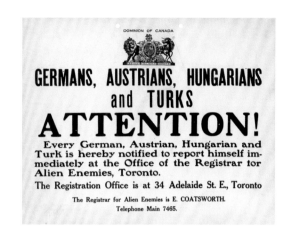

DOMINION OF CANADA

GERMANS, AUSTRIANS, HUNGARIANS and TURKS
ATTENTION!

Every German, Austrian, Hungarian and Turk is hereby notified to report himself immediately at the Office of the Registrar for Alien Enemies, Toronto.

The Registration Office is at 34 Adelaide St. E., Toronto

The Registrar for Alien Enemies is E. COATSWORTH.
Telephone Main 7465.

"enemy aliens" and policy-makers had to decide what to do about any threat they posed to national security. At the immediate outset of the war the fear of the alien spiked as people worried how German-Canadians would respond. (One, Joachim Ribbentrop, a wine merchant in Ottawa and one of the most eligible bachelors in the capital, fled immediately by train to New York, then made his way home to Germany and into uniform; he survived the war and later served as Adolf Hitler's foreign minister.) There was a widespread, if unfounded, fear that armed Germans from the United States would cross the border to invade Canada.

As time passed, these immediate fears subsided. Aliens were required to register with authorities, but for the most part they were left alone. As the war dragged on, however, and casualties mounted, the public began to rethink its tolerant attitude toward the estimated 120,000 "aliens" in their midst. In Toronto, Montreal and Winnipeg, German-owned businesses came under attack from angry mobs. When word reached Victoria that fifteen local people, including the son of James Dunsmuir, a former premier, were among the *Lusitania* victims, a crowd of liquor-fuelled patriots smashed up the German Club. Armed guards had to be posted at Government House for fear that the mob might take its anger out on the wife of the lieutenant-governor, who was a member of a German family. In Ottawa, when a mysterious fire destroyed the Centre Block of the Parliament Buildings early in February 1916, killing seven people, it was widely believed that the Kaiser's saboteurs were responsible.

As public opinion turned and hardened against them, more and more Germans, Austrians and other central Europeans found themselves without work. The pre-war recession had been hard on immigrant labourers who had been brought to Canada to take unskilled jobs in the mines, logging operations and construction camps of the resource hinterland. Many had lost their jobs in the economic downturn; now they were the victims of wartime para-

A public notice posted in Toronto that required all "enemy aliens" to report to the authorities to be registered. For years the government had been urging people from these countries to immigrate to Canada. Now suddenly the newcomers found themselves viewed with suspicion and living in fear of internment.

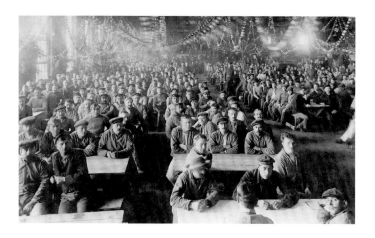

Christmas at a Canadian internment camp, 1916. Decorative streamers hang from the ceiling but there is nothing on the tables and not a happy face in sight. As the photograph indicates, most internees were men, though women and children sometimes joined them. Most of the men were put to work at menial jobs.

noia. Large numbers congregated in the cities in search of work, creating real concern for the Borden government that Canada was on the verge of widespread civil unrest. The government's response was to create a network of internment camps for enemy aliens. By the end of 1915 there were fourteen camps across the country holding more than seven thousand men, the majority of them civilians who posed no real threat to the country. Internees were herded like animals into tents and makeshift barracks, confined behind barbed wire and guarded by armed soldiers. In some cases they were joined by their wives and children who had no other means of support. Most of these men were set to work as cheap labour on land and road clearing, in mines and on railway construction.

Meanwhile, anti-alien sentiment continued to flourish in the broader society. In Toronto, city council voted to fire any employee of German, Austrian or Turkish background who was not a naturalized Canadian. In May 1916 the town of Berlin,

Ontario, changed its name to Kitchener to disassociate itself from the enemy. A year later, when someone suggested switching back, riots erupted in protest. Calls were heard regularly to strip aliens of their jobs or to deport them without cause. In April 1917, as casualty reports reached Toronto from the Easter battle at Vimy Ridge, a mob of angry returned soldiers gathered on Yonge Street and began smashing up cafés believed to be owned by "aliens" and roughing up their customers who looked "foreign." The commanding officer of the Toronto district finally dispatched a troop of soldiers to enforce the law. Afterwards, it was the aliens who were blamed for the riot. Under the pressures of war, Canadians drew an increasingly strict line between "us" and "them." Enemy aliens were demonized and victimized, no matter how long they had been in Canada.

Another way that ethnic divisions in Canadian society revealed themselves was in recruitment policy. While the publicity campaign to support the war effort

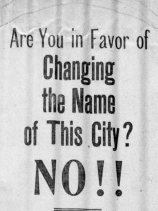

Are You in Favor of Changing the Name of This City?

NO !!

This is a time when our Dominion and Provincial Parliaments and many municipal and other public bodies are putting off their elections, and the discussion of many other matters, so that all may work harmoniously together in the defence of the British Empire. This vexed question should not have been brought before our people at this time.

We do not wish to reflect upon the motives of the citizens who first launched this agitation, but their arguments are weak and intemperate and their actions high handed and wanting in that spirit of justice and fair play which is supposed to be characteristic of every true Briton.

Our city has always had the reputation of being the most loyal, peaceable, law abiding and thriving community in the Dominion of Canada. The discussion of this question has created bitter feelings, and led to scenes of discord and lawlessness which were never before known here. For all this the citizens who first started the movement to change the name of our city are directly or indirectly responsible.

We are told that the move is patriotic and for that reason should have the support of our citizens. We believe to add one single recruit to the ranks of the 118th battalion, or to pay one single dollar to the Patriotic or to the Red Cross funds, is more patriotic and of more real help to the British Empire to-day than to change the name of the city.

We are told that if we do not change the name BERLIN, our manufacturers will have to close down and the grass grow in the streets of our city. To-day our manufacturers are nearly all busier than they have ever before been in their history. Many are working over time. Some of them with their best efforts are not able to fill the orders they already have on their books. There is not a single mechanic or laborer in our city to-day, able and willing to work, who is not employed at good wages. Our mechanics have the reputation of turning out the most reliable goods in the Canadian market. So long as they keep up that reputation the name "BERLIN" will be no handicap either to them, or to the manufacturers who employ them.

The citizens who are active in this effort to change the name, assume the right to insult and brand as disloyal and pro-German every one who does not agree with their views. Our citizens who are opposed to the change of name are just as loyal to the British Empire, and more loyal to the city in which they live and prosper, than the most violent agitator who tries to change its name and injure its reputation.

To vote Yes would be to plead guilty to the stigma of disloyalty, which these agitators are trying to fasten upon you and your city.

Show your confidence in the city of BERLIN and the loyalty of the people by going to the polls on Friday next, the nineteenth, and voting

NO!

THE COMMITTEE.

Before the war the Ontario town of Berlin, a centre of German settlement in the province, was called "the German capital of Canada." In August 1914 a bronze bust of Kaiser Wilhelm in one of the city's parks was thrown into a nearby lake, and soon German-language instruction was suspended in schools. Eventually the board of trade convinced the city council that the name Berlin was hurting business and giving the impression that the town sympathized with the enemy cause. Although some opposed changing the name, as this message from the "No Committee" shows, Berlin officially became Kitchener, in honour of the late Lord Kitchener, on September 1, 1916.

called on all Canadians to do what they could, not all Canadians received equal treatment when they stepped forward. As one historian sardonically notes, "killing Germans was the privilege of white troops." Blacks, Asians and members of Canada's First Nations all wanted to fight. The young men from these minority communities shared the mainstream Canadian enthusiasm for the cause and the thirst for adventure, and they also hoped that by volunteering they might win for their communities the full rights of citizenship they had been denied so far. Instead, the military establishment rebuffed them. There was no official government policy to exclude minorities, but there didn't have to be. Recruitment was left up to the individual units and with few exceptions they rejected minority volunteers. When they were allowed to join, members of minorities usually ended up in non-combat roles; for example, the No. 2 Construction Battalion (Coloured) based in Nova Scotia and consisting of Black recruits. Apparently, when the recruitment

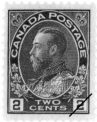

England's King George V depicted on a two-cent stamp. In response to the anti-German sentiment felt in all the Allied countries during the war, George V changed the name of the British royal family from Saxe-Coburg and Gotha to Windsor in 1917.

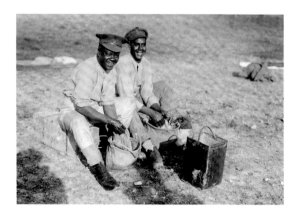

Members of the all-Black No. 2 Construction Battalion from Nova Scotia do their laundry during a break in the action. About one thousand Black soldiers served in the Canadian Expeditionary Force, mostly in the No. 2 Battalion, building roads, railways and defences.

poster insisted that "Canada Needs You" it did not mean anyone with a foreign accent or a minority skin colour.

——————

PRIME MINISTER BORDEN HAD PROMISED that Canada would contribute half a million soldiers to the war, but by the end of 1916 the country had just short of three hundred thousand men and women in uniform. Of the few thousand who were still signing up each month, not many volunteered to join the infantry, where the need was greatest. By May 1917 monthly casualty rates were more than double the rate of new recruitment. Reluctantly, Borden recognized that the voluntary system had wrung as many young men as possible out of the country; it was time to plan for compulsory service. He knew it was a policy that might tear the country apart, but he believed the emergency in Europe made the risk necessary. Canada would be disgraced in the eyes of the world if it did not shoulder its share of the burden. Canadians would be ashamed in their own eyes if they did not keep faith with the thousands of men and women who had already given their lives for the cause.

Conscription was terribly unpopular in Quebec, where the war had never taken on the aspect of a holy crusade as it had in English-speaking Canada. Anti-conscriptionists snaked through the streets of Montreal in loud protest marches, threatening violence and secession if compulsory service was introduced. At the same time, French-English relations were at a low point anyway because of attempts by the Ontario government to limit the teaching of French in its schools. The "Ontario Schools Question," as it has become known to historians, aggravated tensions between French and English and made many Québécois wonder why they should fight for a country that would not recognize their basic rights.

But conscription was unpopular outside Quebec as well, particularly with some labour groups and farmers. Labour activists argued that working people had already been asked to bear a disproportionate share of the war burden. "No conscription of manpower without conscription of wealth" was their rallying cry, by which they meant that the wealth of the elites and the profiteers should be "conscripted," or taxed, to ensure that the burden of fighting the war was more evenly distributed. Farmers argued that they needed their sons at home helping with the harvest, which produced the food that was so vital to the war effort.

Borden attempted to avoid a French-English split over the issue by inviting Liberal leader Wilfrid Laurier to join a coalition government that would introduce conscription as a united front. After mulling over his options, Laurier refused, calculating that he would lose all credibility in his home province. The coalition went ahead without him, with several anglophone Liberals and independents joining Borden's Unionist government. With a federal election looming in December 1917, and conscription in the balance, Borden engineered a brazen manipulation of the electoral process to

WARTIME PROPAGANDA ROUTINELY made use of alleged German atrocities to maintain public anger against the enemy. A notable instance was the "Crucified Canadian." In May 1915 rumours emerged from the front that German soldiers in Belgium had pinned a young Canadian officer to a barn door with bayonets, then stabbed him repeatedly. Obviously symbolic of Christian sacrifice, the story of the crucified soldier was intended to demonize "the Hun"

and sanctify the suffering of Canadian troops. As historian Paul Maroney has pointed out, the image was emblematic of the nation as a whole, sacrificing the blood of its young men in a noble cause.

Did the event actually take place? No one knows for sure. No body was found and different eyewitness accounts contradicted one another. Sometimes the victim was a British soldier; sometimes the setting was a tree, not a barn door. As recently as 2002 a British filmmaker claimed to have un-

earthed fresh evidence that the "crucifixion" had taken place and that the victim was Sgt. Harry Band from Ontario. Band did die near Ypres in 1915 and his body was never recovered.

In 1918 British artist Francis Derwent Wood made a bronze sculpture depicting the brutal murder, titled *Canada's Golgotha*, Golgotha being the site of Jesus's crucifixion. The piece was part of a post-war Canadian War Memorials exhibition but was withdrawn when the German government

objected that the episode had never been verified and the Canadian government could not prove beyond a doubt that it had taken place. The sculpture passed into the control of the National Gallery after the war, along with the rest of the War Memorials collection and in 1930, at the request of the Defence Department, it was put in permanent storage. The work has been displayed since, but remains controversial.

THE CRUCIFIED CANADIAN

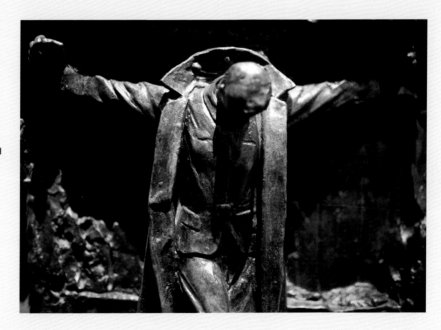

Canada's Golgotha, a bronze sculpture by Francis Derwent Wood. The piece was displayed in public for the first time since the war in 1992 at the Canadian War Museum.

...ion drew closer and the debate grew more heated, recruitment posters and handbills like these began emphasizing the shame of being forced to serve and encouraging the few men still not in uniform to step forward and do the right thing voluntarily.

No person may point the finger of scorn if you join the **Princess Pats** before

CONSCRIPTION

Ask for the Guards' Depot tor the Pats at the Base Recruiting Office

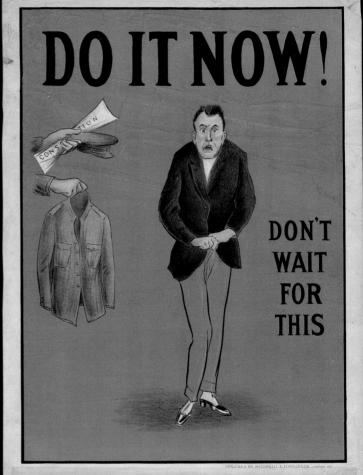

DO IT NOW!

DON'T WAIT FOR THIS

DESIGNED BY McCONNELL & FERGUSSON LONDON ONT

WHERE TO ENLIST

IN THE

142ND BATTALION

CANADIAN OVERSEAS CONTINGENT

"LONDON'S OWN"

Central Recruiting Station, Dominion Savings Building, Richmond and King Streets.

East End Recruiting Station, 781 Dundas Street, Near East End Town Hall.

Hamilton Road Recruiting Station, Old Egerton Street Baptist Church, Hamilton Road and Egerton Street.

Or the Armouries, Dundas Street.

OR WRITE FOR INFORMATION TO

CITIZENS' RECRUITING ASSOCIATION

Board of Trade Rooms, City Hall

This Unionist poster from the December 1917 federal election makes the spurious claim that a vote for Laurier was a vote for an enemy victory. It shows the German Kaiser toasting Laurier's supposedly defeatist war policy. The election, with its claims and counterclaims of patriotism and treason, was one of the most vicious in Canadian history.

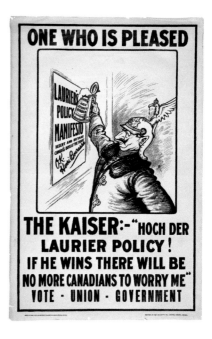

increase the chances of his success. First of all, his government passed the Military Voters Act, which gave the vote to all members of the armed forces no matter how long they had lived in Canada, including women and Aboriginals, two groups that had not possessed the franchise to that point. Military voters were asked simply to select their political party of choice, which could then assign the ballots to any constituency it wanted. (It was estimated that in the ensuing election Borden's Unionists won at least fourteen parliamentary seats by manipulating the military vote in this way.) Next the government forced the Wartime Elections Act through Parliament. This legislation gave the vote to all female relatives of servicemen while at the same time taking the vote away from conscientious objectors and from people who were born in an enemy country and had become naturalized Canadians since 1902. The result was that tens of thousands of people lost the right to vote.

The ensuing election campaign was one of the bitterest in Canadian history.

Though it might have been necessary to win the war, conscription was far from popular. Borden did not dare venture into Quebec for fear of a violent reception, and even in Ontario he was often hounded from the platform by anti-conscription crowds. When it looked as though farmers were going to vote against him, Borden suddenly, two weeks before voting day, decided to exempt farmers' sons from the draft. On the other side, Laurier was vilified as a traitor and a friend of the Kaiser. "Every Hun sympathizer from Berlin to the trenches... wishes success to Laurier," warned the Unionist cabinet minister, Sir George Foster. In Toronto, war veterans beat up voters who openly declared their support for the Liberal leader.

Unsurprisingly, the Unionist government won the 1917 election and conscription was secure. The Unionists took 153 seats, of which only three were in Quebec. The Laurier Liberals held on to eighty-two seats, of which only twenty were not in Quebec. (One of the losing Liberals was the forty-three-year-old labour consultant

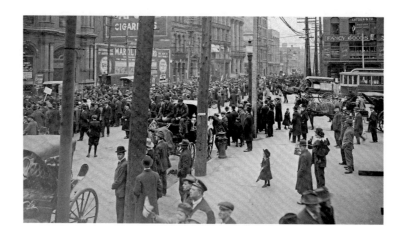

This anti-conscription parade in downtown Montreal on May 24, 1917, passed off without violence. Not so an event in Quebec City, where street battles and rioting during Easter 1918 resulted in the deaths of four demonstrators.

William Lyon Mackenzie King, who paid for his loyalty to Laurier with a defeat in a Toronto-area riding; less than two years later he would take over as leader of the Liberal Party and eventually become the longest-serving prime minister in Canadian history.) The cost of conscription was a deeply divided country, not only along the French-English fault line but also along the urban-rural and labour-capital divides. The most blatant manipulation of the electoral process for political gain in Canadian history left a bad taste in the mouths of many Canadians who believed that the war was being used to justify draconian policies.

The election result did not end unrest in the country. The following spring police looking for draft evaders in Quebec City touched off riots that required troops to be called in from Ontario. On April 1, four civilians died when the soldiers fired on a crowd. If conscription was used to find more soldiers, it was also used to get anti-war pacifists and radicals out of circulation. The most notorious case in

western Canada was Ginger Goodwin, a labour activist in British Columbia and outspoken opponent of the war. A thin, frail man, suffering from an ulcer and debilitating lung disease, he had nevertheless been classified fit for service under the new law. Most of Goodwin's friends thought the authorities were out to railroad him into the army to rid themselves of a troublesome agitator. Instead of reporting for duty, Goodwin took to the hills around Comox Lake on Vancouver Island with several other draft evaders, hiding out in abandoned hunting shacks and surviving on food slipped to them by local sympathizers. On July 27, 1918, in a confrontation with the provincial police, he was shot and killed. The special constable who pulled the trigger was acquitted on charges of manslaughter, but the incident left many questions unanswered. On August 2, the day of Goodwin's funeral, the Vancouver labour movement called for a protest strike. Streetcar drivers, stevedores, shipyard workers, garment workers and the building trades all walked off

The Union government was a coalition of Conservatives and some Liberals formed to push through conscription. These three posters are from the federal election of December 17, 1917. The Unionists draped themselves in the "flag of freedom" and won an overwhelming victory.

For those who could not afford to buy a Victory Bond – the smallest denomination was $50 – the government issued war savings stamps. The stamps sold for twenty-five cents each and could be affixed to a certificate and eventually redeemed in the same manner as a bond. Children in particular were encouraged to contribute to the war effort by buying stamps. These posters suggest that the stamps would ensure prosperity in the present and the future.

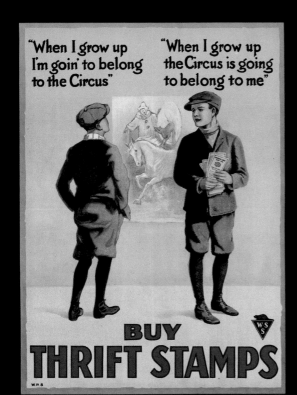

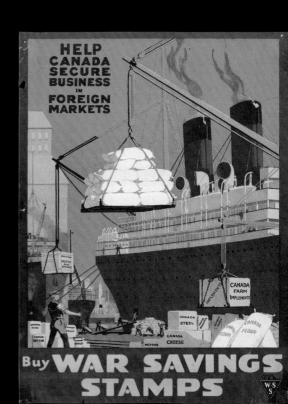

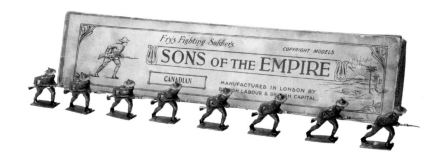

Children were encouraged to learn about and support the war in many ways, including in their play. The Fry company sold this "Sons of the Empire" set of toy Canadian soldiers.

the job, bringing the city to a halt. It was British Columbia's first general strike and indicated how unpopular conscription was with many working people. In the end, conscription was not a crucial factor in the war. About one hundred thousand more men were enrolled in the army but only slightly more than twenty-four thousand reached the front before peace was declared on November 11, 1918. The disunity stirred up by conscription was a heavy price to pay for such small military gain. Still, Borden was not to know that the war would not drag on for years, requiring every bit of manpower Canada could muster.

_____

THE WAR ALSO BROUGHT SOME SIGNIFICANT discomforts to the daily life of most Canadians. Of course these were minor when compared to the ultimate sacrifice being asked of the men and women in uniform. Nonetheless, disruptions to life on the home front were not insignificant and ate away at public morale and support for

the war. The cost of living rose steadily during the war years – 8 percent in 1916 and a whopping 18 percent the next year – riding an inflationary wave fuelled by the production of war goods and the expansion of exports. Wages did not keep pace, so most working people saw a noticeable decline in their standard of living. The weekly budget for the average family was $7.96 when the war began; by war's end it was $13.49. Domestic supplies of key products needed in the war effort grew scarce. By the winter of 1916–1917, for instance, there was a con-tinent-wide shortage of coal. Manufacturers had first call on dwindling supplies while stockpiles for home heating got smaller and smaller. So-called heatless days became a regular occurrence. In early 1918, during an extreme cold spell in Ontario, the shortage was so dire that Toronto schools closed their doors and the government imposed a three-day work stoppage for all business and industrial activity. People who went to work did so bundled up in overcoats and scarves.

It was not all doom and gloom on the home front. The war brought an end to the pre-war recession and a boost to Canadian productivity. Manufacturers received millions of dollars' worth of contracts to produce a wide variety of goods – from underwear to bullets – necessary to keep a modern army in the field. The sudden expansion of war industries provided thousands of new jobs, many of them taken for the first time by women who entered the labour force in large numbers to make up for the men who were absent overseas. Women received much lower wages for the same work, but the war provided them with an opportunity to fill jobs that had traditionally been closed to them.

In the hurry to outfit an instant army, a series of equipment failures – boots that disintegrated in the mud, rifles that jammed during the heat of the action, trench shovels that didn't dig properly – led to charges of profiteering and political patronage. The war profiteer became as familiar a figure of public scorn as the shirker or the dreaded Hun. The propaganda campaign

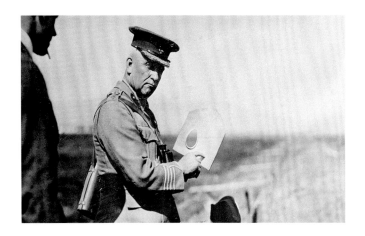

Sir Sam Hughes, minister of militia and defence from 1911 to 1916, holding a MacAdam shovel. The shovel was the brainchild of Hughes's secretary, Ena MacAdam, and was patented by Hughes under her name, though it was often called the Hughes shovel as well. In practice the shovel turned out to be useless. It did not stop gunfire from even the smallest handgun and was inefficient at digging and had to be scrapped. Hughes's desire to provide his "boys" with Canadian-made equipment was admirable in principle but seldom successful.

The boots leaked, vehicles lacked spare parts, military belts were irregular and the trench equipment was unusable. The manufacture of munitions was the subject of scandal. And perhaps worst of all in Hughes's eyes, the Ross rifle had to be replaced with a British gun. Eventually Hughes's methods discredited him, even in the eyes of his government colleagues, and he was dropped from the cabinet.

drummed into the public mind the message that sacrifice was a prerequisite of victory. It seemed unconscionable that anyone should appear to be getting rich from the conflict.

One businessman who came to symbolize the greed of the profiteer was Joseph Flavelle, president of the William Davies Company, Toronto's largest meat packer. Flavelle was a deeply religious Methodist who led an abstemious personal life and believed strongly in public service. During the war he served as the unpaid chair of the Imperial Munitions Board, the agency that purchased British munitions in Canada. It was widely agreed that he did an admirable job straightening out the affairs of the board, which in its original incarnation as the Shell Committee had been plagued by incompetence and corruption. It is ironic, therefore, that Flavelle was implicated in one of the worst profiteering scandals of the war and that he was held up to ridicule ("His Lardship") and abuse as one of the country's leading plutocrats.

Flavelle's meat packing business did

very well out of the war, selling bacon to the British and tinned "bully" beef for the men in the trenches. Historian Tim Cook recounts that of all the brands of bully beef handed out to the men, the Davies brand was considered the worst. Nonetheless, company profits more than tripled. In the summer of 1917 a federal government report seemed to indicate that the Davies company had made a killing on its sales of bacon. Press reports blundered in their interpretation of the findings, making them seem much more damning than they were, and suddenly Flavelle was tarred as a hypocrite millionaire making a fortune from the suffering of others. The public was furious. "I can truly say that I never before met with such widespread rage over any other scandal," remarked one Ottawa politician. The *Christian Guardian*, the journal of Flavelle's own Methodist Church, expressed public opinion: "There is a general feeling abroad in Canada...that the man or the corporation which comes out of this war richer than when they went into it... have failed

This letter from Wallace Shipyards Ltd. was in response to the government's request that women be given jobs in the marine industries. As the letter indicates, Wallace Shipyards, based in North Vancouver, was less than enthusiastic about the request, arguing that women did not have "the necessary constitution to stand this extremely heavy work." Nonetheless, the war did offer women expanded opportunities in the workforce.

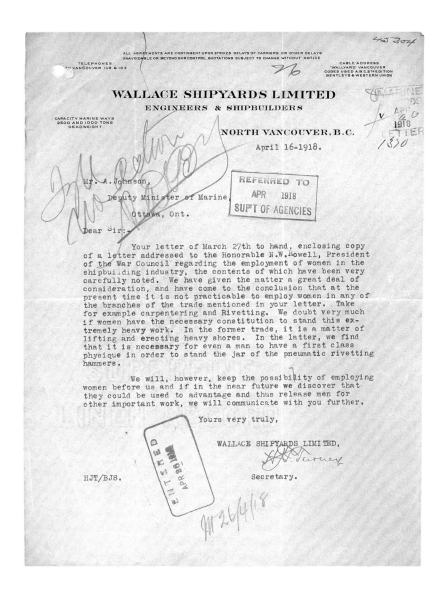

to exhibit true patriotism." Customers boycotted Davies stores and editorialists vilified Flavelle in the daily press. In the end a government inquiry ruled that the Davies company was simply conducting legitimate business. But it didn't really matter. Flavelle, and war profiteers generally, continued to be held in contempt for making millions while young Canadians fought, and died, in the trenches for $1.10 a day.

————————

EASTER 1917. VIMY RIDGE IN NORTH-EASTERN France, near the town of Arras a few kilometres from the border with Belgium. German troops had occupied the low escarpment overlooking the Allied lines since the beginning of the war. Three times British and French troops had tried to win it back and three times they had failed. The long, low ridge had already cost both sides three hundred thousand in casualties. Protected by a web of machine gun nests, deep trenches, barbed wire and concrete, it was considered one of the most

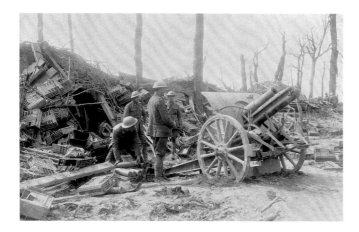

Members of the 17th Battery, Canadian Field Artillery, fire a captured German gun at the retreating enemy at Vimy Ridge. The victory was the most storied in Canadian history.

impregnable German positions along the entire front line. The commander of the French army believed it could not be captured. Yet that was the assignment given to the Canadian Corps as part of a British-French assault on the German lines.

The Canadians began the attack at first light on April 9, Easter Monday. Behind a massed artillery and machine gun barrage, fifteen thousand Canadian infantrymen broke from their trenches and advanced toward the ridge. On the night of April 12, after four days of fierce fighting, a pounding artillery barrage and countless acts of personal courage, the last German position fell and Vimy Ridge was in possession of the Allies.

Vimy Ridge was celebrated as an extraordinary Canadian victory, one of the most important victories of the war. In the first blush of victory it seemed as if the door was open for an unstoppable offensive that would drive the enemy from the field of battle. It was the first time that all four divisions of the Corps had gone into battle together and it was

agreed that the soldiers had acquited themselves like champions. Prime Minister Borden, who was in London for meetings, reported in his diary "All newspapers ringing with praise of the Canadians." "Canadians Lead in Triumph" was the headline in the Toronto *Globe*. "Well Done Canada" praised the *New York Tribune*. Desperate for good news, the Allies took encouragement from the Canadian success. Who could resist glowing with pride that their soldiers had played such a crucial role in the war? As historian Tim Cook notes, "Vimy was more than just a battlefield victory." It was a turning point for the army; as Cook writes, Vimy was "the point where it moved from an amateur to a professional warfighting force." Buoyed with confidence, the Canadian Corps went on to experience success after success against the enemy. More than that, Vimy seemed also to be a turning point for the nation. It became a symbol of what Canadians could achieve together. From the confusion and sacrifice of battle, Canada emerged with a new sense

of its own identity and a new stature on the world stage. Canada had succeeded where other larger, older nations had failed. The nation had come of age at Vimy.

That was the legend that grew up in the aftermath of battle. The reality, as usual, was something different. The Germans had been driven from Vimy Ridge but at an extreme cost. "As we looked back up that ridge in the early dawn we witnessed a scene never to be forgotten," one soldier wrote. "The entire face of the hill was covered with German green and Canadian khaki. Men lay out there in that blood-soaked field, some dead, some dying." The toll of casualties from this single battle was 3,598 Canadians dead, another 7,000 wounded. More men died on April 9, 1917, than on any other day in Canadian military history. It was a remarkable victory but it led to no great breakthrough. The French and British attacks had not gone well. After suffering terrible losses, French soldiers actually mutinied and refused to engage in any more attacks. The

Prime Minister Robert Borden (seated, fourth from left) meets with other members of the Imperial War Cabinet in London. The cabinet was created by British Prime Minister David Lloyd George in the spring of 1917 to coordinate the Empire's military policy. Borden was adamant that Canada's contribution to the war should be recognized by greater autonomy on the world stage.

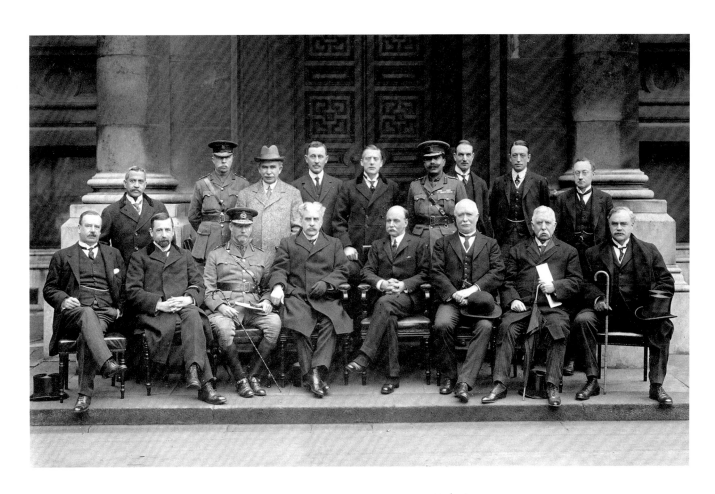

BELOW Casualties lie on the battlefield following a Canadian charge. As Canadians added up the enormous costs of each battle, the naive enthusiasm of the war's early months was long forgotten.

RIGHT Members of the 29th Infantry Battalion advancing across "No Man's Land" through barbed wire and heavy German fire at the Battle of Vimy Ridge, April 1917.

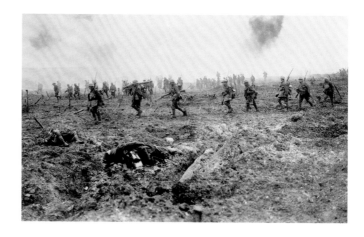

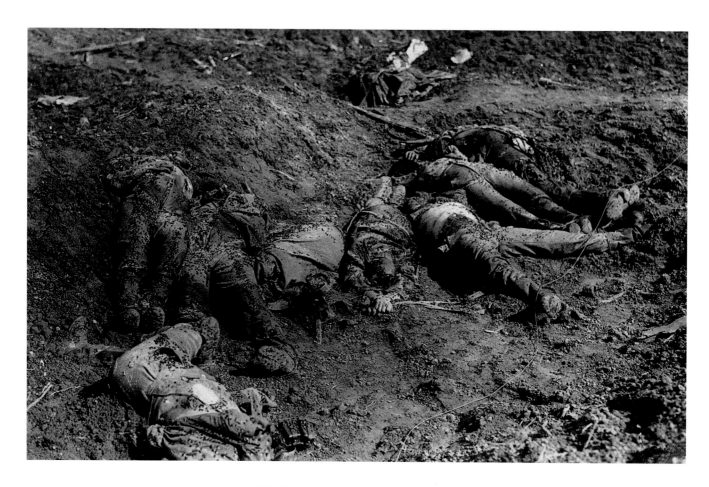

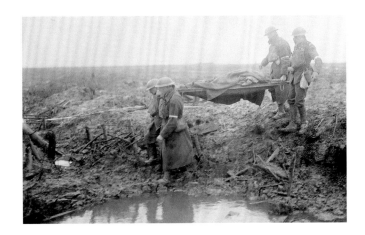

enemy simply withdrew to a new line and the fighting continued.

In fact, Vimy was a prelude to a low point in the war when a pessimist had grounds for believing that all might yet be lost. In the summer of 1917 the Western Front continued to degenerate into a zone of attrition with its attacks and counter-attacks, its mud and gas, its relentless death toll. In the fall the horrible debacle at Passchendaele claimed 275,000 more casualties for the Allies, 15,000 of them Canadians. The objective "isn't worth a drop of blood," the Canadian commander, Arthur Currie, had told his superiors. Yet the operation went ahead. Canadian soldiers won another victory, but overall the battle failed to achieve an end to the military stalemate. In November the Bolsheviks took power in Russia and began the process of withdrawing from the Eastern Front. Back home, the devastating explosion in Halifax harbour on December 6, 1917, was followed eleven days later by the rancorous, dispiriting federal election. Then, in the spring, came the deadly

anti-conscription riots in Quebec. There seemed reason to believe that the war would go on for another year or two. Ypres, Courcelette, St. Eloi, Vimy, Arras, Passchendaele; one by one the names of the battles accumulated like answers to some grim geography lesson. What might finish it, nobody knew.

At the end of March 1918 the Germans launched their "peace offensive" on the Western Front, hoping with one giant effort to overrun the Allies and end the war. But Allied lines held and, as it turned out, the Germans were more weakened by their offensive than the Allies, who that September counterattacked in a long, brutal campaign that came to be called the Hundred Days. To the surprise of almost everyone, the enemy gave way, though not without fierce resistance that led to 45,835 Canadian casualties. Frederick Varley, the war artist and founding member of the Group of Seven, was with the troops during this nightmarish final chapter. He wrote home to his wife: "You in Canada... cannot realize at all what war

A wounded Canadian soldier is carried over muddy terrain back to an aid post during the Battle of Passchendaele, November 1917. The battlefield was situated in a low-lying area reclaimed from marshy lands by an elaborate drainage system. Once shelling started, flooding turned the whole battlefield into a swamp, greatly complicating the evacuation of wounded soldiers.

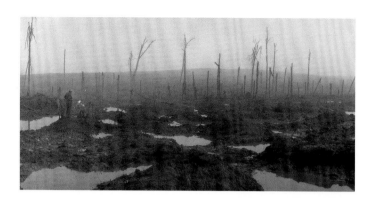

A lone soldier looks down on the bleakness of Passchendaele after the battle, November 1917. The soldier's posture parallels that of the central figure in the poster opposite.

is like. You must see it and live it. You must see the barren deserts war has made of once fertile country... see the turned-up graves, see the dead on the field, freakishly mutilated – headless, legless, stomachless, a perfect body and a passive face and a broken empty skull – see your own countrymen, unidentified, thrown into a cart, their coats over them, boys digging a grave in a land of yellow slimy mud and green pools of water under a weeping sky. You must have heard the screeching shells and have the shrapnel fall around you, whistling by you... until you've lived this... you cannot know."

Finally, at 11 a.m. on November 11, the guns fell silent and the slaughter ended.

THE GREAT WAR OCCUPIES A SPECIAL place in Canadian mythology. At least one historian has called it the most important event in the country's history. It seemed to signify a breakthrough. Because of Canada's contribution to the war, the country moved from colony to nation, recognized for the first time by others and by itself as an independent, mature state. Canadians, said Prime Minister Borden, were filled "with an impelling sense of nationhood never before experienced." The success and the sacrifice of its soldiers gave Canada the right to be taken seriously. It was no longer a minor league player in the world, but an equal partner in Empire. The Great War was our "war of independence," writes Tim Cook, in the sense that it conferred a hard-won autonomy, first on the battlefield, then at the peace talks and finally in the post-war world. As examples of our new stature, Canadian diplomats signed the 1919 peace treaty separately from Great Britain and later occupied their own seats at the League of Nations. More than that, argues Cook, the war brought a large number of Canadians from disparate backgrounds and provinces together for the first time in a shared experience that produced a deeper appreciation for a shared nationality.

During the war, as the number of Canadians killed and wounded mounted and

THIS VICTORY BONDS POSTER features lines from "In Flanders Fields," one of the most famous poems written during the Great War. The poet was a young medical officer from Guelph, Ontario, John McCrae, who penned his poem in the aftermath of the Battle of Ypres, Easter 1915. He had lost a friend in battle the day before. The story goes that McCrae wrote three stanzas of the poem on a piece of paper in a few spare minutes. Then, unhappy with his attempt, he threw away the paper and went back to work tending the wounded. The scrap of paper was recovered and sent to the British magazine *Punch* where it appeared on December 8, 1915.

> *In Flanders fields the poppies blow*
> *Between the crosses, row on row...*

McCrae died of pneumonia at a field hospital in France early in 1918. The next year a book, *In Flanders Fields and Other Poems*, was published in Canada where it topped the bestseller list.

> *If ye break faith with those who die*
> *We shall not sleep, though poppies grow*
> *In Flanders fields*

Canadians were encouraged to keep faith with their war dead by doing whatever they could to make their sacrifice meaningful; in this case by buying bonds to raise money to support the war effort.

IN FLANDERS FIELDS

Another lone soldier looks down on the results of war. Rather than thinking about the terrifying desolation of Passchendaele seen in the opposite photograph, this soldier looks down on the poppy-covered grave of a lost comrade.

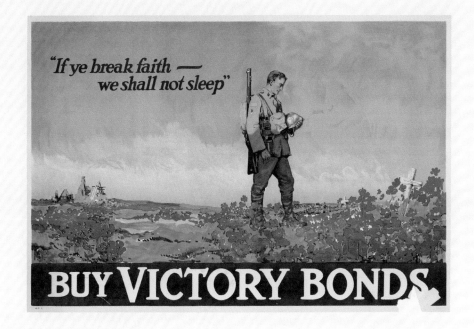

Trench art. Although made of copper and brass shell casings or gun parts, these souvenirs of war were not produced in the trenches. Instead they were crafted behind the lines by soldiers, civilian artisans, prisoners of war and commercial manufacturers. The copper letter opener (centre front) was fashioned as a gift for a friend, while the items behind the letter opener (left to right) were crafted for other practical and decorative purposes: a vase is inscribed "Lens 1918"; a jar with a lid is marked "Cambrai"; military badges cover a brass shell casing; a match holder is etched with "Ypres"; and a picture frame is shaped like a maple leaf.

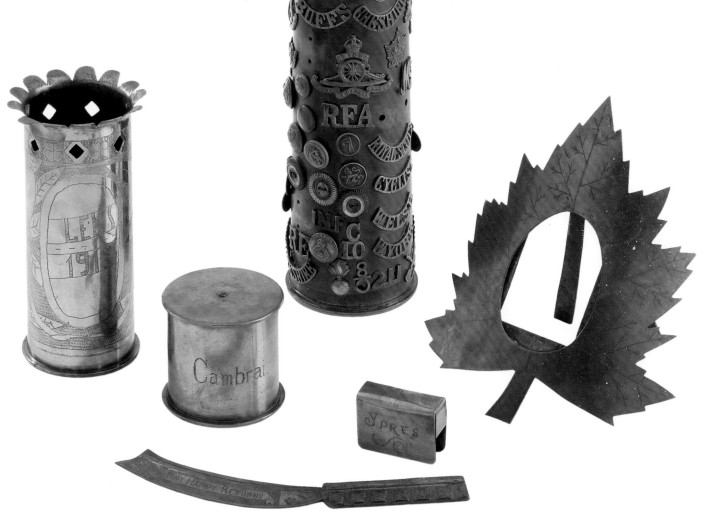

During the war many Canadians answered this poster's call to fight in defence of the British Empire. When the Empire was threatened, so was Canada. However, Canadians eventually came to see themselves as equal partners in the fight and the country emerged from the war with a new confidence and maturity.

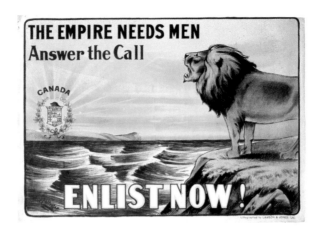

THE EMPIRE NEEDS MEN
Answer the Call
CANADA
ENLIST NOW!

the list of battlefield accomplishments for Canadian soldiers lengthened, the message of the propaganda campaign had changed. In the beginning the conflict was presented in old-fashioned terms as a fight for Empire. Canada was in it because the Mother Country needed help. We were not so much an ally as a faithful family retainer. It was Britain's struggle and we were lending a hand. This message was reflected in the iconography of the earliest propaganda produced, which contained images of the British lion and the British flag and calls to come to the aid of the Empire. By mid-war, however, the propaganda message had been nationalized. The war had become a fight in which Canada was participating as an equal partner. Canadian soldiers had proven to be equal to, in some cases superior to, the armies of other nations. The losses the Canadian Corps sustained, the victories it won, the effort Canadians made on the home front to sustain the struggle, all transformed the Great War into Canada's war as much as anyone else's.

Given the censorship imposed on information about the war, Canadians did not have a realistic sense of what was actually happening in Europe. How could they have? In most cases, the authorities feared such knowledge might erode the popular support that was needed to continue the struggle. The government did not usually lie to the public. Instead, it supplied "good news" stories and partial truths. Missing the full story, the public thought of the war in terms of familiar heroic stereotypes. Canadian soldiers were gallant warriors engaged in a noble crusade against a savage enemy. The Allies were on a mission to save civilization from the barbaric Hun. But there was nothing heroic about the Western Front and the awful slaughter that took place there. One of the long-term casualties of World War I was the old-fashioned notion of war as an ennobling enterprise. In the aftermath of the war, as people gained a deeper knowledge of the conflict and a distance from its urgency, the romantic view was replaced by a revulsion

against what had happened. Instead of a heroic victory in a great cause, the war seemed more like an inglorious waste of a generation of young men led to slaughter by callous generals and calculating politicians. Only in the past few years has the revisionist wheel come full circle and many Canadians have rediscovered their respect for the veterans of the Great War and what they accomplished.

Can the propaganda effort in favour of the war be said to have had an effect? As so often with historical questions, the answer is both yes and no.

On the one hand, Canadian society was divided by events that occurred during the war. Conscription set French against English and was deeply resented by the labour movement and farmers. The voices of minorities and pacifists were silenced. The conflict exacerbated inequalities in the economy and brought a great deal of hardship to people on the home front. It was a disturbed, agitated society that emerged from the war, as witnessed by the civil unrest that followed in the winter and

Thus did Canada answer the call. From the workshops and the offices of her cities, from the lumber camps of her forests, from the vast wheatfields of the West, from the farms and orchards of the East, from the slopes of the Rockies, from the shores of Hudson Bay, from the mining valleys of British Columbia, from the banks of the Yukon, from the reaches of the St. Lawrence, the manhood of Canada hurried to arms.

– SIR MAX AITKEN MP, *Canada in Flanders*, January 1916

OPPOSITE Recruiting posters often exhorted young men to defend their wives, sisters and mothers by joining the army. This detail is from a poster designed by the Montreal artist Hal Ross Perrigard (1891–1960). It is modelled on the famous 1871 portrait of his mother by the American painter James McNeill Whistler. By the time Perrigard borrowed it, the image of "Whistler's Mother" had come to represent womanhood in general and would have sent a powerful message of "family values" that needed defending.

spring of 1919. And it was not just Canadian society that was divided. Individuals also felt conflicted within themselves, relieved that the war was over and proud that the country seemed to have achieved so much, yet appalled at the magnitude of the loss and confused as to how it could be made meaningful.

On the other hand, Canadians as a whole rallied enthusiastically to the cause and sustained their support through five long years of war. In his study of wartime Toronto, historian Ian Miller concludes that Canadians well understood the cost of the war and willingly paid it. Of course, the fact that most Canadians backed the military effort cannot be attributed solely to the propaganda campaign waged by the government. By and large, Canadians were already patriotic imperialists; they did not need posters, poems and rallies to tell them that the war needed to be won. Still, the Great War propaganda played an important role by presenting images of the conflict that persuaded Canadians they were engaged

in a death struggle with a barbaric foe. If they had believed in anything less, they might not have seen the need to carry on.

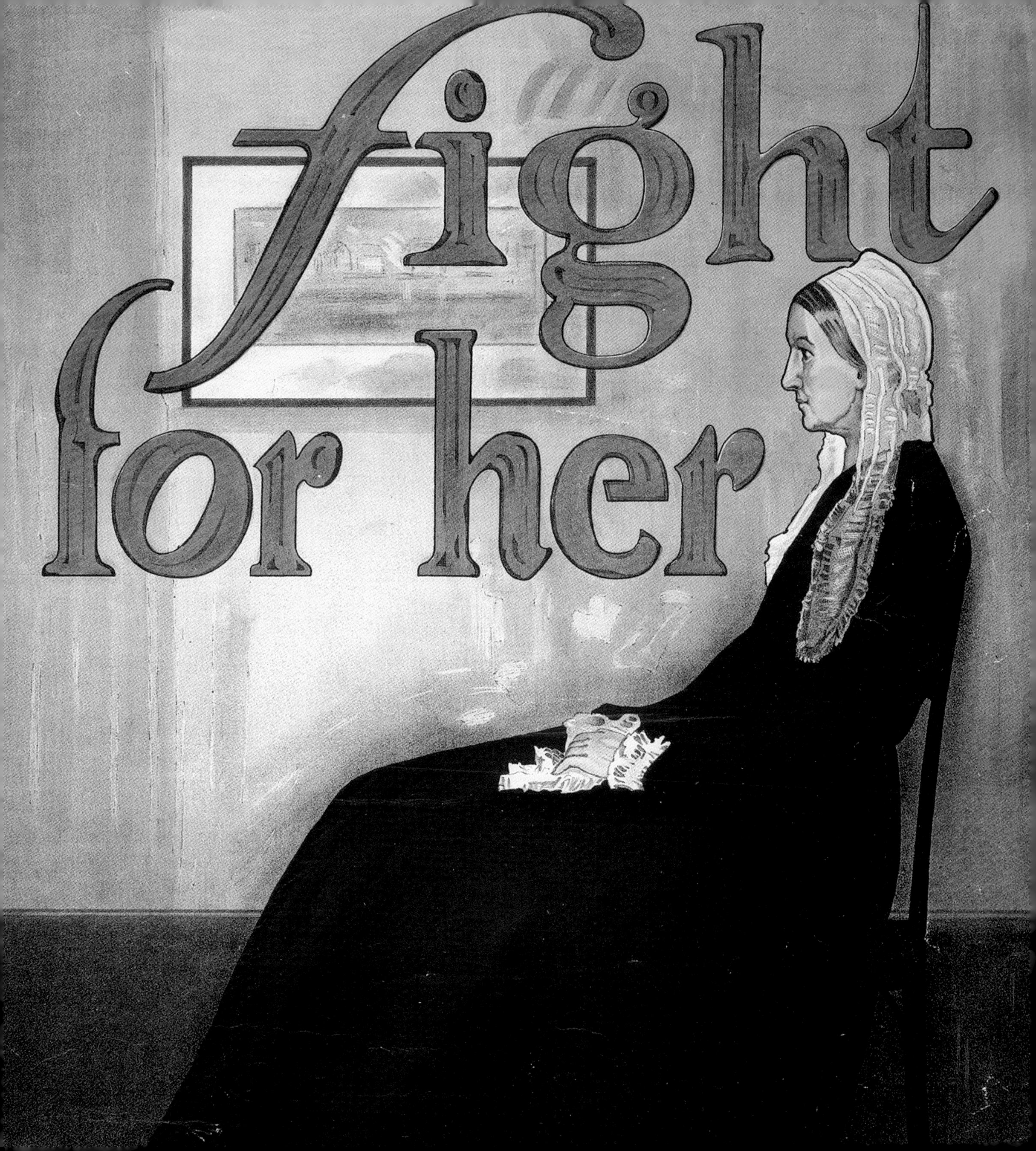
fight
for her

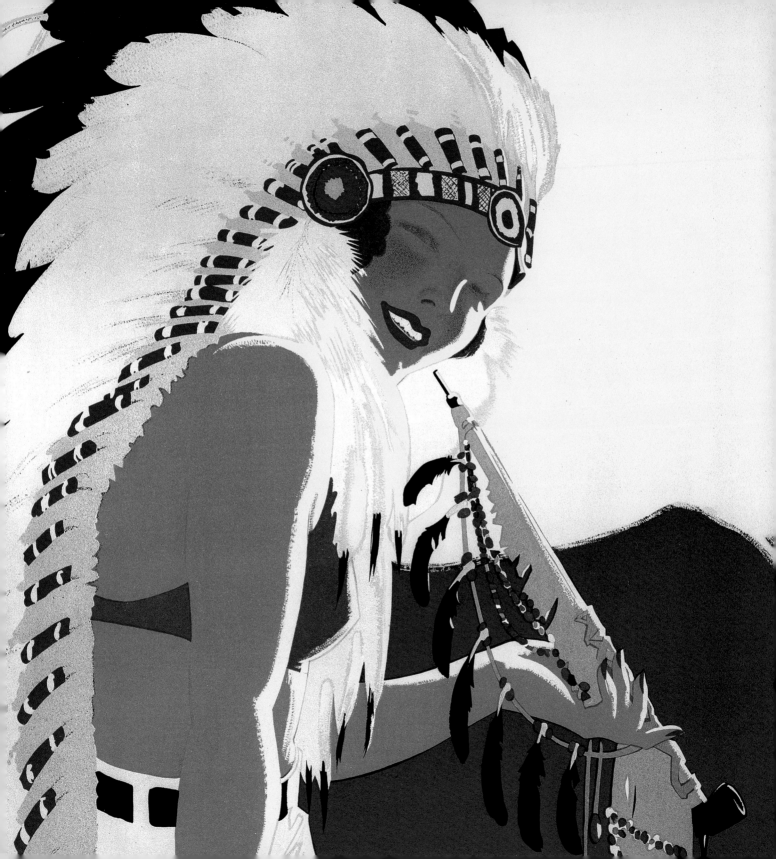

COME TO CANADA:
Selling Canada to Tourists

CHAPTER THREE

Since we can't export the scenery, we will have to import the tourists.
– WILLIAM VAN HORNE

IN 1889 THE ENGLISH ARTIST EDWARD Roper visited Canada. Settled comfortably in his berth aboard a passenger car on the newly completed transcontinental railway, Roper travelled from Montreal all the way to Vancouver, taking breaks along the way to chat with new immigrants, to fish and hunt in the backwoods, and to hike in the Rocky Mountains. Roper was no stranger to the country. He had lived in Ontario with his family as a youth and had visited the West on other occasions. This time he was particularly interested in seeing the country through the eyes of the tourist. "I know of no more delightful mode of travelling than by 'sleeper' on the CPR," he observed in the book he wrote about his adventures, *By Track and Trail: A Journey Through Canada*. More generally he gave an unqualified thumbs-up to Canada as a tourist destination.

> To tourists, to those desiring a glorious holiday, I would say, go to Canada; go camping on the lakes, the back lakes of Ontario; to Muskoka, amongst the One Thousand Islands on the St. Lawrence, or the Ten Thousand Islands in Georgian Bay, Lake Huron. Go to Penetanguishene and hire a yacht there and spend some weeks cruising and camping, fishing and shooting in the season... Or take your camping kit and go by CPR to Calgary or a station or two west of it, and there begin to camp, going by easy stages through the mountains to the coast.

By the time Edward Roper published this enthusiastic advice, Canada had been on the itinerary of travellers from Europe and the United States for at least a generation. From the middle of the nineteenth century, British hunters and adventurers came in search of big game and manly sport. A few of these visitors wrote magazine articles and books about their experiences, introducing British readers to a Canadian North and West that were remote, exotic and picturesque, with a whiff of danger. Probably the most influential of these

OPPOSITE This detail from a Canadian Pacific Railway poster advertising tourism in the Canadian Rockies invokes the image of the alluring "Indian Princess." Exotic Aboriginal people and stunning wilderness landscapes were two of the attractions the tourist industry used to sell Canada as a travel destination.

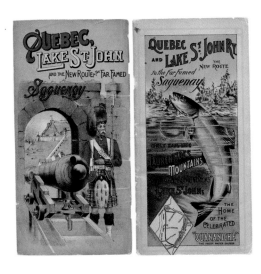

Many smaller railways produced creative and interesting materials to bring tourists to their own corner of Canada – in this case the Saguenay River Valley north of Quebec City. In 1906 the Quebec and Lake St. John Railway promoted its line as "the New Route to the Far-Famed Saguenay." While the brochure content included schedules, maps and other practical details, the cover images promised magnificent fishing and cultural experiences.

imperialist explorers was William Francis Butler, the British military officer who had travelled west to Red River in 1870 with the force dispatched to pacify the Metis. Asked by his superiors to investigate conditions in the North-West, Butler travelled by horseback across the plains as far as the Rocky Mountains. His popular account of the expedition, published in 1872 as *The Great Lone Land*, went through seventeen editions before he died in 1910, and reinforced the prevailing view that Canada, or at least western Canada, was an untouched wilderness. To a significant degree this view is still held by the many foreign hunters and sport fishers who visit the Canadian hinterland each year in search of animal trophies.

The sights of eastern Canada were more accessible to early travellers than the "wild" West. The massive fortress of Quebec City with its historic Old Town along the river attracted visitors wishing to experience the colonial roots of the continent. "Quebec is perhaps the most romantic spot in the British Empire,"

enthused one magazine writer in 1908. The Huron at Lorette, north of the city, and the Iroquois at Kahnawake, outside Montreal, carried on a profitable trade in handicrafts with tourists in search of souvenirs of the original inhabitants. With the advent of steamboat excursions, the picturesque Thousand Islands section of the St. Lawrence River became a popular part of a "Northern Tour" that culminated at Niagara Falls, the number one tourist attraction in North America, where the first hotels opened in the 1820s.

All of this was travel at a leisurely pace indulged in for the most part by well-to-do excursionists with plenty of time as well as plenty of money. Then came the transcontinental railway, transforming the experience of travel. No longer an adventure for a wealthy few, travel for travel's sake became affordable for the middle classes. There was one problem. As the Canadian Pacific pushed west across the plains and into the mountains, it ran ahead of its market. The railway preceded settlement, rather than following it.

BELOW At Niagara Falls, always a popular tourist destination, the first *Maid of the Mist* was launched in the mid-nineteenth century to carry passengers across the river. It soon began offering sightseeing excursions and has been in continuous operation serving tourists ever since.

RIGHT As tourist sites developed across the country, souvenir markets such as Walker's Indian Bazaar at Niagara Falls became a staple. Visitors were enthralled by the apparent exoticism of Aboriginal cultures and eager to buy "curiosities."

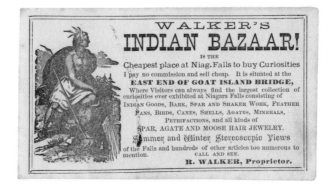

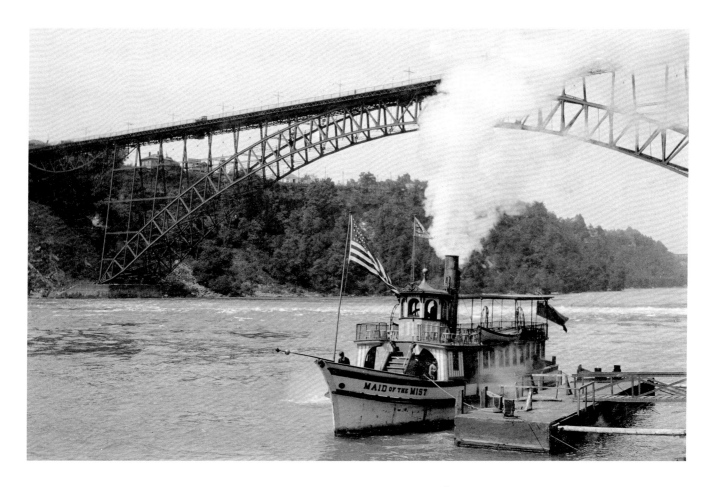

The World's Columbian Exposition, also known as the Chicago World's Fair, was held in 1893 to celebrate the 400th anniversary of Christopher Columbus's arrival in the New World in 1492. The CPR took part in the fair, exhibiting a full-size train, including a first-class day coach, dining car and sleeper. The cars contained maps of the CPR rail lines and photographs and paintings of the picturesque Canadian landscape. An astonishing twenty-seven million people visited the fair, many of whom would have been exposed to the CPR advertising.

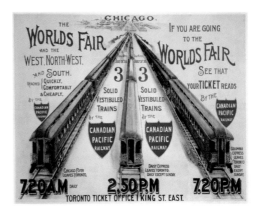

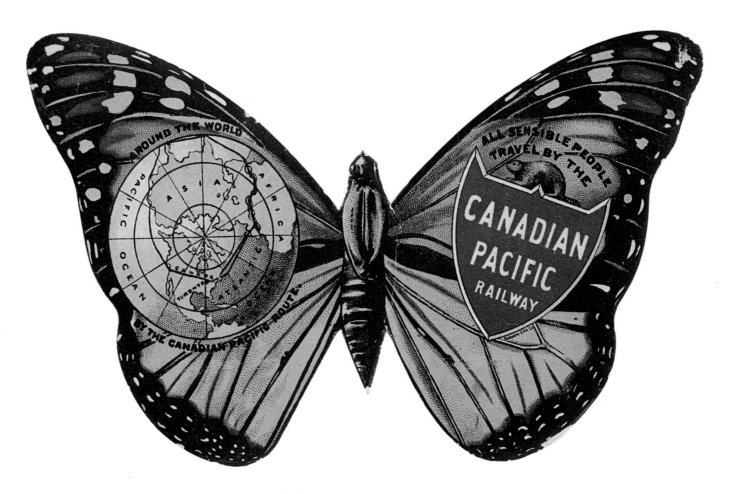

These toy figures of railway workers – a baggage handler and a station agent – date from the early twentieth century and suggest the general level of interest there was in rail travel.

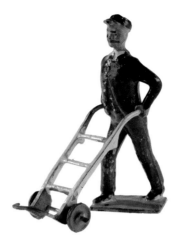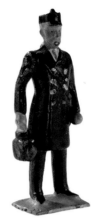

In the mid-1880s, when the last spike was driven, the prairie population boom was still a decade in the future. If the railway was going to profit, passengers were going to have to be convinced to travel on it. As CPR general manager William Van Horne remarked, "Since we can't export the scenery, we'll have to import the tourists." And so the Canadian Pacific, supported by the government, began a mammoth campaign to convince travellers that they must visit Canada, and especially western Canada.

CANADIAN PACIFIC USED A VARIETY OF promotional techniques to sell Canada to tourists. The company's publicity department produced a flood of posters, pamphlets, maps and books in a variety of languages for distribution throughout Europe and across the United States. While initially most of this material was aimed at potential homesteaders, the company also targeted the tourist trade and made strenuous efforts to promote Canada, and

particularly the Rocky Mountain West, as an attractive region for visitors.

The railway's very first promotional giveaway was a brochure featuring a magazine article written by the former governor general, Lord Lorne, and illustrated by his wife, Princess Louise, the daughter of Queen Victoria. "Nowhere can finer scenery be enjoyed from the window of a car than upon this line," Lorne declared. This pioneering effort was followed up by a second brochure that promised the sightseer "mighty rivers, vast forests, boundless plains, stupendous mountains and wonders innumerable; and yet you shall see all in comfort, nay in luxury." If adventure tourism was more your interest, the copywriter added, "and if you have lived in India, and tiger hunting has lost its zest, a Rocky Mountain grizzly will renew your interest in life." This brochure, and others that followed, were the big guns deployed by a small army of passenger and ticket agents whose job it was to drum up business for the line.

To help market Canada as a scenic destination, the CPR engaged the Montreal firm of William Notman and Son to take photographs of the mountain and prairie sections of the line. The CPR distributed these images widely in its promotional material, while the Notman company retained the right to sell individual photographs as postcards, prints and in viewbooks on the trains, at the stations and in the hotels. The CPR publicity department also persuaded painters to use the West, and particularly the mountains, as subject matter. Travelling on free passes provided by the company, these "railway artists" produced a steady stream of canvases that revealed to the world the beauty and majesty of the Canadian landscape. Painters such as John Hammond, Lucius O'Brien, John Fraser, Thomas Mower Martin and F.M. Bell-Smith made many excursions into the mountains at company expense and some of their work turned up as illustrations in publicity materials. William Van Horne – a talented amateur painter and

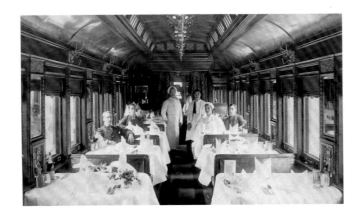

The mahogany interior of the dining car "Buckingham," complete with starched linens, silver and crystal, was typical of the style of accommodation for first-class passengers on CPR transcontinental trains in the 1890s. This particular photograph was taken by the Vancouver firm of Trueman and Caple, founded by a Canadian (R.H. Trueman) and an Englishman (Norman Caple), who did a lot of work for the railway between 1890 and 1893.

collector himself – recognized early on that art could be used to serve the purposes of commerce.

To increase the number of visitors, the CPR also made efforts to provide every comfort for the touring public. While immigrants travelling west had to be content with the plain wooden seats and spartan service aboard the colonist cars, first-class travellers luxuriated in the plush, upholstered armchairs of the parlour cars and ate in the dining cars on white linen tablecloths with gleaming silverware. Sleeping cars were panelled with carved mahogany and fitted with brass lamps and metal fixtures. Much was made in the advertising of the company's determination to spare no expense to ensure that tourists might enjoy the spectacular Canadian scenery in elegance and comfort. The whole experience was like "a first-class hotel on wheels," one writer enthused. For those travellers who were in a hurry, the CPR launched the Imperial Limited, a passenger train that made the trip from Montreal to Vancouver in just over four days.

DESPITE THE MANY COMFORTS PROVIDED, early train travel was not entirely free of danger and inconvenience. On his 1889 trip across the country Edward Roper had to disembark and cross a narrow wooden bridge on foot in the middle of a blizzard because rising water had made the route impassable for the train. Back on board, Roper was sitting in his coach when a boulder rolled down a hillside and smashed through a window – the harbinger of a rock slide that pelted the train, threatening to knock it off the track into a canyon. No sooner had Roper and his fellow passengers got underway again than they ran into a forest fire that threatened to burn up the wooden trestles. Then there were snow slides near Rogers Pass and Revelstoke that delayed the train yet again. It was with enormous relief that Roper rolled into Vancouver, several days late. Of course, these were the kinds of incidents that the CPR omitted from its brochures.

As well as rock slides, fire and snow, the CPR had to contend with some tech-

THE CANADIAN PACIFIC BEGAN passenger service aboard its transcontinental line on June 28, 1886, a "Red Letter Day for Canada" as one of the company posters proclaimed. Prime Minister John A. Macdonald had hoped to be aboard this inaugural train when it left the Montreal station, but official business kept him at work for a few more days. As a result it was late in the evening of Saturday, July 10, when the prime minister, his wife Agnes, his personal secretary Joseph Pope, a police guard and two attendants boarded their special train in Ottawa and embarked for Port Moody, which was then the transcontinental's Pacific terminus.

The cross-country expedition took two weeks. As well as giving Macdonald his first look at the country he had done so much to create, the trip served as a campaign tour. Macdonald was anticipating a general election – one that would eventually be called for the following February – and took advantage of the opportunity to get the bandwagon rolling. The party travelled only by daylight and made lengthy stops at Winnipeg and Regina. At Gleichen, near Calgary, a group of Blackfoot chiefs, including Crowfoot, waited to meet the prime minister. There Macdonald presented the old chief with a dark suit of broadcloth and silk, an acknowledgement that Crowfoot was in mourning for his adopted son Poundmaker, who had died a few days earlier.

Afterwards, as the train wound its way through the mountains, Macdonald and his wife ventured out onto the buffer bar, or cow-catcher, at the front of the engine to marvel at the deep canyons and snow-capped peaks.

From Port Moody the prime minister travelled by steamer to Victoria, where he and Agnes stayed for two weeks. It was his first visit to British Columbia, even though he had been elected to Parliament for a Victoria seat in 1878 after he lost a by-election in his hometown of Kingston.

Macdonald and his party made their way back across the country in the same leisurely manner, stopping often along the way to make speeches and shore up political support among the locals. The trip finally ended early on the morning of August 30 when the train arrived in Ottawa after travelling for fifty days and covering close to 10,000 kilometres.

SIR JOHN A. SURVEYS HIS RAILWAY

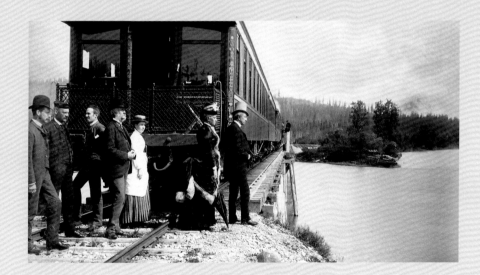

Prime Minister John A. Macdonald and his wife Agnes (right) pause during their cross-Canada trip in 1886 to admire a view across the Stave River near Mission, BC, east of Vancouver.

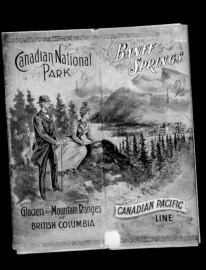

Canadian National Park

BANFF SPRINGS

Glaciers and Mountain Ranges of BRITISH COLUMBIA

CANADIAN PACIFIC LINE

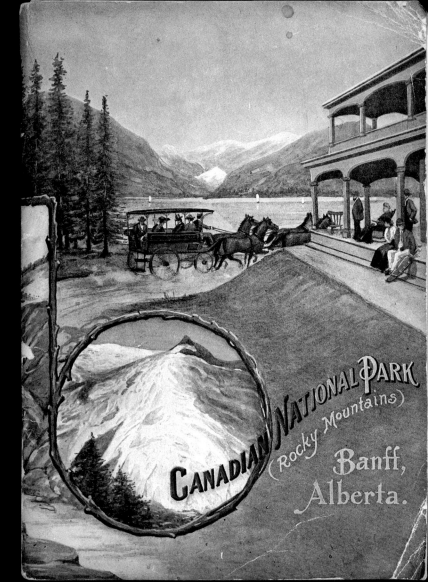

CANADIAN NATIONAL PARK
(Rocky Mountains)
Banff, Alberta.

Visitors bathe in the original hot springs at Banff. Construction of the railway reached the area in 1883 and the government set aside the springs as reserve land two years later. It was the beginning of Banff National Park. At the time it was believed that a swim in the sulphur springs was good for what ailed you, whether it was rheumatism, gout or a hangover.

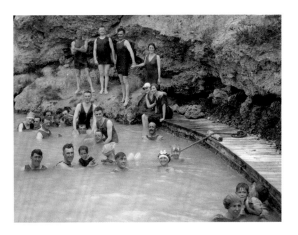

nology and infrastructure limitations. Once a train reached the mountains it had to shed its dining cars, which were too heavy to be pulled up the steep inclines. As an alternative, the company constructed a series of restaurant stops – Mount Stephen House, Glacier House and Fraser Canyon House – to provide meals and accommodations for any passengers wishing to stop over. More ambitiously, the company in 1888 opened a luxury hotel at Banff in the heart of the Rockies. Built to resemble a Scottish castle, the Banff Springs was the first of a chain of luxury, Château-style hotels that later included the Château Frontenac (1893) in Quebec City and the Empress in Victoria (1908).

The federal government collaborated with the CPR in turning the Canadian landscape into a profit centre. Railway survey crews had come across hot springs in the vicinity of what is now Banff and in 1887 the government designated some of the land around the springs as Rocky Mountains Park, later renamed Banff

National Park, Canada's first national park. Within a decade several more reserves were established for later development as national parks. The founding of these mountain parks was motivated less by conservationist ideals than by a desire to promote tourism in the Rocky Mountain West. "I do not suppose in any portion of the world there can be found a spot... which combines so many attractions and which promises in as great a degree not only large pecuniary advantage to the Dominion, but much prestige," Prime Minister Macdonald told the House of Commons. "Nothing attracts tourists like national parks," agreed J.B. Harkin, the Commissioner of Dominion Parks. The early promoters saw the western scenery as a commodity, a natural resource that could be sold just as other natural resources were sold. The CPR touted them as the most spectacular alpine scenery in the world. Why go to Europe when Canada was, as Van Horne put it, "1001 Switzerlands Rolled into One"? The company even went so far as

to appropriate ownership of the mountains, describing them in publicity material as the "Canadian Pacific Rockies." Harkin made this "capitalization of the landscape" explicit in one of his annual reports. In 1915 alone, he calculated, sixty-five thousand foreign visitors came to Rocky Mountains Park and spent a total of more than $16 million in Canada. Using a simple formula, the commissioner worked out that tourism brought in more money per acre of scenery than the country's wheat exports.

The federal government also partnered with the railway to conduct tours of the country by selected "opinion makers." One example was a tour by delegates to the congress of the Chambers of Commerce of the Empire, which met in Montreal in 1903. Following their meetings, delegates were invited to participate in a six-week rail tour of Canada, from the Maritimes through Quebec and Ontario all the way to British Columbia, largely paid for by the Canadian government. The railway made a special train available

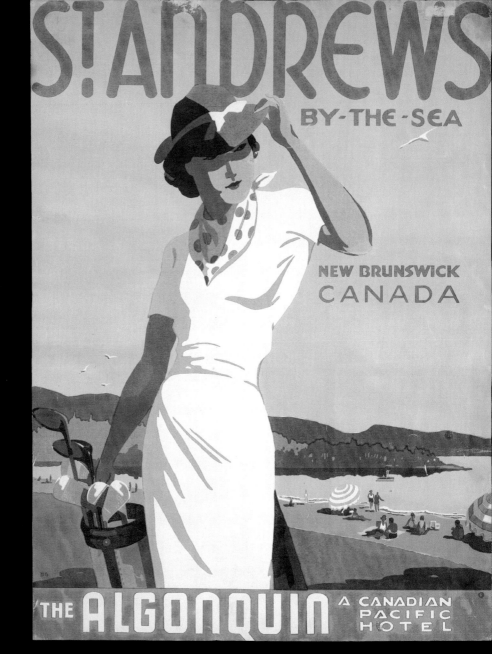

St. Andrews, New Bruns-
wick, on the Bay of Fundy,
has been a popular tourist
destination since the late
nineteenth century, and
Canadian Pacific has had
a long association with
the town. Railway pre-
sident William Van Horne
vacationed at a summer
home on nearby Ministers
Island and the company
operated the luxurious
Algonquin Hotel in St.
Andrews from 1903 to
1970. The poster dates
from 1937.

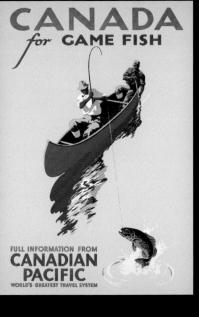

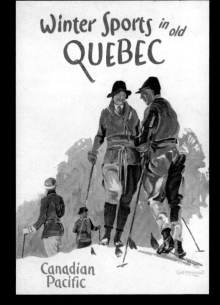

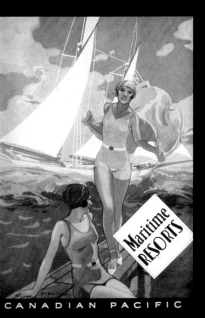

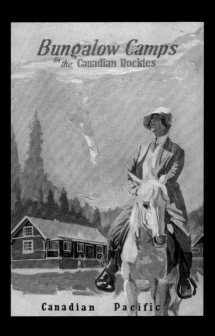

Canadian Pacific marketed a wide range of travel experiences, from fishing and swimming in the Maritimes, to skiing in Quebec and horseback riding in the Rockies. The railway also created its own chain of hotels and resorts to serve the tourists enjoying these experiences, and its art department produced a steady stream of gorgeous posters containing romanticized images of the country.

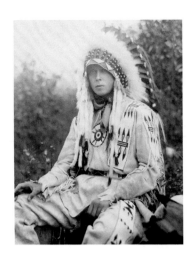

His Royal Highness the Prince of Wales in full regalia as Chief Morning Star of the Stoney Indians in Banff during his tour of Canada in 1919. He became King Edward VIII early in 1936 but abdicated eleven months later in order to marry Wallis Simpson, an American divorcee.

and official photographers accompanied the tour to produce scenic photographs for the delegates. Clearly it was in the government's interest to do whatever it could to support the railway's promotional efforts. What was good for the CPR was good for Canada.

One particular tourist gave a tremendous boost to the reputation of the CPR as a first-class travel experience. In September 1901, the Duke of York arrived in Quebec City with his wife, Princess Mary, to begin a five-week cross-country-and-back-again tour. The Duke was the grandson of Queen Victoria – who had died earlier in the year – and the son of the new monarch, Edward VII. He would eventually accede to the throne himself in 1910 as King George V. The royal party, with accompanying British journalists, travelled aboard a special train prepared by the CPR, a nine-car "palace on wheels" boasting all the latest mod cons, including padded rubber bathtubs, electric lights and telephone communications between cars. Conductors were expected

to wear black neckties and gloves and all along the route the company laid on special welcomes at the different stations. The tour produced columns and columns of positive publicity for the CPR, and for Canada, in newspapers around the world. Likewise in 1919, when the Prince of Wales, the future King Edward VIII, toured Canada in what a Calgary paper called "the most palatial train that has ever been assembled in North America," and again in 1939, when King George VI and Queen Elizabeth visited, it was the CPR that benefited from the sort of publicity only royalty could produce.

———

IF CANADA WAS "SOLD" TO TOURISTS AS a spectacular wilderness where visitors could experience nature in all its majesty, it was also promoted as "Indian Country," every bit as exotic for its native inhabitants as the depths of Africa or a remote island in the South Pacific. Indigenous people had been part of the attraction of Canada to outsiders since

JOHN HAMMOND WAS ALREADY A successful painter and the principal of an art school in Saint John, New Brunswick, when he met William Van Horne and became part of the CPR campaign to promote western Canada as a tourist destination. In 1891 Hammond made the first of many cross-Canada, all-expenses-paid rail trips to paint the western landscape. The following year he hired a guide and travelled on horseback and by foot into the area around Yoho, country too remote for most tourists. Hammond painted his impressions on small wooden panels, which he then worked up into larger canvases back in the studio.

Hammond's field trips on the CPR continued into the new century. On occasion he travelled with company vice-president David McNicoll in a special car with a living room, kitchen and dining room, and two bedrooms, each complete with bath. "So on these tours we had a royal time," he wrote. His paintings appeared as part of the company's exhibits at the 1893 World's Fair in Chicago, the Paris Exposition in 1900, and other international exhibitions. A series of murals that he painted for the walls of the company's head office in Trafalgar Square in London in 1905 established his claim to being pre-eminent among the railway artists.

The murals were his last work for the CPR. Hammond, by then sixty-two years old, retired from the peripatetic life of a mountain painter to his teaching position at Mount Allison University in Sackville, New Brunswick. He continued to paint and exhibit until his death in 1939.

A MOUNTAIN PAINTER

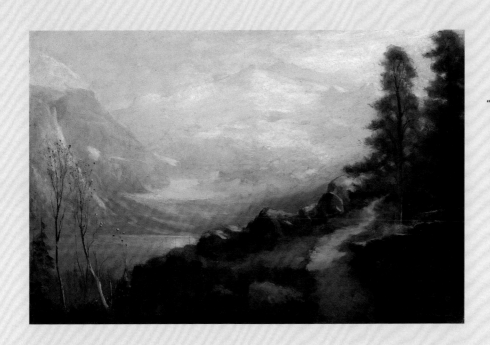

"Banff," one of the oil paintings done by John Hammond during the period that he travelled and sketched on behalf of the CPR.

A 1926 poster by the art-
ist Wilfred Langdon Kihn
promotes Banff Indian
Days. Indian Days began
when a rock slide blocked
the CPR main line near
Banff. Wanting to occupy
the stranded passengers,
the railway manager in-
vited a group of Stoney
people from Morley to
provide entertainment.
The impromptu event
evolved into the annual
Indian Days. Langdon
Kihn (1898–1957) was an
American artist who spe-
cialized in painting por-
traits of North American
Aboriginals.

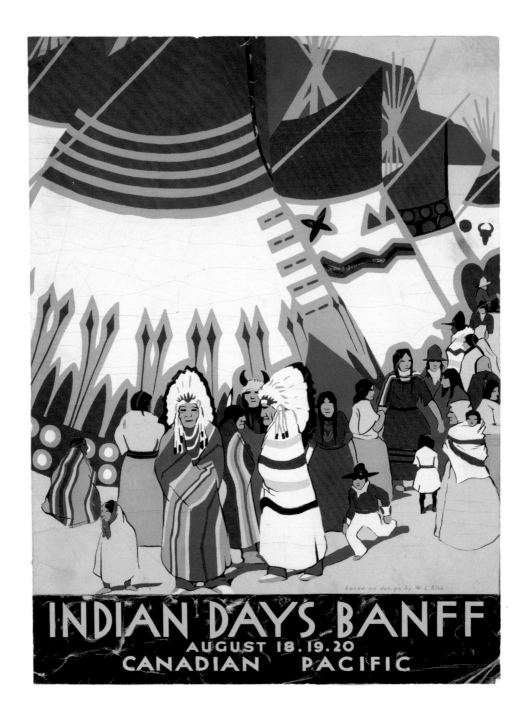

Chicken dancers from the Stoney First Nation perform at Banff Indian Days in 1941, with the Banff Springs Hotel looming in the background. The celebration of Indian Days was discontinued in 1978 but was revived more recently by the Stoney.

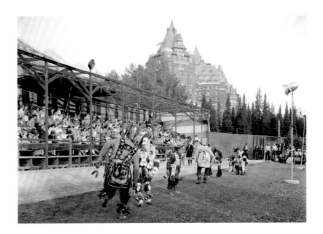

the earliest explorers arrived to trade for furs. During the eighteenth century, British colonial officials routinely paid visits to First Nations villages where they purchased souvenirs and witnessed dances and ceremonies. (Anthropologists call these displays "staged ethnicity" and they remain a part of the tourist experience in Canada to the present day.) In 1860, when Queen Victoria's eighteen-year-old son Albert, the Prince of Wales, made the first royal visit to Canada, Aboriginal people played a prominent role in many of the receptions staged to welcome the prince. Visitors to Niagara Falls seldom failed to include the Tuscarora Nation village on the American side as part of their itinerary.

This pattern of exploiting the outsider's fascination with North America's indigenous people was continued by the CPR. When the British writer Douglas Sladen crossed Canada by rail in 1894 he noted that "the Indians and the bears were splendid stage properties to have at a station where both the east and west

bound trains... stop for lunch." Following the invention of roll film by George Eastman, snapshot photography came into widespread use. During the 1890s, tourists armed with brand new Kodak cameras took advantage of every opportunity to "Kodak the Indians" as they crossed the country. "The average passenger would as soon think of going without his anti-bilious medicines as without a camera," remarked Sladen. "Whenever you stop at a station," he went on, "all the steps getting down are packed with people taking pot shots with Kodaks. American children learn Kodaking before they learn to behave themselves."

Recognizing the marketability of indigenous people, the CPR inaugurated Banff Indian Days, an annual summer festival featuring aspects of local First Nations culture, in 1894. Each summer the railway sponsored a similar pageant in Desbarats, Ontario, with actors in costume performing scenes from a version of Longfellow's popular long poem "Hiawatha." Photographs of Aboriginal

people and their villages were popular with travellers wishing to take home mementoes of their exotic experiences. Canada's "Wild Indians" were promoted as every bit as exciting for tourists as the tribes of darkest Africa, yet a lot easier to access by way of the railway.

The campaign to attract tourist traffic for CPR trains eventually did more than promote access to exotic people and stunning landscapes. Over time Canadians came to see the railway as much more than an iron road between points on a map. They began to see it as the enterprise that "created" Canada, rather than vice versa. Books written about the line portrayed the backers of the CPR as "empire builders," not simple businessmen. The completion of the railway "made Canada possible," the argument ran. "The construction of the Canadian Pacific consummated Confederation," the company even boasted in one of its early publications. Without the line, it was said, the North-West would have fallen into the grasping hands of the United

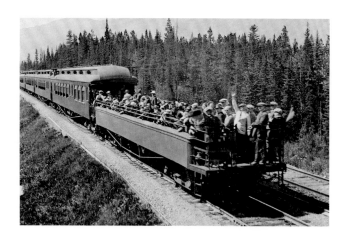

Travellers on a CPR train admire the mountains from an open-air observation car at Field, BC, in 1924.

States; without the line, western grain would not have reached its markets and new settlers would never have populated the plains. George Ham, the company publicist, was expressing conventional wisdom when he marvelled that the line "magically transformed a widely scattered Dominion into a prosperous and progressive nation." The Canadian Pacific was not just a railway; it was, as Pierre Berton dubbed it, a "National Dream."

Whether or not the railway deserves the credit it has received for making Canada possible, it definitely played a leading role in imagining the country into existence. Prior to World War I, it was impossible to see the country except by rail. Travellers rode on CPR trains, stayed at CPR hotels and had what they saw interpreted by CPR promotional literature. The company produced the images that gave most people their first look at the Canadian landscape. So Canada became "The Last, Best West," the granary of the British Empire, an untamed wilderness inhabited by exotic tribes

and rustic pioneers. All these familiar images of nationality were created by the CPR as part of its corporate strategy to develop the western hinterland as a profit centre.

And it worked. The CPR's multi-faceted marketing campaign, reinforced by the efforts of government immigration officials who were already selling the West as a sunny paradise full of wild game and fertile farmland, resulted in a significant increase in the number of people visiting Canada. In his book on tourism and the CPR, E.J. Hart used the expanding number of first-class sleeping and dining cars as a measure of the increase in tourist traffic. During the first decade of transcontinental passenger service, the number of these cars doubled and the revenue they produced for the railway tripled. By 1913 the CPR alone was carrying 15.5 million passengers a year and two other transcontinental rail lines – the Canadian Northern, built by entrepreneurs William Mackenzie and Donald Mann, and the Grand Trunk

CANADIAN PACIFIC ASPIRED TO make its transcontinental railway part of a travel service that spanned the globe. To this end the company chartered its first steamships in 1887 and initiated passenger service across the Pacific from Hong Kong and Japan to Vancouver. Four years later the company launched its Empress fleet of speedy luxury liners carrying passengers between Canada's Pacific Coast and various ports in the Far East. In fact the Pacific crossing was just one leg in an around-the-world cruise offered by the company. For $600, passengers could board an Empress liner in Liverpool, England, and travel through the Mediterranean and the Suez Canal, across the Indian Ocean to Singapore, China and Japan and on to Vancouver where they boarded a transcontinental train for the trip across Canada. The final leg of the voyage across the Atlantic to Britain was arranged by the CPR but utilized vessels owned by other companies. Then, in 1903, CPR completed this missing link when it began offering its own passenger service between Canada and Liverpool as well.

The Dominion was an integral part of this imperial highway (known as the "All-Red" route, a reference to the member countries of the British Empire, coloured red on the map). As an article in the Canadian Gazette put it, the railway "makes Canada Britain's half-way house to the Far East."

Canadian Pacific's integrated transportation system handled hundreds of thousands of immigrants and tourists each year.

In 1915 the company organized its steamship service as Canadian Pacific Ocean Services, later the Canadian Pacific Steamship Company. The service was aimed at the middle-class tourist with a yen to see the exotic sights of Canada and the East.

TAKING THE ALL-RED ROUTE TO THE ORIENT

This poster advertising the "All-Red" route illustrates how Canadian Pacific created a total experience for the traveller, integrating "steamships, trains, hotels" in a trip that spanned the globe.

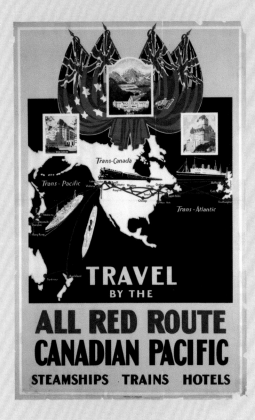

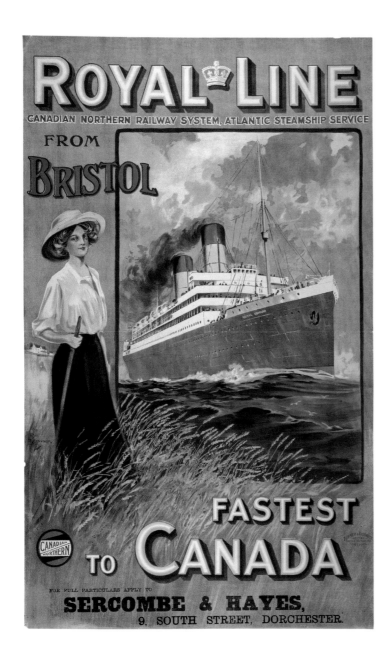

The Royal Line was one of the shipping companies that brought immigrants to Canada, sailing from Bristol, England, and connecting with the Canadian Northern Railway. The Canadian government paid a bonus to steamship ticket agents for each immigrant in three specified categories: farmers, farm labourers and domestics. The line also contributed to the development of tourism in Canada and profited from European interest in the remote and marvellous Canadian frontier.

Pacific – were set to begin service to the West Coast within two years. Many of these millions of train passengers were new immigrants, of course, but many were tourists from abroad or elsewhere in Canada, eager to experience the country they had seen and read about in the railway's promotional literature.

FOLLOWING WORLD WAR I, THE AUTO-mobile arrived in Canada with a rush and challenged the railways' monopoly on the tourist trade. There had been motor vehicles before the war but only a few thousand. British Columbia, for instance, had just four thousand licensed automobiles in 1912; Nova Scotia a mere 911. In Prince Edward Island the mainly agricultural population so disliked cars that it was illegal to drive one until 1913; even then, motorized vehicles were allowed on the road only three days of the week. Suspicion changed to enthusiasm during the 1920s when the motor car stopped being a curiosity owned by a few adven-

By the 1920s the motor car was well established as a necessary part of middle-class life in Canada. This photograph shows the corner of Sunnyside Drive and Keele Street in Toronto in April 1922. Already traffic had become heavy enough to require a traffic cop.

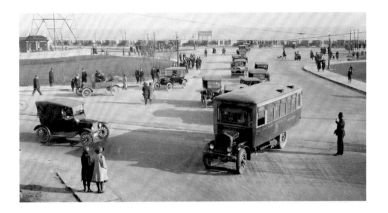

turous souls and instead became a necessary part of middle-class life. By 1930 there were a million registered automobiles in the country, population ten million, and Canada boasted the third-largest per capita rate of car ownership in the world. The motorization of society was happening at an even faster pace south of the border in the United States, the source of most tourists visiting Canada. There the number of registered vehicles rose from eight million to twenty-three million during the 1920s. By 1925, two million American-owned motor cars were entering Canada annually, accounting for an estimated $150 million worth of tourist spending. The Depression of the 1930s slowed the flow of tourists but by no means halted it. In 1933, seven million tourists entered Ontario from the United State and nationwide tourist spending amounted to $120 million, down from pre-Depression numbers but still significant.

Government expenditure on roads rose along with the number of motor vehicles using them. Most of the new

thoroughfares headed south to the border to provide access for American motorists who wished to visit the scenic wonders of Canada, but domestic road building was a high priority for government as well. By the middle of the 1920s the provinces collectively were spending more on highways than any other single item in their budgets. During the Depression, federal public works projects, part of Prime Minister R.B. Bennett's "New Deal," pumped tens of millions of dollars into road construction. One by one the gaps in the cross-Canada highway system were filled in. In June 1940, for example, the Big Bend Highway connected Golden to Revelstoke through the mountainous interior of British Columbia and for the first time it was possible to travel by car from Alberta to the Pacific on an all-Canadian route. In the same year another Depression-era relief project, the Banff–Jasper Highway, opened the magnificent central Rockies to the motoring tourist. Then, in 1942 crews completed a 246-kilometre stretch of gravel road between

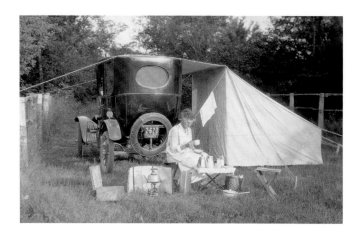

Hearst and Geraldton in northern Ontario that was the final link in a network of highways, most of them still unpaved, that spanned the country. Finally, motorists could drive across Canada without the inconvenience of having to dip south of the border to follow American routes.

Along with roads, the inter-war period also saw the development of basic infrastructure for motor tourists. There had always been hotels, of course, but many motorists preferred simply to go "gypsying," which meant pitching a tent by the side of the road and camping out under the stars. Auto camps, some of them operated free by municipalities eager to attract the wandering auto-tourist, evolved into cottage camps where travellers slept in separate cabins, and then into the first motels where sleeping units were part of a single building. In the summer of 1963, Edward McCourt, a professor of literature at the University of Saskatchewan, drove across Canada on a holiday with his wife Margaret. In the book that he wrote about the excursion, McCourt looked back to

an earlier era and its "quaint little motels of yesteryear, each unit complete with pot-bellied stove, broken-down bed, naked overhead bulb, and privy in the bushes out back." He had fond memories of these early way stations with their invitations to Amble Inn or Bide-a-Wee, though he was happy enough to have a modern room in which to rest his weary bones after a day's hard driving.

———

DURING THE 1920S AND 1930S, AT THE same time travel by road was accelerating, the involvement of the railways in tourism intensified. During the pre–World War I economic boom the CPR had lost its monopoly on rail travel when the Grand Trunk Pacific and the Canadian Northern pushed their way from eastern Canada to the Pacific. Both of these new transcontinental lines ran into immediate financial difficulties as the cost of building far exceeded the revenue they could produce, and by 1923 the federal government had merged their operations

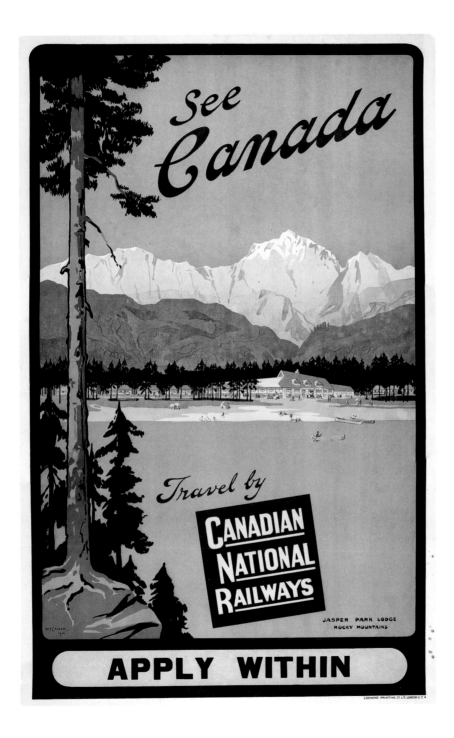

The federal government created Canadian National Railways following World War I from a merger of two other transcontinental lines, the Canadian Northern and Grand Trunk Pacific. In Jasper National Park, CN built Jasper Park Lodge, which opened in the summer of 1922 as a complex of small bungalows. A year later the main lodge, shown in this poster, opened. According to CN, its lodge was the largest single-storey log structure in the world.

A "musical souvenir" of a visit to the Muskoka Lakes, a vacation land in south-central Ontario. By the time this song by E.B. Sutton appeared in 1903, Muskoka had several resort hotels and a reputation for picturesque scenery. Sutton himself built the Bala Bay Inn in 1910.

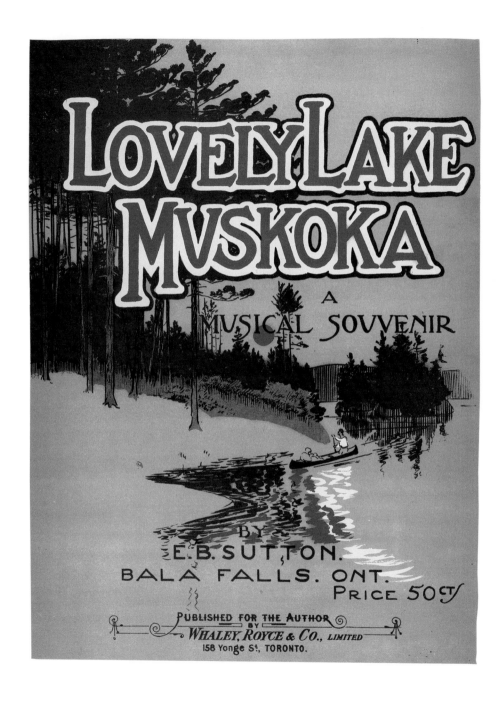

LEFT This sheet music cover from 1914 contains many of the conventional tropes of tourist literature: the moonlit lake, the canoe and an Indian "princess." Jack Caddigan and Chick Story were American songwriters who often collaborated.

RIGHT Another piece of sheet music, this time from 1912, makes the familiar association between Canada and the wild outdoors. One of the trio of campers sharing a story around the moonlit fire appears to be a Mountie.

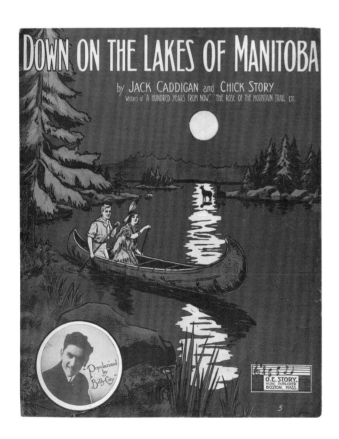

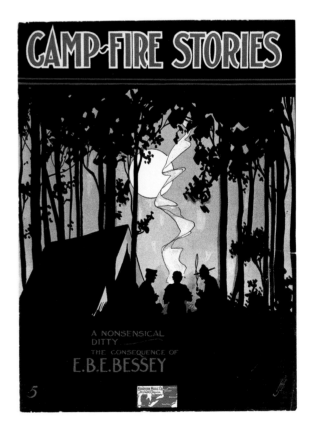

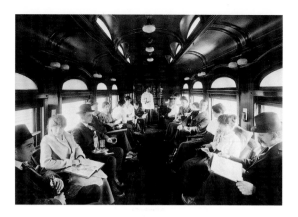

The club car aboard a Canadian Northern train, where passengers enjoyed refreshment and convivial conversation as they sped through the Canadian landscape. Canadian Northern ran into financial difficulties during World War I and became part of the government-owned Canadian National system.

into a single, state-owned line, the Canadian National Railway (CNR). Whatever their financial problems, these short-lived lines, and later the CNR, used the same sort of promotional schemes the CPR relied on to attract passengers. In 1914, for example, the Grand Trunk Pacific invited Sir Arthur Conan Doyle, author of the Sherlock Holmes stories, on a tour in his own luxuriously appointed rail car in hopes of attracting visitors to Jasper National Park, established seven years earlier. Doyle did not fail his hosts, writing in a British magazine that "Jasper Park is one of the great national playgrounds and health resorts which the Canadian government with great wisdom has laid out for the benefit of the citizens."

During the 1920s the CNR and the federal parks branch collaborated on developing Jasper as a tourist centre, a northern equivalent of Banff, where the CPR still dominated. CNR was a publicly owned enterprise in a precarious financial position and the government was feeling the pressure to turn it into a money-maker.

Therefore Ottawa had every interest in encouraging the railway's efforts to attract tourist traffic. Led by its dynamic new president Henry Thornton, the railway established Jasper Park Lodge, a resort hotel complete with golf course, which boosters expected would rival the Banff Springs. Thornton promoted a scenic triangle route for tourists, utilizing the western rail lines belonging to CN's original two partners. Beginning in Jasper, travellers could follow the route of the old Canadian Northern down the Fraser Canyon to Vancouver, where they could board a CNR-owned coastal steamer for a cruise north through the Inside Passage to Prince Rupert. They could then meet the former Grand Trunk Pacific line, which would carry them eastward along the Skeena River, through Prince George and back to Jasper.

As the CPR had done, CN promoted western Canada as "Indian Country" to appeal to tourists' taste for the exotic. The railway took advantage of the fact that a large number of totem poles re-

Early tourists belonged to a privileged social class and brought along their own accoutrements to make themselves comfortable when travelling by sea or rail. This nineteenth-century French-made travel kit contains fifty-four items, including drinking cups, hairbrushes and razors. There is even room for a buttonhook, a ruler, a pen and a whetstone; in short, everything that a "civilized" traveller might need. The box itself is walnut trimmed with copper and leather, and many of the articles are made of silver and ivory.

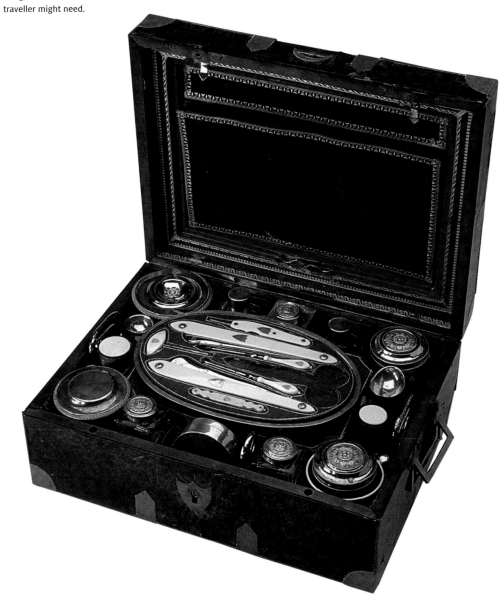

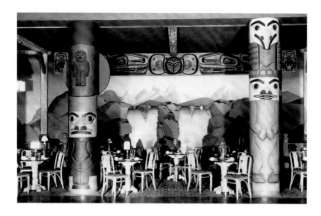

The Jasper Room at the Château Laurier in Ottawa, circa 1930, designed by the artist Edwin Holgate and evoking the material cultures of the Pacific Coast First Nations.

mained in the Gitksan villages visible from the train as it ran along the Skeena River. The large-scale looting of coastal villages by museum collectors during the nineteenth century had removed most of the Aboriginal artifacts, including many giant totem poles. By 1920 hardly any poles remained, and those that did were rapidly deteriorating. This made the Skeena River poles especially interesting, so with the arrival of the railway they became a major tourist attraction. One writer in a Montreal newspaper figured they were the most photographed objects in Canada after Niagara Falls. First Nations populations were declining at the time and it was widely believed that Canada's indigenous people were disappearing, doomed by disease, poverty and the encroachment of "civilization." In this context, totem poles took on added significance for tourists, who believed they were witnessing the poignant demise of cultures that would soon be extinct.

CN recognized the value of the Skeena poles and took a leading role in their preservation. The railway was supported in this effort by federal agencies such as the Parks branch, the Indian Department and the Victoria Memorial Museum (the forerunner of today's Canadian Museum of Civilization), which were concerned with the heritage and anthropological value of the poles. Restoration work began in 1925, beginning with poles that were actually within sight of the rail line. During the summer of 1926 the railway sponsored visits to the Skeena by artists A.Y. Jackson and Edwin Holgate, who came to sketch the area much as the CPR's railway artists had been sent to paint the Rockies thirty years earlier. CN also commissioned Holgate to design a "Totem Pole Room" for dining and dancing in its Ottawa hotel, the Château Laurier. The room was decorated with columns resembling totem poles along with large murals and Aboriginal masks and designs.

CPR too continued to promote tourism by being a patron of the arts in the inter-war period, giving passes to members of the Group of Seven to visit different

BELOW Ans'pa yaxw, or Kispiox, which means "hiding places" in the Gitksan language, is one of the villages on the Skeena River. It was originally a winter village with eleven longhouses facing the Skeena and was the site of more than twenty totem poles, some of which dated back to as early as 1880. The people of Ans'pa yaxw experienced a dramatic loss in population because of the various epidemics that followed contact with Europeans. Today the community is home to about fifteen hundred people.

RIGHT Tourists visiting the totem poles at Kitwanga on the Skeena River in northern British Columbia.

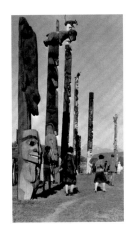

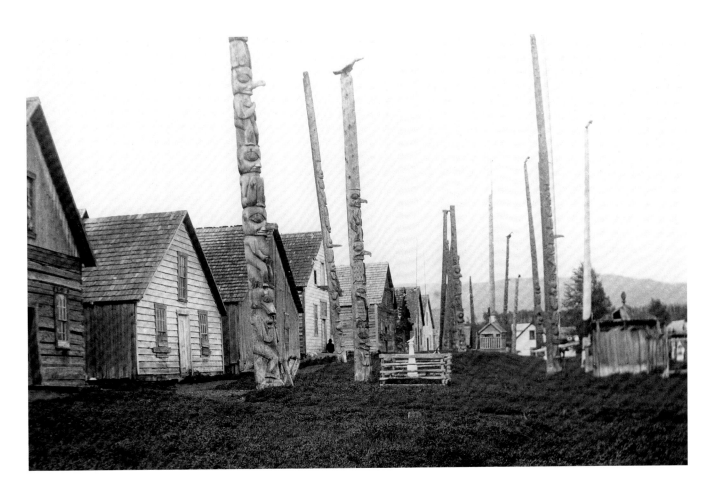

AS THE POLES CARVED BY INDIG- enous people on Canada's Pacific coast began to disappear from their original settings, they became valued as a link with the country's First Nations cultures. Before and after contact, poles were carved by many nations and for many different purposes: to recount legends, to illustrate clan relationships and to commemorate notable events. Over the years these tree-sized sculptures gradually went from having cultural significance to being part of the British Columbia tourism "brand."

In Vancouver, Stanley Park was originally home to village sites belonging to the Squamish people. After the park was established in 1886, its Squamish inhabitants were removed to other locations. Once the local Aboriginal presence was erased, members of the city's Art, Historical and Scientific Association came up with the idea of locating a model Indian village in the park. Originally they hoped to transport a village from the north coast down to the city, but in 1925 this plan ran into opposition from the Squamish. Given that the park was their traditional territory, they did not want the site occupied by structures associated with another culture.

Instead, the association began placing totem poles at the site. The Squamish did not carve poles at that time, so they were acquired from Kwakwaka'wakw villages on northern Vancouver Island. Later more poles were added until today the collection of poles at Brockton Point is one of the city's major tourist attractions.

THE POLES IN STANLEY PARK

Every year more than three million people visit the totem poles in Vancouver's Stanley Park, making them the province's number one tourist attraction.

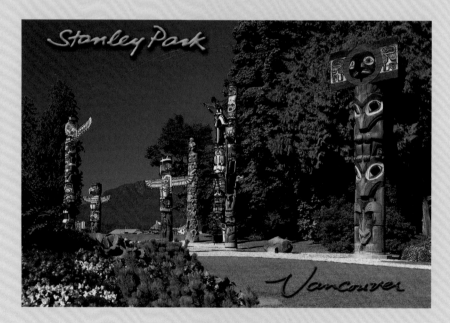

Bon Echo Inn was located in what is now Bon Echo Provincial Park in eastern Ontario. The rustic inn was purchased in 1910 by Flora Denison and her husband Howard. Flora was a feminist and a supporter of the arts and made the inn a retreat for the artistic avant-garde, as did her son Merrill Denison who inherited the resort in 1921. This 1924 poster features a painting by A.Y. Jackson, a member of the Group of Seven. The inn closed in 1928.

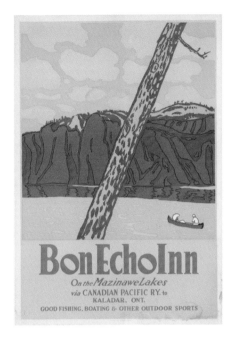

parts of Canada, then using some of their paintings in promotional material. In 1922 the company invited an American painter, Langdon Kihn, to paint on the Stoney Reserve at Morley, Alberta. The railway purchased several of Kihn's paintings and used them to illustrate a book, *Indian Days in the Canadian Rockies*, written by anthropologist Marius Barbeau. The book was commissioned with the expectation that it would help promote the annual Banff Indian Days celebration and bring visitors to the area.

The Skeena River project was initiated by the government and the railway with similar expectations, although it did not always enjoy the acceptance of the local Gitksan people. Outsiders may well have thought of northern British Columbia as "Indian Country," but the Gitksan who lived there saw no need to market their culture as a tourist attraction. "They are unfavourably disposed toward white men in general," reported Harlan Smith of the Victoria Memorial Museum, "and particularly toward Government officials."

After all, continued Smith, it was white settlers who were pushing the Gitksan off their land, white canneries that were devouring the salmon, white loggers who were cutting up the best timber. By the time restoration came to an end in 1930, only about a third of the poles had been "rescued." From an anthropological point of view, the project had mixed results, but in terms of tourism promotion it was a huge success and CN gained a great deal of publicity by advertising itself as "the railway to totem pole land."

————————

HISTORIAN IAN MCKAY HAS IDENTIFIED the 1920s as a period when government intervened to promote tourism in an especially aggressive way. Once Ottawa became a proprietor of its own transcontinental railway, Canadian National, it had a strong interest in selling Canada as a travel destination. But tourism was about more than railways. In 1929 revenue from tourism was estimated to be almost $310 million and governments, both federal and

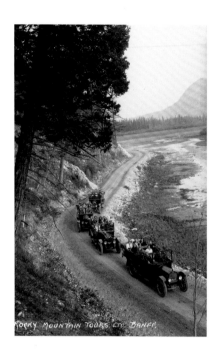

provincial, recognized that travel was an industry that produced substantial economic benefits. As a result they supported it by building highways for motor tourists, supporting national parks and encouraging new ethnic "traditions," all of which was expected to make Canada a more accessible and interesting place to visit.

Direct federal government involvement in tourism promotion came during the 1930s when the promise of visitor spending seemed to offer one way out of economic difficulties. In the spring of 1934 the Canadian Senate created a special committee to investigate the possibilities that tourism offered. Tourism revenues had been falling precipitously since the onset of the Depression. In its report the Senate committee optimistically predicted that an invigorated tourism industry could result in annual revenues of half a billion dollars. It recommended an "emergency" campaign to lure visitors to Canada and suggested that the national government create its own travel bureau to encourage tourism across the country. Within months just such an agency, the Canadian Government Tourist Bureau, was up and running, promoting Canada as a destination both abroad and domestically. The bureau's first director was Leo Dolan, a thirty-nine-year-old journalist from New Brunswick who had been heading up that province's Bureau of Information and Tourist Travel. The new federal bureau acted as a clearing house for distributing information to prospective visitors, published promotional literature and road maps (two of its popular publications were *Canada Your Friendly Neighbour Invites You!* and *Canada Calls You*), maintained a library of photographs, promoted road building and the creation of more national parks, and produced a campaign to educate Canadians about the importance of being friendly hosts. The message was "Tourism is everybody's business."

Provincial governments were active tourism promoters long before Ottawa got involved. In Nova Scotia the government encouraged the invention of a handicraft "tradition" and a Scottish

LEFT During the mid-1930s the Bureau of Information and Tourist Travel published this 48-page booklet, *Canada Your Friendly Neighbour Invites You*, to attract American visitors. The cover painting, done by Jack Bush, later a leading abstract expressionist, features many stereotypical Canadians: lumberjacks, fiddlers, Mounties, farmers and fishermen.

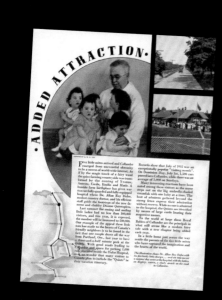

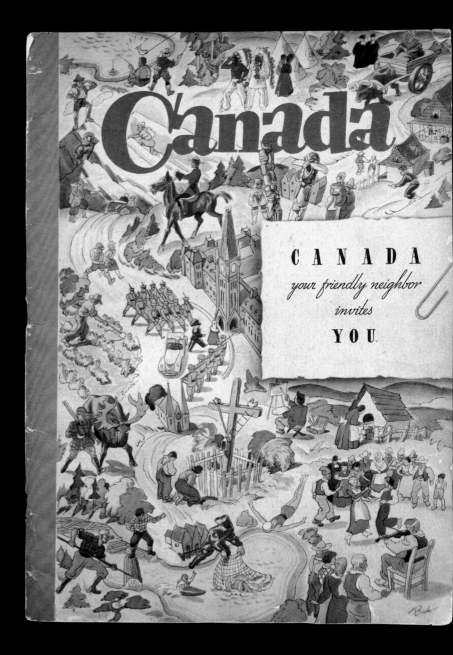

ABOVE One of the twenty articles in the booklet told the story of the Dionne Quintuplets, the "Royal Babies of Callander," who drew huge numbers of tourists to this town north of Toronto. At the Quintland theme park visitors could watch the dark-haired little girls at play and buy souvenir plates, plaques and dolls.

BELOW The BC Electric Railway Company began running open-air observation cars through Vancouver in 1909. They remained a favourite way to tour the city for over forty years. This one is at the corner of Hastings and Main Street in 1910, with City Hall (left) and Carnegie Library in the background.

RIGHT Butchart Gardens near Victoria, BC, was a former limestone quarry transformed into a public garden by cement manufacturer Robert Butchart and his wife Jennie. This photograph shows the tea house. The elaborate gardens remain a popular tourist attraction.

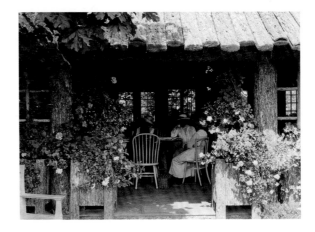

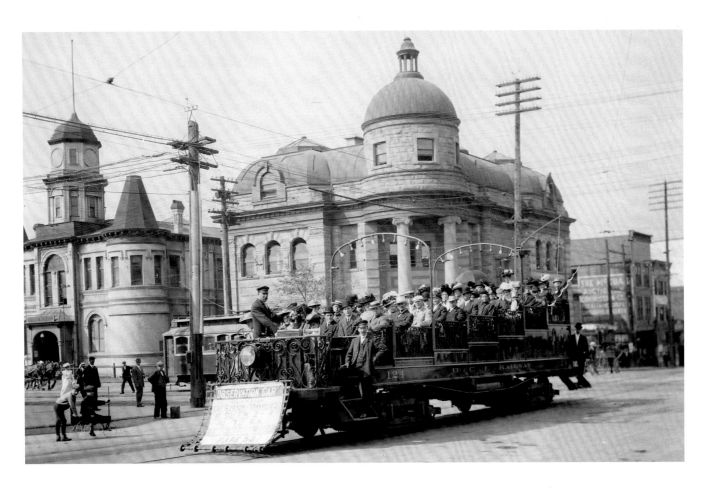

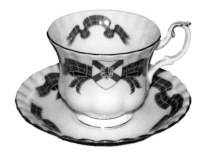

The Nova Scotia tartan was the first provincial tartan in Canada. It is supposed to reflect the contribution of the Scots to the founding of Nova Scotia and the pioneer settlement of the province. The tartan adorns any number of items, including this Royal Albert bone china tea cup and saucer designed and produced by the Royal Doulton Company in England.

ethnicity – "tartanism" – to provide the province with an identity that might appeal to visitors. During the 1920s and 1930s, historian Ian McKay argues, rug hooking and weaving were invigorated with public support. "Crafts in Nova Scotia," he writes, "were not so much the continuation of age-old traditions handed on through the generations as they were the products of a conscious state policy of meeting the expectations of tourists, who came to the province expecting to find quaint, handmade articles that were somehow 'typical' of Nova Scotia." A similar phenomenon occurred in Quebec, where the provincial Department of Agriculture was heavily involved in encouraging the production of craft goods such as rugs, blankets and carvings. Aside from their intrinsic merits, traditional handicrafts appealed to members of the touring public, who liked to think they were seeing the last remnants of authentic folk cultures before they were swept away by industrial modernism. It was not just Aboriginal people who were thought to be vanishing; so too were the old rural ways of life. Souvenirs of craft goods made by local people gave a shot in the arm to rural economies while providing visitors with a glimpse into what they considered an ideal past.

Regarding the "Scottishness" that went along with the Nova Scotia handicraft "tradition," one might assume that the province's official tartan could be traced back to the earliest Scottish migrants who came to Cape Breton from the Highlands in the late eighteenth century. In fact, the Nova Scotia tartan was designed in 1953 by an Englishwoman, not a Scot at all, in response to a desire on the part of tourism promoters to add another layer to the province's Scottishness. Soon the design was appearing on all manner of clothing and other goods and was being used on official occasions as a symbol of the province. Historians have called this phenomenon the "invention of tradition" and the tourism industry is one of its most industrious practitioners. Tourists appreciate heritage. They like to think that they are seeing the essence of the place they are visiting, that they are having an authentic cultural experience. It is easier to "sell" a region to visitors if the experience can be boiled down to a few simple images that seem to convey the essence of a place. In Nova Scotia, argues McKay, that essence has been its Scottishness.

At the same time Nova Scotia was elaborating its Scottish personality, a nascent tourism industry was taking shape at the other end of the country in British Columbia. There the provincial government created a Bureau of Information in 1900 and two years later both Victoria and Vancouver had their own tourist associations. These were alliances of local merchants and real estate agents who combined to promote the Pacific Coast as a tourist destination. As historian Michael Dawson points out, early boosters were interested in luring visitors to British Columbia mainly as a way of impressing them with the province's investment opportunities. Later, tourism, and the

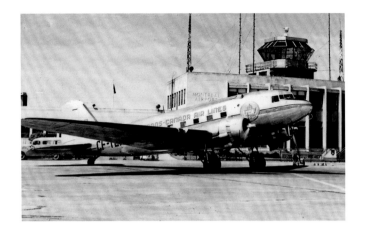

The age of aviation brought new opportunities for tourist promotion. Trans-Canada Airlines was created as a subsidiary of the government-owned Canadian National Railway and launched its first flight on September 1, 1937, between Vancouver and Seattle. Prior to TCA, no large national airline existed in Canada. In 1939 the company began offering passenger service between Vancouver and Montreal and two years later it added scheduled flights to Europe. Above, the former grand lady of aviation, the Douglas DC-3, at Dorval Airport in Montreal, circa 1940.

spending it engendered, became ends in themselves. During the 1920s, British Columbia joined with neighbouring American states to promote tourism to the Pacific Northwest generally. British Columbia was touted as "The Switzerland of America" and the region as a whole was marketed as "The World's Greatest Out of Doors." Victoria discovered its "British-ness" and began highlighting a "tea and crumpet" milieu that would attract visitors who wished to experience Jolly Olde Englande in a North American setting. By 1937 British Columbia had its own government agency: the Bureau of Industrial and Tourist Development, later the British Columbia Government Travel Bureau. Advertising campaigns emphasized the wild beauty of the coast and the recreational possibilities of the mountainous interior, usually with a totem pole somewhere in the foreground. Early slogans used to sum up life in British Columbia included "The Evergreen Playground," "Always Cool, Never Cold," and "The Playground of North America." In

reality, of course, British Columbia was not a playground. It was a resource frontier with an economy that relied on exploiting the same natural environment that the tourism industry was marketing as pristine and inviting. But just as Nova Scotia sold its Scottish identity, British Columbia sold itself to tourists as a place barely removed from the wilderness, a place to encounter exotic First Nations people and unspoiled nature within easy reach of civilized comforts.

———

A KEY FIGURE IN THE HISTORY OF TOURISM promotion in Canada was John Murray Gibbon. Officially Gibbon was chief publicist for Canadian Pacific; unofficially he was much more. With his connection to the CPR and links to a variety of literary groups, he was the leading cultural entrepreneur in Canada during the inter-war period. He encouraged the crafts movement, launched folk festivals, wrote books and radio programs, and celebrated the Canadian wilderness.

JOHN MURRAY GIBBON WAS ONE of the 240,000 Scots who came to live in Canada between 1901 and the outbreak of World War I. Unlike most of his fellow immigrants, he was already an expert on his new country, and he did more to influence Canada's sense of itself than almost anyone else during the inter-war period.

Gibbon was born on his father's tea plantation in Ceylon in 1875 and returned home for his education, which ultimately included a degree from Oxford University. He was a respected journalist, well connected in literary circles, when he joined the publicity office of the CPR in London in 1907. On his first visit to Canada he'd become fascinated with the country and made himself something of an expert on its culture and history. Before the CPR even moved him to its Montreal headquarters in 1913, Gibbon had produced a book about the country, *Scots in Canada*.

In Montreal Gibbon was named the CPR's chief publicity agent with responsibility for the company's advertising and public relations. For more than three decades he was a tireless ambassador for the railway and a promoter of Canadian culture. He was the founding president of the Canadian Authors Association, the organizer of countless artistic events and the author of more than thirty books, one of them a history of the CPR. Historian Ian McKay calls him "one of the principal figures in imagining the Canadian community in the 1920s and 1930s." Gibbon died in Montreal in July 1952.

MEET MR. CANADA

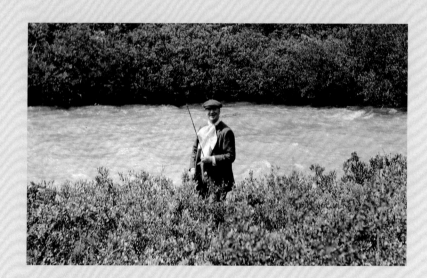

John Murray Gibbon travelled widely across the country promoting the railway and the arts. Here he is at White Man's Pass on the upper Kootenay River during a 1923 fishing expedition.

These posters advertise two of the folk festivals sponsored by Canadian Pacific and originated by the company's chief publicist John Murray Gibbon in 1926. Gibbon thought that folk culture was a vehicle to promote understanding between Canada's ethnic and linguistic communities. Of course, he also saw an opportunity to promote the CPR and its hotels.

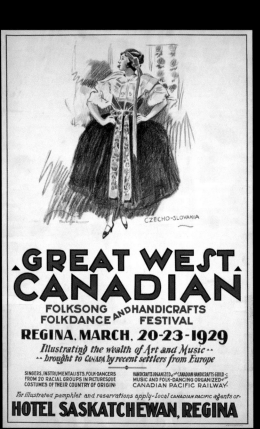

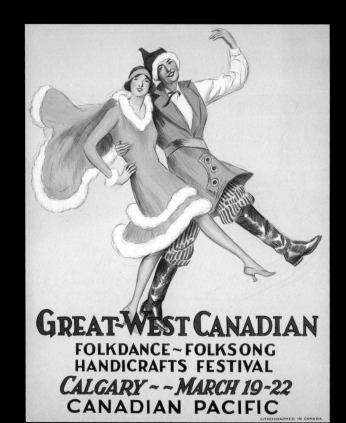

John Murray Gibbon liked to go trail riding in the western mountains and in 1924 he launched the Trail Riders of the Canadian Rockies to promote this form of athletic tourism. When the Trail Riders turned out to be a great success he created a parallel group for walkers in 1933, the Sky Line Trail Hikers of the Canadian Rockies. The honorary president of the hikers was CPR chief executive Edward Beatty. This 1936 poster features the art of Norman Fraser.

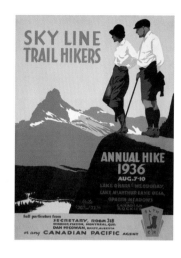

Beginning in 1926, Gibbon staged a series of festivals at the company's major hotels featuring the arts and crafts of different cultural groups. The first of these festivals was in Quebec City, where the company was opening a refurbished wing of the Château Frontenac. This event featured a performance by the well-known Québécois folksinger, Charles Marchand, and was such a success that it evolved into an annual New Canadian Folksong and Handicraft Festival at the hotel. Gibbon, who was a proponent of biculturalism long before it became state policy, hoped to use folk culture to promote better understanding between French and English in Canada. But his ambitions went beyond helping bridge the bicultural divide. During the following years Gibbon extended the company's roster of festivals by launching a Scottish Highlands Gathering at the Banff Springs Hotel, a New Canadian Festival featuring a variety of ethnic performers at the Royal Alexandra Hotel in Winnipeg and a Sea Music Festival in Vancouver. Publicity for the Winnipeg event announced that it would feature "15 Racial Groups in picturesque songs, dances and costumes" and would reveal that non-British immigrants "have a fine gift of music and artistry for the making of the Canadian nation." The literature that accompanied the festivals drove home the point that diversity was creating a new Canada where all "races" made a contribution.

During the Depression Gibbon's festivals became the basis for a radio program called "Canadian Mosaic" and in 1938 he published a book by the same name that described Canada as a mosaic of the many ethnic groups he had been featuring at the CPR-sponsored events. Gibbon's book, which won a Governor General's Award, surveyed the history and culture of the different "racial groups" that he thought made up Canadian society. "The Canadian people today presents itself as a decorated surface," he wrote, "bright with inlays of separate coloured pieces... and so the ensemble may truly be called a mosaic." If he was not the first person to use the word in this context, Gibbon was the first to transform it from a description into an ideal. For Gibbon, the mosaic was a positive metaphor for the manner in which Canadians should live together, welcoming differences and celebrating diversity, and the CPR folk festivals were manifestations of this ideal. Forty years before Prime Minister Pierre Trudeau instituted multiculturalism as an official policy in 1971, Gibbon was promoting his folk-arts approach to ethnic relations, in which cultural groups were encouraged to retain their distinctive customs in order to make Canada a livelier, more colourful place for Canadians to live, and for tourists to visit.

Of course, the mosaic described by Gibbon was more myth than reality. In the 1930s Canada was not a place of equal opportunity where all ethnicities were welcome: the immigration of Chinese people was banned; Canadians of First Nations and Asian descent did not have the vote; anti-Semitism was widespread and acceptable to the majority. Canada

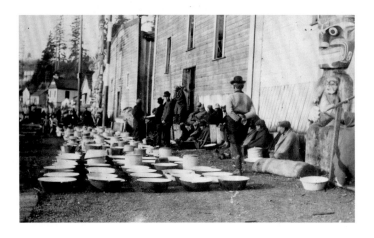

The idealized image of Canada as a "mosaic" of many cultures living harmoniously together did not include First Nations people, who were marginalized economically and socially and had many of their cultural practices suppressed. For example, in 1884 the federal government banned the potlatch, a ceremony belonging to West Coast Aboriginal groups. Missionaries and government agents claimed the potlatch encouraged waste and anti-social behaviour. Many Aboriginals went on potlatching anyway, as this photograph of a ceremony in Alert Bay, circa 1912, shows. The government finally rescinded the ban in 1951.

was still, during Gibbon's lifetime, a "white man's country." His book, *Canadian Mosaic,* made no mention of the contributions of Asian or Black Canadians and seems to have shared the racialist assumption that these groups could not be assimilated into mainstream society. Still, through the work of Gibbon and the CPR, the mosaic was established as the dominant metaphor that Canadians began to invoke when they described their society. In this sense the CPR, in its desire to attract tourists, might be said to have initiated Canada's policy of official multiculturalism.

———

JOHN MURRAY GIBBON'S INFLUENTIAL book was subtitled "The Making of a Northern Nation." This was another image that tourism promoters relied on: "The True North, strong and free," as it appeared in the pages of a James Curwood story or in the Klondike poems of Robert Service or in the canvases of the Group of Seven. "Our art is founded on a long

and growing love and understanding of the North," wrote Lawren Harris, the Group's acknowledged leader. It makes no difference that for most members of the Group, as for most Canadians, "north" usually meant Algonquin Park or Georgian Bay, areas now considered well within the boundaries of Ontario's cottage country. What is important is that the Group reinforced the idea that the authentic, even official, Canadian landscape was a rough wilderness of tree, rock and sky, not a pastoral view of field and parkland.

The Group of Seven landscape was the view of Canada that tourism promoters used most often. In an article in the *Canadian Magazine* in 1900 titled "Canada and the tourist," J.A. Cooper wrote that the "thousands of lakes and rivers afford plenty of sport for the seeker after pleasant excitement, her vast forest preserves are still well stocked with the finest game in the world, and the natural beauty of the many regions, which the prosaic hand of civilization has not yet touched, affords

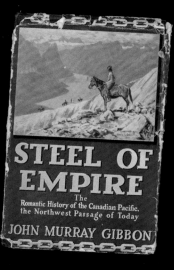

STEEL OF
EMPIRE
The
Romantic History of the Canadian Pacific,
the Northwest Passage of Today
JOHN MURRAY GIBBON

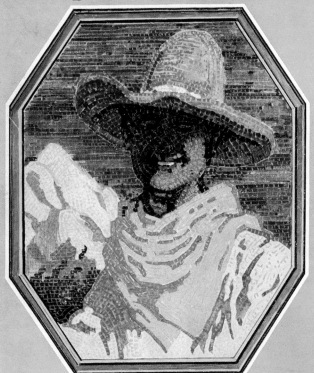

CANADIAN
MOSAIC

THE MAKING
OF A
NORTHERN NATION
JOHN MURRAY GIBBON

The CPR promoted Canada, especially western Canada, as "a paradise for sportsmen." Both the back (left) and front (right) covers of this publication emphasize the wilderness of wonders awaiting the adventure tourist. The back cover features a grizzly bear by noted American wildlife artist Carl Rungius. The front cover features an image by Philip R. Goodwin, another American illustrator who specialized in painting the outdoors.

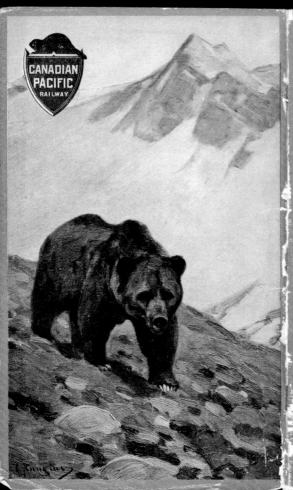

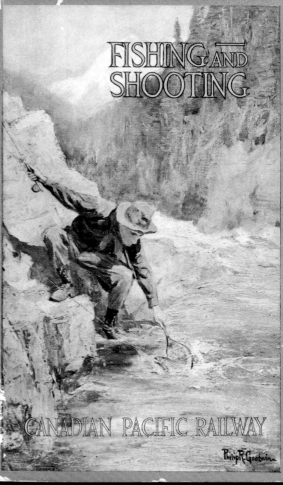

A party of guests sets out from the Château Lake Louise for a trail ride, circa 1914. The first CPR hotel at the lake was little more than a rustic log cabin. It was replaced by a larger structure in 1894 and eventually became far grander than the Château shown here.

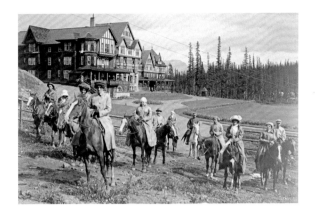

rest to the tired man or woman of the world." Cooper touched on several basic elements of a visit to Canada: the healing hand of nature, the opportunity to witness wild animals in an unspoiled setting, the experience of a safe, tame wilderness ("pleasant excitement") within easy reach of the major cities. These were the benefits of a trip to Canada, which was often presented as a rest cure as much as a vacation. In an article in *Saturday Night* magazine in 1936, the historian and political commentator Frank Underhill referred to this "cult of the North." It was, he wrote, "pure romanticism at its worst," pointing out that most Canadians aspired to a city lifestyle, not a rough shack in the backwoods. A fixation on northernness rather than the realities of contemporary urban life promoted escapism, he grumbled. But Underhill's was a minority view. When Canadians sought to sell their country to visitors, they instinctively reached for northern and nature themes.

Before World War II, most visitors to Canada were sports tourists: fishers and hunters and outdoors enthusiasts. It made sense to appeal to their love of the wild outdoors, whether the mountains of western Canada, the fishing lakes of northern Ontario and Quebec, or the salmon rivers of British Columbia and New Brunswick. But even with the rise of family travel in the post-war era, Canada was still sold as a wilderness destination. In 1949 the Canadian Government Travel Bureau's newsletter, *Travel News*, identified a list of things that were "purely suggestive" of Canada. The list included moccasins, a bush pilot, a Hudson's Bay Company blanket, an elk's head, a canoe and "the painting of a Canadian autumn landscape when done by a Canadian artist of a generation ago" (that is, a member of the Group of Seven). These were the things that said "Canada" to the average visitor, and each of them had a connection to the idea of northernness. Is it any wonder that many foreigners to this day persist in believing that Canadians live in ice houses and play hockey, outside, year-round?

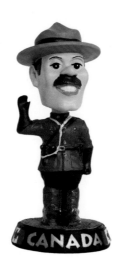

The red-coated Mountie has long been a convenient Canadian identifier. This bobble-head doll, made in China under licence from the RCMP, was purchased at a souvenir shop in downtown Vancouver.

MUCH OF THE MYSTIQUE OF THE NORTH has been associated with Canada's red-coated Mounted Police. The Mounties are a northern police force and most of their heroic tales (for example, the St. Roch, the Lost Patrol, the Mad Trapper) are about northern adventures. They are as identifiably Canadian as John Bull is British or IKEA is Swedish.

Canada is the only country in the world that has transformed its national police force into a tourist attraction. Members of the Royal Canadian Mounted Police, standing guard in their gaudy scarlet outside public buildings, are photographed at least as often as Niagara Falls or the *Bluenose II*. The Mountie is a ubiquitous attendant at public events. So familiar is the image of stern-faced moral rectitude that the force was able to strike a deal with the Disney corporation in 1995 to market it. Mounties are the face of Canada for most people around the world. "How often have we... heard visitors ask 'Where are the Mounties?'" noted a tourism promoter in 1937. They

symbolize Canada, said another, "just like Uncle Sam symbolizes the United States." In 1938 the Canadian Government Tourist Bureau produced a sixty-page, full-colour promotional booklet, *Canada Calls You*, spilling over with illustrations and information for the tourist. What image appeared on the cover? A Mountie with the Rocky Mountains in the background. In 1952 the Mountie was one of four symbols that a federal-provincial tourism conference decided might represent Canada in all advertising for tourists. (The other three were the maple leaf, the crown and the Union Jack; unanimity could not be reached and so the idea of adopting a single symbol was dropped.) When members of the Monty Python comedy troupe dressed as red-coated Mounties and posed in front of a mountain backdrop to sing their famous "I'm a Lumberjack" song, no one had to be told where they were or who they were impersonating. In other words, in the eyes of Canadians and of the world, the Mounted Police represent Canada.

Historically, members of the force were their own best publicists. The origins of the RCMP go back to 1873 when the federal government created the North West Mounted Police, a frontier force sent to protect the First Nations from American whisky traders and to pacify the prairie West in preparation for the expected influx of white settlement. Their success on this mission became part of our cultural mythology. Thanks to the Mounties, Canada is a "peaceable kingdom"; according to the myth, Canadians are law-abiding and deferential to authority because authority, symbolized by the Mountie, is just and benign. Part of the appeal of the Mounties as a national symbol is that they differentiate Canadians from our neighbours to the south. Unlike the United States, we tell ourselves, Canada had no "wild west," no ingrained history of violence, and that was because of the Mountie. The Mountie of legend has a Boy Scoutish quality that is as basic to our national personality as flag-waving is to the Americans or

BELOW Another postcard full of images used to represent and to sell Canada: the noble Indian, the northern wilderness, the bountiful prairie, hunting, fishing and, of course, the ubiquitous Mountie and the maple leaf.

RIGHT The cover from this 1938 government tourism brochure shows a Mountie striding purposefully across an iconic landscape of mountains and lakes. There was no more representative symbol of the country than a member of our own souvenir police force.

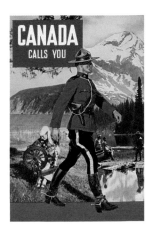

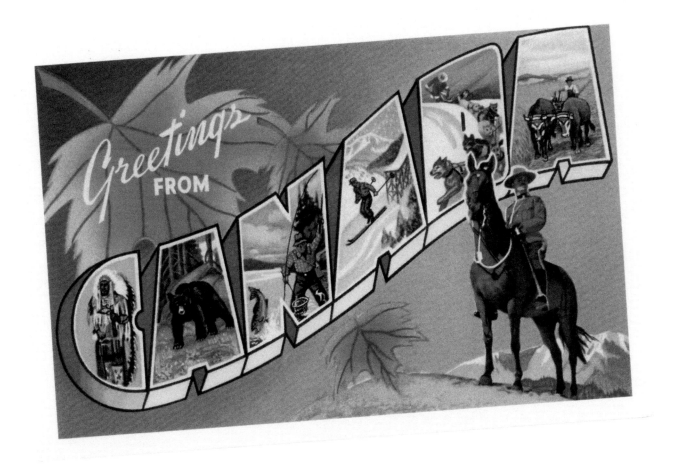

Among the most popular comic book Mounties was Sergeant Preston, who battled northern criminals along with his faithful sled dog Yukon King. Set during the Klondike gold rush of the 1890s, the Preston story began as a radio series where the sergeant's familiar "On King! On you huskies!" thrilled a generation of young listeners. During the 1950s Dell Comics published twenty-nine issues of a comic book version of the story. This one dates from early in 1956. Sergeant Preston was also a television series from 1955 to 1958.

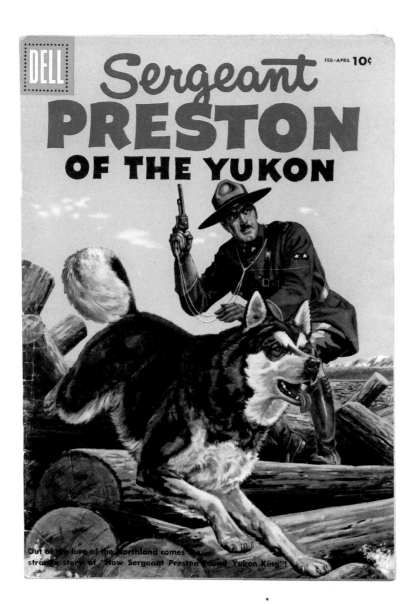

the stoic stiff upper lip is to the British.

The heroic legend of the Mountie emerged from the pages of the many memoirs, histories and dime novels that were written about the force. The adventures of the frontier police force that "always got its man" proved irresistible to popular writers, who churned out Mountie books by the hundreds. "The scarlet tunic! What a story!" gushed one author in *Chums*, a British adventure magazine for boys. In 1935 the American adventure novelist Zane Grey loaned his name to a popular comic strip, King of the Royal Mounted, which appeared in North American newspapers for twenty years. At the same time Hollywood exploited the image. Pierre Berton calculates in his book, *Hollywood's Canada,* that close to half of all the movies Hollywood has made about Canada feature Mounties in the leading role. "To an international audience," writes Berton, "Canada and the mounted police are inseparable." The first Mountie movie, a silent film called *The Cattle Thieves*, was released in 1909.

Another comic book Mountie was Dave King, a.k.a. King of the Royal Mounted. He was the invention of Steven Slesinger, an American pop culture entrepreneur. Slesinger developed the character of King of the Royal Mounted, then licensed the byline of Zane Grey, the popular writer of pulp westerns, as a way to attract readers. This Dell comic is from 1938. In the 1940s the series became a movie serial as well. The American public had an insatiable appetite for fast-paced adventure stories featuring Canadian lawmen.

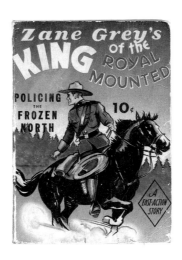

In 1922 alone the industry produced twenty-three features starring the Canadian redcoats, "the most dapper police organization in the world" according to the publicity for one of them. The most famous Mountie movie of all was *Rose Marie*, a 1936 feature starring Nelson Eddie as the crooning cop and Jeanette MacDonald as his love interest. Berton recounts how MGM executive Louis B. Mayer brought all his influence to bear so that actual members of the RCMP could be used as extras in the film. Later the fictional Mountie moved onto American television, most notably as Sergeant Preston of the Yukon, a mid-1950s CBS series that recast the legend of the Mountie for a younger generation. "No matter what the cause," intoned the narrator, "nor how remote the region, the North West Mounted Police stood true to their motto, 'Uphold the Right.'" These examples may seem whimsical, even trivial, but they illustrate how pervasively the image of the Mountie imprinted itself on popular culture.

Pierre Berton makes the point several times in his book that the RCMP shunned publicity and only very reluctantly allowed itself to be dragged into the Hollywood spotlight, but this is disingenuous. The force may have disliked publicity that misrepresented its history or made it look foolish, as Hollywood tended to do, but in general the Mounties co-operated with any promoters who wished to make them an essential part of the Canadian identity. The RCMP also never shied from burnishing its heroic public image. A case in point would be the Musical Ride, the regularly staged public display of precision drills and equestrian skills used to remind us of the force's historical roots on the western frontier.

In truth, the modern RCMP has little to do with the romance of the original mounted force. Its history is more complicated than that. In its early years the force survived several near-death experiences as the government debated whether it continued to serve any useful purpose. At the end of World War I the force, by then renamed the Royal North-West Mounted Police, again verged on dissolution as many of its members had resigned to join the armed forces. It seemed to Ottawa that a second police agency, the Dominion Police, which had been active in eastern Canada since 1868, might as well take over national jurisdiction. However, at the end of the war, as the force was about to be relegated to history, a wave of national paranoia gripped the country. Canadians feared that Bolshevik-inspired elements in the labour movement were plotting to overthrow the government and install a made-in-Moscow regime in Ottawa. Far-fetched as this sounds today, it seemed all too real to authorities in 1919. One of the ways they responded to the perceived threat was to give the Mounties the task of gathering secret intelligence about the activities of left-wing political groups and labour unions. So effective was the newly invigorated force in carrying out this job that in 1920 the government combined it with the Dominion Police

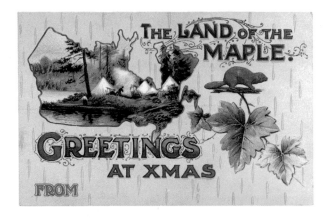

to create a single new force, the Royal Canadian Mounted Police. Ever since, the Mounties have traded on their historic roots as backwoods policemen pursuing their man on dogsled and horseback to produce an image of the stalwart defender of the right. But this reading of history conveniently ignores the force's modern origins as a domestic spy agency working clandestinely to stamp out legal, if radical, political activity.

––––––––

THE BRITISH SOCIAL SCIENTIST BENEDICT Anderson coined the term "imagined community" to describe the modern nation state. According to Anderson, a country finds its identity and promotes unity through shared images. Canada is a northern wilderness. Canada is a cultural mosaic. Canada is a peaceable kingdom. These are just three of the images that Canadians believe describe themselves and their society. Another word for these images would be myths, not because they are untrue but because they express important cultural ideals and values. They seem to explain our history and give meaning to our national existence.

From the beginning, tourism has played a central role in the development of many of Canada's organizing myths. In their quest for visitors, the railways and the government produced picture-postcard images that over time came to represent the nation. As a relatively young country, Canada needed a way of asserting itself in the world, of projecting an identity. To a large degree, the CPR provided these defining narratives and traditions, presenting folkloric images of Old Quebec and wilderness images of prairies and western mountains. The image of the red-coated Mountie was added to the mix, along with the tragic image of the noble but vanishing Indian, and pretty soon the country had a set of symbols that seemed to say "This is Canada."

These images were then used by tourism promoters in posters, brochures, books, photographs, even movies, and presented to travellers as Canada. Obviously it was a partial version of the country, one designed to attract the interest of people seeking novelty, relaxation, diversion and adventure. Canada was much more than its Rocky Mountains or its noble police force. Nonetheless, many of the images that were created to sell Canada to tourists became indelible components of the way Canadians came to understand themselves.

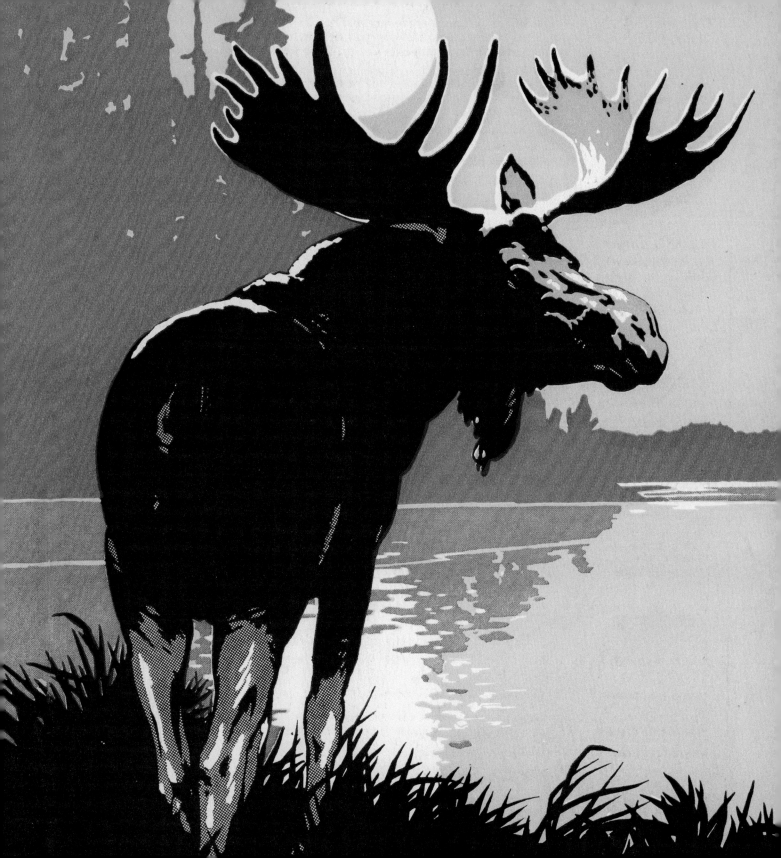

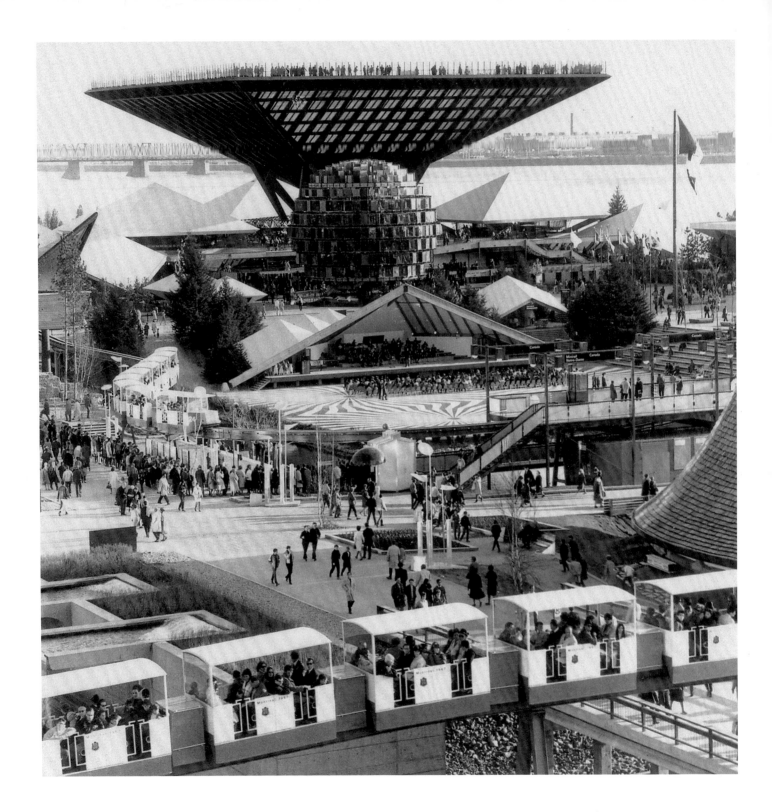

CREATING CANADA

Love of country is an act of the imagination.
– MICHAEL IGNATIEFF

IN 1967 CANADA HOSTED ITS OWN COMING-OUT PARTY. ONE HUNDRED YEARS
after Confederation Canadians celebrated their centennial with a blowout
from coast to coast to coast. In an atypical display of national pride and enthusiasm, communities came together to build hundredth-birthday presents to
themselves, ranging from the ordinary (new community centres and skating
rinks) to the whimsical (a landing pad for UFOs) and everything in between.
At the centre of the festivities was Expo 67, a Category One world exposition
held on two islands in the middle of the St. Lawrence River at Montreal. It was a
huge success, more so than anyone had dared to dream. Expo changed the way
Canadians thought about themselves and the way other people thought about
Canada, at least for a little while. "Expo '67 is an outrageous, lunatic, wondrous
dream come to reality," announced the *Montreal Star* on opening day, April
28, 1967. More than fifty million visitors poured through the gates before they
closed six months later. The fair made the cover of *Life* magazine and *Paris
Match*; the most popular television host of the time, Ed Sullivan, came to Montreal to broadcast one of his Sunday evening shows. For Canadians, it was a
chance to strut their stuff on an international stage, a way of attracting worldwide attention. Suddenly the country seemed like a modern, urban, sophisticated, fun place. This was the selling of Canada on a grand scale.

Forgotten in all the excitement of the fair's success was the fact that it
almost didn't happen at all. Originally the international governing body turned
down Canada's application in favour of the Soviet Union, which would be celebrating its fiftieth anniversary in 1967. But then the USSR withdrew and Canada
got its chance. It was a daunting challenge, too daunting for some. As preparations lurched from crisis to crisis, many people suggested Canada should

OPPOSITE The Expo 67 fairgrounds
in Montreal. The inverted pyramid
was the centrepiece of the Canada
Pavilion. It was called Katimavik,
"meeting place" in the language of
the Inuit. Its exuberant futuristic
design reflected the optimism and
pride of the Centennial celebrations.

follow the Russian example and throw in the towel. But Montreal's mayor, Jean Drapeau, would have none of it. In many ways it was his dogged refusal to say "non" that made the fair a reality.

Afterwards, the second thoughts and indecision were forgotten. According to the pundits, Expo 67 represented the rebirth of Canadian pride and national unity. Journalist Peter Newman wrote that the success of the fair proved "we could do anything." It was the greatest thing Canadians had ever done as a nation, he pronounced. The country seemed to have found the self-confidence and maturity it had been searching for its entire history. And because the fair took place in Quebec with the enthusiastic involvement of the rest of Canada, it seemed to portend an era of good feeling between the "founding peoples."

Unhappily, the deepening unity crisis between French and English required more than a World's Fair to resolve. Once again, the image the country had of itself did not correspond to reality. In Quebec, the era of modernization known as the Quiet Revolution had grown noisy in a hurry with several bombings by members of the extremist Front de Libération du Québec (FLQ). Expo may have marked a resurgence of Canadian nationalism, but 1967 was also the year that broadcaster/politician René Lévesque quit the Quebec Liberal Party to form his own separatist party (later the Parti Québécois). Within three years Canada would be plunged into its worst political nightmare, the October Crisis of 1970, with its kidnappings and political assassination. The image of a peaceful, tolerant, law-abiding country would be smashed by the reality of armed soldiers in the streets and the disappearance of fundamental civil rights. And then, in May 1980, just thirteen years after the warm glow of the centennial celebrations filled Canadians with pride, came a referendum in Quebec asking voters if they wished the province to seek political independence from Canada. The "No" side won, but obviously the consensus that had made Expo 67 such a success no longer existed.

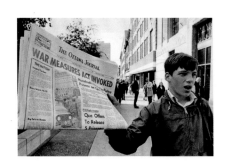

The October Crisis of 1970 and the invocation of the War Measures Act by the federal government shattered the optimistic view that Canada was a peaceful, united country. The poet Al Purdy wrote about this period: "the little eddy that is my life/ and all our lives quickens/ and bubbles break as we join/ the mainstream of history."

BETWEEN 1880 AND THE 1930S, THREE GREAT SALES CAMPAIGNS TRANSFORMED the way Canadians thought about themselves and the way outsiders thought about Canada. If Benedict Anderson is right that nations are "imagined communities," then these campaigns provided the raw material for nationhood. Each of them produced images that expressed what Canadians believed to be fundamental and true about their country. And yet in each case the images turned out to be misleading, an idealized portrait rather than a realistic snapshot, just as Canadians in Centennial Year believed they were united behind a proud, invigorated nationalism, only to be shocked a few years later to discover the French-English divide was deeper than ever.

At the end of the nineteenth century and the beginning of the twentieth,

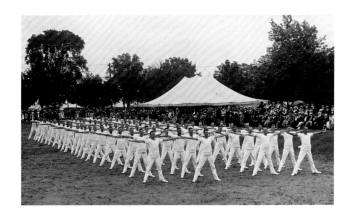

Canada was a young country in search of a destiny. What was the purpose of the political arrangement that had been made in 1867? Was it simply a marriage of convenience for the separate colonies that combined to form a new country? Or did the Dominion have a unique purpose? Many countries find the answer to such a question in their history. But as a new country, Canada did not have much history; no dramatic storyline of war and revolution was available to provide meaning. Instead, Canadians looked to their landscape for their identity and to develop what one critic has called a "wildercentric" view of their nationality. The stark, northern wilderness, it was argued, imparted a set of characteristics that came to be recognized as uniquely Canadian. This idea found its popular expression in the art of the Group of Seven and the adventure stories of James Curwood. Exotic images of northernness played a large role in the version of Canada that was marketed to tourists.

Many Canadians were content to rest comfortably in the familiar embrace of Great Britain. At the turn of the century Canada was a British country with British institutions and a population that was more than 50 percent British in heritage with strong psychological ties to the Mother Country. But as the years passed the makeup of the population changed and the issue of autonomy became more pressing, especially with the war experience. The search for an independent path became the core of a new narrative of Canada that depicted World War I as our war of independence. Canadian soldiers proved on the battlefield that Canada was no one's colony and deserved an equal place among the nations of the world.

Like all propaganda campaigns, those mounted to sell Canada to immigrants, to sell the Great War to Canadians, and to sell Canada to the world

World War I recruits doing calisthenics in front of a crowd at the Canadian National Exhibition Camp in Toronto in 1915. The experience of the war, to which Canada made such an important contribution, created a new sense of nationality in the country.

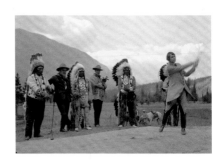

ABOVE A party of First Nations chiefs golfing at Banff sometime before World War II. The humour of this photograph lies in the way it subverts conventional tourist images of how Indians were supposed to behave. The "noble Indian" played a central role in the campaigns to brand Canada.

OPPOSITE A Royal Canadian Mountie dressed in full ceremonial regalia greets a pair of tourists at Banff in 1930. The photographer, Reinhold Palenske, was an American artist often employed by the CPR to illustrate its promotional material. Palenske may have been an American but it was images like this one, of Mounties and mountains, that presented an idealized version of Canadianness.

involved deception of some kind, whether by actual lies or by the omission of inconvenient truths. New immigrants to Canada were told about the free land and the healthy climate; they were not told about the rigours of life on the frontier. During World War I new recruits were told about the atrocities committed by the enemy; they were not told about the horrors of trench warfare. Tourists visiting Canada were encouraged to photograph the exotic Aboriginal people; they were not told how these same people had lost their land and were subsisting on meagre handouts.

The process of "selling Canada" to Canadians and to outsiders generated a wide variety of visual and written materials evoking dominant images of the country. These images promoted an idealized version of Canada: a Canada of fruitful farmland and happy families, of loyal soldiers and supportive wives and mothers, of stupendous scenery, wide open spaces, picturesque Native people and colourful, well-integrated ethnic groups; a country united in determination against common enemies. At the same time it papered over many of the social problems that disturbed the country. The difficulties facing many of Canada's First Nations were obscured by Indians in feathered headdress and buckskin performing for the "Kodaking" tourist crowds, and the prejudices directed at different cultural groups were drowned out by the music of dance festivals and folk carnivals. The ideal version of the country was flattering to Canadians but it was a false basis on which to build a national identity.

In the end the campaigns to sell Canada had both positive and negative results. On the plus side, they helped to attract hundreds of thousands of new settlers to the country at a time when Canada desperately needed more people to boost its population and develop its resources. They rallied the populace in support of the government during the war and helped to create a tourist industry that contributed significantly to the national economy. And they also contributed to the development of a set of characteristics that came to be recognized as distinctively Canadian; a Canadian identity if you will. The negative results of these campaigns were equally significant. They can be found mostly in the distance that lay between the images employed and the harsh realities the campaigns obscured. By creating a sense of the country that was both misleading and exclusive, these advertising efforts saddled Canada with a set of stereotypes that survive to this day – the real legacy of the three great campaigns to sell Canada.

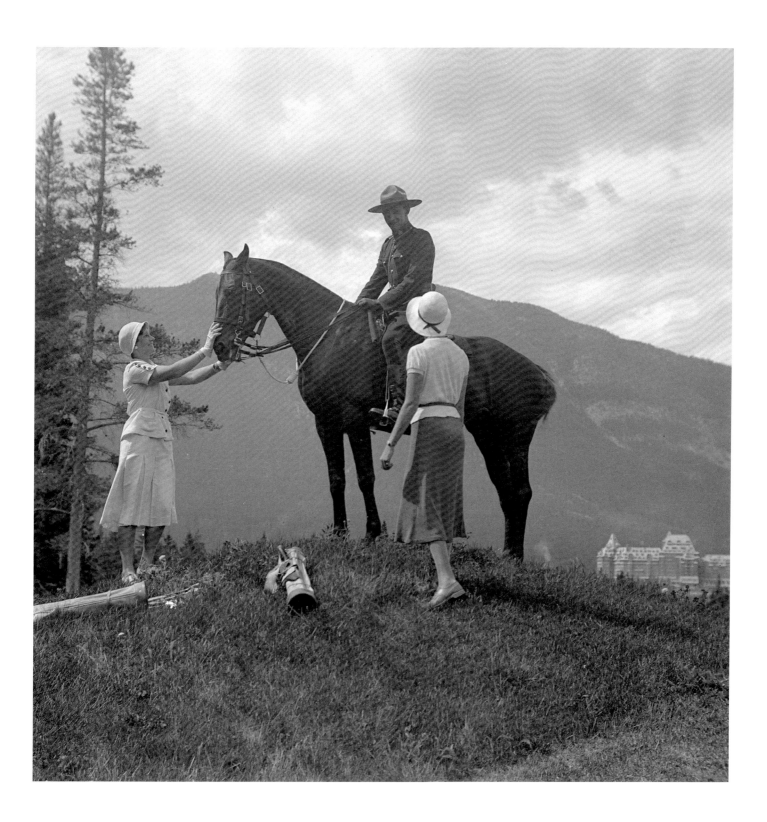

SOURCES

PROLOGUE

The information about James Oliver Curwood comes from his autobiography, *Son of the Forests* (New York: Doubleday, Doran and Co., 1930). Curwood's career is also sketched by Pierre Berton in his *Hollywood's Canada: The Americanization of Our National Image* (Toronto: McClelland & Stewart, 1975).

CHAPTER ONE

The changing perceptions of western Canada are detailed in R. Douglas Francis, *Images of the West: Changing Perceptions of the Prairies, 1690–1960* (Saskatoon: Western Producer Prairie Books, 1989) and Douglas Owram, *Promise of Eden: The Canadian Expansionist Movement and the Idea of the West 1856–1900* (Toronto: University of Toronto Press, 1980). An excellent general history of the prairie West is Gerald Friesen, *The Canadian Prairies: A History* (Toronto: University of Toronto Press, 1984). The comments by William Francis Butler are from his classic *The Great Lone Land* (London: S. Low, Marston, Low & Searle, 1872; reprint: M.G. Hurtig, Edmonton, 1968). The organization of early immigration promotion is described in Patrick Dunae, "Promoting the Dominion: Records and the Canadian Immigration Campaign, 1872–1915," *Archivaria* 19 (Winter 1984–85). The great post-1896 immigration wave has been widely documented. For a general introduction, see Pierre Berton, *The Promised Land: Settling the West, 1896–1914* (Toronto: McClelland and Stewart, 1984). John Dafoe's study, *Clifford Sifton in Relation to His Times* (Toronto: The Macmillan Company, 1930), is still valuable, though it has been superseded by David J. Hall's superb two-volume biography *Clifford Sifton: The Young Napoleon 1861–1900*, volume 1 (Vancouver: UBC Press, 1981) and *Clifford Sifton: A Lonely Eminence 1901–1929*, volume 2 (Vancouver: UBC Press, 1985).

Sifton's immigration policies in particular are described in Hall's, "Clifford Sifton: Immigration and Settlement Policy, 1896–1905" in Howard Palmer, ed., *The Settlement of the West* (Calgary: University of Calgary, 1977): 60–85. For the role of the CPR in immigration promotion, see John A. Eagle, *The Canadian Pacific Railway and the Development of Western Canada* (Montreal: McGill-Queen's University Press, 1989). The efforts to attract American settlers to Canada are documented in Harold Troper, *Only Farmers Need Apply* (Toronto: Griffin House, 1972). For an analysis of immigration propaganda, see Klaus Peter Stich, "'Canada's Century': The Rhetoric of Propaganda," *Prairie Forum* (April 1976): 19–30; also R. Douglas Francis, "The Ideal and the Real: The Image of the Canadian West in the Settlement Period" in Richard C. Davies, ed., *Rupert's Land: A Cultural Tapestry* (Waterloo, ON: Wilfrid Laurier University Press, 1988), Ronald Rees, *New and Naked Land: Making the Prairies Home* (Saskatoon: Western Producer Prairie Books, 1988) and David C. Jones, "It's All Lies They Tell You: Immigrants, Hosts and the CPR" in Hugh A. Dempsey, ed., *The CPR West* (Vancouver: Douglas & McIntyre, 1984): 107–124. Stanley Triggs, *William Notman: The Stamp of the Studio* (Toronto: Art Gallery of Ontario, 1985) describes the work of the Notman photographic firm. The controversy over the North Atlantic Trading Company is analyzed in Jaroslav Petryshyn, "Canadian Immigration and the North Atlantic Trading Company 1899–1906: A Controversy Revisited," *Journal of Canadian Studies* (Fall 1997): 55–77. The importation of domestic servants is described in Marilyn Barber, *Immigrant Domestic Servants in Canada* (Ottawa: Canadian Historical Association Booklet #16, 1991); Magda Fahrni, "'Ruffled' Mistresses and 'Discontented' Maids: Respectability and the Case of Domestic Service, 1880–1914," *Labour/Le Travail* 39 (Spring 1997): 69–97; and Ellen Scheinberg, "Bringing 'Domestics' to Canada: A Study of

Immigration Propaganda" in Sharon Anne Cook, Lorna R. McLean and Kate O'Rourke, eds., *Framing Our Past: Canadian Women's History in the Twentieth Century* (Montreal: McGill-Queen's University Press, 2001): 336–342. For the Doukhobors, see George Woodcock and Ivan Avakumovic, *The Doukhobors* (Toronto: Oxford University Press, 1968).

CHAPTER TWO

Charles Gordon's reminiscence is from his autobiography, *Postscript to Adventure: The Autobiography of Ralph Connor* (Toronto: McClelland and Stewart, 1975). Many other first-hand accounts of the war are collected in Daphne Read, ed., *The Great War and Canadian Society: An Oral History* (Toronto: New Hogtown Press, 1978) and in Ian Hugh Maclean Miller, *Our Glory and Our Grief: Torontonians and the Great War* (Toronto: University of Toronto Press, 2002). The events of the war, both at home and in Europe, are related in Desmond Morton and J.L. Granatstein, *Marching to Armageddon: Canadians and the Great War 1914–1919* (Toronto: Lester & Orpen Dennys, 1989) and in Tim Cook's two volumes, *At the Sharp End: Canadians Fighting the Great War, 1914–1916* (Toronto: Viking Canada, 2007) and *Shock Troops: Canadians Fighting the Great War, 1917–1918* (Toronto: Viking Canada, 2008). Many of the posters used in the propaganda campaign are in Marc H. Choko, *Canadian War Posters: 1914–1918, 1939–1945* (Laval, QC: Éditions du Méridien, 1977) and Joseph Darracott, ed., *The First World War in Posters* (New York: Dover Publications, 1974). Canadian propaganda efforts are described in Jeffrey A. Keshen, *Propaganda and Censorship During Canada's Great War* (Edmonton: University of Alberta Press, 1996). Max Aitken's activities are chronicled in Tim Cook, "Immortalizing the Canadian Soldier: Lord Beaverbrook and the Canadian War Records Office in the First World War" in Briton C. Busch, ed., *Canada* and the Great War (Montreal: McGill-Queen's University Press, 2003): 46–65. Recruitment is the subject of Paul Maroney's article, "'The Great Adventure': The Context and Ideology of Recruiting in Ontario, 1914–17," *Canadian Historical Review* (March 1996): 62–98, while the internment operation is described in Desmond Morton, "Sir William Otter and Internment Operations in Canada During the First World War," *Canadian Historical Review* (March 1974): 32–58. Professor Morton has also written a study of military families during the war, *Fight or Pay: Soldiers' Families in the Great War* (Vancouver: UBC Press, 2004). The work of the war artists is the subject of Maria Tippett's *Art at the Service of War: Canada, Art, and the Great War* (Toronto: University of Toronto Press, 1984) and Dean F. Oliver and Laura Brandon's *Canvas of War: Painting the Canadian Experience, 1914–1945* (Vancouver: Douglas & McIntyre, 2000). The section on Joseph Flavelle relies on Michael Bliss, *A Canadian Millionaire* (Toronto: Macmillan, 1978). Jonathan Vance considers the memorialisation of the war in *Death So Noble: Memory, Meaning, and the First World War* (Vancouver: UBC Press, 1997), while James W. St. G. Walker studies "Race and Recruitment in World War I: Enlistment of Visible Minorities in the Canadian Expeditionary Force," *Canadian Historical Review* (March 1989): 1–26.

CHAPTER THREE

The pioneering work in Canadian tourism history is E.J. Hart, *The Selling of Canada: The CPR and the Beginnings of Canadian Tourism* (Banff, AB: Altitude Publishing, 1983). More recent studies include Patricia Jasen, *Wild Things: Nature, Culture, and Tourism in Ontario, 1790–1914* (Toronto: University of Toronto Press, 1995), Michael Dawson, *Selling British Columbia: Tourism and Consumer Culture 1890–1970* (Vancouver: UBC Press, 2004), Karen Dubinsky, *The Second Greatest Disappointment: Honeymooning and Tour-*

ism at Niagara Falls (New Brunswick, NJ: Rutgers University Press, 1999), Ian McKay, *The Quest of the Folk: Antimodernism and Cultural Selection in Twentieth-Century Nova Scotia* (Montreal: McGill-Queen's University Press, 1994), Ian McKay and Robin Bates, *In the Province of History: The Making of the Public Past in Twentieth-Century Nova Scotia* (Montreal: McGill-Queen's University Press, 2010) and C. James Taylor, *Jasper: A History of the Place and Its People* (Markham, ON: Fifth House, 2009). Two accounts of Victorian travel in Canada are Edward Roper, *By Track and Trail: A Journey through Canada* (London: W.H. Allen & Co., 1891) and Douglas Sladen, *On the Cars and Off* (London: Ward, Lock and Bowden Ltd., 1895). The life of Lord Lorne is chronicled in Robert Stamp, *Royal Rebels: Princess Louise and the Marquis of Lorne* (Toronto: Dundurn Press, 1988). Stamp has also described several of the royal tours in "Steel of Empire: Royal Tours and the CPR" in Hugh A. Dempsey, ed., *The CPR West* (Vancouver: Douglas & McIntyre, 1984): 275–290. One of the railway artists is profiled in George F.G. Stanley, "John Hammond: Painter for the CPR," also in Hugh Dempsey, ed., *The CPR West*. The role of the automobile and highway building in stimulating tourism is expanded upon in Daniel Francis, *A Road for Canada: The Illustrated Story of the Trans-Canada Highway* (Vancouver: Stanton, Atkins & Dosil, 2006). Edward McCourt's account of a cross-Canada road trip is in *The Road Across Canada* (Toronto: Macmillan of Canada, 1965). The story of the Skeena River totem poles is told in David Darling and Douglas Cole, "Totem Pole Restoration on the Skeena, 1925–30: An Early Exercise in Heritage Conservation," *BC Studies* (Autumn 1980): 29–48 and in Ronald W. Hawker, *Tales of Ghosts: First Nations Art in British Columbia, 1922–61* (Vancouver: UBC Press, 2003). The origins of the Canadian Government Tourist Bureau are described in Alisa Apostle, "Canada, Vacations Unlimited:

the Canadian Government Tourist Industry, 1934–1959," PhD thesis, Queen's University, 2003, and in Philip Goldring, "Inventing a Friendly Neighbour," *Canada's History* (Dec. 2010–Jan. 2011): 30–33. The image of the Mountie in Canadian history is discussed in Daniel Francis, *National Dreams: Myth, Memory and Canadian History* (Vancouver: Arsenal Pulp Press, 1997) and Michael Dawson, *The Mountie from Dime Novel to Disney* (Toronto: Between the Lines, 1998).

CONCLUSION

The idea of a "wildercentric" identity is discussed in John O'Brian and Peter White, eds., *Beyond Wilderness: The Group of Seven, Canadian Identity, and Contemporary Art* (Montreal: McGill-Queen's University Press, 2007).

DANIEL FRANCIS

CREDITS & PERMISSIONS

Every reasonable effort has been made to trace and contact all holders of copyright and to credit sources correctly. In the event of omission or error SA&D Publishers should be notified so that a full acknowledgment may be made in future editions.

ABBREVIATIONS

AM	Archives of Manitoba
AO	Archives of Ontario
CPR	Canadian Pacific Railway Archives
CSTM	Canada Science & Technology Museum
CTA	City of Toronto Archives
CVA	City of Vancouver Archives
CWM	Canadian War Museum
GA	Glenbow Archives
GM	Glenbow Museum
LAC	Library and Archives Canada
MM	McCord Museum
MUL	Rare Books and Special Collections McGill University Library
NGC	National Gallery of Canada
NYPL	New York Public Library
PAA	Provincial Archives of Alberta
RBCM	Royal BC Museum
UBC	University of British Columbia, Chang Collection
UWL	University of Washington Libraries, Special Collections
VPL	Vancouver Public Library
WDM	Western Development Museum
WMCR	Whyte Museum of the Canadian Rockies

DUST JACKET

Front left: CPR BR196; centre: MUL WP1.M2.FI; right CPR A636.

FRONTISPIECE

LAC C-63256

TITLE PAGE
CPR NS8454

CONTENTS PAGE
NYPL 495066

PROLOGUE
p.2, p.3 and p.4: private collection; p.5: left: private collection; right: LAC C-137813

CHAPTER 1
p.6: CPR A6199; p.8: GA NA-1149-6; p.9: LAC E008072637; p.10/11: GA G3471 B5 1880 C212; p.12: LAC C-081677; p.13: LAC C-011068; p.14: LAC NLC16301; p.15: LAC PA-124866; p.16: AM P4453AF.3; p.17 top: LAC C-075938; bottom: LAC C-079517; p.18: LAC C-056946; p.20 left: GA poster-22; right: LAC C-137979; p.21 top: CPR NS16354; bottom: GA NA-2294-23; p.22: MM N-0000.25.1056; p.23: MM M970.92.1.1-4; p.24: LAC PA-027943; p.25: LAC C-063434; p.26: LAC E010938594; p.28: LAC C-052819; p.29: LAC NLC-11361; p.30: LAC C-004745; p.31: LAC PA-011543; p.32: LAC C-009671; p.33 top: LAC PA-160539; bottom: LAC C-075991; p.34: LAC C-056088; p.35: LAC C-037957; p.36: LAC C-053796; p.37: LAC C-085854; p.38 top: LAC C-089531; bottom: LAC C-089538 and LAC C-089539; p.40: LAC PA-012761; p.41: LAC E006154733; p.42: LAC PA-122664; p.43 left: LAC C-137960; right: LAC C-137978; p.44: LAC C-80108; p.45: LAC C-144748; p.47 top: GA NA-2181-3; bottom: GA NA-2181-2; p.48 top: GA NA-4514-10; bottom: GA NA-118-27; p.49: GA NA-1043-1; p.50: CPR A6019; p.51 left: CPR BR196; right: CPR BR195; p.52: LAC PA-117283; p.53: LAC C-015020; p.54: LAC NLC012993; p.55: LAC PA-020910; p.56: GA NA-938-1; p.57: PAA P457; p.58: LAC NLC-3572; p.59 left: LAC NLC-4041; right: LAC NLC-6870; p.60: GM C-30420 A-E/H-J/BC-BH; p.61: private collection; p.62: UBC EX-4-32; p.63: LAC PA-040745; p.64: LAC C-014118; p.65: VPL 136; p.66: VPL 39046; p.67: LAC C-137978

CHAPTER 2
p.68: CWM 20010129-0729; p.70: CTA fonds 1244, item 729; p.71: LAC C-095392; p.72: LAC C-095285; p.73 left: LAC E010697051; right: LAC C-095380; p.74 top: CTA fonds 1244, item 721; bottom: CTA fonds 1244, item 992; p.75 top: AO 10004817; bottom: CWM 19390002-687; p.76: LAC e010696451; p.77: LAC e010697485; p.78 top: CWM 19990128-008; bottom: CTA fonds 1244, item 821; p.79: GA NA-3496-2; p.80: CTA fonds 1244, item 952, p.81: top, left to right: CWM 20030334-006, CWM 20030334-016, CWM 20030334-001, CWM 20030334-020; bottom: LAC C-098670; p.82: LAC E010696729; p.83: CTA fonds 1244, Item 726; p.84 top: CTA fonds 1244, item 732; bottom: CWM 19880212-093; p.85 top: CWM 19730061-002; bottom: GA NA-1567-4; p.86: CWM 19940018-001pub; p.87: LAC C-004755; p.88 left: CWM 20030334-037; right: LAC E010697273; p.89 top: AO 10004800; bottom: LAC C-097748; p.90: CWM E-1981O561-001; p.91: MUL WPI.R34.FRI; p.92: LAC E010697134; p.93 left: LAC C-095281; right: LAC C-095280; p.94: LAC C-055111; p.95: LAC CSM7244-1C; p.96: LAC PA-023014; p.97: CWM Canadian Daily Record, January 16, 1917; p.98: GA M-5756-26; p.99: CWM 19740049-001; p.100: LAC C-095268; p.101: AO 10022025; p.102: LAC C-014104; p.103 left: LAC E000000566; right: LAC POS-000160; p.104: CWM 19920044-725; p.105: Owen Byrne; p.106 left: LAC E010696980; right: LAC C-095736; p.107: LAC C-093224; p.108: LAC C-006859; p.109 left: LAC E010697151; right top: LAC E010697155; right bottom: LAC E010697156; p.110: left: LAC E010697256; right: LAC E010697263; p.111: CWM 19860157-008; p.112: LAC PA-202396; p.113: LAC E000000237; p.114: LAC PA-001018; p.115: LAC C-000241; p.116 top: LAC PA-001020; bottom: AO 10004778; p.117: LAC PA-002107; p.118: LAC PA-040141; p.119: LAC E010697283; p.120: GM C-10638, C-10652, C-10683, C-32300 A-B, C-49710, R1903.2; p.121: LAC C-095742; p.123: LAC C-095738

CHAPTER 3
p.124: CPR A6539; p.126: **LAC NLC003045**; p.127 top: LAC E010775198; bottom: LAC PA-020795; p.128 top: CPR A6331; bottom: CPR A18111; p.129 left: MM M976.73.11; right: MM M976.73.3; p.130: CPR A189; p.131: GA NA-4967-132; p.132 left: CPR A20297; right: WMCR 13.113-C16; p.133: WMCR V465PD1097; p.134: CPR A6126; p.135 top left: CPR A6695; top right: CPR BR172; bottom left: CPR BR176; bottom right: CPR BR85; p.136: LAC PA-022267; p.137: NGC 6077; p.138: CPR A6145; p.139: GA NA-1241-655; p.140: LAC PA-122000; p.141: CPR A6024; p.142: GA Poster-15; p.143: LAC PA-084782; p.144: LAC PA-086290; p.145: LAC C-137967; p.146: LAC CSM-07134; p.147 left: LAC CSM-1401; right: LAC CSM-918; p.148: LAC C-034305; p.149: MM M966.144.4.1; p.150: CSTM CN003257; p.151 top: RBCM AA-00054; bottom: UWL NA3370; p.152: private collection; p.153: UBC 4032; p.154: WMCR V263/NA3473; p.155: left and right: private collection; p.156 top: WMCR V465/PD2-157; bottom: LAC PA-009530; p.157: private collection; p.158: CSTM CN000264; p.159: WMCR V465/PD3–121; p.160 left: CPR A6264; right: CPR A6187; p.161: CPR A6776; p.162: CVA IN P113.2; p.163 left and right: private collection; p.164 left: CPR BR124-2; right: CPR BR124-1; p.165: CPR NS1498; p.166: private collection; p.167: top and bottom: private collection; p.168: private collection; p.169: private collection; p.170: private collection; p.171: CPR BR117

CONCLUSION
p.172: LAC E001096693; p.174: The Canadian Press/Peter Bregg; p.175: CTA fond1244, item 777d; p.176: WMCR V263/NA-3284; p.177: CPR NS23257

LIBRARY AND ARCHIVES CANADA CATALOGUING IN PUBLICATION

Francis, Daniel
    Selling Canada / Daniel Francis.

Includes bibliographical references and index.
ISBN 978-0-9809304-4-3

1. Canadian immigration literature.
2. World War, 1914–1918 – Canada – Propaganda.
3. Tourism – Canada – Marketing – History.
I. Title.

FC49.F73 2011   325.7109   C2011-904817-5

Stanton Atkins & Dosil Publishers
Mailing address
2632 Bronte Drive
North Vancouver, BC
Canada, V7H 1M4

www. s-a-d-publishers.ca

Edited by: Barbara Tomlin
Proofread by: Eva van Emden
Designed by: Roberto Dosil
Colour preparation by: Ernst Vegt
Printed in Canada by: Friesens

This book's title is set in Gotham, a typeface family designed by Tobias Frere-Jones released in 2000. The chapter headings, text, sidebars and captions are set in Milo Serif and Milo Medium, a typeface family designed by Mike Abbink released in 2009.

FIRST EDITION / FIRST PRINTING

MIX
Paper from
responsible sources
FSC® C016245